OBSTETRICS AND GYNECOLOGY FOR POSTGRADUATES

Volume 1

OBSTETRICS AND GYNECOLOGY FOR POSTGRADUATES

Volume 1

General Editors

SABARATNAM ARULKUMARAN PhD, FRCOG, FRCS
Professor and Head of Obstetrics and Gynecology
St George's University of London
London, UK

SARALA GOPALAN FRCOG, PhD, FAMS
Formerly Professor and Head, Department of Obstetrics and Gynecology
Postgraduate Institute of Medical Education and Research (PGIMER)
Chandigarh, India

PRATAP KUMAR MD, DGO, FIMCH
Professor and Head of the Department of Obstetrics and Gynecology
Kasturba Medical College
Manipal, India

Universities Press

UNIVERSITIES PRESS (INDIA) PRIVATE LIMITED

Registered Office
3-6-747/1/A & 3-6-754/1, Himayatnagar, Hyderabad 500 029, India
email: info@universitiespress.com, www.universitiespress.com

Distributed by
Orient Blackswan Private Limited

Registered Office
3-6-752 Himayatnagar, Hyderabad 500 029, India

Other Offices
Bengaluru / Bhopal / Bhubaneshwar / Chennai / Ernakulam / Guwahati
Hyderabad / Jaipur / Kolkata / Lucknow / Mumbai / New Delhi / Noida / Patna

First published 1994
Reprinted 1995, 1996, 1999, 2001
Second Edition 2003, Reprinted 2006
Third edition 2009
Reprinted 2011, 2013, 2014

ISBN 978 81 7371 661 4

Cover design
Binita Desai

Cover and book design:
© Universities Press (India) Private Limited 2009

Typeset by
Trinity Designers and Typesetters
Chennai 600 041

Printed at
Baba Barkha Nath Printers
New Delhi

Published by
Universities Press (India) Private Limited
3-6-747/1/A & 3-6-754/1, Himayatnagar, Hyderabad 500 029, India

Preface to the third edition

The first two editions of *Obstetrics and Gynecology for Postgraduates* were brought out under the distinguished editorship of Professor SS Ratnam from Singapore, Professor K Bhasker Rao from Chennai and one of the current editors, Professor Sabaratnam Arulkumaran who then worked in Singapore but is currently Head of Obstetrics and Gynecology at St. George's Medical School, University of London. With the passing away of Professor SS Ratnam and the retirement of Professor K Bhasker Rao, a decision was taken to bring in two new editors with distinguished careers in obstetrics and gynecology. Professor Sarala Gopalan, formerly Head of the Postgraduate Institute of Obstetrics and Gynecology, Chandigarh and Professor Pratap Kumar, Head of the Department of Obstetrics and Gynecology from the Manipal University kindly agreed to help.

A distinct difference from the previous editions is that the chapters on obstetrics are in the first volume and those on gynecology in the second. This is a deviation from the past 16 years, where we had both obstetrics and gynecology in the two volumes, with 20 chapters in obstetrics and 20 in gynecology in each volume. We have maintained the number of chapters in each volume at 40.

The other major difference has been for the editors to divide the chapters based on their expertise. We commissioned well known authors and edited their respective chapters with the help of the authors. This provided more freedom to the authors to express their views, backing it with strong evidence. This approach has expanded the contents of each chapter compared to the previous editions; they are much richer in quality and quantity.

The field of obstetrics and gynecology has seen major advances starting from obstetric and gynecological ultrasound by Ian Donald in the 1960s and in vitro fertilisation in the 1970s by Steptoe and Edwards. In addition to these there have been major advances in developing new hormones and new types of operative procedures. Not only have new medicine and new technology advanced the field, but also the culture of evidence-based medicine has added greatly to it. Having protocols and guidelines have unified our views and have enhanced safe practice in this specialty. It is not an easy task to be up to date with all the current literature. These two volumes have made an attempt to synthesise recently available, acceptable and appropriate management in different settings. We believe that these volumes will enable postgraduates and clinicians to provide the best care possible in women's health.

Needless to say, there might be questions on best or acceptable practice. The editors and the publishers welcome comments so that errors, if any, can be rectified in the subsequent reprints or edition. Since the editorial work was divided amongst the three editors, there may be some overlap of the contents in different chapters. This is deliberately left as it is to provide continuity of the subject in each individual chapter.

The publishers have taken great pains to bring these two volumes with a new format, more pictures, readable type, and new layout. We are most grateful to them. We hope that readers will benefit from these two volumes.

SABARATNAM ARULKUMARAN
SARALA GOPALAN
PRATAP KUMAR

Preface to the second edition

It has been a source of great satisfaction and pleasure to the editors that the first edition of this book was extensively used by postgraduates not only in India but also in many parts of Asia. We are also happy that the book has been particularly useful to students preparing for examinations. The book has undergone several reprints and we are happy to present this revised edition.

While the editors recognise that it would not be possible to cover all aspects of obstetrics and gynecology, and women's health in a comprehensive manner, we have attempted to cover all the major aspects of the discipline in the two volumes of the book. Most of the chapters in this volume have been extensively revised and new chapters on operative vaginal deliveries, tropical diseases and thyroid disorders have been included to make the volume more complete and to assist postgraduate students and practising clinicians in updating their knowledge and keeping pace with current advances.

The editors have made special efforts to identify contributors with interest in a particular subject area so as to make their chapter authoritative. The contributors belong to different parts of Asia. Every chapter of the book has been edited, independently and jointly by the editors and despite all efforts to make the book as comprehensive as possible we do recognise that the reader will need to refer to published articles to further update their knowledge in a particular subject area.

We hope to deal with the advances in reproductive health, obstetrics and gynecology, and in awareness of women's health, particularly with relevance to socioeconomic status, in the new edition of the second volume.

We hope that this edition of volume 1, will be as relevant to and popular among postgraduate students and practising clinicians as the earlier edition.

1999

SS RATNAM
K BHASKER RAO
S ARULKUMARAN

Preface to the first edition

Although many books have been written on obstetrics and gynecology and a number of monographs appear regularly, there is a dearth of books for postgraduates with particular reference to Asian countries. This book does not attempt to cover basic information that is available in standard textbooks but aims to address current topics with emphasis on issues of controversy and advances that have taken place in recent times.

The editors have made a special effort to identify contributors with interest in the particular subject so as to make it authoritative. With this in mind, the editors have looked beyond India for contributors and fifty per cent of the contributions have come from outside. Every chapter has been edited by the three General Editors independently and jointly, and it is hoped that the book will serve as a textbook for postgraduates preparing for the higher examinations as well as serve as a reference book for practising obstetricians and gynecologists.

This volume covers a wider range of subjects spanning obstetrics and gynecology. It is not possible to cover all aspects of the discipline in one volume and the editors hope to bring out the second volume soon to address subjects of interest that have not been included in this volume and where advances have taken place and where controversies still persist.

1992

SS RATNAM
K BHASKER RAO
S ARULKUMARAN

Contents

Contributors

Akhila Vasudeva MD
Assistant Professor, Department of Obstetrics and Gynecology
Kasturba Medical College
Manipal, India

Amarnath Bhide MD, MRCOG
Consultant, Department of Obstetrics and Gynecology
Fetal Medicine Unit,
St. George's Hospital,
London, United Kingdom

Amita Suneja MD, FIMCH, MNAMS
Professor, Department of Obstetrics and Gynecology
University College of Medical Sciences and Guru Tegh Bahadur Hospital
Delhi, India

Asmita Muthal Rathore MBBS, MD, MRCOG
Professor, Department of Obstetrics and Gynecology
Maulana Azad Medical College and Loknayak Hospital
New Delhi, India

Baskaran Thilaganathan PhD FRCOG
Consultant and Director
Fetal Medical Unit
St. George's Hospital NHS Trust
London, United Kingdom

K Bhasker Rao
Formerly Director, Institute of Obstetrics and Gynaecology, Chennai and
Consultant Obstetrician and Gynecologist,
Vijaya Hospitals
Chennai, India

Deepika Deka
Professor, Department of Obstetrics and Gynecology
All India Institute of Medical Sciences
New Delhi, India

Gita Radhakrishnan MD
Professor, Department of Obstetrics and Gynecology
University College of Medical Sciences and Guru Tegh Bahadur Hospital
Delhi, India

Gowri Ramanathan MBBS, MRCOG
Special Registrar
St George's Hospital
London, United Kingdom

Hema Diwaker MD
Diwaker's Hospital
Bengaluru, India

Inusha Panigrahi MD, DM
Assistant Professor, Department of Pediatrics, Postgraduate Institute of Medical Education and Research
Chandigarh, India

Jasvinder Kalra MD
Additional Professor, Department of Obstetrics and Gynecology
Postgraduate Institute of Medical Education and Research
Chandigarh, India

Jayaraman Nambiar M MBBS, DGO, MD
Associate Professor, Department of Obstetrics and Gynecology
Kasturba Medical College
Manipal, India

Jyothi Shetty MBBS, MD
Associate Professor of Obstetrics and Gynecology
Kasturba Medical College
Manipal, India

Kiran Guleria
Reader, Department of Obstetrics and Gynecology
University College of Medical Sciences and Guru Tegh Bahadur Hospital
Delhi, India

Madhuchanda Dey MBBS, MRCOG (UK), Diploma in Obstetric Ultrasound (RCOG/RCR-UK)
Specialist Registrar in Obstetrics and Gynecology
Singleton Hospital
Swansea, United Kingdom

Muralidhar V Pai MD
Professor and Head, Department of Obstetrics and Gynecology
Melaka Manipal Medical College
Melaka, Malaysia

Nalini Arora MD, DNB, MNAMS, FIMSA
Associate Professor, Department of Obstetrics and Gynecology
Institute of Postgraduate Medical Education and Research
Kolkata, India

Narayanan R MD, DGO, MNAS, FICS, FICOG
Former Professor and Head, Department of Obstetrics and Gynecology
St John's Medical College and Hospital
Bengaluru, India

Narayan Jana MD, DNB, MRCOG, MFFP, MAMS, FIMSA, FICOG
Associate Professor of Obstetrics and Gynecology
Institute of Postgraduate Medical Education and Research
Kolkata, India

Niraj Krishnamurthy Yanamandra MBBS, MD, MRCOG
Senior Registrar, Department of Obstetrics and Gynecology
St George's Hospital
London, United Kingdom

Parvathi Bhat MD DNB
Associate Professor, Department of Obstetrics and Gynecology
Kasturba Medical College
Manipal, India

Prashanth K Adiga MD
Assistant Professor, Department of Obstetrics and Gynecology
Kasturba Medical College
Manipal, India

Pratap Kumar MD, DGO, FIMCH
Professor and Head, Department of Obstetrics and Gynecology
Kasturba Medical College
Manipal, India

Rajeshwari G Bhat MD
Associate Professor, Department of Obstetrics and Gynecology
Kasturba Medical College
Manipal, India

Ramkumar Venkateswaran MBBS, MD
Professor and Head, Department of Anesthesiology
Kasturba Medical College
Manipal, India

Rani Akhil Bhat MD
Associate Professor, Department of Obstetrics and Gynecology
Kasturba Medical College
Manipal, India

Rashmi Bagga MD, DNB
Additional Professor, Department of Obstetrics and Gynecology
Postgraduate Institute of Medical Education and Research
Chandigarh, India

Renu Saxena MBBS, MD
Professor and Head, Department of Hematology
All India Institute of Medical Sciences
New Delhi, India

Reva Tripathi MBBS, MD
Professor, Department of Obstetrics and Gynecology
Maulana Azad Medical College and Loknayak Hospital
New Delhi, India

Sabaratnam Arulkumaran PhD, FRCOG, FRCS
Professor and Head of Obstetrics and Gynecology
St George's University of London
London, United Kingdom

Sachin Ajmera
Consultant Gynecologist
Mumbai, India

Sanjay B Rao MD, DNBE, FCPS, DGO, DFP, MICOG
Specialist Registrar in Obstetrics and Gynaecology,
Severn,Wessex and Peninsula Deanery,
Bristol, United Kingdom

Sarala Gopalan FRCOG, PhD, FAMS
Formerly Professor and Head, Department of Obstetrics and Gynecology
Postgraduate Institute of Medical Education and Research
Chandigarh, India

Sathisha Nayak MBBS, MD, DNB
Associate Professor, Department of Obstetrics and Gynecology
Melaka Manipal Medical College
Melaka, Malaysia

PK Shah MD, DGO, DFP, FCPS
Professor and Unit Head, Department of Obstetrics and Gynecology
LTM Medical College and LTMG Hospital
Mumbai, India

Shripad Hebbar MD
Associate Professor of Obstetrics and Gynecology
Melaka Manipal Medical College
Melaka, Malaysia

Shanthi Sairam MRCOG
Academic Department of Obstetrics and Gynecology
Fetal Medical Unit
St. George's Hospital
London, United Kingdom

Shashikala K Bhat MD
Assistant Professor, Department of Obstetrics and Gynecology
Melaka Manipal Medical College
Melaka, Malaysia

V Sivanesaratnam MBBS, FRCOG, FICS, FACS, FAMM
Consultant Gynecologic Oncologist
University of Malaysia Medical Centre
University of Malaysia Specialist Centre
Kuala Lumpur, Malaysia

Shyamala Guruvare MD
Associate Professor, Department of Obstetrics and Gynecology
Kasturba Medical College
Manipal, India

Soma Mukherjee MBBS, MRCOG, DGO, DNB, MNAS, FICOG, FICMCH, RCOG/RCR Dip Advanced Obstetric Ultrasound
Clinical Lecturer in Obstetrics and Gynecology
Fetal Medical Unit
St. George's University of London
London, United Kingdom

Stergios K Doumouchtsis Phd MRCOG
Senior Specialist Registrar in Obstetrics and Gynecology
St George's Hospital
London, United Kingdom

Suchitra N Pandit B Pharm, MD, DNBE, DGO, DFP, MRCOG, MICOG
Associate Professor and Unit in Charge, Department of Obstetrics and Gynecology LT Medical College Hospital,
Mumbai, India

Sujatha Janakiraman MBBS, MD, DGO, DNB (Obstetrics and Gynecology)
Assistant Professor, Department of Obstetrics and Gynecology
Melaka Manipal Medical College
Melaka, Malaysia

Tulika Singh MBBS, DGO, MRCOG
Senior Registrar, Department of Obstetrics and Gynecology
Queens Hospital,
Essex, United Kingdom

K Uma Devi MD, DGO, MNAMS, MRCOG, PGDMLE, PGDHM
Professor and Head of the Department (Obstetrics and Gynecology)
MS Ramaiah Medical College
Bengaluru, India

Vanita Jain MD, DNB
Professor, Department of Obstetrics and Gynecology
Postgraduate Institute of Medical Education and Research
Chandigarh, India

Vanita Suri MD
Professor, Department of Obstetrics and Gynecology
Postgraduate Institute of Medical Education and Research
Chandigarh, India

Vani Ramkumar MBBS, MD
Professor, Department of Obstetrics and Gynecology
Kasturba Medical College,
Manipal, India

Vijay C Pawar MD, FCPS, DGO,
Senior Registrar
LT Medical College Hospital,
Mumbai, India

1

Reproductive Health in Developing Countries

K Bhasker Rao

Introduction

When the state of women's health in developing countries is under discussion, 'reproductive health (RH)' is a better choice of term than 'maternal health', because it encompasses the health of women from childhood and adolescence through the reproductive epoch and the post-menopausal period.

Reproductive health is defined as a state of complete physical, mental and social well-being, and not merely the absence of illness or disease, in relation to the reproductive processes, systems and practices at all stages of life (World Health Organization 1994).

Thus, RH encompasses human sexuality, fertility control, safe motherhood and child survival, and prevention and treatment of reproductive tract infections, besides menopausal problems and prevention and treatment of genital cancer.

Human Sexuality

Human sexuality influences thoughts, emotions, actions and interactions contributing to the motivation to seek love, contact, warmth, intimacy, peace and happiness. If both partners practise responsible sexual behaviour, the chances of an unwanted pregnancy or any disease are significantly reduced and there is good sexual health. Unsafe sexual behaviour at any age leads to reproductive ill health.

Adolescent Health

Adolescence is the most critical period of life when nutrition, physical activity (sports) and education (including sex education) are needed to prepare men and women for professional, social and reproductive life later on. With reproductive maturation resulting from endocrinological changes at this period of life, any sexual misadventure may lead to an unwanted pregnancy, unsafe abortion or sexually transmitted diseases (STDs), early dropping-out from school and problems relating to juvenile delinquency (Table 1.1).

There is a global need for adolescent-friendly sexual and reproductive health services, and counselling on sexuality, family planning, pregnancy and post-abortal issues.

Fertility Control

In the last five decades, uncontrolled fertility and declining death rates have contributed to population explosion. There has also been an increase in the life expectancy at birth, slightly more so for girls than for boys. This demographic revolution has in

TABLE 1.1: CHALLENGES TO ADOLESCENT HEALTH IN DEVELOPING COUNTRIES

Adolescents form 20–25% of the population in the developing world
Globally, 10% of all births occur in the adolescent age group
Maternal mortality at age <18 years is 2–4 times higher than at 18–25 years
Annually, 1 to 4.4 million adolescents undergo abortions, most of which are unsafe
Each year, 5% of adolescents acquire curable STDs (excluding viral infections)
Every year, of the estimated 333 million new STD cases in the world, 111 million occur in young people (<25 years)
Globally, over 50% of all new HIV infections are seen in the 15–24 age group

(Source: WHO Tech Rep Series No. 886, 1999)

turn necessitated a contraceptive revolution. With population education and increased acceptance of contraception during these five decades, there has been a decline in the total fertility rates (TFR) from 5–6 in the 1950s to as low as 1.8–2 by the turn of the twenty-first century in most developing countries.

From Table 1.2 it can be seen that the key to good reproductive health is female literacy or education—the higher the female literacy the greater the contraceptive acceptance, the smaller the family and the lower the reproductive mortality rates. In China and India, metal-bearing intrauterine devices (IUDs) are more acceptable than oral or injectable hormonal contraceptives. Again, in these two countries, sterilisation accounts for 25–30% of all acceptors. Globally, there is a marked decline in the number of vasectomies and this explains why in about 5 million sterilisations reported annually in India, only 3–4% are vasectomies. In China, the recently introduced 'no scalpel' method of vasectomy is trying to reverse this trend.

Emergency or post-coital contraception: This is extremely useful in preventing pregnancy after an unprotected coitus (or in cases of rape) and has helped to eliminate millions of unwanted pregnancies and unsafe abortions. A single dose of L-norgestrel 1.5 mg, or mifepristone (RU 486) 10 mg, taken orally within five days (120 hours) of unprotected coitus is effective in preventing pregnancy in 98.5% of cases (Hertzen et al 2002).

ABORTIONS: Globally, 13% of all maternal deaths are due to unsafe abortions and most of those who survive suffer from reproductive ill-health due to pelvic inflammatory disorders (PID). According to the United Nations Population Division, 98% of the world's 193 countries allow abortion to save the life of the woman, 62% to preserve her physical and mental health, 43% in cases of rape or incest, only 39% for fetal impairment, 32% for socioeconomic reasons and 27% upon request (UNFPA 1999; Lancet 2002). The liberalisation of abortions alone is not an adequate measure. If abortion facilities are not easily accessible, unsafe abortions may continue to take their toll on the life and health of these women, as seen in India, where even 30 years after passing the most liberal abortion laws, thousands of young lives are still lost annually due to unsafe abortions (Rao 2000).

Repeated abortions are harmful but abortion facilities are necessary when contraception fails. The best way to reduce

Table 1.2: Fertility control and RH (1995-2000)					
Country	*Secondary School Enrollment (F) %*	*Contraceptive Prevalence %*	*Total Fertility Rate*	*Maternal Mortality Rate*	*Under-5 Mortality Rate (F)*
Afghanistan	12	2	6.9	1500	257
Bangladesh	13	49	3.1	850	116
India	39	45	3.2	437	97
Malaysia	65	48	3.2	43	13
Myanmar	30	17	2.4	580	104
Pakistan	17	18	5.0	340	104
Singapore	65	74	1.7	10	6
Sri Lanka	78	66	2.1	30	20
Thailand	56	74	1.7	200	33

(Source: UNFPA 1999)

abortions is to prevent unwanted pregnancies by making family planning services easily accessible.

SAFE MOTHERHOOD

In developing countries, one out of six women in the age group of 15–44 years, dies due to maternal disorders. Other important causes of death in this group are tuberculosis (10%), suicide (7%), war (4.4%), road accidents (3.7%) and HIV (3.4%) (Murray and Lopez 1997).

Accurate estimation of maternal mortality depends mainly on a sound vital registration system and precise reporting of maternal deaths. There is significant under-reporting and misclassification of these deaths.

Globally, of an estimated 515,000 maternal deaths in 1995, only 206 (0.4%) were reported from the developed region (WHO 1996). Though the maternal mortality rate (MMR) in the world is estimated to be about 400 per 100,000 live births, it varies widely from 830 per 100,000 in Africa to 330 in Asia, compared to 24 in Europe. Thus, we find that it is as low as 20 per 100,000 in the developed regions, and 440 in the developing regions (20 times that for the developed regions). Over 75% of global maternal deaths are reported from the developing countries of just two continents—Asia and Africa. China, with a population larger than that of India accounts for only 6% of global maternal deaths compared to 25% in India, because of its higher literacy and contraceptive acceptance rates resulting in a much lower TFR (Table 1.3). It may again be seen that the higher the female literacy and contraceptive acceptance, the smaller the family and the lower the risk of maternal death.

However, the most important predictor of maternal death in a country is the percentage of deliveries getting skilled care.

Life-time Risk of Maternal Death

Globally, this risk is 1 in 60 pregnancies. In the developing countries, the risk is higher (about 1 in 48 compared to 1 in 1800 in the developed region). It is highest in south-central Asia—1 in 35. In Afghanistan it is 1 in 7 compared to 1 in 4900 in Singapore (WHO 1996).

Maternal Morbidity

For each maternal death there are at least five

'near-deaths' due to severe morbidity (Baskett 2000). For each maternal death, it is estimated that there are 15 cases of morbidity (Dutta et al 1980; de Barnis et al 2000). Morbidity may include PID, chronic pelvic pain, infertility, genital prolapse and, worst of all, urinary and fecal incontinence (Mala 2003). In the African region alone, about 50,000 to 100,000 cases of obstetric fistulae are reported to occur annually (International Committee on Incontinence 2000). Shah (1991) estimates that in the developing countries of Asia, its incidence is about 0.5–2% of gynecological admissions.

Causes of Maternal Deaths: In most developing countries, 80% of the deaths are due to direct obstetric causes, and 20% to associated causes. The leading direct causes are hemorrhages (25%), infections (15%), unsafe abortions (13%), eclampsia and pre-eclampsia (12%), obstructed labour (8%) and others (7%) (WHO 1999). Tetanus, though easily preventable, still accounts for 2–7% of maternal deaths in Bangladesh and India (Rochat and Akhtar 1999; MOH India 1999).

Amongst the associated causes of maternal deaths, anemia, malaria and viral hepatitis complicating pregnancy are common. Globally, over 50% of pregnant women are anemic, and in South Asia this figure is even higher. Many of them suffer from nutritional anemia worsened by helminthiasis and malaria, and this is responsible for 10–15% of maternal deaths in developing countries (Guidotti 2000). Most cases of falciparum malaria are seen in Africa (south of Sahara), though the disease is also prevalent in India, Myanmar and Thailand and accounts for 10,000 maternal deaths globally. Cerebral malaria complicating pregnancy carries a fatality rate of over 30% (Kocher et al 1999). Chemoprophylaxis, twice in the course of pregnancy, has not only helped to reduce these maternal deaths but has also contributed to the reduction of the LBW rates in Malawi (WHO 2000).

The factors contributing to maternal mortality are discussed below:

(i) The better the care during pregnancy and labour, the safer the delivery and the mother's health. In the developing world, only 66% get prenatal care, 45% deliver in institutions and 50% access skilled care during delivery. Skilled care includes doctors, nurses

TABLE 1.3: MATERNAL MORTALITY RATES

Country	% Literacy >15 Years (Female)	Total Fertility Rate	Skilled Care at Delivery (%)	MMR per 100,000 Births	IMR per 1000 Births
Bangladesh	26	3.1	13	850	79
China	77	1.8	67	115	41
India	38	3.1	43	437	72
Malaysia	79	3.2	96	43	11
Sri Lanka	87	2.1	94	30	18
Singapore	86	1.7	100	10	5
Thailand	92	1.7	71	200	29
Sweden	100	1.6	100	7	5

(Source: UNFPA (1999) and WHO (2001))

and midwives and excludes traditional birth attendants (TBAs) (WHO 1997). The high maternal death rates in South Asian countries may be explained by poor maternity care as only one in two get prenatal care, one in four have institutional delivery and less than a third get skilled attention during delivery. Of the maternal deaths, 25% occur in pregnancy, 15% intrapartum and 50–70% postpartum (of these, almost 50% occur in 24 hours and two-thirds in the first week). The commonest causes of maternal deaths are hemorrhage, sepsis and unsafe abortion. Annually, it is estimated that there are 46 million induced abortions of which 40% or 18 million are unsafe and are responsible for 68,000 maternal deaths (WHO 2005).

In Sri Lanka, the MMR declined from 1500 in 1945–50 to 30 in 1994, by increasing the coverage of skilled care to 94% by training a large number of midwives and also by providing facilities for early referral of obstetric emergencies to first referral centres (WHO 1999).

(ii) The MMR is not only influenced by the number of women receiving skilled assistance but also by ensuring provision of facilities for tackling obstetric emergencies with the least delay (Abou Zahar et al 2001). The emergency cesarean rate should be between a minimum of 5% and an optimum of 15%. In the sub-Saharan region, a very low rate of less than 1.5% explains the high MMR, as such facilities are few and far between and rapid transport is not available to reach such centres in time (Dumont et al 2001).

(iii) Three crucial delays are also significant contributors (Kurian et al 2000):

- Delay in deciding to seek help on the part of the patient or relatives
- Delay in reaching the care (usually due to lack of transport)
- Delay in treating the emergency at the facility for lack of blood etc.

Steps to Reduce Maternal Mortality

As multiple causes are responsible for maternal deaths, multiple strategies are required to reduce the MMR:

- Better education, including health education of women, since this ultimately contributes to better reproductive health.
- By proper health education, an awareness has to be created in the community that a small (and well-spaced) family promotes reproductive health. Each pregnancy requires care from the time the periods are missed, and should also be booked in advance for safe delivery with a skilled person or institution. The community should also be educated about when, where and how to reach the nearest first referral hospital (FRH) in an emergency (Mala et al 2000).
- Unwanted pregnancies can be prevented by making effective contraception and safe abortion facilities available.
- Pregnancy complications may be prevented by good quality prenatal care (including tetanus immunisation and prophylaxis against anemia and malaria), with not more than 4–5 visits till delivery, as described in the WHO multicentric trial (Villar et al 2001).
- A skilled attendant can provide complete intranatal care—this, along with backup of transport for prompt referral to the first referral unit for emergency obstetric care, can contribute significantly.
- Guidelines for management of common obstetric problems can be made available, such as
  - Prevention of PPH with oxytocics including carboprost, and 'PPH drill' to manage it.
  - Prevention of eclampsia by parenteral

magnesium sulphate prophylaxis as advocated in the MAGPIE trial (2002) and to treat eclampsia with magnesium sulphate as recommended by the Eclampsia Collaborative Trial Group (1995).
  - o Use of partography to prevent prolonged or obstructed labour.
  - o Use of broad-spectrum antibiotics to prevent and combat sepsis.
- Audit of all maternal deaths and 'near-deaths', with periodic reports of recommendations as to their prevention, as has been done by the UK Confidential Enquiry (1998).

Quantified reduction in maternal mortality is one of the important developmental goals of the United Nations and it is hoped that by 2015 all developed countries will have an MMR below 60 per 100,000 live births (Lancet 2002).

CHILD SURVIVAL

The newborn is perhaps the most vulnerable to trauma, anoxia and death around birth. It was estimated that globally about 2.45 million newborns die each year due to perinatal causes. The perinatal mortality rate (PMR), which by definition includes all stillbirths and first-week deaths among 1000 births, varies from a low rate of 5–9 per 1000 births for Western Europe (Graafmans et al 2001) to a moderate range of 20–40 for most developing countries and a high of over 40 in Brazil, Egypt, India, Nigeria and Pakistan (WHO 1996) (Table 1.4). The important causes of PMR are birth trauma and anoxia, sepsis and prematurity. Bangladesh and India have the highest rates of low birth weight infants contributing to a high infant mortality rate. Good prenatal and intranatal care with strengthening of essential neonatal care including prevention of neonatal hypoxia and hypothermia is important; breastfeeding and immunisation help reduce perinatal and infant mortality rates.

Out of 136 million births annually, including 3.3 million stillbirths, about 10.6 million children die before the age of five years: most of these are from poor socioeconomic conditions. Much of this under-5 mortality is avoidable.

Prevention of malnutrition, prevention and prompt treatment of pneumonia (19%), diarrhea (18%), malaria (8%), measles (3%) and neonatal conditions like prematurity, birth anoxia and infections (37%) contribute to reduction of under-5 mortality rates (WHO 2005). The reduction of child mortality by two-thirds by 2015 is one of the important millennial goals of the UN.

REPRODUCTIVE TRACT INFECTIONS

Poverty and permissiveness are contributors to unsafe sexual practices; this has resulted in a marked increase in reproductive tract infections (RTI) all over the world. According to the WHO (1999), 333 million new cases of STDs were reported worldwide during 1995. The spectrum of STDs has changed in the last three decades. Out of 30 STDs caused by bacteria, parasites and viruses, the commonest was chlamydiasis (89 million) followed by gonorrhea (62 million) and syphilis (12 million). Chlamydial infections have been reported in 2.6% of women and 2% of men in China; 6–8% of women with PID and 18–20% of women suffering from STD in China and in Thailand, most of them with coexisting gonococcal disease (Ramachandran 2002; Beyrer 2003). In rural Bangladesh, chlamydial and gonococcal infections were seen only in 0.5% of women (Hawkes et al 2002). Unfortunately, most women suffering from chlamydiasis are asymptomatic or have very mild symptoms; however, recurrent

Table 1.4: Vital statistics pertaining to child survival in some Asian countries compared to Sweden

Country	HDI Rank 2002	LBW (%) (1995–2000)	PMR 1996	IMR 2000	Under-5 MR 2000	MMR (1999)
Bangladesh	145	30	>40	54	82	350
China	96	6	20–40	32	40	55
India	124	26	>40	69	96	540
Japan	9	7	<10	4	4	8
Malaysia	59	9	20–40	8	9	41
Myanmar	127	16	20–40	78	110	230
Sri Lanka	89	17	20–40	17	19	60
Singapore	25	8	10	4	4	6
Indonesia	110	9	20–40	35	48	380
Thailand	70	7	20–40	25	29	44
Sweden	2	4	4.5	3	4	5

(Japan and Singapore are considered developed countries)
HDI rank = Human Development Index assigned by UNDP in 2002.

infections often lead to reproductive ill-health—ectopic pregnancy, infertility, PID and chronic pelvic pain. In the presence of coexisting pyogenic infection, it may result in peritonitis, septic shock or death.

Besides bacterial infections, STDs may also be caused by viruses like HBV, HPV, HSV-2 and, most importantly, by HIV.

HIV/AIDS AND REPRODUCTIVE HEALTH

UNAIDS estimated that in late 2001 approximately 40 million persons worldwide were living with HIV/AIDS, besides 5 million new cases and 3 million deaths due to AIDS occurring that year. Stover et al (2002) predicted that HIV infections will increase by 25% by 2005 with at least 45 million new cases by 2010 due to its spread in Russia, China, India and Nigeria. In Africa, heterosexual spread has resulted in over 28 million persons getting infected. With sero-positivity rates varying from 5% to 30% among women attending prenatal clinics (see Table 1.5) and with mother-to-child transmission rates of 25–45% (due to breastfeeding), about 19,000 children acquire the infection daily. Of these, 35–60% die before the age of two years. The mothers survive for a median of nine years after early infection. By 2001, over 12 million children in Africa were orphaned. The UN has now stepped in with measures to reduce the transmission rates by 50% by 2010 (Dabis and Ekpini 2002).

In Asia, the spread occurs by infected needles among drug addicts, besides the heterosexual route. In Thailand, since 2001, an intensive campaign has helped in antenatal prophylaxis with zidovudine to HIV-positive mothers (from 34 weeks through labour and oral prophylaxis with ZDV for the newborn, in addition to formula feeds for a year). This has helped reduce vertical transmission rates to a large extent (Amornvichet et al 2002). Though 19 drugs are approved by the FDA for anti-retroviral therapy, for those

Table 1.5: Incidence/Prevalence of HIV/AIDS (2004)

Region	*Adults and Children Living with HIV/AIDS*	*Adults and Children Newly Infected with HIV/AIDS*	*Adult Prevalence (%)*	*Adult and Child Deaths Due to AIDS*
Sub-Saharan Africa	25.4 million	3.1 million	7.4	2.3 million
North Africa & Middle East	540,000	92,000	0.3	28,000
South & Southeast Asia	7.1 million	890,000	0.6	490,000
East Asia	1.1 million	290,000	0.1	51,000
Oceania	35,000	5,000	0.2	700
Latin America	1.7 million	240,000	0.6	95,000
Caribbean	440,000	53,000	2.3	36,000
Eastern Europe & Central Asia	1.4 million	210,000	0.8	60,000
Western & Central Europe	610,000	21,000	0.3	6,500
North America	1.0 million	44,000	0.6	16,000
TOTAL	39.4 million (35.9–44.3 million)	4.9 million (4.3–6.4 million)	1.1% (1.0–1.3%)	3.1 million (2.8–3.5 million)

** The proportion of adults (15–49 years of age) living with HIV/AIDS in 2004, using 2004 population numbers (Joint United Nations Programme on HIV/AIDS (UNAIDS): AIDS Epidemic Update, December 2004.)*

women with HIV-1 RNA, less than 1000 copies/ml monotherapy with ZDV during the second and third trimester is still the best option (with transmission rates of only 1% compared with 9.8% in the controls). But in those with a higher viral load, combination therapy (with 2 nucleoside analogues with a protease inhibitor) is preferred (Perinatal HIV Guidelines Working Group 2002). The current guidelines recommend initiation of HAART in asymptomatic HIV-infected persons with CD4+ T lymphocyte count of less than 200 cells/cubic mm (with treatment considered in those whose counts are between 200 and 350 cell/cubic mm (Reynolds et al 2003). Preventive measures include health education, use of condoms, vaccines, use of sterile syringes and needles for IV drug users, universal testing for HIV and ways to reduce vertical mother-to-child transmission such as counselling and therapy with artificial infant-feeding.

MENOPAUSAL PROBLEMS

During the last 50 years there has been a gradual increase in the longevity of life at birth, with more women living up to 75 years and beyond. Thus, we find that an increasing number of women survive to over a third of their lifespan beyond menopause. Thus, when they 'add years to life' it is necessary for us to help them 'add life to years.' Some of them may need hormone replacement therapy for a short period. With ageing, there is an increased risk of genital prolapse, genital cancer, and cardiovascular and cerebrovascular diseases (Rao 2002).

CANCER OF THE REPRODUCTIVE ORGANS

The common sites of cancer in the reproductive organs in the order of frequency are the cervix, breast, ovary and uterine corpus. Worldwide, there are about 1.4 million cases of cervical cancer annually and 3–7 million cases of severe cervical dysplasia. Increase in the incidence of cervical cancer in developing countries may be due to early marriage and sexual activity, multiple partners and HPV infections. Though its incidence can be reduced by 80% by cytological screening of sexually active women every 3–5 years, alternative screening methods like visual inspection with acetic acid and HPV testing have been found to be extremely useful and cost-effective in developing countries, where the cytological methods were not found to be technically feasible (Sankaranarayanan et al 2001). However, recent trials with vaccines against HPV types 16 and 18 have been encouraging (Koutsky et al 2002). Breast cancer is familial and is likely to be seen in nulliparous women and in those who have been on OCP and HRT for over 5–10 years. Monthly self-examination of breasts and mammographic screening every three years is useful. Trials are underway for chemical prophylaxis against breast cancer and surgical prophylaxis in selected cases of hereditary breast cancer (King et al 2001; Haber 2002). At present there is no cost-effective screening methodology available for early detection of ovarian cancer.

GENDER INEQUITY

Gender inequity contravenes human rights and adversely affects reproductive health. In some developing countries, discrimination against women is lifelong, coexisting with female feticide, infanticide, domestic violence, bride-burning, gang rape and forced prostitution in spite of stringent laws.

The 1994 Declaration of the International Conference on Population and Development (ICPD), Cairo, provides for gender equity, empowerment of women and elimination of all forms of discrimination against women. It assures women the right to sexual health and control of their own fertility to decide the number and spacing of their children and the right to safe motherhood. As most developing countries are signatories to this declaration, they are committed to restore gender equity so that women can enjoy reproductive health as much as men.

It is hoped that with better education, empowerment, gender equity and well-organised community reproductive health care services available to them in developing countries, women will enjoy better reproductive health by 2010.

References

Abou Zahr C and E Royston. 1991. *Maternal mortality: A global factbook*. Geneva: World Health Organization.

Abou Zahr C and T Wardlaw. 2001. Maternal mortality at end of the decade: Signs of progress? *Bull World Health Org* 79:561–573.

Amornwichet P, A Teeraratkul and RJ Simonds. 2002. Preventing mother to child HIV transmission: The first Year of Thailand's National Program. *JAMA* 288:245–248.

Baskett TF and J Sternadale. 1998. Maternal intensive care and near miss maternal deaths. *Br J Obstet Gynaecol* 105:921–927.

Beyrer C. 2003. Hidden epidemic of sexually transmitted diseases in China. *JAMA* 289:1303–1305.

Confidential Enquiry into Maternal Deaths in the UK (1994–96). Report of 1998. Norwich: Her Majesty's Stationery Office.

Dabis F and ER Ekpini. 2002. HIV-1/AIDS and maternal and child health in Africa. *Lancet* 359: 2097–3004.

Datta KK, RS Sharma, PMA Rasack et al. 1980. Morbidity pattern amongst rural pregnant women in Rajasthan. *Health Pop Prospect Iss* 3:282–292.

De Barnis L, A Dumont, D Bouillin et al. 2000. Maternal morbidity and mortality in two different populations of Senegal. *Br J Obstet Gynaecol* 107:68–74.

Dumont A, L deBernis, B Bouvier-Colle et al. 2001. Cesarean section rate for maternal indication in sub-Saharan Africa. *Lancet* 358:1328–1334.

Eclampsia Trial Collaborative Group. 1995. Which anticonvulsant for women with eclampsia? *Lancet* 345:1455-1463.

Graafmans WC, J Richardus, A Macfarlane et al. 2001. Comparability of published perinatal morality rates in West Europe. *Br J Obstet Gynaecol* 108:1237–1245.

Guidotti RJ. 2000. Anemia in pregnancy in developing countries. *Br J Obstet Gynaecol* 107:437–438.

Haber D. 2002. Prophylactic oophorectomy to reduce the risk of ovarian and breast cancer in carriers of BRCA mutations. *N Engl J Med* 346:1660–1661.

Hill K, C Abou Zahr and T Wardlaw. 2001. Estimates of maternal mortality for 1995. *Bull WHO* 79:182–193.

Hawkes S, C Morison and J Chakraborty. 2002. Prevalence of reproductive tract infections in rural Bangladesh. (Matlab region) *Bull World Health Org* 80:180–188.

International Scientific Committee on Incontinence. 2000. Assessment and treatment of incontinence. *Lancet* 355:2153–58.

King MC, S Wieand, K Hale et al. 2001. Tamoxifen and breast cancer incidence among women with inherited mutations in BRCA-1 and BRCA-2. *JAMA* 286:251–256.

Kocher DK, I Thanvi et al. 1999. Mortality trends in falciparum malaria. *J Assoc Phys India* 47: 774–777.

Koutsky LA et al. 2002. A controlled trial of HPV 16 vaccine. *New Engl J Med* 347:1645–1651.

Kurian J, Rao KB, Mala V. 2000 Maternal mortality and morbidity in developing countries. Paper presented at the plenary session of the Asia Oceania Congress of Obstetrics and Gynecology, Singapore, 14 July 2000.

Lancet. 2002. News (UNFPA) *Lancet* 360:64

Magpie Trial Collaborative Group. 2002. Do women with pre-eclampsia benefit from magnesium sulphate? *Lancet* 359:1877–1890.

Mala V, Kurian J, Rao KB. 2000. Maternal mortality in developing countries. Proceedings of the World Conference on Women's Health, Kolkata, 9-12 Nov 2000, p 110.

Mala V and Rao KB. 2003. Incontinence in women. In *Obstetrics and Gynecology for Postgraduates*, eds SS Ratnam, KB Rao, S Arulkumaran, Vol 2, 2nd edn. Chennai: Orient Longman Pvt Ltd, p 375–397.

Ministry of Health. 1996. Annual Report on Special Schemes 1994–95. New Delhi: Ministry of Health and Family Welfare, p 17.

Murray CJL and AD Lopez. 1997. Mortality by cause for 8 regions of the WHO. *Lancet* 349: 1271–1276.

Perinatal HIV Guidelines Working Group. 2002. Summary of Updated Recommendations from the Public Health Service Task Force to reduce perinatal HIV-1 transmission rates in the US. *Obstet Gynecol* 99:1117–1126.

Population Reference Bureau. 2004. World Population Data sheet, p 1

Ramachandran P. 2002. Reproductive tract infections. In *Obstetrics and Gynecology for Postgraduates*, eds SS Ratnam, KB Rao, S Arulkumaran, Vol.2, 2nd edn. Chennai: Orient Longman Pvt Ltd.

Reynolds SJ, JG Bartlett, TC Quinn, C Beyrer and RC Bollinger. 2003. Antiretroviral therapy where resources are limited. *N Engl J Med* 348(18):1806–1809.

Rao KB. 2000. Reproductive Health of Women in India: A review for the last 50 years. *J Obstet Gynecol India* 50:99–103.

Rao KB. 2003. Aging in women and its consequences. In *Obstetrics and Gynecology for Postgraduates*, eds SS Ratnam, KB Rao, S Arulkumaran, Vol 2, 2nd edn. Chennai: Orient Longman Pvt Ltd., p 433–445.

Rochat R and HH Akther. 1999. Tetanus and pregnancy related mortality in Bangladesh. *Lancet* 354:565.

Sankaranarayanan R, AM Budukh and R Rajkumar. 2001. Effective screening programmes for cervical cancer in low- and middle-income developing countries. *Bull World Health Org* 79:954–961.

Shah KP. 1991. Obstetric fistulae WHO/MCH/MSM /91.5. Geneva: World Health Organization.

Stover J, N Walker, GP Garnett et al. 2002. Can we reverse the HIV/AIDS epidemic with an expanded response? *Lancet* 360:73–77.

UNDP. 2002. 12th Annual Human Development Report. New York: Oxford University Press, pp 162–177.

UNFPA. 1999. *The state of the world population: 6 Billion, A time for choices*. New York: UNFPA.

Villar J, H Ba'aqeel, G Piaggio et al. 2001. WHO antenatal care randomised trial for the evaluation of a new model of routine antenatal care. *Lancet* 357:1551–1564.

von Herzen H, G Piaggio, J Ding et al 2002. Low dose mifepristone and two regimens of levonorgestrel for emergency contraception: A WHO multicentre randomised trial. *Lancet* 360(9348):1803–1810.

World Health Organization. 1994. Health, population and development. Geneva: World Health Organization, WHO/FHE/94.1.

World Health Organization. 1996. Revised 1990 estimates of maternal mortality WHO/UNICEF, Geneva: World Health Organization.

World Health Organization. 1996. Adolescent health and development. *Tech Rep Series No* 886.

World Health Organization. 1996. Available data on perinatal mortality. Geneva: World Health Organization.

World Health Organization. 1997. *Global coverage of maternity care*, 4th edn. Geneva: World Health Organization.

World Health Organization. 1999. World Health Report: Causes of maternal deaths, latest available year 1999. Geneva: World Health Organization, p 97–104.

World Health Organization. 1999a. Reduction of maternal mortality Joint statement of WHO, UNFPA, UNICEF and World Bank. Geneva: World Health Organization, p 20.

World Health Organization. 1999. b. Annual Technical Report 1998 WHO/UNDP/UNFPA of HRP. Geneva: World Health Organization, p 186–190.

World Health Organization. 2000. WHO Expert Committee on Malaria, 20th Report, *Tech Comm Report* Series no. 892. Geneva: World Health Organization, p 42.

WHO, UNICEF, UNFPA Statement. 2004. Geneva: World Health Organization.

World Health Organization Annual Report. 2005. Geneva: World Health Organization

2

Recurrent Pregnancy Loss

Vanita Jain

Recurrent pregnancy loss (RPL) is one of the most frustrating problems in reproductive medicine because the cause is often unknown and there are few evidence-based diagnostic and treatment strategies.

Definition

Recurrent pregnancy loss is defined as the occurrence of three or more consecutive losses of clinically recognised pregnancies prior to the 20th week of gestation

Types

RPL may be primary or secondary. ***Primary RPL*** refers to repeated miscarriages in which a pregnancy has never been carried to viability. ***Secondary RPL*** implies that a live birth has occurred at some time.

Incidence

The incidence of sporadic loss of a clinically recognised pregnancy is approximately 15%. About 2% of pregnant women experience two consecutive pregnancy losses and 0.4–1.0% suffer three consecutive pregnancy losses. This incidence is greater than that which can be reasonably attributed to chance alone, since the theoretical risk of three consecutive pregnancy losses is 0.34% (Alberman 1988).

Etiology

The cause of RPL can be determined in only 50% of patients. The causative factors include genetic and anatomical abnormalities, and endocrine, immunological, thrombophilic and environmental factors.

Genetic factors: Abnormalities of chromosome number or structure are a common cause of pregnancy loss. About 3–5% of couples with RPL show major chromosomal rearrangement (against 0.7% of the general population). These abnormalities could be balanced translocations or inversions (Franssen et al 2005). Balanced translocations are the most common inborn parental chromosomal abnormality contributing to RPL. As the number of miscarriages increases, the prevalence of chromosomal abnormality decreases and the chance of recurring maternal cause increases (Ogasawara et al 2000). If the karyotype of the miscarried pregnancy is abnormal, there is better prognosis in the next pregnancy (Carp et al 2001).

Anatomical abnormalities: Anatomical abnormalities of both the uterine body and the cervix may lead to RPL. These abnormalities may be congenital or acquired. Anatomical abnormalities may be responsible for 10–50% of RPL cases (Hill 1999). The prevalence of uterine malformations appears to be higher in women with late miscarriages than in with women who suffer early miscarriages, but this may be related to the cervical weakness that is frequently associated with uterine malformation.

Congenital anomalies: Congenital uterine anomalies are present in 10–15% of women with RPL as against 7% of all women (Harger et al 1983). It is difficult to assess the exact contribution that congenital uterine anomalies make to recurrent pregnancy loss as the prevalence and reproductive implications of uterine anomalies in the general population have not been clearly established. Pregnancy loss, may be related to impaired uterine distension or abnormal implantation. The septate uterus is the most common uterine abnormality associated with RPL and is known to have the poorest reproductive outcome (Homer et al 2000). The miscarriage rate in women with untreated septate uterus is greater than 60% (Heinonen et al 1982). The mechanism by which a septate uterus causes pregnancy loss is not clearly understood, but poor blood supply to the septum leading to poor implantation is one possibility. The longer the septum, the worse the prognosis (Buttram and Gibbons 1979). Congenital anomalies of the uterine arteries may also contribute to pregnancy loss through impaired blood flow to the implanted conceptus.

Acquired anomalies: These anomalies include leiomyomas and intrauterine adhesions. Submucous leiomyomas protrude into the endometrial cavity and can impede normal implantation as a result of their position. Intrauterine adhesions or synechiae lead to pregnancy loss because there is insufficient endometrium to support fetoplacental growth.

Cervical incompetence: Cervical incompetence (or cervical insufficiency) is a cause of recurrent mid-trimester pregnancy loss, rather than early abortion. Traditionally, the cervix has been considered either completely competent or incompetent; diagnostic criteria and therapeutic modalities were based upon this concept. However, it is likely that cervical incompetence represents a spectrum of diseases with multiple causes, involving both congenital and acquired factors. There is a tendency to assume that cervical weakness is the cause of the mid-trimester miscarriage, however, since it is the most common cause; obstetricians should guard against this.

Antiphospholipid antibodies Antiphospholipid syndrome (APS) refers to the association between antiphospholipid antibodies (aPL) and adverse pregnancy outcome or vascular thrombosis. Adverse pregnancy outcomes include

(a) three or more consecutive miscarriages before ten weeks of gestation
(b) one or more morphologically normal fetal deaths after the tenth week of gestation and
(c) one or more preterm births before the 34th week of gestation due to severe pre-eclampsia, eclampsia or placental insufficiency (Wilson et al 1999).

APS is the only condition proven to be a causal factor of RPL. It has been associated with both recurrent early miscarriage and repetitive late fetal death (>10 weeks of gestation). Antiphospholipid antibodies are present in 15% of women with recurrent miscarriage. By comparison, the prevalence of aPL in women with a low-risk obstetric history is less than 2% (Pattison et al 1993). In women with recurrent miscarriage associated with aPL, the live birth rate in pregnancies with no pharmacological intervention may be as low as 10%.

Endocrinologic factors: These factors include progesterone deficiency, diabetes mellitus and thyroid disease. Progesterone is essential for successful implantation and maintenance of pregnancy. Therefore, disorders related to impaired progesterone production or action (for example, luteal phase defect, hyperprolactinemia and polycystic ovary syndrome) are likely to affect pregnancy outcome. However, serum progesterone concentrations are not predictive of pregnancy outcome (Ogasawara et al 1997), nor is there evidence to support the use of exogenous progesterone supplementation to prevent early miscarriage (except possibly in the setting of an inadequate luteal phase.) (Goldstein et al 1989). However, the existence of luteal phase defect, method of diagnosis, relationship with miscarriage and treatment are controversial issues.

Hyperprolactinemia: Normal circulating levels of prolactin may play an important role in maintaining early pregnancy. However, the role of hyperprolactinemia as a risk factor for recurrent miscarriage is debatable and the evidence is conflicting (Li et al 2000).

Polycystic ovary syndrome: The prevalence of polycystic ovaries, identified using pelvic ultrasound criteria, is significantly higher among women with recurrent miscarriage (41%) when compared with the general population (22%) (Rai et al 2000). The spontaneous abortion rate in women with polycystic ovary syndrome (PCOS) is 20–40%, which is higher than the baseline rate in the general obstetric population (10–20%) (Glueck et al 2002). The mechanism for increased pregnancy loss in these patients is unknown, but may be related to elevated serum luteinising hormone (LH) levels, high testosterone and androstenedione concentrations and/or insulin resistance. Polycystic ovary morphology itself does not predict an increased risk of future pregnancy loss among ovulatory women with a history of recurrent miscarriage who conceive spontaneously.

Diabetes mellitus: Women with diabetes who have high hemoglobin A_{Ic} levels in the first trimester are at risk of miscarriage and fetal malformation (Hanson et al 1990). The increased rate of spontaneous abortions in poorly controlled diabetic women is thought to be secondary to hyperglycemia, maternal vascular disease and possibly immunological factors. There is no increased risk of miscarriage in women with well-controlled diabetes mellitus (Mills et al 1988).

Thyroid disorders: Hypothyroidism has been associated with RPL. Even in euthyroid patients, the presence of antithyroid antibodies might be associated with RPL.

Immunological factors: Various immunological factors such as HLA incompatibility between couples, the absence of maternal leucocytotoxic antibodies, the absence of maternal blocking antibodies and endometrial immunity have been linked with RPL. It has been suggested that immune effector cell dysfunction (defects in the imunosuppressive factors, cytokines and growth factors at the local maternofetal interface) may be implicated in the pathogenesis of implantation failure and recurrent early pregnancy loss (Johnson et al 1999). However, this is a research field and the association and methods of treatment require further clarification. At present it is difficult to assess the role of immunological factors in reproductive failure (Kallen and Arici 2003).

Thrombophilic factors: The abnormalities of the uteroplacental circulation seen in thrombophilias can cause late fetal loss, intrauterine growth restriction, placental abruption and pre-eclampsia. A link with early pregnancy loss is less clear (Hohlagschwandtner et al 2003).

Advancing maternal age: Advancing maternal age is associated with a higher rate of pregnancy loss of both normal and abnormal conceptuses (Nybo Andersen et al 2000). Advanced age adversely affects ovarian function, giving rise to a decline in the number of good quality oocytes, resulting in chromosomally abnormal conceptions that rarely develop further. It is also associated with a higher rate of pregnancy loss of normal conceptuses. This is probably because of uterine factors (for example, diminished endometrial receptivity) and reduced endocrine function in this age group.

Environmental factors and stress: There is no evidence from well-designed studies showing a relationship between RPL and environmental agents, occupational factors or stress.

Male factor: Women whose male partners have semen with poor sperm morphology (fewer than 4% normal forms) may have recurrent pregnancy loss (Plouffe et al 1992).

Infection: No infectious agent has been proven to cause RPL. For an infective agent to be implicated, it must be capable of persisting in the genital tract and avoiding detection or must cause insufficient symptoms to disturb the women. Toxoplasmosis, rubella, cytomegalovirus, herpes and listeria infections do not fulfill these criteria. The presence of bacterial vaginosis in the first trimester of pregnancy has been reported as a risk factor for second trimester miscarriage and preterm delivery, but the evidence for an association with first trimester miscarriage is inconsistent (Ralph et al 1999).

Unexplained RPL: A significant proportion of cases of recurrent miscarriage remain unexplained, despite detailed investigation. Women with unexplained RPL have a greater incidence of elevated day 3 serum follicle stimulating hormone (FSH) and estradiol (E_2) levels than women with a known cause of RPL (Trout and Seifer 2000) that may be related to poor quality oocytes with inherent chromosomal compromise.

Evaluation for RPL

Indication for evaluation: Evaluation of healthy women is not recommended after a single first trimester or early second trimester spontaneous miscarriage, as they are relatively common events. The risk of another pregnancy loss after two consecutive miscarriages is 24–29%; after three or more miscarriages, it is 31–33% (Stirrat 1990). Therefore, evaluation and treatment of RPL can reasonably be started after two consecutive miscarriages (ACOG 2001), especially when fetal cardiac activity has been identified in previous losses or when the woman is more than 35 years old or the couple is subfertile. The minimum diagnostic work-up of couples with RPL consists of a complete medical, surgical, genetic and family history, and a physical examination.

History

Past obstetric history: This is the most important aspect of history taking in a patient with RPL. The history should include a description of the gestational age and characteristics of all previous pregnancies. RPL typically occurs at a similar gestational age in consecutive pregnancies and the most common causes of RPL vary by trimester. For example, spontaneous abortions related to chromosomal and endocrine defects tend to occur earlier in gestation than losses due to anatomical or autoimmune abnormalities. It is important to note if embryonic/fetal cardiac activity was ever detected. A history of subfertility or infertility should also be taken.

Menstrual history: Abnormalities in cycle length may be due to endocrine dysfunction.

Family history: History of RPL or birth defects in the family may suggest a genetic cause.

Medical history: History suggestive of thyroid disorders, glucose intolerance, androgenic disorders or other autoimmune disorders should be elicited. Additional history includes a history of galactorrhea (suggesting hyperprolactinemia), uterine instrumentation (suggesting Asherman syndrome), birth defects or karyotypic abnormalities (suggesting genetic factors) and exposure to environmental toxins or drugs and venous thrombosis (suggesting an inherited thrombophilia or antiphospholipid antibody syndrome).

Physical Examination

Physical examination should include a general physical assessment with attention to signs of endocrinopathy, for example, hirsutism, galactorrhea and thyroid disorders. A pelvic examination should be done to identify any cervical laceration or uterine malformation and to detect signs of estrogenisation of mucosal tissues.

Laboratory Evaluation

Karyotype: Chromosomal abnormalities detectable in parents may be considered an indirect indicator of fetal karyotype (Hassold et al 1988). Many experts also recommend obtaining a karyotype of the abortus or products of conception. A normal karyotype suggests that a maternal environmental factor is the cause of pregnancy loss. However, cytogenetic testing is expensive and karyotyping of the abortus may be reserved for patients who have undergone treatment in the index pregnancy since it provides useful information for counselling and future management (Carp et al 2001).

Uterine assessment: Anatomical causes of RPL are typically diagnosed using hysterosalpingography (HSG) or sonohysterography. Hysteroscopy, laparoscopy or magnetic resonance imaging (MRI) can also be performed as needed, but are more expensive (except for MRI) and more invasive than sonohysterography. These modalities provide information about the type and extent of underlying pathologies such as submucous myomas, uterine malformations, intrauterine adhesions and tubal patency. The routine use of hysterosalpingography as a screening test for uterine anomalies in women with recurrent miscarriage is questionable. It is associated with patient discomfort, carries a risk of pelvic infection and radiation exposure and is not more sensitive than the non-invasive pelvic ultrasound assessment of the uterine cavity with (or without) sonohysterography (Soares et al 2000). Transvaginal ultrasound (TVS) is useful in diagnosing a septate uterus, especially during pregnancy (Homer et al 2000). It also provides information about the presence and location of uterine myomas, the possibility of cervical incompetence and assessment of fetal viability; it is the investigation of choice especially during pregnancy. Magnetic resonance (MR) imaging is useful for distinguishing between a septate and bicornuate uterus suspected on ultrasonography or HSG. It is less invasive and less costly than laparoscopy for this purpose. Costly and invasive investigations, such as hysteroscopy and laparoscopy, are usually reserved for patients who have had a non-diagnostic evaluation of RPL or those in whom intrauterine pathology is strongly suspected.

Cervical incompetence: Many tests have been described to make the diagnosis of cervical incompetence in the non-pregnant woman. These inlcude hysterography, pulling through of inflated balloon catheters and passing cervical dilators through the cervix without resistance. However, there is currently no satisfactory objective test that can identify women with cervical weakness in the non-pregnant state. The diagnosis is usually based on a history of late miscarriage preceded by spontaneous rupture of membranes or painless cervical dilatation. Transvaginal ultrasound assessment of the cervix during pregnancy may be useful in predicting preterm birth in some cases of suspected cervical weakness (Owen et al 2001).

Antiphospholipid antibody syndrome: This syndrome is diagnosed by the presence of one or more antiphospholipid antibodies (anticardiolipin antibodies or lupus anticoagulant) in a patient with RPL. Both tests should be done twice, 6–8 weeks apart, because a low- to mid-positive level can be due to viral illness and revert to normal. The anticardiolipin antibody titre is considered elevated if medium or high titres of both IgG and IgM isotypes are found in the blood (Roubey 2000). The detection of the lupus anticoagulant is generally based on an activated partial thromboplastin time, kaolin plasma clotting time or dilute Russell viper venom test time (Vinatier et al 2001). In detection of lupus anticoagulant, the dilute Russell's viper venom time (dRVVT) test is more sensitive and specific than either the activated partial thromboplastin time (aPTT) or the kaolin clotting time (KCL) tests.

Hypercoagulable state: The benefit of evaluation for inherited thrombophilia in women with early RPL is not clear unless the patient has a personal or family history of thrombosis. A meta-analysis found that factor V Leiden mutation, activated protein C resistance, protein S deficiency, and prothrombin G20210A mutation were associated with early recurrent fetal loss (Rey et al 2003). Based on the available evidence, assessment for these thrombophilias is justified in women with RPL.

Thyroid function: Thyroid function should be assessed in women with clinical manifestations of underlying thyroid disease. Screening for subclinical thyroid dysfunction appears to be appropriate since most studies report an increased risk of abortion in women with subclinical hypothyroidism (Abalovich et al 2002; Christiansen et al 2005).

Evaluation of ovarian reserve: Evaluation of ovarian reserve using a day 3 follicle stimulating hormone (FSH) concentration can be considered in the evaluation of RPL. Adequate ovarian reserve is established using a cycle day 3 FSH concentration less than 15 mIU/ml. High day 3 serum estradiol concentrations of over 80 pg/ml are also associated with reduced oocyte numbers (Trout and Seifer 2000).

Additional tests: may be indicated in women with clinical manifestations suggestive of a medical disorder. However, testing for these disorders should not be a part of the routine evaluation of women with RPL.

Tests not indicated

Infection screen: Routine TORCH screening is not indicated in women with RPL (Summers 1994; Regan and Jivraj 2001).

Antinuclear antibody: The pregnancy outcome of women with and without antinuclear antibody (ANA) is the same. Current available data does not support testing women with RPL for ANA (ACOG 2001).

Thyroid antibodies: Routine screening for thyroid antibodies in women with recurrent miscarriage is not recommended.

Diabetes: Screening for diabetes mellitus should be limited to women with clinical manifestations of the underlying disease. Only poorly controlled diabetes is associated with spontaneous abortion.

Progesterone: Progesterone concentrations are not predictive of future pregnancy outcome and its estimation is not indicated (Ogasawara et al 1997).

Endometrial biopsy: This test has been shown not to be predictive of fertility status and is not recommended.

MANAGEMENT

Many treatments have been proposed to improve pregnancy outcome in women with RPL. Choice of therapy depends on the underlying cause of RPL. Emotional support is important in caring for these couples, and may enhance therapeutic success (Liddell et al 1991).

Genetic Abnormality

Couples with chromosomal abnormalities should be referred to a geneticist for counselling (Tharapel et al 1985). They should receive information regarding the probability of having a chromosomally normal or abnormal conception. The magnitude of these risks varies according to the specific chromosomal abnormality. The options available for these couples are antenatal genetic studies, such as amniocentesis or chorionic villus sampling, *in vitro* fertilisation (IVF) with preimplantation genetic diagnosis (PGD), gamete donation (egg or sperm), surrogacy and adoption. The choice depends on the specific abnormality.

Anatomical abnormality: No randomised trial assessing the benefits of surgical correction of uterine abnormalities on pregnancy outcome has been performed. Observational studies have shown a significant reduction in abortion rates after repair of bicornuate uteri, hysteroscopic resection of a uterine septum or lysis of adhesions (March and Israel 1981; Heinonen et al 1982). Surgery can be offered to women with a surgically correctable cause of pregnancy loss, such as a uterine septum, intrauterine adhesions, submucosal myoma or bicornuate uterus. The first three conditions can be treated by hysteroscopy, while bicornuate uterus requires transfundal metroplasty. Open uterine surgery is associated with postoperative infertility and carries a significant risk of uterine scar rupture during pregnancy (Jacobsen and DeCherney 1997). These complications are less likely to occur after hysteroscopic surgery (Grimbizis et al 2001). Surrogacy can be considered in women with irreparable uterine defects.

Cervical incompetence: Women with cervical incompetence can benefit from the placement of a cervical cerclage. However, two randomised controlled trials failed to demonstrate any significant improvement in perinatal survival from ultrasound-indicated cervical cerclage, although there was a small decrease in preterm birth and delivery of very low birth weight babies (Althuisius et al 2000; Rust et al 2000; MRC/RCOG 1993). Cerclage is usually done after 14 weeks (to exclude causes of first trimester abortions) and before 24 weeks of gestation. An ultrasound is done before the procedure to confirm a living fetus and to exclude congenital malformations. Procedures done with dilated cervix and bulging membranes (emergency cerclage) are associated with high failure rates. Complications include infection, rupture of membranes and onset of uterine contractions. The procedure used most frequently is McDonald's (Fig. 2.1) and modified Shirodkar's.

Transabdominal cerclage has been advocated in selected women with previous failed transvaginal cerclage and/or a very short and scarred cervix (Anthony et al 1997). A recent systematic review compared abdominal versus vaginal cerclage in women with failed vaginal cerclage in a previous pregnancy (Zaveri et al 2002). This review concluded that abdominal cerclage may be associated with a lower risk of perinatal death or delivery before 24 weeks of gestation, but it may be associated with higher operative morbidity.

Antiphospholipid Antibody Syndrome

In women with recurrent miscarriage associated with APS, the live birth rate in pregnancies with no pharmacological intervention may be as low as 10%. The treatment modalities for this syndrome include low dose aspirin, prednisolone, unfractionated heparin, or low molecular weight heparin given either alone or in combination. Aspirin alone probably does not reduce miscarriage rates (Rai et al 1997). The combination of aspirin with heparin or prednisolone results in a significantly higher number of live births than therapy with aspirin alone (Kutteh 1996). However, the prednisone–aspirin combination is associated with increased incidence of preterm delivery, usually from premature rupture of membranes or pre-eclampsia. A combination of low dose aspirin (81 mg daily) and low dose heparin or low molecular weight heparin (LMWH) appears to be effective in improving pregnancy outcome in women with antiphospholipid syndrome and RPL. The live birth rates for aspirin/heparin and aspirin/enoxaparin groups are similar (Noble et al 2005). Aspirin is initiated in all patients once pregnancy is confirmed with a positive urine pregnancy test. Subcutaneous heparin (5000 units subcutaneously every 12 hours) or LMWH (Dalteparin 5000 units subcutaneously daily or enoxaparin 40 mg subcutaneously daily) is started once a fetal heart beat is established through ultrasonography. Immunotherapy is not recommended for prevention of miscarriage in women with APS.

Endocrinological Factors

Progesterone: Progesterone is widely used as empiric treatment of unexplained RPL. However, its use has not been shown to conclusively influence pregnancy outcome in women with RPL (ACOG 2001; Oates-Whitehead et al 2003). It can be administered orally (50–100 mg twice daily or micronised progesterone 100 mg 2–3 tablets per day) or intravaginally (progesterone in gel or micronised progesterone). It is typically started three days after the LH surge, so as not to inhibit ovulation, and continued until 10 weeks of gestation, when placental progesterone production should be fully functional.

Luteal phase defects: A variety of therapies have been proposed for treatment of luteal phase deficiency. However, the value of these interventions has not been proven.

Polycystic ovary syndrome: PCOS is associated with a high abortion rate. This may be due to insulin resistance. Treatment of insulin resistance with metformin in women with PCOS is associated with a reduction in pregnancy loss (Jakubowicz et al 2002; Glueck et al 2002). However, no randomised trials have been conducted to establish the effectiveness of metformin for the prevention of early pregnancy loss, and metformin is not an FDA-approved drug for use during pregnancy. Pre-pregnancy pituitary suppression of LH among ovulatory women with recurrent miscarriage and polycystic ovaries, who hypersecrete LH, does not improve the live birth rate (Clifford et al 1996).

Hyperprolactinemia: In patients with hyperprolactinemia, treatment with bromocryptine has been associated with a

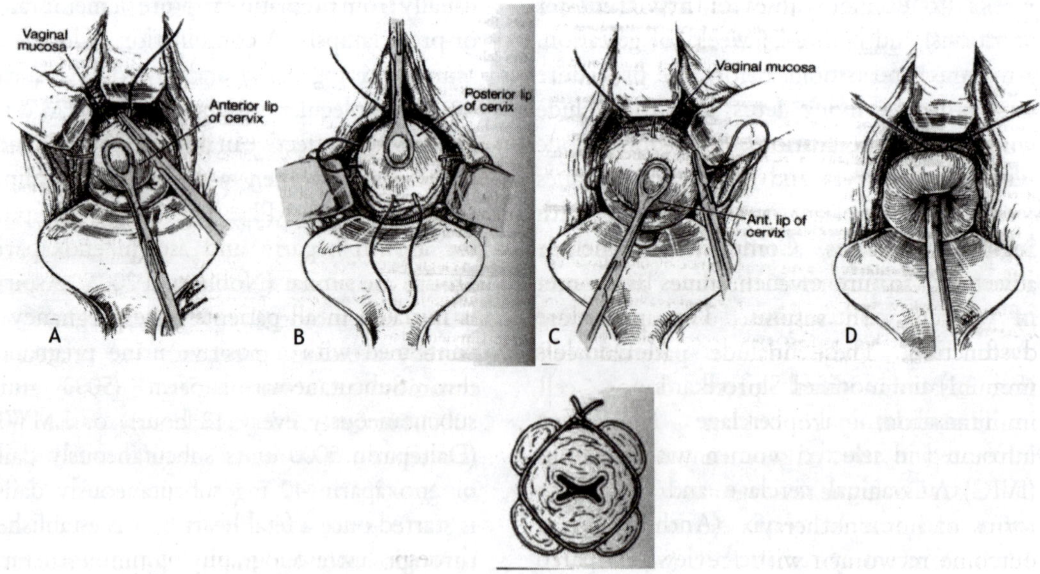

Figure 2.1: McDonald cerclage for cervical incompetence

A, B, C: Placement of monofilament non-absorbable #2 suture around the cervix at the level of the internal os.
D: Tightening of suture with a small dilator *in situ*

higher rate of successful pregnancy (Hirahara et al 1998).

Human chorionic gonadotropin: A Cochrane review of women with RPL concluded that hCG therapy was associated with a reduced risk of miscarriage, particularly in women with oligomenorrhea (Scott and Pattison 2000). However, there was insufficient evidence to recommend the use of hCG to prevent pregnancy loss in women with a history of unexplained RPL.

Clomiphene citrate: Clomiphene citrate increases the follicular number, and therefore serum estradiol levels, which leads to an increase in the number of corpora luteal and a higher midluteal progesterone concentration. It has been tried in women with inadequate luteal phase with results similar to that of progesterone (Murray et al 1989).

Thyroid dysfunction and diabetes mellitus: Women with overt thyroid disease or diabetes should be treated medically to get their disease under control. Empirical treatment of euthyroid and normoglycemic women is not recommended.

Immunological Factors

Several immunological treatments have been advocated to improve the live birth rate in women with suspected immunological dysfunction. These include paternal cell immunisation, third party donor cell immunisation, trophoblast membrane infusion and intravenous immune globulin (IVIG). A Cochrane review found that various forms of immunotherapy did not improve outcome in women with RPL (Scott 2003). Thus, immune therapy for RPL should be considered experimental.

Corticosteroids: Administration of corticosteroids for treatment of RPL is not recommended because of uncertain efficacy and an increase in complications such as preterm premature rupture of membranes, gestational diabetes and maternal hypertension (Laskin et al 1997).

Infection

The Cochrane review has shown that for women with a history of previous preterm birth or late trimester abortion, detection and treatment of bacterial vaginosis, early in pregnancy, may prevent a further preterm birth (Brocklehurst et al 2000).

Unexplained RPL

Many empirical therapies have been tried in women with unexplained RPL. In evaluating the success of these therapies one must remember that the chance of a live birth after three unexplained RPLs is over 50% with no intervention (Scott 1994). Treatment that has been offered to these couples includes:

In vitro fertilisation (IVF) and preimplantation genetic diagnosis (PGD): Embryos of women with unexplained RPL have a higher incidence of aneuploidy than embryos obtained from healthy women (Hassold 1988). Preimplantation genetic diagnosis can identify and transfer only chromosomally normal embryos, thereby avoiding pregnancy loss related to chromosomal abnormalities (Egozcue et al 2000). However, this is a technically demanding procedure and experience is still limited.

Oocyte donation: Poor quality oocytes may be responsible for many of the pregnancy losses (Remohi et al 1996). Ovum donation can overcome this problem.

Management in Pregnancy

Women with a history of RPL who become pregnant may be at higher risk of recurrent loss, developing fetal growth restriction and premature delivery (Jivraj et al 2001). The greatest risk of recurrent loss occurs during the period in the current pregnancy that corresponds to that up to the time of the miscarriage of the previous pregnancy. In women with APS, aspirin plus heparin

TABLE 2.1: Causative factors, available investigations and management options for recurrent pregnancy loss

Etiological Factor	*Evaluation*	*Management*
Genetic	Parental karyotype Karyotype of abortus	Genetic counselling IVF, PGD Genetic evaluation Adoption
Anatomic	Transvaginal sonography Sonohysterography Hysterosalpingography MRI Hysteroscopy Laparoscopy	Surgical correction
Cervical incompetence	Transvaginal sonography	Cervical cerclage
Antiphospolipid anti-body syndrome	Anticardiopipin antibody IgG and IgM Lupus anticoagulant	Low dose aspirin + Heparin
Endocrinology PCOD Thyroid	 TSH	 Metformin Clomiphene
Thrombophilia	Factor V Leiden mutation Activated protein C resistance Protein S Prothrombin G20210A	Heparin
Infection	Cultured for bacterial vaginosis	Metronidazole
Unexplained Ovarian reserve Empirical treatments	 Day 3 FSH	 Clomiphene Progesterone Human chorionic gonadotrophic IVF, PGD Oocyte donation

IVF In vitro fertilisation, PGD Preimplantation genetic diagnosis, FSH Follicle stimulating hormone, MRI Magnetic resonance imaging, TSH Thyroid stimulating hormone

treatment substantially improves the chance of live birth but these pregnancies remain at high risk of complications during the three trimesters including repeated miscarriage, pre-eclampsia, fetal growth restriction and preterm birth (Backos et al 1999). Obstetrical management depends on the underlying cause of RPL, if known.

The causes, investigations and management options of RPL are summarised in Table 2.1.

Prognosis

The chance of a live birth following RPL, excluding antiphospholipid syndrome and cervical incompetence, is 70–85% regardless of treatment. Fetal loss rates after sonographic demonstration of fetal cardiac activity have been reported to be 5–22% in women with RPL compared to 3–6% in controls (Bricker and Farquharson 2002). The prognosis for successful pregnancy is better with secondary RPL than primary RPL (Paukku et al 1999).

References

Abalovich M, S Gutierrez, G Alcaraz et al. 2002. Overt and subclinical hypothyroidism complicating pregnancy. *Thyroid* 12:63–68.

Alberman E. 1988. The epidemiology of repeated abortion. In *Early Pregnancy Loss: Mechanisms and Treatment,* ed RW Beard and F Sharp, 9–17. London: RCOG Press.

Althuisius SM, GA Dekker, HP van Geijn, DJ Bekedam and P Hummel. 2000. Cervical incompetence prevention randomized cerclage trial (CIPRACT): study design and preliminary results. *Am J Obstet Gynecol* 183:823–829.

American College of Obstetricians and Gynecologists. 2001. Management of recurrent early pregnancy loss. *ACOG Practice Bulletin no. 24*. Washington, DC: American College of Obstetricians and Gynecologists.

Anthony GS, RG Walker, AD Cameron, JL Price, JJ Walker and AA Calder. 1997. Transabdominal cervico-isthmic cerclage in the management of cervical incompetence. *Eur J Obstet Gynecol Reprod Biol* 72:127–130

Backos M, R Rai, N Baxter, IT Chilcott, H Cohen and L Regan. 1999. Pregnancy complications in women with recurrent miscarriage associated with antiphospholipid antibodies treated with low-dose aspirin and heparin. *Br J Obstet Gynaecol* 106:102–107.

Bricker L and RG Farquharson. 2002. Types of pregnancy loss in recurrent miscarriage: implications for research and clinical practice. *Hum Reprod* 17:1345.

Brocklehurst P, M Hannah and H McDonald. 2000. Interventions for treating bacterial vaginosis in pregnancy. *Cochrane Database Syst Rev* CD000262.

Buttram VC Jr and WE Gibbons. 1979. Müllerian anomalies: a proposed classification (an analysis of 144 cases). *Fertil Steril* 32:40.

Carp H, V Toder, A Aviram, M Daniely, S Mashiach and G Barkai. 2001. Karyotype of the abortus in recurrent miscarriage. *Fertil Steril* 75:678–682.

Christiansen OB, AM Nybo Andersen, E Bosch et al. 2005. Evidence-based investigations and treatments of recurrent pregnancy loss. *Fertil Steril* 83:821.

Clifford K, R Rai, H Watson, S Franks and L Regan. 1996. Does suppressing luteinising hormone secretion reduce the miscarriage rate? Results of a randomised controlled trial. *BMJ* 312:1508–1511.

Egozcue J, J Santalo, C Gimenez et al. 2000. Preimplantation genetic diagnosis. *Mol Cell Endocrinol* 166:21.

Franssen MT, JC Korevaar, NJ Leschot et al. 2005. Selective chromosome analysis in couples with two or more miscarriages: case-control study. *BMJ* 331:137.

Glueck CJ, P Wang, N Goldenberg and L Sieve-Smith. 2002. Pregnancy outcomes among women with polycystic ovary syndrome treated with metformin. *Hum Reprod* 17:285–288.

Goldstein P, J Berrier, S Rosen et al. 1989. A meta-analysis of randomized control trials of progestational agents in pregnancy. *Br J Obstet Gynaecol* 96:265.

Grimbizis GF, M Camus, BC Tarlatzis, JN Bontis and P Devroey. 2001. Clinical implications of uterine malformations and hysteroscopic treatment results. *Hum Reprod Update* 7:161–174.

Hanson U, B Persson and S Thunell. 1990. Relationship between haemoglobin A1C in early type 1 (insulin-dependent) diabetic pregnancy and the occurrence of spontaneous abortion and fetal malformation in Sweden. *Diabetologia* 33:100–104.

Harger JH, DF Archer, SG Marchese et al. 1983. Etiology of recurrent pregnancy losses and outcome of subsequent pregnancies. *Obstet Gynecol* 62:574.

Hassold T, PA Jacobs and D Pettay. 1988. Cytogenetic studies of couples with repeated spontaneous abortions of known karyotype. *Genet Epidemiol* 5:65.

Heinonen PK, S Saarikoski and P Pystynen. 1982. Reproductive performance of women with uterine anomalies. *Acta Obstet Gynecol Scand* 61:157.

Hill JA. 1999. Recurrent pregnancy loss. In *Kistner's Gynecology and Women's Health,* 7th ed, ed KJ Ryan, RS Berkowitz, RL Barbieri and A Dunaif, 396. St Louis: Mosby.

Hirahara F, N Andoh, K Sawai et al. 1988. Hyperprolactinemic recurrent miscarriage and result of randomized bromocriptine treatment trials. *Fertil Steril* 70:246.

Hohlagschwandtner M, G Unfried, G Heinze et al. 2003. Combined thrombophilic polymorphisms in women with idiopathic recurrent miscarriage. *Fertil Steril* 79:1141.

Homer HA, TC Li and LD Cooke. 2000. The septate uterus: A review of management and reproductive outcome. *Fertil Steril* 73:1.

Jacobsen LJ and A DeCherney. 1997. Results of conventional and hysteroscopic surgery. *Hum Reprod* 12:1376–1381.

Jakubowicz DJ, MJ Iuorno, S Jakubowicz et al. 2002. Effects of metformin on early pregnancy loss in the polycystic ovary syndrome. *J Clin Endocrinol Metab* 87:524.

Jivraj S, B Anstie, YC Cheong et al. 2001. Obstetric and neonatal outcome in women with a history of recurrent miscarriage: a cohort study. *Hum Reprod* 16:102.

Johnson PM, SE Christmas and GS Vince. 1999. Immunological aspects of implantation and implantation failure. *Hum Reprod* 14:26–36.

Kallen CB and Arici A. 2003. Immune testing in fertility practice: truth or deception? *Curr Opin Obstet Gynecol* 15:225.

Kutteh WH. 1996. Antiphospholipid antibody associated recurrent pregnancy loss: Treatment with heparin and low dose aspirin is superior to low dose aspirin alone. *Am J Obstet Gynecol* 174:1584.

Laskin CA, C Bombardier, ME Hannah et al. 1997. Prednisone and aspirin in women with autoantibodies and unexplained recurrent fetal loss. *N Engl J Med* 337:148.

Li TC, MD Spuijbroek, E Tuckerman, B Anstie, M Loxley and S Laird. 2000. Endocrinological and endometrial factors in recurrent miscarriage. *BJOG* 107:1471–1479.

Liddell HS, NS Pattison and A Zanderigo. 1991. Recurrent miscarriage—outcome after supportive care in early pregnancy. *Aust NZ J Obstet Gynaecol* 31:320.

March CM and R Israel. 1981. Gestational outcome following hysteroscopic lysis of adhesions. *Fertil Steril* 36:455.

Mills JL, JL Simpson, SG Driscoll et al. 1988. Incidence of spontaneous abortion among normal women and insulin-dependent diabetic women whose pregnancies were identified within 21 days of conception. *N Engl J Med* 319:1617.

MRC/RCOG Working Party on Cervical Cerclage. 1993. Final report of the Medical Research Council/Royal College of Obstetricians and Gynaecologists multicentre randomised trial of cervical cerclage. *Br J Obstet Gynaecol* 100:516–523.

Murray DL, L Reich and EY Adashi. 1989. Oral clomiphene citrate and vaginal progesterone suppositories in the treatment of luteal phase dysfunction: a comparative study. *Fertil Steril* 51:35.

Noble LS, WH Kutteh and N Lashey et al. 2005. Antiphospholipid antibodies associated with recurrent pregnancy loss: prospective, multicenter, controlled pilot study comparing treatment with low-molecular-weight heparin versus unfractionated heparin. *Fertil Steril* 83:684.

Nybo Andersen AM, J Wohlfahrt, P Christens et al. 2000. Maternal age and fetal loss: population based register linkage study. *BMJ* 320:1708.

Oates-Whitehead RM, DM Haas and JA Carrier. 2003. Progestogen for preventing miscarriage. *Cochrane Database Syst Rev* CD003511

Ogasawara M, K Aoki, S Okada and K Suzumori. 2000. Embryonic karyotype of abortuses in relation to the number of previous miscarriages. *Fertil Steril* 73:300–304.

Ogasawara M, S Kajiura, K Kantano et al. 1997. Are serum progesterone levels predictive of recurrent miscarriage in future pregnancies? *Fertil Steril* 68:806.

Owen J, N Yost, V Berghella, E Thom, M Swain, GA Dildy III et al. 2001. National Institute of Child Health and Human Development, Maternal-Fetal Medicine Units Network. Midtrimester endovaginal sonography in women at high risk for spontaneous preterm birth. *JAMA* 286: 1340–1348.

Pattison NS, Chamley LW, McKay EJ, Liggins GC and Butler WS. 1993. Antiphospholipid antibodies in pregnancy:prevalence and clinical association. *Br J Obstet Gynaecol* 100:909–913.

Paukku M, M Tulppala, M Puolakkainen et al. 1999. Lack of association between serum antibodies to Chlamydia trachomatis and a history of recurrent pregnancy loss. *Fertil Steril* 72:427.

Plouffe L, EW White, SP Tho et al. 1992. Etiologic factors of recurrent abortion and subsequent reproductive performance of couples: Have we made any progress in the past 10 years? *Am J Obstet Gynecol* 167:313.

Rai R, H Cohen, M Dave and L Regan. 1997. Randomized controlled trial of aspirin and aspirin plus heparin in pregnant women with recurrent miscarriage associated phospholipid antibodies (or antiphospholipid antibodies). *BMJ* 314:253.

Rai R, M Backos, F Rushworth and L Regan. 2000. Polycystic ovaries and recurrent miscarriage: a reappraisal. *Hum Reprod* 15:612–615.

Ralph SG, AJ Rutherford and JD Wilson. 1999. Influence of bacterial vaginosis on conception and miscarriage in the first trimester: Cohort study. *BMJ* 319:220–223.

Regan L and S Jivraj. 2001. Infection and pregnancy loss. In *Infection and Pregnancy,* 291–304. London:

RCOG Press.

Remohi J, E Gallardo, M Levy et al. 1996. Oocyte donation in women with recurrent pregnancy loss. *Hum Reprod* 11:2048.

Rey E, SR Kahn, M David and I Shrier. 2003. Thrombophilic disorders and fetal loss: a meta-analysis. *Lancet* 361:901.

Roubey RA. 2000. Update on Antiphospholipid Antibodies. *Curr Opin Rheumatol* 12:374.

Rust OA, RO Atlas, KJ Jones, BN Benham and J Balducci. 2000. A randomized trial of cerclage versus no cerclage among patients with ultrasonographically detected second-trimester preterm dilatation of the internal os. *Am J Obstet Gynecol* 183:830–835.

Scott JR and N Pattison. 2000. Human chorionic gonadotrophin for recurrent miscarriage. *Cochrane Database Syst Rev* CD000101.

Scott JR. 1994. Recurrent miscarriage: overview and recommendations. *Clin Obstet Gynecol* 37:768.

Scott JR. 2003. Immunotherapy for recurrent miscarriage. *Cochrane Database Syst Rev* CD000112.

Soares SR, MM Barbosa dos Reis and AF Camargos. 2000. Diagnostic accuracy of sonohysterography, transvaginal sonography, and hysterosalpingography in patients with uterine cavity diseases. *Fertil Steril*; 73:406–411.

Stirrat GM. 1990. Recurrent miscarriage. *Lancet* 336:673

Summers PR. 1994. Microbiology relevant to recurrent miscarriage. *Clin Obstet Gynecol* 37:722–729.

Tharapel AT, SA Tharapel and RM Bannerman. 1985. Recurrent pregnancy losses and parental chromosome abnormalities: a review. *Br J Obstet Gynaecol* 92:899.

Trout SW and DB Seifer. 2000. Do women with unexplained recurrent pregnancy loss have higher day 3 serum FSH and estradiol values? *Fertil Steril* 74:335.

Vinatier D, P Dufour, M Cosson and JL Houpeau. 2001. Antiphospholipid syndrome and recurrent miscarriages. *Eur J Obstet Gynecol Reprod Biol* 96:37.

Wilson WA, AE Gharavi, T Koike, MD Lockshin, DW Branch, JC Piette et al. 1999. International consensus statement on preliminary classification criteria for definite antiphospholipid syndrome: report of an international workshop. *Arthritis Rheum* 42:1309–1311.

Zaveri V, F Aghajafari, K Amankwah and M Hannah. 2002. Abdominal versus vaginal cerclage after a failed transvaginal cerclage: a systematic review. *Am J Obstet Gynecol* 187:868–872.

3

Prenatal Diagnosis of Congenital Malformations

Madhuchanda Dey | Tulika Singh | Amar Bhide

Chromosomal Anomalies

Chromosomal anomalies are a major cause of perinatal death and childhood handicap. They involve the inheritance of extra genetic material or deletion of essential genetic material. Anomalies that affect the autosomes are more common than those that affect the sex chromosomes. The vast majority of them are lethal and result in spontaneous miscarriage. Sex chromosomal anomalies are rarely suspected prenatally but may be incidentally discovered if karyotyping is done for other reasons. X chromosomal anomalies are relatively benign compared to analogous autosomal anomalies. Absence of one X chromosome, although it leads to a specific syndrome (Turner's syndrome), is relatively benign. Absence of an autosome is invariably lethal.

About 15%–20% of all recognisable pregnancies terminate in spontaneous miscarriage, and over half of these are caused by chromosomal abnormalities. The risk of chromosomal anomalies decreases with increasing gestational age. For example, the rate of fetal death in Trisomy 21 between 12 weeks and term is 30% and between 16 weeks and term is 20%. Similarly, for Trisomies 18 and 13, the rate for intrauterine lethality between 12 and 40 weeks is about 80%. For Turner's syndrome, the prevalence is about 1 in 1500 at 12 weeks, 1 in 3000 at 20 weeks and 1 in 4000 at 40 weeks. Polyploidy affects approximately 2% of recognised conceptions, but it is also highly lethal and thus rarely observed in live births. The prevalence of polyploidy at 12 and 20 weeks of gestation is approximately 1 in 2000 fetuses and 1 in 250,000 fetuses, respectively.

In the early 1970s, about 5% of pregnant women in the UK were aged 35 years or more and this group contained about 30% of the total number of fetuses with Trisomy 21 (Down syndrome). In subsequent years, especially in developed countries, there was an overall tendency for women to get pregnant at an older age. Now, about 15% of pregnant women in the UK are 35 years or older and this group contains about 50% of the total number of fetuses with Trisomy 21.

The goal of screening is to detect or define the risk for disease in the population. Diagnostic testing is intended to identify or confirm an affected individual, whereas screening is intended to identify populations with an increased risk for a specific disorder and for whom diagnostic testing may be warranted.

An ideal perinatal screening test should fulfil the following criteria:

- Identify common or important fetal disorders
- Be cost effective and easy to perform
- Have a high detection rate and a low false-positive rate
- Be reliable and reproducible
- Test for conditions for which a diagnostic test exists
- Be positive early enough in gestation to permit safe and legal options for pregnancy termination if desired

Down syndrome is the most commonly identified genetic form of mental retardation and the leading cause of specific birth defects and medical conditions. Many developed countries have adopted policies for screening for the more common trisomies (21, 18 and 13) and research continues to be carried out to improve detection rates for these chromosomal abnormalities while reducing the false-positive rate.

Screening Parameters

The screening parameters used to identify the population at high risk are maternal age, ultrasound at 11–14 weeks using nuchal translucency, maternal serum biochemical testing, anomaly scan in the second trimester and a combination of these options.

Screening Based on Maternal Age The incidence of common autosomal trisomies (21, 18 and 13) increases with advancing maternal age. In contrast, the incidence of Turner's syndrome (45 X), which is caused by the loss of the paternally derived X chromosome, is unrelated to maternal age. Until recently, the sole basis for identifying high-risk women was age. This led to the policy of offering amniocentesis to all women at or above a certain age (typically 35 or 37 years). However, use of maternal age as the only screening test has shown poor results. At best, only 30% of fetuses with Down syndrome could be detected when older women (5% of the pregnant population in the UK in 1970) were offered prenatal diagnosis with amniocentesis. Currently, maternal age is used in combination with one or more of the other screening tests for prenatal risk assessment for trisomies (Table 3.1).

Screening using Ultrasound in the First Trimester The realisation that fetuses affected by common autosomal trisomies showed ultrasound evidence of fluid accumulation behind the neck was a big step towards prenatal screening for chromosomal abnormalities. This fluid accumulation was termed nuchal skinfold thickness in the second trimester and nuchal translucency (NT) in the first trimester (Fig. 3.1). The Fetal Medicine Foundation in the UK should be credited for i) developing a reproducible technique for NT measurement, ii) developing computer software to integrate maternal age and NT for individual risk assessment, iii) providing training on a large scale and iv) carrying out continued audits. NT combined with maternal age leads to a 75% detection rate at a 5% false-positive rate. The following figure shows nuchal translucency measurement at 11–14 weeks.

It was soon recognised that over 60% of fetuses affected with Down syndrome do not have a detectable nasal bone on ultrasound at 11–14 weeks. Down syndrome fetuses also show ultrasound evidence of tricuspid regurgitation and an abnormal ductus venosus blood flow pattern. Maternal age and the ultrasound information can be combined to assess the risk of Trisomy 21 for an individual.

TABLE 3.1: RISK OF TRISOMY 21 (1/NUMBER) BASED ON MATERNAL AND GESTATIONAL AGE

	Gestation (weeks)			
MA (years)	*12*	*16*	*20*	*40*
20	898	1053	1175	1527
21	887	1040	1159	1507
22	872	1022	1140	1482
23	852	999	1114	1448
24	827	969	1081	1406
25	795	933	1040	1352
26	756	887	989	1286
27	710	832	928	1206
28	655	768	856	1113
29	593	695	776	1008
30	526	617	688	895
31	457	536	597	776
32	388	455	507	659
33	322	378	421	547
34	262	307	343	446
35	210	246	274	356
36	165	193	216	280
37	128	150	168	218
38	98	115	129	167
39	75	88	98	128
40	57	67	74	97
41	43	50	56	73
42	32	38	42	55

Screening using Serum Biochemistry

The use of maternal serum biochemisty in screening for Down syndrome is an off-shoot of the maternal serum alpha-fetoprotein (AFP) programme for screening for neural tube defects. It was realised that the AFP levels are abnormally low in mothers carrying fetuses with Down syndrome. It was also noted that mothers carrying Down syndrome fetuses have abnormally high levels of β-hCG. This realisation led to the search of other potential biomarkers, and several were identified. The commonly used ones include AFP, free beta-human chorionic gonadotrophin (β-hCG), pregnancy associated placental protein-A (PAPP-A), unconjugated estriol (uE3) and Inhibin A. A combination of AFP and free β-hCG (double test) or AFP, free β-hCG and uE3 (Triple test) have been used for Down syndrome screening. Biochemical screening in the second trimester is carried out between 15 and 22 weeks of gestation. At 11–14 weeks of gestation, the maternal serum

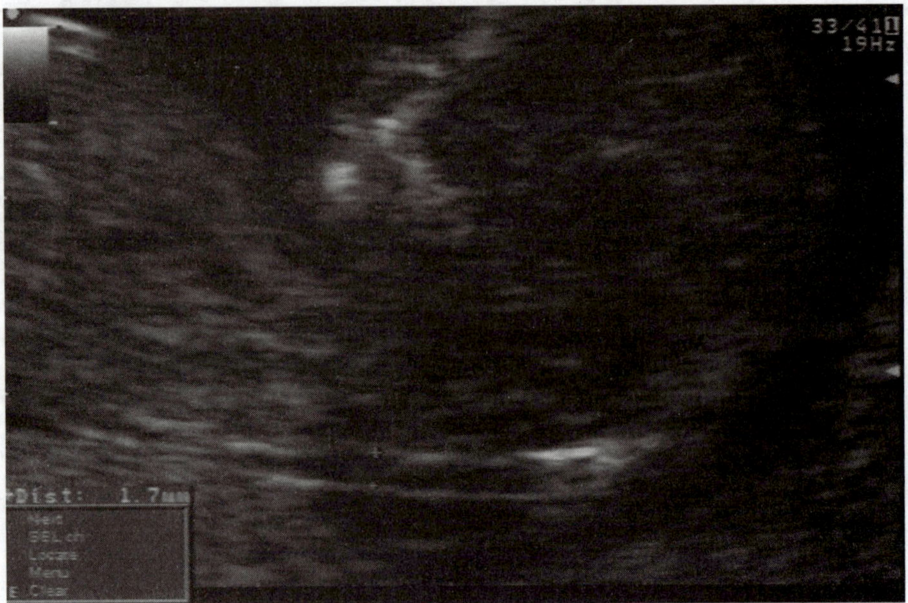

FIGURE 3.1: ULTRASOUND MEASUREMENT OF NUCHAL TRANSLUCENCY

concentration of free β-hCG is higher in Trisomy 21, whereas PAPP-A is lower than in chromosomally normal pregnancies. The detection rate of Trisomy 21 by first trimester biochemical screening alone is 60% for a screen-positive rate of 5%. Various factors such as maternal weight, insulin-dependent diabetes, twin pregnancies, ethnic origin, smoking, parity and assisted reproduction (ovulation induction and IVF) influence the levels of serum markers.

The detection rates for the various biochemical screening tests in the second trimester are given in Table 3.2.

ULTRASOUND FOR PRENATAL DIAGNOSIS

Ultrasound has been used for prenatal diagnosis of fetal congenital anomalies since the early 1970s. The main advantage of ultrasound is its lack of demonstrable adverse effects on the fetus. Major congenital anomalies affect about 2% of fetuses and infants and have a significant impact on perinatal and infant mortality and morbidity. The majority of these

TABLE 3.2: PERFORMANCE OF THE DIFFERENT TESTS IN DETECTION OF TRISOMY 21

Test	*Detection Rate (%)*	*False-positive Rate (%)*
Double test	60	5
Triple test	81	6.9
Quadruple test	84	5.7
Combined test	83	5
Integrated test	90	2.8

(Data from the SURUSS study)

abnormalities occur in the low-risk group and hence ultrasound screening programmes are now routinely offered as a part of antenatal care to all pregnant women.

Fetal anomaly screening helps in identifying anomalies that are incompatible with life, fetal conditions associated with high morbidity and conditions which are amenable to intrauterine therapy. Prenatal diagnosis reduces the prevalence of severely disabling conditions and helps in planning the management of pregnancies that would require specialist care.

Ultrasound Screening in the Second Trimester

Several ultrasonographic features have been described in the second trimester that could possibly assist in the detection of fetuses with chromosomal abnormalities. These can be classified into two categories. The first category comprises major fetal structural abnormalities associated with Trisomy 21, namely congenital heart defects, ventriculomegaly and duodenal atresia. The other category comprises many minor sonographic appearances called 'soft markers', which may be present in normal fetuses, but have been found in association with abnormal karyotypes (Table 3.2).

Soft markers are minor, usually transient ultrasound features which may indicate a risk of serious fetal abnormality but which in themselves are probably inconsequential. The presence of two or more markers makes the possibility of abnormal karyotype more likely, although some markers such as NT have a significant association with chromosomal abnormalities even when they occur alone. On the other hand, absence of these markers in a high-risk population could reduce the risk of chromosomal abnormalities by up to 50%. The use of second trimester ultrasound as a primary screening method for Trisomy 21 is not yet justified. The performance of screening could be improved by producing a risk estimate for chromosomal abnormalities based on the presence or absence of a combination of ultrasound markers.

The problem with using multiple markers is that the false-positive rate can be very high (estimated at 10–18%). In addition, information on the extent to which these markers may not be independent of each other, and may falsely increase the risk, is awaited.

Screening using Serum Biochemistry and Scan in the First Trimester (Combined Test) At 11–14 weeks of gestation, the maternal serum concentration of free β-hCG is higher in Trisomy 21 whereas PAPP-A is lower than in chromosomally normal pregnancies. The detection rate of Trisomy 21 by first trimester biochemical screening alone is 60% for a screen-positive rate of 5%. When serum screening in first trimester is combined with NT measurement in the first trimester (combined test), the detection rate for Trisomy 21 is 90%, with a false-positive rate of 5%. Examination of the nasal bone combined with fetal NT and maternal serum screening in the first trimester can achieve a Trisomy 21 detection rate of more than 95%.

There is no significant association between fetal NT and maternal serum free β-hCG or PAPP-A in either Trisomy 21 or chromosomally normal pregnancies and therefore the ultrasonographic and biochemical markers can be combined to provide more effective screening than either method individually.

An important development in biochemical analysis is the introduction of a new technique (random access immunoassay analyser

TABLE 3.3: ULTRASOUND SOFT MARKERS OF CHROMOSOMAL ABNORMALITIES

Choroid plexus cyst	Sandal gap
Echogenic focus in the heart	Increased nuchal thickness
Short femur	Rocker-bottom feet
Mild renal pelvic dilatation	Clinodactyly
Choroid plexus cyst	Brachycephaly
Echogenic focus in the heart	Short nasal bone
Echogenic bowel	Two-vessel cord
Small for gestational age (SGA)	

using time-resolved, amplified-cryptate emission), which provides automated, precise and reproducible measurements within 30 minutes of obtaining a blood sample. This has made it possible to combine biochemical and ultrasonographic testing as well as to counsel in one-stop clinics for early assessment of fetal risk (OSCAR).

In summary, screening for chromosomal abnormalities in the first trimester with the combined test offers the highest detection rates. Those women, who do not have the facility for NT, can be offered a Quadruple test in the second trimester with similar detection rates.

DIAGNOSTIC TESTS

The indications for invasive prenatal diagnosis include diagnosis of chromosomal disorders:

- In the presence of a positive screen test based on age, biochemical or nuchal translucency screening
- In the presence of increased risk as with a previous affected pregnancy or parental translocations
- In the presence of fetal structural abnormalities suspicious of chromosomal anomalies

Definitive prenatal diagnosis of chromosomal abnormalities requires cytogenetic analysis of cells obtained by one of the invasive procedures—chorion villus sampling, amniocentesis or fetal blood sampling (FBS).

AMNIOCENTESIS

Amniocentesis is the most common prenatal invasive procedure carried out in fetal medicine throughout the world. It is generally performed after 15 weeks of gestation, using aseptic techniques under continuous ultrasound guidance. The risk of fetal loss following an amniocentesis is quoted as 1% above the background rate of miscarriage. This is derived from the only randomised controlled trial of mid-trimester amniocentesis versus conservative management (Tabor et al) published in 1986. Amniotic fluid contains fetal cells, which are cultured and used for karyotyping.

Chorionic Villous Sampling The other method of prenatal diagnosis is chorionic villous sampling (CVS). This is gaining popularity as it can be carried out in the first trimester and the results are available earlier to allow surgical termination of pregnancy, should the karyotype be abnormal. Unfortunately, there are no studies that compare CVS with no testing. Only one trial compared transabdominal CVS with amniocentesis and it found similar total pregnancy loss. Randomised trials comparing

CVS by any route with second trimester amniocentesis showed an excess pregnancy loss of 3%. However, several experts believe that the procedure-related fetal loss rates following amniocentesis and CVS are probably very similar.

Fetal Blood Sampling Fetal blood sampling (FBS) is technically difficult before 18–20 weeks and is associated with a higher risk of miscarriage than amniocentesis or CVS. The advantage of FBS is that a full karyotype can be obtained faster (within 5–7 days) from the leucocytes. Fetal blood sampling for diagnosis of chromosomal abnormalities has limited applicability in clinical practice, particularly with the availability of rapid aneuploidy testing (RAD).

Karyotyping The traditional method of karyotype uses cultured cells, and takes about 10–14 days. The chromosomes cannot be seen in interphase nuclei. They are visible only in cells in the process of division (metaphase). It is necessary to stimulate cell division using phyto-hemagglutinin, and then halt it in metaphase using colchicine before observing cells under the microscope to determine the karyotype. The procedure not only takes a long time, but is also labour-intensive, requiring highly skilled cytogeneticists. Karyotyping has proved to be highly reliable for diagnosis of numerical chromosome abnormalities (aneuploidy) and large structural rearrangements (>5–10 million base pairs, Mb) in fetal cells. The diagnostic accuracy of karyotyping cultured amniotic fluid cells has been found to be 99.4–99.8% and that of CVS 97.5–99.6%.

Rapid Aneuploidy Typing More recently, many techniques in molecular biology have been applied to prenatal diagnosis to provide quicker results. These techniques are grouped together as rapid aneuploidy diagnosis (RAD). Fluorescent in-situ hybridisation (FISH) is a technique in which fluoresecent probes specific for chromosomes 13, 18 and 21 can be applied to interphase nuclei. Fluorescence can be seen with the help of a fluorescence microscope, and the presence of two signals in a cell is indicative of disomy. The probes for different chromosomes can be colour-coded. Identification of three signals of a colour suggests trisomy for that chromosome. The presence of three signals in a cell for all the coloured probes is indicative of triploidy.

Quantitative fluorescent polymerase chain reaction (QF PCR) has replaced the use of FISH in many laboratories. In this technique, DNA sequences specific to chromosomes 13, 18, 21, X and Y are amplified using the PCR technique. The DNA sequences are highly polymorphic short tandem repeats (STRs) or microsatellites that are specific to chromosomes. It is possible to identify the copy numbers of each of these chromosomes using QF PCR. For each probe used, two peaks of fluorescence activity with a peak height or area ratio of about 1:1 will be produced from samples obtained from normal heterozygous fetuses (diallelic normal). The samples from trisomic fetuses will usually demonstrate either three peaks with a ratio of 1:1:1 (trisomic triallelic) or two peaks with a ratio of 2:1 or 1:2 (trisomic diallelic) for each informative probe. If four or more probes are used for every chromosome, very few samples will remain non-informative. The advantages of this technique are that it can be used on interphase cells, results can be obtained in one or two days and the process is fully automated, thus making it cost-effective. The disadvantages of these techniques are that they may not detect small deletions not mapped by the markers, structural rearrangements may be missed and abnormalities of chromosomes other than the ones tested for will be missed.

Debate continues on the use of RAD as a stand alone or as an adjunct to karyotyping. The controversy is due to the small residual risk of a chromosomal abnormality (both balanced or unbalanced) when RAD reports a normal result. An estimate of this risk was 0.9%, and in 0.4% of these the chromosomal abnormality was deemed to be clinically significant. A reasonable option is to perform only RAD and supplement it with conventional karyotype only in a selected group of women. In the setting of Down syndrome screening using NT, the policy of performing conventional karyotype only in cases with NT >4 mm resulted in 99% detection of all chromosomal abnormalities, and conventional karyotype was needed only in 10.1% of cases. This has financial and ethical implications and therefore needs to be carefully analysed before universal guidelines are developed.

In comparative genomic hybridisation (CGH), a comparison is made between a control genome and the patient's sample on an array of genomic fragments. The genomic fragments can cover the entire human genome. Thus, it can overcome many limitations of other RAD techniques. It is a comprehensive, high-resolution, genome-wide technique, easily amenable to automation. However, at least at present the costs are high.

The Anomaly Scan

Timing of the scan The timing of the anomaly scan is an important aspect of prenatal screening. It should be undertaken at a gestational age when technical ability and organ development allows complete assessment of fetal anatomy and also provides sufficient time to undertake diagnostic tests and termination of pregnancy if the parents so wish.

Most screening programmes recommend anomaly scans at 18–22 weeks. However, in an unselected population second-trimester scan is easier to perform and less likely to require additional scans at 20–22 weeks compared to a scan at 18 weeks (Schwarzler et al 1999).

Recommended strategy for the anomaly scan A complete anomaly scan consists of a systemic review of the fetus, the placenta, cord and amniotic fluid. Table 3.1 shows the components of a complete fetal anomaly scan.

Effectiveness of screening The overall effectiveness of prenatal diagnosis is directly related to its sensitivity in identifying congenital anomalies and thereby reducing perinatal mortality and morbidity.

The RADIUS trial (1994) compared pregnant women who underwent routine scanning (15–22 weeks and 31–35 weeks) with those who had scans only when indicated. Although the detection rate of anomalies was 35% in the screened group versus only 11% in the control group, the overall sensitivity was 17% and had no significant effect on perinatal outcome. However, this trial was reported more than ten years ago. Equipment quality, skills and training of sonographers and knowledge about screening have significantly improved since then. Later studies like the Eurofetus Study (1999) and the EUROCAT Study (2005) reported a higher detection rate of 61.4% and 64%, respectively. The Eurofetus Study also reported a higher detection rate for major abnormalities than for minor abnormalities (73.7% versus 45.7%). It was also higher for abnormalities of CNS (88.3%) and urinary tract (84.8%) compared to cardiovascular (38.8%) and musculo-skeletal system (18%).

The EUROCAT Study is the most recent study assessing the frequency with which severe structural abnormalities are detected in Europe. In the period 1995-1999, data were collected from 17 European population-based registries of congenital malformations. It included all live births, fetal deaths and terminations of pregnancy. As many as 68% of the anomalies were diagnosed at a gestational age of less than 24 weeks.

Table 3.2 shows the detection rate for individual malformations.

The EUROCAT study shows a wide variation in the rate of prenatal diagnosis across Europe. This is probably due to variations in screening policies and skills, women's attitude towards screening and differences in laws regarding the upper limit of the gestational age for pregnancy termination.

Central Nervous System Abnormalities

Neural tube defects include anencephaly, encephalocele and spina bifida; of these anencephaly and spina bifida account for 95% of cases. The diagnosis of neural tube defects is made using ultrasound.

In anencephaly there is absence of a cranial vault with subsequent degeneration of the exposed brain. It can be reliably diagnosed at the scan taken at 11–14 weeks. It is a uniformly fatal condition. Detection of spina bifida is facilitated by the presence of intracranial findings in the second trimester—the 'lemon' sign (scalloping of frontal bone) and 'banana' sign (abnormal shape of cerebellum with obliteration of the cisterna magna) (Fig. 3.2). These features are seen in almost all cases of spina bifida. Intelligence may be normal in spina bifida, but surviving infants are often severely handicapped with lower limb paralysis and incontinence.

Encephaloceles are cranial effects with herniated fluid filled or brain-filled cysts affecting mainly the occipital region (75%). In most cases the sac contains parts of the brain and the prognosis is poor. In rare cases, the sac contains only CSF, in which case the prognosis is good.

Ventriculomegaly (lateral ventricle diameter of 10 mm or more) is seen in 1% of pregnancies. The causes are multi-factorial including chromosomal and genetic abnormalities, intrauterine hemorrhage, congenital infections, and may sometimes be unexplained. Holoprosencephaly is a rare cerebral abnormality resulting from incomplete cleavage of the forebrain. It is typically associated with midline facial defects like cyclopia, proboscis midline clefts and chromosomal anomalies like Trisomy 13. Dandy–Walker malformations is associated with abnormalities of the cerebellar vermis,

Table 3.4: Components of fetal anomaly scans

Complete review of the fetus should include

- Head shape + internal structures - cavum pellucidum, cerebellum, ventricular size at atrium (<10 mm)
- Spine—longitudinal, transverse and coronal views
- Abdominal shape and contents at the level of stomach, kidneys and umbilicus
- Renal pelvis (<5 mm AP measurement)
- Thorax at level of four-chamber cardiac view and outflow tracts
- Longitudinal axis—abdominal-thoracic appearance
- Upper limbs—three bones and hand
- Lower limbs—three bones and foot
- Face and lips

TABLE 3.5: EUROCAT STUDY—DETECTION RATES FOR INDIVIDUAL MALFORMATIONS.

Malformations	*Detection rate*
Anencephaly	94%
Encephalocele	79%
Spina bifida	68%
Hydrocephalus	77%
Transposition of great arteries	27%
Hypoplastic left heart syndrome	57%
Limb reduction defects	36%
Bilateral renal ageneis	78%
Diaphragmatic hernia	52%
Exomphalos	77%
Gastoschisis	89%

cystic dilatation of the fourth ventricle and enlargement of the cisterna magna and is associated with chromosomal abnormalities like Trisomy 13 and 18 and triploidy as well as congenital infections.

Ultrasonography can also diagnose abnormalities in the shape of the head, like craniostenosis.

Facial Abnormalities Proper evaluation of the face is important in the diagnosis of genetic disorders and syndromes. This can be accomplished with coronal, sagittal and transverse views of the face. The facial abnormalities that can be identified on scan include facial clefting, hypo- or hypertelorism, microphthalmia, micrognathia, frontal bossing and flattened profile. The detection rate varies from 17% to 50%—the lowest for isolated cleft palate and the higher for combined cleft lip and palate. However in specialist centres, the detection could be as high as 75%.

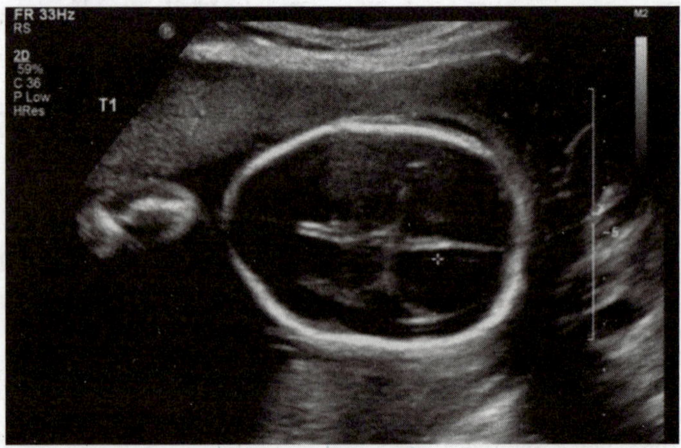

FIGURE 3.2: SPINA BIFIDA—NOTE THE PRESENCE OF A 'LEMON SIGN'. ALSO NOTE THE ABNORMAL SKULL SHAPE AND ENLARGED LATERAL VENTRICLES.

The sagittal view of the face aids in the diagnosis of micrognathia which could be associated with genetic syndromes like Teacher Collin syndrome, chromosomal abnormalities like Trisomy 18 and triploidy. Frontal bossing is seen in conditions like thanatophoric dysplasia and achondroplasia. A flattened face is associated with Trisomy 21.

Cardiac Abnormalities Congenital heart defects (CHD) are the most common congenital abnormalities. Approximately half of these are lethal or require surgery. It affects about 5–10 per 1000 livebirths and in 30 per 1000 stillbirths. However, the antenatal detection rate among the general obstetric population remains low. The Eurofetus study showed a global sensitivity of CHD detection of 34% which is significantly low when compared to CNS abnormalities (88%) and urogenital malformations (89%). The detection rate is higher for major rather than minor abnormalities and also for CHD associated with other abnormalities compared to isolated CHD.

The ideal time for screening a low-risk person for CHD is around 20 weeks (Allan 2003), but women at increased risk of congenital heart defects such as those with family or personal history of heart defects, maternal diabetes or collagen disease, increased nuchal thickness should have fetal echocardiography at 12–14 weeks.

When scanning for cardiac defects, views of the four chambers of the heart and outflow tracts increases the detection sensitivity (Fig. 3.3). Identification of the four chambers of the heart being normal, rules out abnormalities of the mitral and tricuspid valves, hypoplastic left heart, co-arctation, Ebstein anomaly and sub-membranous ventricular septal defect. Normal offset of the crux excludes atrioventricular septal defect. A normal aortic outflow tract excludes double outlet right ventricle, aortic stenosis and Fallot's tetralogy. Abnormal pulmonary artery outflow tract is seen in double outlet right ventricle and pulmonary stenosis. A normal crossover of the aorta seen in the three-vessel view excludes transposition of great arteries—prenatal diagnosis enables immediate postnatal intervention and improves outcome.

Pulmonary Abnormalities Pulmonary abnormalities that may be detected antenatally include cystic adenomatoid malformation of the lung, congenital diaphragmatic hernia, lung sequestration and pleural effusion. Cystic adenomatoid malformation (CAM) of the lung is found in 1 in 1000 births. It is a developmental anomaly arising from overgrowth of the terminal bronchioles. The ultrasound scan demonstrates a hyper-echogenic pulmonary tumour which could be macrocystic (CAM-I), mixed (CAM-II) or microcystic (CAM-III). Lesions are unilateral in 85% of cases. Bilateral disease is lethal due to progressive fetal hydrops. Lung sequestration is a condition when part of the lung develops without connection to airways and are supplied by blood vessels arising directly from descending aorta which can be demonstrated by colour Doppler. Large lung sequestrations can act as an arteriovenous fistula leading to heart failure and hydrops.

Congenital diaphragmatic hernia (CDH) affects about 1 in 4000 fetuses. About 50% of affected fetuses have associated chromosomal abnormalities (Trisomy 18 and 13) or genetic syndromes (deLange and Marfan). There could be associated cardiac and cranio-spinal abnormalities (Fig. 3.4). In 85% of cases, the hernia is on the left side. The stomach and intestines are the common herniating organs. Prognosis is poor in the presence of intrathoracic herniation of the liver. The herniated mass leads to mediastinal shift, lung hypoplasia, pulmonary hypertension and, in rare cases, hydrops. Fetal pleural effusions can occur in association with fetal hydrops or may be isolated. The prognosis depends on the duration and degree of effusion.

Abdominal Wall Defects Retraction of the midgut into the abdominal cavity occurs at 10–12 weeks. A normal cord insertion into the anterior abdominal wall seen at the scan excludes abdominal wall defects like exomphalos and gastroschisis.

Exomphalos results from the failure of normal embryonic regression of the midgut from the umbilical stalk into the abdominal cavity. The herniated part is covered by the peritoneum and amnion and the umbilicus is inserted at the apex of the defect. About half of the cases are associated with chromosomal abnormalities like Trisomy 13 and 18 or cardiac defects.

Gastroschisis results from evisceration of the fetal intestine through a para-umbilical wall defect. The umbilical cord is normally inserted. Associated chromosomal abnormalities are rare.

Gastrointestinal Tract Abnormalities Upper gastrointestinal tract obstruction is usually associated with polyhydramnios, presenting usually after 25 weeks of gestation. Persistent absence of stomach or an abnormally small stomach bubble increases the suspicion of esophageal atresia, especially in presence of polyhydramnios. However, 90% of cases of esophageal atresia are associated with tracheo-esophageal fistula which allows fluid to enter the stomach, thus making diagnosis difficult. A 'double bubble' can be seen in duodenal atresia, and 30% of cases with duodenal atresia are associated with Trisomy 21. Lower gastrointestinal tract abnormalities are generally not detectable prenatally.

Renal Tract Abnormalities The kidneys can be visualised from week 9 of gestation.

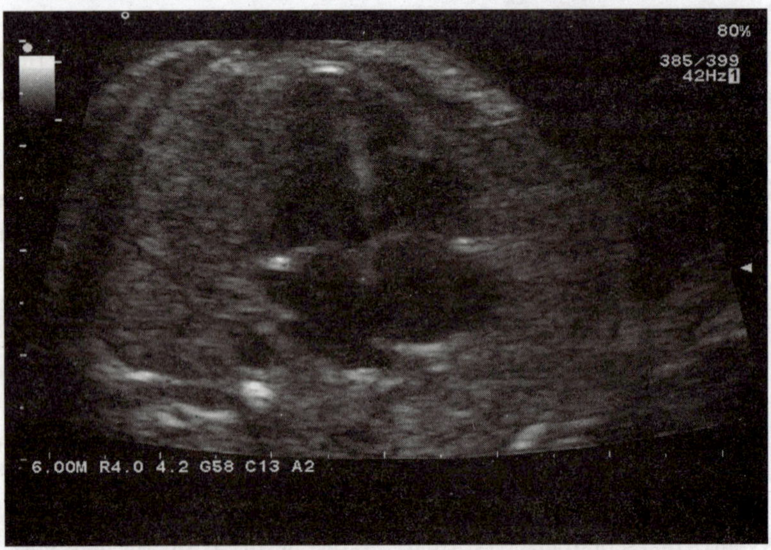

FIGURE 3.3: NORMAL FOUR-CHAMBER VIEW OF THE FETAL HEART

The bladder can be seen in 90% of fetuses at 13 weeks. Abnormalities of the renal tract include bilateral or unilateral renal agenesis, polycystic kidney disease and obstructive uropathies. Bilateral renal agenesis presents with anhydramnios and fetal bladder. (The colour Doppler scan fails to demonstrate the renal arteries.) It is a universally fatal condition. Unilateral renal agenesis is difficult to diagnose prenatally as there are no major features like anhydramnios or absent bladder. The colour Doppler will demonstrate unilateral absence of renal artery. The prognosis is normal. Infantile polycystic kidney disease can be diagnosed by demonstrating bilateral enlarged and hyper-echogenic kidneys. It is a fatal condition. Obstructive uropathy can affect the uretero-pelvic junction, uretero-vesicle junction and the urethra leading to dilatation of the urinary tract above the obstruction. Complete obstruction in early life leads to renal hypoplasia and dysplasia.

Skeletal Abnormalities Skeletal dysplasias are rare. Skeletal abnormalities often involve the limbs—these may be absent or of abnormal length, shape or degree of mineralisation. Ultrasound diagnosis is based on identification of these abnormalities in the limbs, skull, ribs and vertebral bodies. The common fatal dysplasias are thanotophoric dysplasia and osteogenesis imperfecta. Prenatal diagnosis should be complemented by postmortem or postnatal radiological skeletal survey to aid proper counselling on recurrence in subsequent pregnancies.

Fetal Hydrops Fetal hydrops is characterised by abnormal accumulation of fluid in skin and body cavities (pleural, pericardial or ascitic). Hydrops could be of two kinds—immune or non-immune. Non-immune hydrops is more common (seen in 80% of hydrops cases) and is associated with trisomies 13, 18 and 21, Turner syndrome and triploidy, fetal infections and

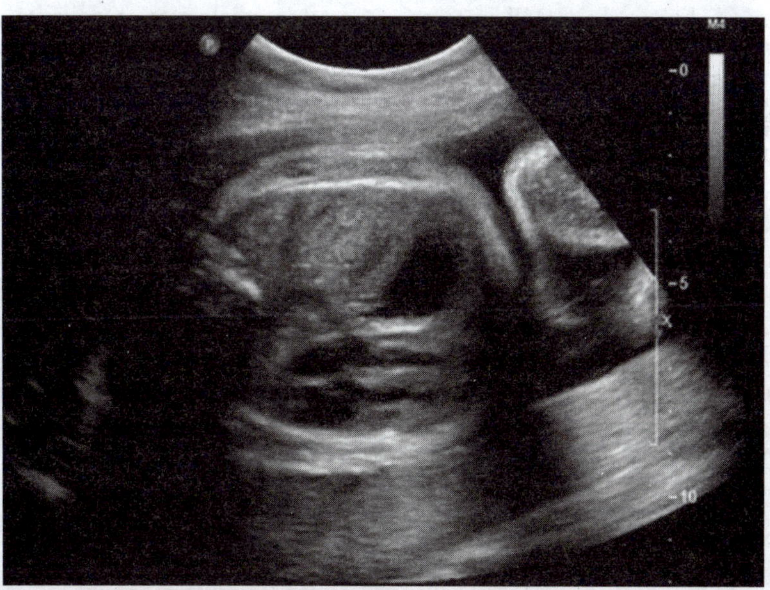

FIGURE 3.4: CONGENITAL DIAPHRAGMATIC HERNIA. NOTE THE FETAL HEART AND THE STOMACH IN THE SAME TRANSVERSE SECTION.

anemia. In cases of hydrops it is important to exclude structural anomalies. Fetal therapy is used successfully to reverse some forms of non-immune and immune hydrops.

Placental and Cord Abnormalities

Chorioangiomas are a rare form of vascular tumour of the placenta. Smaller tumours (<5 cm) are usually benign. Larger tumours can act as fetal arteriovenous anastomosis resulting in hyperdynamic circulation leading to high-output cardiac failure. In one per cent of fetuses, there may be a two-vessel cord resulting from absence of one umbilical artery. It is associated with fetal malformations and intrauterine growth retardation in up to 50% of cases.

Role of MRI in Prenatal Diagnosis

Ultrasound remains the primary imaging modality for prenatal diagnosis. However, fetal magnetic resonance imaging (MRI) could be a useful adjunct to ultrasound to confirm or exclude certain abnormalities. MR imaging is considered safe in pregnancy as it does not use ionising radiation. Due to better soft-tissue contrast, additional investigation by MRI may extend the sonographic diagnosis mainly of fetal CNS abnormalities. MRI can differentiate between white and grey matter and can also visualise the brain surface and sulci. MRI can help in counselling of parents and assist in planning further management.

Summary Prenatal diagnosis by ultrasound is now well-established as an important part of routine antenatal care. More commonly, it reassures parents that their offspring are normal. With increasing expertise and technical advancement, a large proportion of congenital anomalies can be detected antenatally. This allows appropriate counselling of parents and offers them the option of termination of pregnancy where necessary. It also enables the clinician to plan appropriate antenatal and postnatal care through involvement of a multi-disciplinary team of fetal medicine specialists, neonatologists, pediatric surgeons, fetal cardiologists, geneticists and perinatal pathologists.

References

Bui TH. 2007. Prenatal cytogenetic diagnosis: gone FISHing, BAC soon! *Ultrasound Obstet Gynecol* 30:247–251.

Ewigman BG, JP Crane, FD Frigoletto, ML LeFevre, RP Bain and D McNellis. 1993. Effect of prenatal ultrasound screening on perinatal outcome. RADIUS Study Group. *N Engl J Med* 329: 821–827.

Garne E, M Loane, H Dolk et al. 2005. Prenatal diagnosis of severe structural congenital malformations in Europe. *Ultrasound Obstet Gynecol.*25:6–11.

Grandjean H, D Larroque and S Levi. 1999. The performance of routine ultrasonographic screening of pregnancies in the Eurofetus Study. *Am J Obstet Gynecol* 181:446–54.

Nicolaides KH, S Cicero and V Heath. 2002. Increased fetal nuchal translucency at 11–14 weeks. *Prenat Diagnosis* 22: 308–315.

Nicolaides KH. 2003. Screening for chromosomal defects. *Ultrasound Obstet Gynecol* 21:313–321.

RCOG. 2000. Ultrasound Screening. Supplement to Ultrasound Screening for Fetal Abnormalities. Royal College of Obstetricians and Gynaecologists:London (www.rcog.org.uk).

Spencer K, CE Spencer, M Power, A Moakes and KH Nicolaides. 2000. One-stop clinic for assessment of risk for fetal anomalies: a report of the first year of prospective screening for chromosomal anomalies in the first trimester. *Br J Obstet Gynecol* 107:1271–1275.

4

Prenatal Care

Vanita Jain | Sarala Gopalan

Prenatal care is a series of interventions administered to a pregnant woman during the course of her pregnancy with the goal of improving her chances of a favourable outcome. The concept of prenatal care was first formally recommended by Ballantyne in 1902. However, scientific analysis of prenatal care came considerably later with many studies linking increased prenatal care with a decreased chance of adverse pregnancy outcome (Alexander and Cornely 1987). The major goal of prenatal care is to ensure the birth of a healthy baby with minimal risk for the mother.

PRECONCEPTIONAL CARE

Ideally, prenatal care should start long before a woman plans pregnancy. Preconceptional care should be an integral part of prenatal care. Women at risk of potential obstetric or medical complications should consult an obstetrician to ascertain if it is advisable to attempt pregnancy. Many medical disorders (such as diabetes mellitus), and personal habits (such as smoking), could be adequately treated or kept under control before pregnancy is planned. Folic acid supplementation to reduce the risk of neural tube defects is a preconceptional recommendation that applies to all fertile women in the childbearing years. The American College of Obstetricians and Gynecologists (2001) recommends that these women take a folic acid supplement of 400 μg per day.

Number of Prenatal Visits

It is recommended that prenatal care be initiated as soon as there is a likelihood of pregnancy but no later than the second missed period. Traditionally, prenatal visits have been scheduled at intervals of four weeks before 28 weeks, and then every two weeks until 36 weeks, and weekly thereafter in low-risk women. There have been many studies to identify the ideal number of prenatal visits in low-risk women. Hall et al (1980) examined the proportion of routine visits, which resulted in identification of a major problem for the first time. They derived a logical scheme of minimum care for normal primigravidas (10 visits) and normal multigravidas (six visits). Sikorski et al (1996) showed that a reduced visit antenatal programme (seven visits against the traditional 13) led to no difference in the clinical outcome, but the women complained about inadequate time to talk at each visit. The Colorado trial showed no significant difference in 9- and 14-visit schedules, either in clinical outcome or in women's satisfaction with the quality of prenatal care. The Zimbabwe trial (Munjanja et al 1996) showed that an antenatal care programme with fewer, more objectively oriented visits, could be introduced without adverse effects on the main pregnancy outcome.

It should be emphasised that the concept of few routine visits relies strongly on the ability of women to present themselves when unforeseen symptoms develop and on services (emergency or routine) being able to resolve these problems and give advice accordingly. The key issue is not more or less antenatal care or reducing the number of visits, but implementing only those activities proven to be effective; the timing and frequency of visits can then be planned accordingly.

A Cochrane review (Villar 2003) revealed that attempts to provide effective interventions during pregnancy by distributing them in fewer visits than usually recommended could be attempted without risking effectiveness. Such care can be provided by staff other than the obstetrics/gynecology specialist. In light of the available evidence, the four antenatal care visits schedule tested in the largest trials appears to be the minimum that should be offered to low-risk pregnant women.

The current scenario in India is that no more than two in three pregnant women avail of an antenatal check-up, only 44% reported three or more antenatal check-up visits and only a third underwent a check-up within the first trimester of pregnancy (IIPS and ORC Macro 2000). Goals set in the Tenth Plan advocate at least three antenatal check-ups for 90% of pregnant women and universal achievement of complete immunisation for pregnant women.

Components of Prenatal Care

Prenatal care involves confirming the diagnosis of pregnancy, assessment of gestational age, identifying factors posing risk to mother and fetus through interview, physical examination and/or laboratory evaluation, planning prophylactic or intervention strategies based on the factors identified and patient education and counselling (Table 4.1).

Confirm diagnosis of pregnancy: Suspected pregnancy should be confirmed. The earliest signs and symptoms of pregnancy include—absence of expected menses, breast fullness and tenderness, urinary frequency, nausea and fatigue. The 'gold standard' for diagnosis of pregnancy is the detection of the beta subunit of human chorionic gonadotropin (hCG) in blood or urine using immunological techniques. The most sensitive enzyme-linked immunosorbent assays (ELISA) can detect hCG approximately one week after fertilisation. Transvaginal ultrasound can determine fetal viability as early as 5.5–6.5 weeks.

History: Information is collected for assessment of gestational age, which includes menstrual history, dates and results of pregnancy tests, dates and results of examination in early pregnancy and ultrasound done, if any. If there is uncertainty regarding the gestational age, then first trimester or early second trimester ultrasonography can establish the expected date of delivery. Ultrasound measurement of the crown–rump length at 7–14 weeks of gestation is the most accurate technique for

TABLE 4.1: Components of prenatal care
Diagnosing pregnancy
Obtaining information History Examination Laboratory tests
Action Routine medication Based on information Patient education

estimation of gestational age; it is accurate to within 3–5 days.

Additional information includes past medical history, obstetric history, family history, social history including substance abuse, addictions and nutritional assessment. Medical history alerts the obstetrician to a medical or surgical problem requiring attention during pregnancy. An obstetric history consistent with incompetent cervix or one including fetal death near term is likely to alter the prenatal care, such as more frequent cervical assessment or antepartum fetal surveillance. Eliciting family history is important since one can collect information about heritable disorders for which screening or diagnostic tests are available. Social history helps to counsel the patient regarding behavioural modifications if required.

METHOD OF HISTORY TAKING: A randomised trial of three methods of taking antenatal history has been conducted (Lilford 1992). Comparisons were made among a manual system of 29 items routinely used at a University hospital, a structured history of 116 items with a checklist of 31 items with action suggestions for the clinician, and a computer programme in which the patient and midwife face the computer screen and answer 273 possible questions, arranged in a branching format providing clinical action suggestions. Using a structured method of taking antenatal history during the first antenatal visit resulted in more and better information and in improvements in clinical responses. No benefits were found in using the computer to supplement the detailed case notes and checklist.

PHYSICAL EXAMINATION: General physical examination includes recording of height, weight, pulse, blood pressure, presence or absence of edema or jaundice, examination of thyroid, breast, heart, lung, abdomen and nutritional status.

MATERNAL HEIGHT: Routine measurement of maternal height during pregnancy in multigravidas has not been found to be very useful. However, in areas where hospital delivery is not the rule, measurement of maternal height in primigravidas has been used to select those of low stature for hospital birth. The test sensitivity is low but obviously increases with decreasing cut-off levels of height. It is recommended that primigravidas with height less than 145 cm or 4 feet 10 inches should be referred for hospital delivery.

WEIGHT: Excessive weight gain was regarded as one of the cardinal signs of severe pre-eclampsia. However, it has been seen that the sensitivity and specificity of weight gain in prediction of pre-eclampsia is so low that routine weight recording is likely to cause more anxiety than benefit. The significance of weight gain in women with normal or more than average body mass index in prediction of IUGR is also very low (Steer 1993). Thus, the value of weight recording in each antenatal visit is being questioned.

BLOOD PRESSURE: The issue of routine blood pressure measurement in all antenatal care visits is still unresolved. Blood pressure values between 28 and 31 weeks do not accurately predict pre-eclampsia later in the course of pregnancy, despite clear differences in mean blood pressure values between women who remain normal and those who develop pre-eclampsia (Conde-Agudelo 1993). This can be due to the fact that although different, most absolute blood pressure values are usually within the normal range and moderate elevations are usually related to the stress response associated with hospital visits as well as error in measurements (Villar 1989).

However, selecting a subgroup of women for routine blood pressure measurements would create logistic as well as ethical problems. So it is recommended that blood pressure should be recorded at each antenatal visit.

Symphysiofundal height: Between 18 and 32 weeks gestation, there is a good correlation between the gestational age of the fetus in weeks and the height of the uterine fundus in centimetres, when measured as the distance over the abdominal wall from the top of the symphysis pubis to the top of the fundus, with the bladder empty. Routine fundal height measurement has been shown to be helpful in predicting severe intrauterine growth retardation (Jacobsen 1992) and perinatal mortality (Walraven et al 1995) in rural settings. The main advantage of fundal height measurement is its convenience, noninvasiveness and reproducibility.

Symphysiofundal height has been shown to have a good correlation with ultrasonic measurement of biparietal diameter (BPD) and abdominal area (AA). Correlation coefficient of 0.84 for BPD and 0.70 for AA were obtained. The sensitivity (73.1%) and specificity (91.9%) for prediction of IUGR was also very high (Rogers 1985). Thus, measurement of symphysiofundal height at each antenatal visit is recommended. In the third trimester, abdominal examination helps to identify the position and presentation of the fetus.

Fetal heart sounds: The fetal heart is audible by 20 weeks in 80% of women with regular menses. By 21 weeks, audible fetal heart sounds are present in 95% and by 22 weeks in all (Herbert 1987).

Vaginal examination: A randomised control trial showed clearly that routine vaginal examination in all prenatal visits is not justified medically (Buekens 1994). However, it is considered that a full gynecological investigation, including cytological smear and screening for symptomatic 'STDs' and perineal examination for herpetic lesions should be performed once during pregnancy, the timing being flexible. During this examination, evaluation of the cervix, its dilatation and effacement should be observed. Women with cervix dilated >1 cm or effaced >80% should be referred to the hospital or to a specialist for further evaluation (Yawn 1989). The first visit is the best option or if a negative reaction is anticipated from the woman it may be postponed (Bergsjo and Villar 1997). For women with a clinical indication such as pain, bleeding, vaginal discharge or unsure menstrual history and for those who have not had a satisfactory smear within the past three years, a vaginal examination should be done at the booking visit. However, a study from Leeds (O'Donovan 1988) that assessed the value of vaginal examination at hospital booking in the diagnosis of ectopic pregnancy, vaginitis, cervical dilatation and ovarian cyst casts doubt on whether even one routine vaginal examination is justified.

Laboratory evaluation: Certain laboratory investigations are low cost and have many anticipated benefits. They are, thus, advocated routinely during prenatal care. Additional testing can be done for women at risk of specific conditions. The routine tests include hemoglobin, hematocrit, blood group and Rh typing, serological test for syphilis, 1-hour glucose screen following a 50 g oral glucose challenge or random plasma glucose level, urine for albumin and culture of clean-catch midstream sample to identify significant bacteriuria. A hemoglobin or hematocrit should be repeated early in the third trimester. Antibody screening is repeated in unsensitised Rh(D)-negative women and Rh(D) immune globulin administered, as indicated. Voluntary human immunodeficiency virus (HIV) antibody testing with appropriate counselling and consent is encouraged for all women (CDCP 1995). In 2004, the ACOG recommended the use of the opt-out approach to testing, where legally possible. Retesting in the third trimester (around 36 weeks of gestation) is recommended for women at high risk of acquiring HIV infection, in areas of high HIV prevalence, and for women who declined testing earlier in pregnancy. The ACOG recommends screening for hepatitis B antigen (1992). It is recommended that all pregnant women, below 35 years of age with singleton pregnancies, be offered serum screening for Down syndrome using multiple markers. Women who will be 35 years of age at delivery or who are otherwise at increased risk of having a baby with Down syndrome should be offered a diagnostic procedure (ACOG 2003).

The healthcare provider should discuss the interpretation of test results and options for further evaluation. If a disorder is diagnosed, then the natural history of the disorder, risk of disease in the offspring and the woman's reproductive options should be discussed. The decision to conduct screening tests for different diseases must be made on the basis of the prevalence of the disease and available management facilities by proper healthcare authorities and should be incorporated into routine antenatal care.

Ultrasonography: One of the modalities that have revolutionised the practice of obstetrics is ultrasound. It helps doctors view vital organs such as the brain, heart and kidneys, to record bodily measurements with accuracy and to judge fetal well-being. However, there is continuing controversy concerning the issue of universal screening of all pregnancies with ultrasonography. A meta-analysis of randomised controlled trials addressing this issue demonstrated that routine ultrasound screening does not improve the outcome of pregnancy in terms of live births and morbidity, although it has a marginal protective effect for perinatal mortality, mainly by detection of major malformations and abortion in the Helsinki trial (Bucher and Schmidt 1993). The RADIUS trial involving 15,151 pregnant women at low risk of perinatal problems did not demonstrate any improvement in perinatal outcomes, maternal management or outcome from a screening ultrasound as compared with the selective use of ultrasonography on the basis of clinical judgement (Ewigman 1993). Therefore, routine ultrasound evaluation of low-risk pregnancies is not recommended. Routine ultrasound in early pregnancy appears to enable better gestational age assessment, earlier detection of multiple pregnancies and earlier detection of clinically unsuspected fetal malformation at a time when termination of pregnancy is possible. However, the benefits for other substantive outcomes are less clear (Neilson 2003). Currently, the ACOG supports the use of ultrasound when there is a specific medical indication and advises against casual use of ultrasonography during pregnancy (2001). It also stated that routine screening is not mandatory but is reasonable in patients who request it. Thus, it seems both ethical and cost-effective to offer routine screening in the second trimester for detection of fetal anomalies. The examination should be performed at a gestational age that allows for good visualisation of the anatomy, and thus will have a high yield for anomalies.

At the same time, it should be done early enough in gestation to allow completion of prenatal diagnostic procedures (such as fetal karyotype, additional imaging studies) while legal termination of pregnancy is possible, if desired. The optimal timing of second trimester ultrasound screening for fetal anomalies is at 16–20 weeks.

Doppler velocimetry is currently being used as a test of fetal well-being. However, a randomised comparison of routine against highly selective use of Doppler in low-risk women did not demonstrate any benefit or harm for Doppler ultrasound as a routine screening test for all low-risk women (Mason 1993).

Routine prenatal medication: Often practitioners have a tendency to prescribe various supplements during pregnancy. Here, only the role of supplements considered essential is discussed.

Iron and folate: Prenatal iron and folic acid have been the prototypical routine medications given during pregnancy. While there is no doubt about the need for folic acid, the role of iron is less clear. The CDC and the ACOG have recommended supplemental folic acid (400 μg) in the preconceptional and early prenatal period to prevent neural tube defects. The use of iron was justified by calculations based on the typical Western requirement (an average daily absorption of 1 mg of iron and 750 μg of folate) (Kaminetzky 1977). There have been several randomised controlled trials of routine prophylactic iron supplementation during pregnancy as compared with indicated iron treatment, most of them in populations with low prevalence of iron deficiency. These trials concluded that in well-nourished pregnant populations, routine iron supplementation is unnecessary as there was no detectable effect on several maternal, perinatal and long-term outcomes (Mahomed 1993; Hemminki 1995). However, randomised trials did demonstrate a reduction in the proportion of women with hemoglobin < 10 g/dl, increase in circulating ferritin level and a reduction in postpartum blood transfusion with iron supplementation in women from developing countries (Hemminki 1991). Therefore, it is felt that in areas where the prevalence of anemia and folate deficiency is high (> 20%), a situation prevailing in most developing countries, iron and folate supplementation must be provided for every pregnant women. It is expected that this would improve the nutritional status of the mother and reduce the need for blood transfusion. The current recommendation is to increase iron consumption by 15 mg/day (to an RDA of 30 mg/day). A Cochrane review suggests that there is no evidence to recommend routine iron supplementation during pregnancy in well-nourished women despite the improvement in hematological indicators. Likewise, there is no evidence against the provision of routine iron supplementation in populations with high incidence of iron deficiency anemia. In developed countries and in well-nourished populations where anemia is not prevalent, the role of routine iron supplementation is uncertain and further studies to clarify this issue are required (González-Cossío 2004).

Calcium: The Recommended Daily Allowance for elemental calcium is 1000 mg per day in pregnant women. Women whose diet does not provide adequate calcium may benefit by calcium supplementation. Calcium supplementation in the dose of 2 g/day has not been associated with any adverse events.

Micronutrients: Pregnant women in developing countries present with high rates of several micronutrient deficiencies. Because of the possible positive interaction between vitamin A and iron/folate a multiple nutrient intervention, possibly including magnesium and zinc, seems to be justified. However, the scarcity of clinical data available, except for calcium, precludes recommending micronutrient supplementation on a routine basis for the prevention of pregnancy complications (Kulier et al 1998).

Tetanus toxoid: One of the priorities of antenatal care should be to provide tetanus toxoid to mothers who have not been adequately immunised previously. This is provided in two doses, the first between 20 and 22 weeks and the second between 26 and 32 weeks.

Patient education and counselling: The women should be advised regarding nutrition, weight gain, exercise, rest and sexual activity. The danger signals of pregnancy should be explained to the patient. Signs and symptoms to be reported to the healthcare provider should be discussed at each visit, as appropriate for gestational age (for example, vaginal bleeding, ruptured membranes, contractions, decreased fetal activity).

Nutrition: All pregnant women should be encouraged to eat a well-balanced diet (ensuring they match the RDA). Women who typically eat three meals daily consisting of several servings of vegetables, fruits, whole grains, dairy products and a few sources of protein (for example, meat, fish, eggs, dried peas or beans) are likely to have adequate nutrition. The National Research Counsel recommends a 300 kcal per day increase in calories above non-pregnant levels throughout pregnancy.

Work: A woman with an uncomplicated pregnancy may continue to work without interruption until the onset of labour. Working during pregnancy should be limited or contraindicated in some women, such as those with vaginal bleeding, pregnancy-induced hypertension, fetal growth restriction, multiple gestation, prior history of preterm birth, polyhydramnios, short (<3 cm) or dilated cervix before 36 weeks gestation and maternal medical disorders that are unstable or associated with impaired placental perfusion.

Exercise: In the absence of obstetric or medical complications, a pregnant woman may undertake moderate exercises.

Sexual activity: In the absence of pregnancy complications (vaginal bleeding, ruptured membranes), the couple may have sexual intercourse during pregnancy.

Conclusion: The cost of prenatal care is modest compared to the expense of managing serious, preventable complications in the mother, fetus or infant. It has been seen that the frequency of low birth weight infants is much higher in pregnancies without prenatal care and the cost is nearly double for newborn care (Leveno et al 1985). Cost-benefit analysis of Missouri's Medicaid Programme showed a saving of US$ 1.49 on neonatal care for each dollar spent on prenatal care (Schramm 1992). Moore et al showed in a case control study of a low socioeconomic population that for each dollar spent on prenatal care, US$ 3.66 was saved on hospital charges of neonatal care. Thus, it is clear that prenatal care is a cost-effective means for improving the health of the mother and infant and the barriers to care—social, financial and policy-related—must be identified and eliminated.

Although prenatal care is not likely to prevent all maternal deaths, it is still essential for all pregnancies in developing countries. In India, at present only 30% receive some form of antenatal care—this is inadequate. Pregnancy is the only time when women may seek care and accept it. Providing adequate antenatal care in combination with a good referral back-up and optimum emergency obstetric care facilities will reduce maternal morbidity/mortality.

References

ACOG committee opinion number 304. 2004. Prenatal and perinatal human immunodeficiency virus testing: expanded recommendations. *Obstet Gynecol* 104 (5 Pt 1):1119–1124.

ACOG practice bulletin. 2003. Clinical management guidelines for obstetrician–gynecologists. Number 44, July 2003. (Replaces Committee Opinion Number 252, March 2001). *Obstet Gynecol* 102:203.

Alexander GR and DA Cornely. 1987. Prenatal care utilization. Its measurement and relationship to pregnancy outcome. *Am J Prev Med* 3: 243–253.

American College of Obstetricians and Gynecologists. 1992. Hepatitis in pregnancy. *Technical Bulletin No. 174*. American College of Obstetricians and Gynecologists.

American College of Obstetricians and Gynecologists. 2001. Prenatal diagnosis of fetal chromosomal abnormalities. *ACOG Practice Bulletin no. 27*. Washington DC: American College of Obstetricians and Gynecologists.

Ballantyne JW. 1902. Manual of antenatal pathology and hygiene Vol. 1. Edinburgh: William Green & Sons.

Bergsjo P and J Villar. 1997. Scientific basis for the content of routine antenatal care. *Acta Obstet Gynecol Scand* 76:15–25.

Bucher HC and J Schmidt. 1993. Does routine ultrasound screening improve outcome in pregnancy? Meta-analysis of various outcome measures. *Br Med J* 307:13–17.

Buekens P, S Alexander, M Bontsen, B Blondel, M Karminski and M Reid. 1994. Randomised controlled trial of routine cervical examination in pregnancy. *Lancet* 344:841–*844*.

Center for Disease Control and Prevention. 1995. US Public Health Service recommendations for human immunodeficiency virus counselling and voluntary testing for pregnant women. *MMWR* 44: RR–7.

Conde-Agudelo A, JM Behzan, R Lede and E Bergel. 1993. What does an elevated mean arterial pressure in the second half of pregnancy predict? gestational hypertension or preeclampsia? *Am J Obstet Gynecol* 169:509–514.

Ewigman B, J Crane, F Frigoletto, M Le Jeure and the RADIUS Study Group. 1993. Effect of prenatal ultrasound screening on perinatal outcome. *N Eng J Med* 329:821–827.

González-Cossío T. 2004. Routine iron supplementation during pregnancy. RHL commentary (last revised: 21 December 1999). Oxford: *The WHO Reproductive Health Library*, No 7, Update Software Ltd.

Hall MJ, PK Chang and I MacGillivary. 1980. Is routine antenatal care worthwhile? *Lancet* II: 78–80.

Hemminki E and J Merilainen. 1995. Long-term follow-up of mothers and their infants in a randomized trial on iron prophylaxis during pregnancy. *Am J Obstet Gynecol* 173:205–209.

Hemminki E and U Rimpela. 1991. A randomized comparison of routine vs selective iron supplementation during pregnancy. *J Am Coll Nutr* 10:3–10.

Herbert WN, HM Bruninghaus, AB Barefoot and TG Bright. 1987. Clinical aspects of fetal heart auscultation. *Obstet Gynecol.* 69:574–577.

International Institute for Population Sciences (IIPS) and ORC Macro. 2000. National Family Health Survey (NFHS–2), 1998–1999.

Jacobsen G. 1992. Prediction of fetal growth deviation by use of symphysis–fundus height measurements. *Int J Technol Assess Healthcare* 8:152–159.

Kaminetzky HA and H Baker. 1977. Micronutrients in pregnancy. *Clin Obstet Gynecol* 20:363–380.

Kulier R, M de Onis, AM Gulmezoglu and J Villar. 1998. Nutritional interventions for prevention of maternal morbidity. *Int J Gynecol Obstet* 63(3):231–246.

Leveno KJ, FG Cunningham, ML Roark, SD Nelson and ML Williams. 1985. Prenatal care and low birth weight infant. *Obstet Gynecol* 66(5):599–605.

Lilford R, M Kelly, A Baines, S Cameron, M Vave, K Guthrie et al. 1992. Effect of using protocols on medical care; randomized trial of three methods of taking an antenatal history. *Br Med J* 305: 1181–1184.

Mahomed K. 1993. Routine iron supplementation in pregnancy. In *Pregnancy and childbirth module,* eds MW Enkin, MJNC Keirse, MJ Renfrew and JP Neilson, Cochrane database of systematic reviews. Oxford: Cochrane Updates on Disk. Update software.

Mason GC, RJ Lilford, J Porter, E Nelson and S Tyrell. 1993. Randomised comparison of routine versus highly selective use of Doppler ultrasound in low risk pregnancies. *Br J Obstet Gynaecol* 100 (2):130–133.

Munjanja S, G Lindmark and L Nystrom. 1996. Randomised controlled trial of a reduced programme of antenatal care in Harare, Zimbabwe. *Lancet* 348:364–369.

Neilson JP. 2003. Ultrasound for fetal assessment in early pregnancy (Cochrane Review). In *The Cochrane Library*, Issue 4. Chichester: John Wiley & Sons, Ltd.

O'Donovan P, JK Gupta, J Savage, JG Thomson and RJ Lilford. 1988. Is routine antenatal booking vaginal examination necessart fit reasons other than cervical cytology if ultrasound examination is planned? *Br J Obstet Gynaecol* 95:556–559.

Rogers MS and PG Needham. 1985. Evaluation of fundal height measurement in antenatal care. *Aust NZ J Obstet Gynecol* 25:87–90.

Schramm WF. 1992. Weighing costs and benefits of adequate prenatal care for 12,023 births in Missouri's Medicaid program, 1988. *Public Health Rep* 107 (6):647–652.

Sikorski J, J Wilson, S Clement, S Das and N Smeeton. 1996. A randomized controlled trial comparing two schedules of antenatal visits: the antenatal care project. *Br Med J* 312:546–553.

Steer P. 1993. Rituals in antenatal care — do we need them? *Br Med J* 307:697–698.

Villar J, G Carroli, D Khan–Neelofur, G Piaggio and M Gülmezoglu. 2003. Patterns of routine antenatal care for low-risk pregnancy (Cochrane Review). In *The Cochrane Library*, Issue 4. Chichester: John Wiley & Sons Ltd.

Villar J, J Repke, L Markush, W Calvert and G Rhoads. 1989. The measuring of blood pressure during pregnancy. *Am J Obstet Gynecol* 161(4):1019–1024.

Walraven GE, R Mkanje, J van Roosmalen, P van Dongen, H van Asten and W Dolman. 1995. Single pre-delivery symphysis–fundal–height measurement as a predictor of birth weight and multiple pregnancy. *Br J Obstet Gynecol* 102:525–529.

Yawn B and R Yawn. 1989. Pre-term birth prevention in a rural practice. *JAMPA* 262: 230–233.

5

Sonography in First Trimester

P K Shah | Sachin Ajmera

Introduction

Transvaginal sonography (TVS) is the preferred mode of imaging a woman in the first trimester of pregnancy. It can be performed by linear array probes, but frontal radiating sector probes are preferred because one can then evaluate the uterus, pouch of Douglas, cervix and the adnexal regions. A panoramic sector probe is preferred with a scan angle of 250° and acoustic frequency of 5–10 MHz. It can easily view a depth of up to 65 mm.

Recent technological advances in three-dimensional ultrasonography complement conventional evaluation of the developing embryo. In addition, it also presents volume data in a standard anatomical orientation—this is useful to both sonologists and pregnant women (Benoit et al 2002). Three-dimensional power Doppler sonography can study the process of placentation and evaluate the development of the embryonic and fetal cardiovascular systems (Kurjak et al 1999).

Technique of Examination

Most women accept transvaginal scanning, preferring it over the standard transabdominal approach, which requires a full urinary bladder. It should be performed with the same respect for privacy and gentleness of touch as the insertion of a speculum in the vagina. Scanning is performed with the patient in the supine position with her thighs abducted and knees flexed; elevation of the hips may be necessary. The probe should be covered with a condom or a sheath containing a small amount of gel. Additional gel should be placed on the outside of the covered tip. The probe may be inserted by a gentle push posteriorly towards the rectum, while the patient relaxes.

Three basic manoeuvres are possible—advancement or withdrawal along the axis of the vagina, angling by directing the tip from side to side or anterior to posterior, and rotation of the transducer along its axis. After removal of the transvaginal probe, the sheath is removed and the coupling gel wiped off with a damp towel; it may be disinfected.

A systematic approach minimises diagnostic errors. First, the uterus (including the fundus and the cervix) is imaged. Thereafter, the ovaries, adnexae and lateral axes are evaluated and finally, the cul-de-sac is assessed for presence of free fluid. The technique may be modified according to the need of the individual patient.

Sonography

At the end of the fourth week of pregnancy, the products of conception can be detected with high-frequency, state-of-the-art transvaginal ultrasound transducers (Timor-Tritsch et al 1988). A vaginal transducer with a frequency of at least 5 MHz will show the gestational sac, the first definitive sonographic sign of early intrauterine pregnancy. The size threshold for sac detection is 2–3 mm, corresponding to the gestational age of 4 weeks and 2–3 days (Fig. 5.1). At this stage, the chorionic cavity is identified as fluid within the gestational sac. Surrounding the fluid collection is an echogenic rim of tissue, which is the chorionic villi, and the adjacent decidual tissue. The normal gestational sac is located near the fundus and has a round, oval or crescent shape with a smooth, rounded contour (Fig. 5.2). The gestational sac grows at a fairly constant rate of 1 mm per day in diameter during early pregnancy. The sac diameter of >5 mm (five weeks gestational age) can also be detected by transabdominal sonography (Nyberg et al 1987). Abnormality in shape and size is an indicator of poor pregnancy outcome; in such cases, sonographic evaluation should be repeated (Fig. 5.3).

When the mean sac diameter is around 10 mm, it impresses on the central cavity echo complex and is surrounded by two concentric echogenic lines. The inner line represents the chorion along with deciduas capsularis, while the outer line represents the deciduas parietalis. This is also called the double decidual sac sign (Bradley et al 1982) (Fig. 5.4). This sign helps to differentiate between an intrauterine and an ectopic pregnancy; in cases where the yolk sac cannot be visualised on transabdominal sonography and on transvaginal sonography, one may see the pseudogestation sac (Fig. 5.5).

At the beginning of the fifth week, using transvaginal ultrasound, the secondary yolk sac can be discerned within the gestational sac (mean sac diameter 5 mm) (Fig. 5.6). In practice, however, the yolk sac may not always be visualised till five and a half weeks of gestational age (mean sac diameter 8 mm). With transabdominal sonography, the yolk sac should be evident by week 7, when the mean sac diameter is 20 mm (Nyberg et al 1987). It is spherical in shape with a well-defined echogenic rim and a sonolucent centre. The yolk sac gradually increases in diameter from 3.4 mm to 5.5 mm at ten weeks gestational age (Stampone et al 1996). Till Week 8, the yolk sac remains connected to the embryo; thereafter it detaches, but remains visible within the

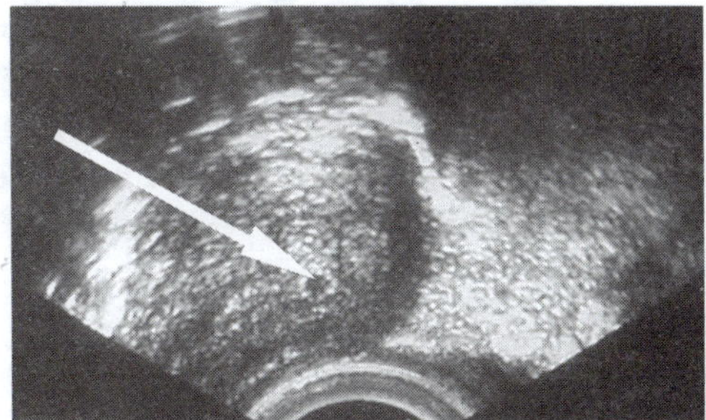

Figure 5.1: Gestational sac 4-5 weeks

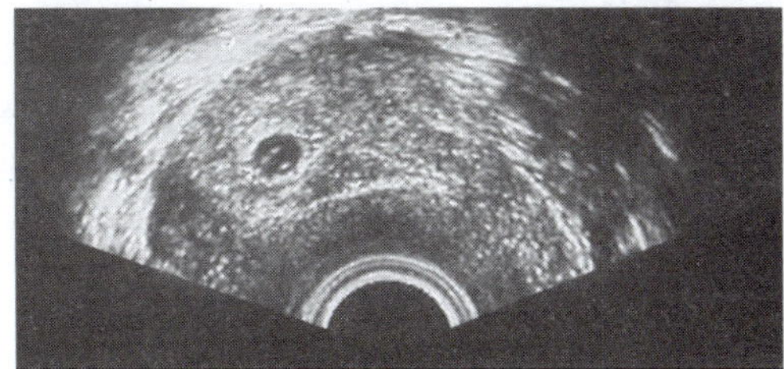

Figure 5.2: Normal gestational sac

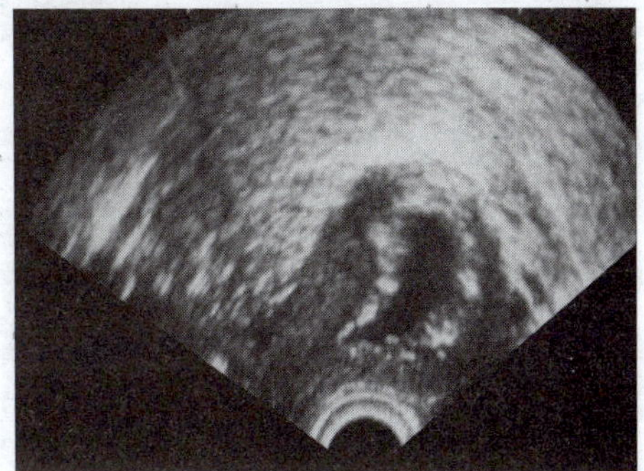

Figure 5.3: Abnormal shape and size of gestational sac

shrinking chorionic cavity. By the end of the first trimester it may no longer be detected by sonography, as the amnion and chorion fuse. Detection of the yolk sac is important for the following reasons:

- It confirms intrauterine pregnancy
- It helps in dating the pregnancy
- It helps to locate the embryonic disc
- An abnormal-appearing yolk sac is associated with early pregnancy failure (Fig. 5.7)

The embryonic disc is detected as an area of focal thickening along the edge of the yolk sac. It can be detected as early as at a gestational age of 5–6 weeks, when it measures 1–2 mm in length.

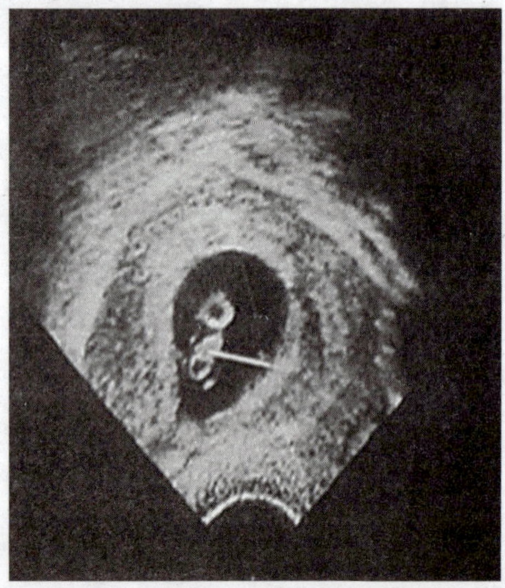

Figure 5.4: Double decidual sac sign

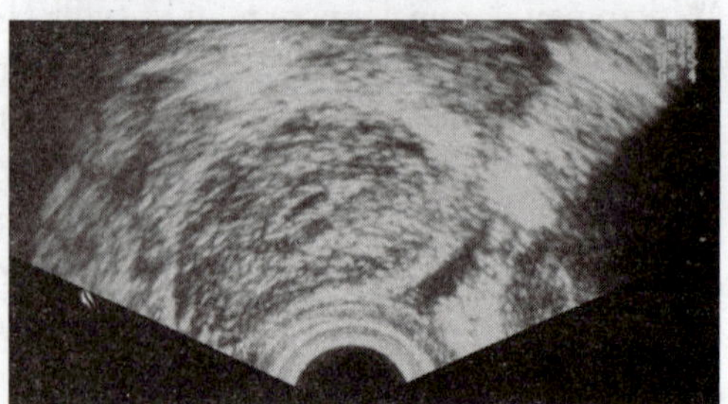

Figure 5.5: Pseudogestation sac

The embryonic period

Embryology: This period lasts from the sixth to the tenth week. During this period, all major internal and external structures begin to form. The developmental stages in the embryo are as given in Table 5.1 (Moore and Persaud 1998).

The crown–rump length increases at the rate of approximately 1 mm per day in Week 6 (Lasser et al 1993), the embryo changes from a flat disc to a three-dimensional, C-shaped structure due to the folding of the cranial and caudal end. Between 7 and 8 weeks, limb buds evolve into paddle-shaped upper and lower limbs (Fig. 5.8). At around 9 weeks, the limbs extend ventrally, the trunk elongates and straightens and midgut herniation can be prominently seen.

Motor activity begins between weeks 7 and

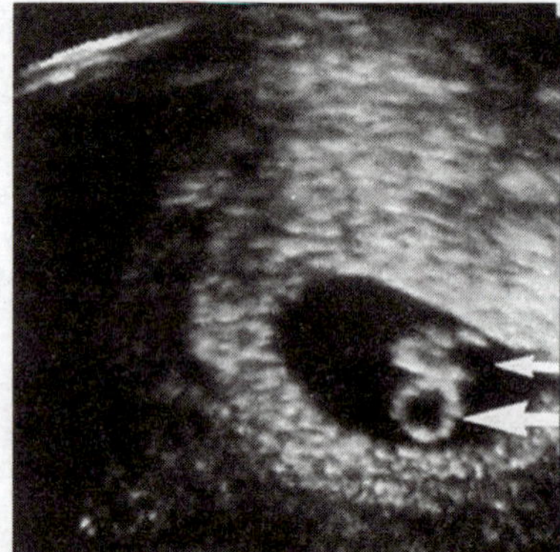

Figure 5.6: Secondary yolk sac

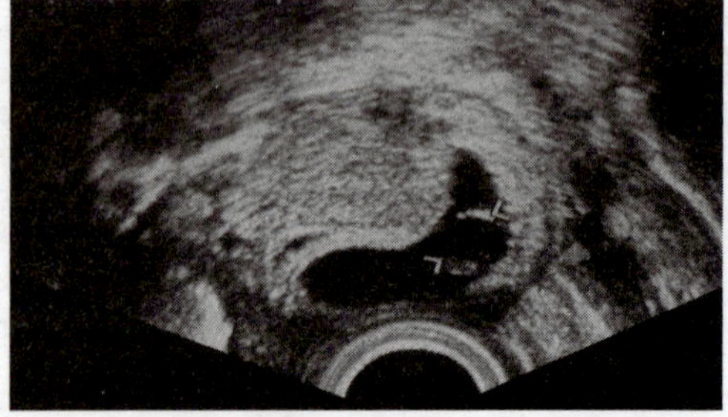

Figure 5.7: Abnormal yolk sac

8 when the spinal reflex pattern has formed. Initially, the nerve fibres are not myelinated and fatigue sets in rapidly. By weeks 8 to 9 embryonic movements can be detected.

The amnion is very thin (0.02–0.5 mm) and is difficult to visualise at week 6 (Bourne 1960) (Fig. 5.9). Occasionally, however, it may be seen when it lies perpendicular to the ultrasound beam. It lies continuous with the embryonic disc opposite to the yolk sac. This appearance is often referred to as the 'double-bleb sign' (Yeh and Rabinowitz 1988). There is a linear relationship between the size of the amniotic cavity and crown–rump length. They increase by 1 mm per day and also have equivalent measurements (Horrow 1992). The amniotic membrane fuses with the chorionic membrane by week 12. After apposition, the amniotic membrane cannot be seen. An abnormally large amniotic cavity relative to the size of the embryo prognosticates poor pregnancy outcome.

The placenta, that is, the chorion frondosum, and the umbilical cord can be identified as early as at eight menstrual weeks (Fig. 5.10). The umbilical cord length correlates with menstrual age. Coiling is an obvious characteristic of the umbilical cord.

With high-frequency probes, it is possible to delineate and observe detailed features,

Table 5.1: Developmental changes in the human embryo

GA (days)	*Length (mm)*	*Main external characteristics*
34–35	1.5–3	Flat embryonic disc
36–37	2.0–3.5	Embryo straight or slightly curved
38–39	2.5–4.5	Embryo curved owing to head and tails fold
40–41	3.0–5.0	Upper limb buds appear
42–44	4.0–6.0	Embryo has C-shaped curve
45–46	5.0–7.0	Upper limbs are paddle-shaped
47–50	7.0–9.0	Hand plates formed; digital rays present. Lower limbs are paddle-shaped
51–54	8.0–11.0	Foot plates formed
55–57	11.0–14.0	Digital rays visible in hand plates
58–60	13.0–17.0	Digital rays clearly visible in foot plates
61–62	16.0–18.0	Limbs extend ventrally. Trunk elongating and straightening. Midgut herniation prominent
63–65	18.0–22.0	Upper limbs longer and bent at elbows. Fingers webbed
66–67	22.0–28.0	Hands and feet approach each other. Fingers are free and longer. Toes are webbed. Stubby tail present.
68–69	23.0–28.0	Toes are free and longer. Eyelids and external ears more developed
70	27.0–31.0	Head more rounded and shows human characteristics. External genitals still have sexless appearance. Distinct bulge still present in umbilical cord, caused by herniation of intestines. Tail has disappeared.

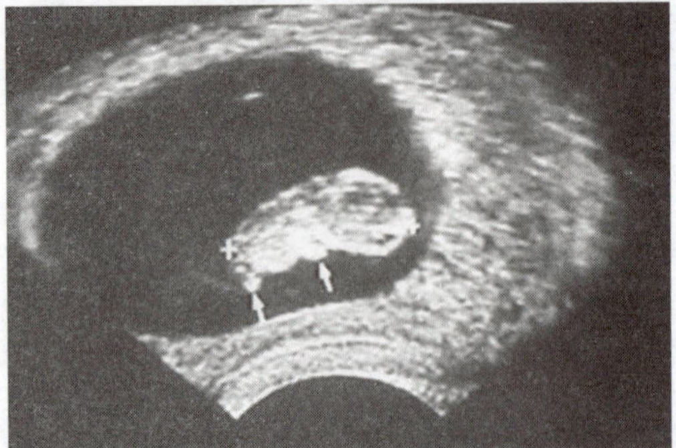

FIGURE 5.8: LIMB BUDS

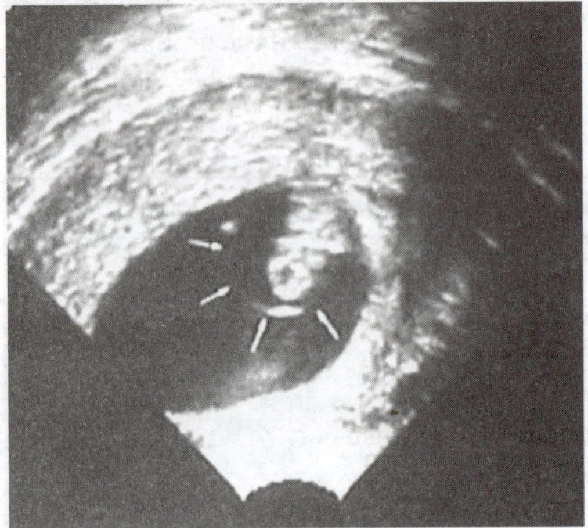

FIGURE 5.9: AMNION AT SIX WEEKS

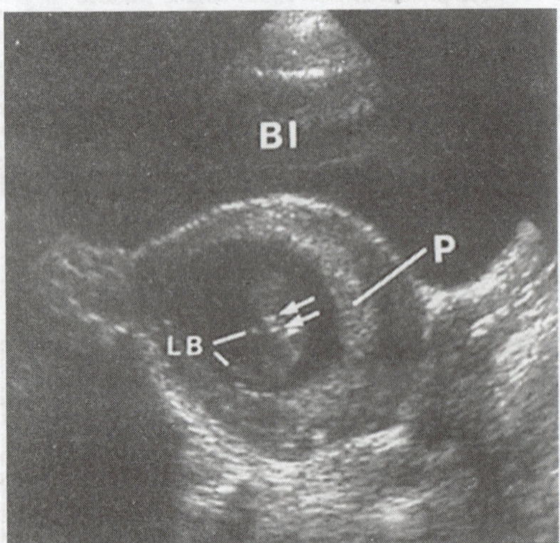

FIGURE 5.10: UMBILICAL CORD

such as the brain vesicles and neural tubes, as early as the beginning of the seventh week of gestation (Merz et al 1995). This, in addition to helping detect congenital anomalies early, also helps in studying the embryology of the fetus (which is not possible even in pathological specimens since the cavities collapse after death).

DEVELOPMENT OF THE CARDIOVASCULAR SYSTEM

The cardiovascular system develops and the heart starts to beat at the beginning of Week 6. At the end of the embryonic period, the crown–rump length measures 30–35 mm.

Sonography: Cardiac activity has been reported at a gestational age of 40 days as soon as the embryo is visualised. In practice, cardiac activity should always be detected when the embryo measures 5 mm or more (Coulam et al 1996). At this period, the gestational age corresponds to 6 weeks/6 weeks 4 days and the mean sac diameter measures 13–18 mm (Levi et al 1988; Coulam et al 1996). The mean embryonic cardiac rate increases from 120 beats per minute at 6 weeks 3 days to a peak of 174 beats per minute at 9 weeks. Subsequently, the heart rate declines to 160 beats per minute at 11 weeks and 146 beats per minute at Week 14. Variability in the heart rate pattern is related to hormonal and neuronal factors. Hence, in an embryo there is almost no variation in the cardiac rate as compared to later gestational age (Schats et al 1990; Montenegro et al 1998).

In embryos with a fetal heart rate of less than 100 beats per minute at 6 weeks 1 day of gestational age and less than 120 beats per minute between 6 weeks 2 days and 7 weeks there is a higher chance of pregnancy failure.

The Fetal Period

Embryology: This period comprises two weeks in the first trimester: the eleventh and the twelfth week. There is continued rapid growth and ongoing organ development.

Sonography: Various fetal structures can be seen and easily identified at this stage. Midgut herniation returns to the abdomen by the end of Week 11 (van Zalen-Sprock et al 1997) (Fig. 5.11). Early congenital anomaly scans are carried out in this period. The various congenital anomalies that can be detected in this period are described later.

Dating the Pregnancy

Since a woman is often not sure of the dates of the menstrual cycle, calculation of gestational age based on menstrual history may be difficult. The best time to date pregnancy (and when it is likely to be most accurate) is in the first trimester, because biological variation is relatively minimal at this stage.

The parameters used to date the pregnancy are gestational sac size and embryonic size. Before the development of the embryo, the gestational sac size closely correlates with the menstrual age. The gestational sac size is best described by the mean sum of three orthogonal dimensions—craniocaudal, anteroposterior and transverse. Gestational age in days can be calculated by adding 30 to the mean sac diameter (Nyberg et al 1987). Between 5 and 11 weeks, gestational age can be easily calculated using this method.

Between 6 and 12 weeks, with the identification of the embryo, the embryonic size or crown-rump length is measured and is considered the most accurate method of pregnancy dating (Daya 1993) (Fig. 5.12). As the embryo grows linearly at the rate of 1 mm per day, the gestational age can be estimated by adding 42 to the crown-rump length in mm (Goldstein and Wolfson 1994; Nyberg et al 1987).

Gestational age in weeks = CRL in cm + 6.5

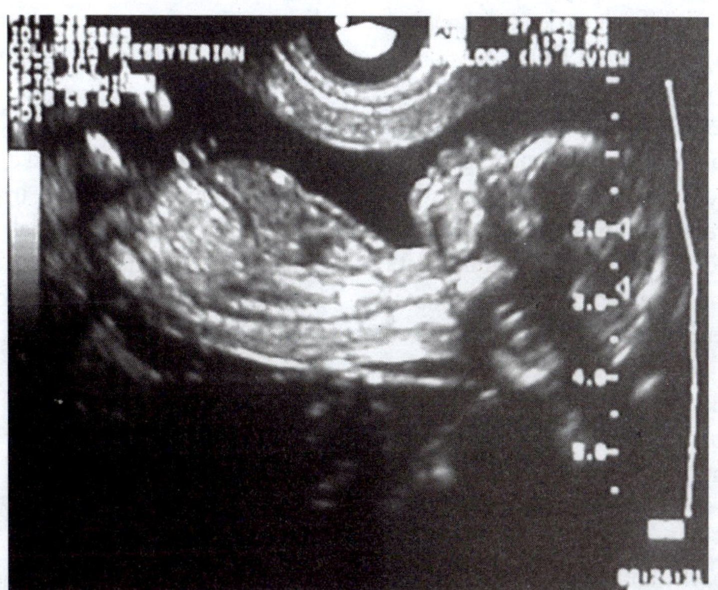

Fig. 5.11: Fetal structures at 11 weeks

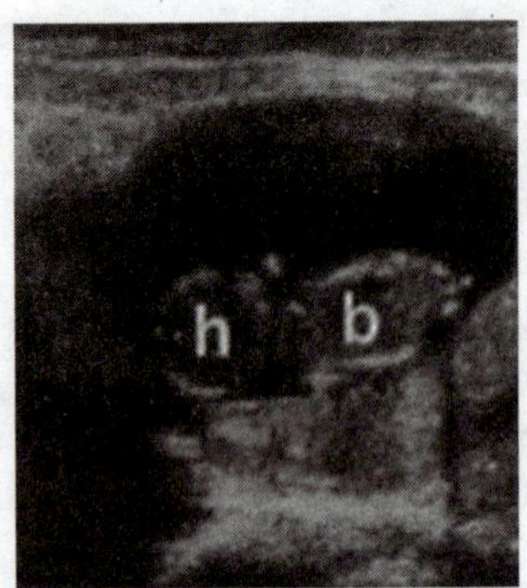

FIGURE 5.12: DATING OF PREGNANCY

DOPPLER SONOGRAPHY IN FIRST TRIMESTER PREGNANCY

In the first trimester, the uterine artery waveform characteristically shows a high resistance flow with a prominent diastolic notch (Colour plate 1). The latter typically disappears in the second trimester and in some cases may disappear as early as at 13 weeks (Coppens et al 1996).

Flow in the subchorionic vessels or spiral arteries is typically pulsatile with a low resistance pattern (Colour plate 2). Doppler flow in the intervillous space is difficult to detect because of very low velocity (Jauniaux 1996).

ROLE OF THREE-DIMENSIONAL SONOGRAPHY

Three-dimensional ultrasound imaging allows imaging from volume sonographic data rather than the conventional planar data. Special probes are used which obtain volume data by acquiring multiple slices of conventional planar data, identifying the location of those slices in space and reconstructing it into a volume. This data is then viewed as a three-dimensional object and displayed using different formats to provide the impression of a three-dimensional structure. In the first trimester, after the acquisition of the data using a vaginal probe, the embryo is rotated into a frontal view, as though facing the sonologist. The uterus can be electronically masked to see the embryo better. When the embryo rotates, the limb and surface features can be seen clearly. Gestational sac volume can be accurately calculated—this may be a marker of pregnancy outcome (Sterner 1994). Nuchal translucency can be accurately measured with minimum errors using this technique.

ABNORMAL FIRST TRIMESTER SONOGRAPHY

Threatened abortion: Sonography will show an embryo with cardiac activity and closed cervical os.

Complete abortion: Sonography will show empty uterus with regular endometrial echoes (Fig. 5.13)

Incomplete abortion: Sonography will show thickened, irregular endometrial echoes or fluid within endometrial cavity (Fig. 5.14).

Embryonic demise: Sonography will show discrete embryo with absent fetal cardiac activity

Blighted ovum: Sonography will show discrepancy in gestational sac development along with little or no embryonic remnant (Fig. 5.15)

Ectopic pregnancy: Sonography will show absent intrauterine sac, thin decidual reaction, weak decidual amplitude, irregular contour; absence of double decidual sac within the uterus and presence of gestational sac in the adnexa points towards ectopic pregnancy (Fig. 5.16).

Subchorionic hemorrhage: A viable fetus may be associated with a sonolucent collection outside the gestational sac. Subchorionic hemorrhage of more than 60 ml is associated with poor outcome. (Fig. 5.17).

Multiple pregnancy: It can be diagnosed as early as 5–6 weeks by transvaginal sonography (Fig. 5.18).

Hydatidiform mole: Snow-storm appearance within the uterus is diagnostic of hydatidiform mole. Assessment of beta-hCG levels would help in further diagnosis and management (Fig. 5.19).

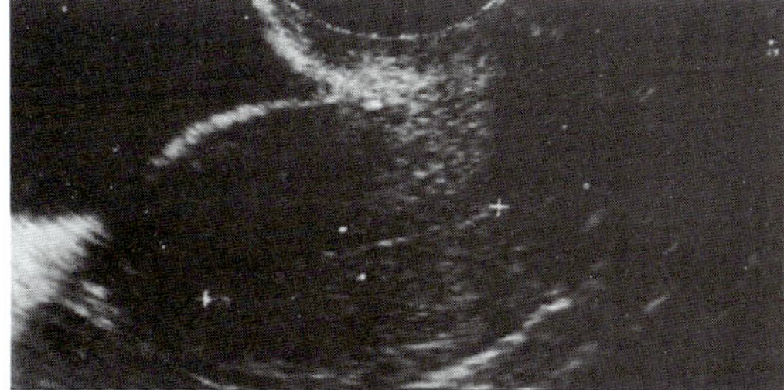

Figure 5.13: Abortion

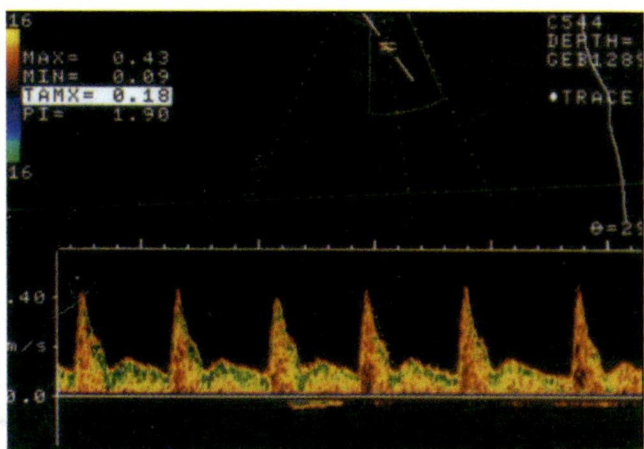

Colour plate 1: Uterine artery waveform

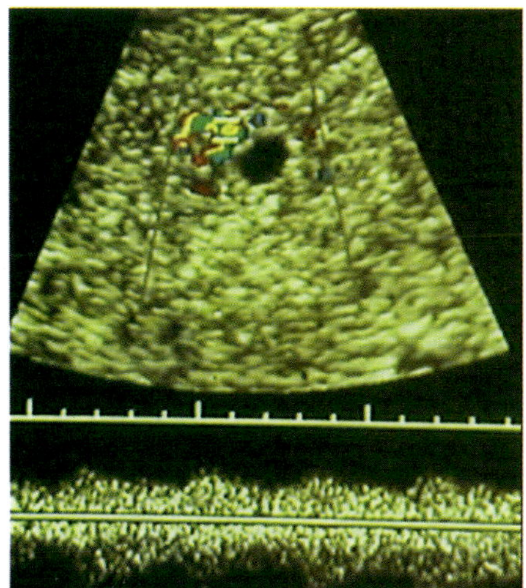

Colour plate 2: Blood flow in spiral arteries

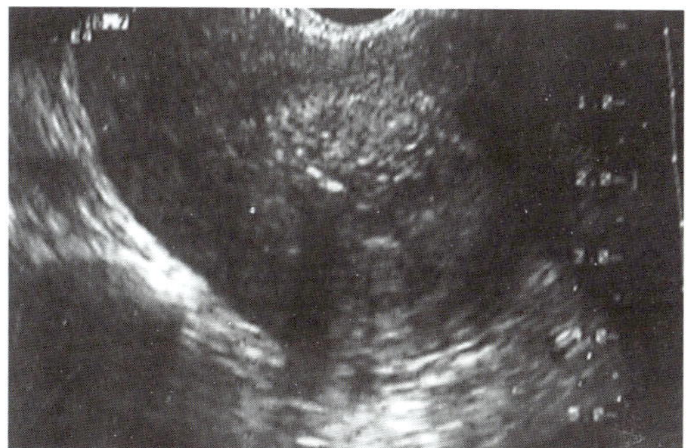

Figure 5.14: Incomplete abortion

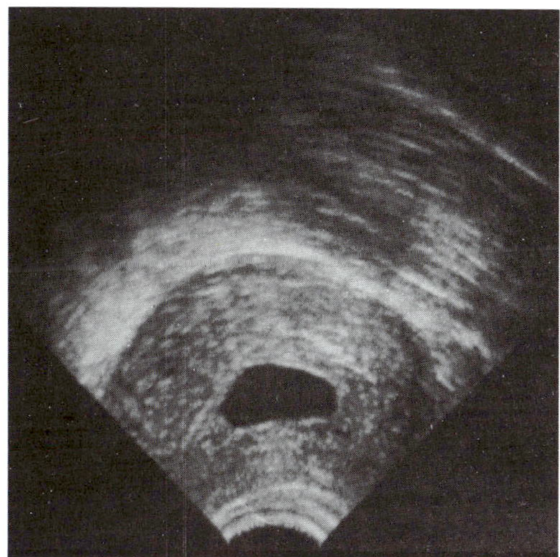

Figure 5.15: Blighted ovum

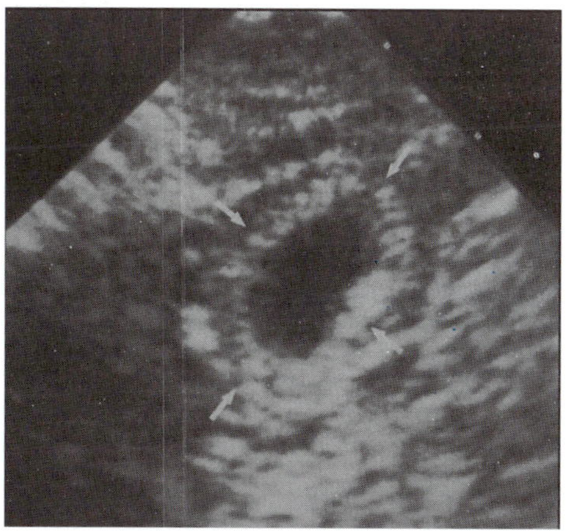

Figure 5.16: Ectopic Pregnancy

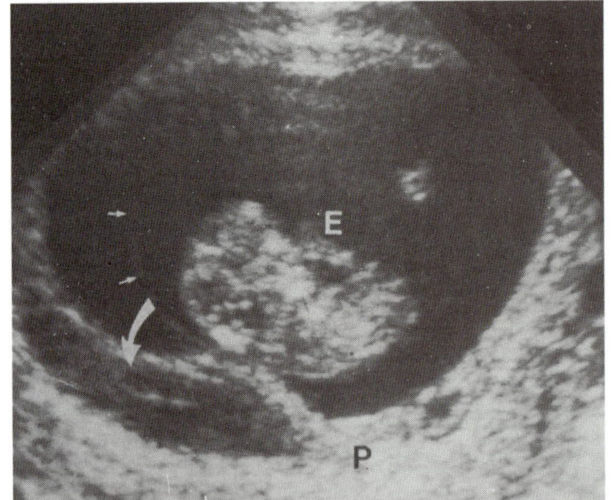

Figure 5.17: Subchorionic hemorrhage

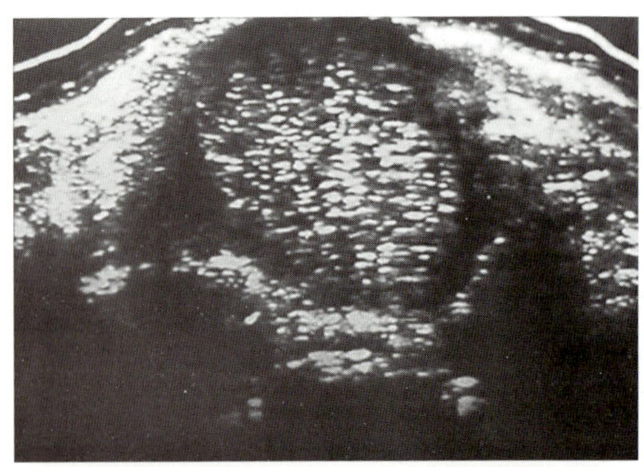

Figure 5.19: Hydatiform mole

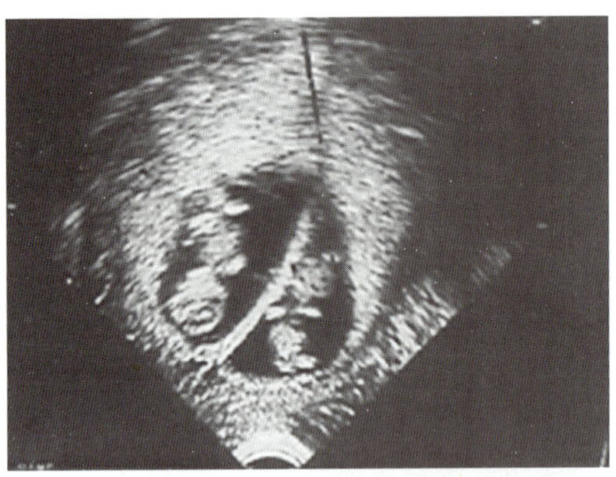

Figure 5.18: Multiple pregnancy

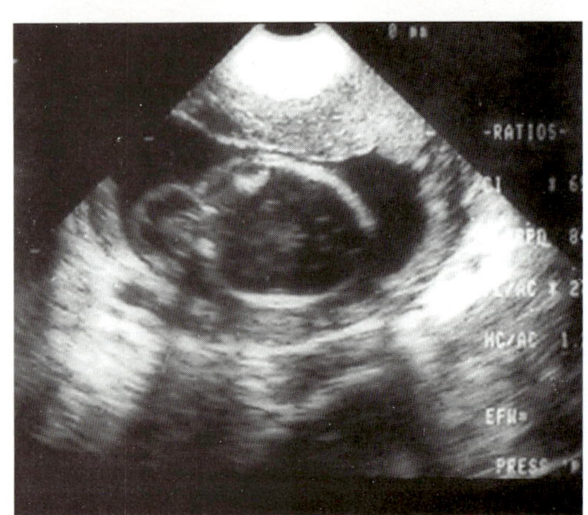

Figure 5.20: Encephalocele

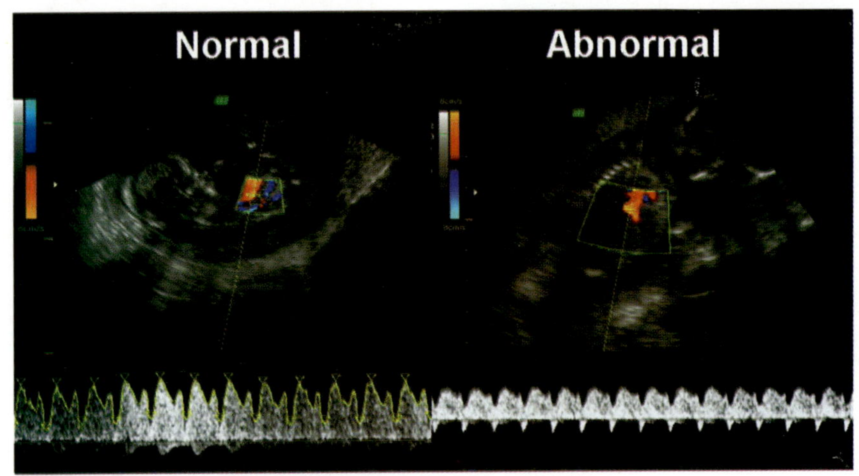

Colour plate 3: Ductus venosus flow

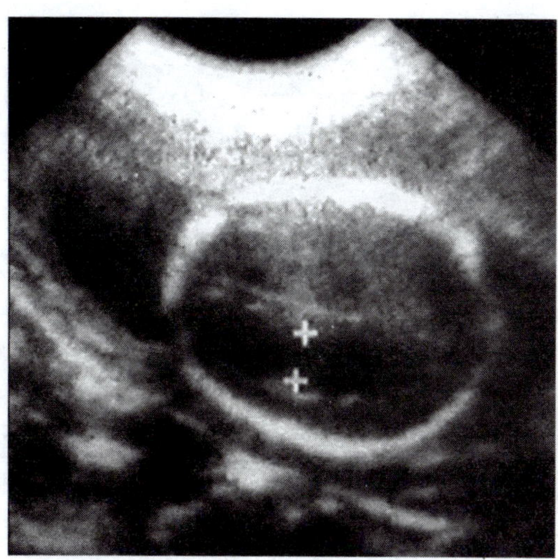

FIGURE 5.21: VENTRICULOMEGALY

Detection of fetal anomalies: It is estimated that about 3–5% of all newborns have congenital anomalies. Birth defects are an important cause of infant deaths. The common causes of birth defects are genetic chromosomal defects (20–25%), fetal infections (3–5%), maternal diseases (about 4%), drugs (< 1%) and defects of unknown origin (65–75%). It is therefore clear that the detection of congenital anomalies is an important part of perinatal management, especially the early detection of such defects.

It is important to establish its early diagnosis so as to enable early termination of the pregnancy, plan the best way of following the development of the fetus or time the delivery and plan for postnatal surgical intervention.

Pregnancy outcome is critically influenced by the timing of exposure of the embryo to teratogens. Very early exposure in the conceptus period (3–5 weeks) typically has an all-or-none result—it may affect several systems or none at all. Exposure during organogenesis or the embryonic period (5–10 weeks) often affects organ development and results in severe congenital anomalies. Exposure during the fetal period has a variable result.

Some of the congenital anomalies that can be easily and reliably detected in the first trimester are:

- *Encephalocele*: This is often associated with microcephaly and can be easily diagnosed because of the presence of brain tissue inside the sac. Encephaloceles carry a neonatal mortality rate of 40% and an incidence of intellectual impairment and neurologic sequelae of 80% (Lorber 1971) (Fig. 5.20).
- *Holoprosencephaly*: It can be detected as early as 11 weeks (Bronshtein and Wiener 1991). There are three major types—alobar, lobar and semilobar. On sonography it is diagnosed by demonstration of single rudimentary cerebral ventricle, presence of dorsal sac and typical facial anomalies (Filly et al 1984). These fetuses have an extremely poor neurological development.
- *Anencephaly*: Sonographic diagnosis depends on the demonstration of absence of cranial vault; hence, it cannot be reliably diagnosed before 10–11 weeks as the calvarium may not have completely calcified then (Fig. 5.22). A prospective study carried out in 1997 concluded that anencephaly can be reliably predicted even at 10–14 weeks of gestation (Johnson et al 1997).
- *Ectopia cordis*: Cardiac herniation through the sternal defect can be detected in the first trimester. It may be associated with omphalocele which is the hallmark of pentalogy of Cantrell (Seahore 1978). Omphalocele, however, cannot be diagnosed before 12 weeks.
- *Conjoined twins*: This is a rare anomaly with a straightforward diagnosis (demonstrated fusion of fetal parts). In first trimester

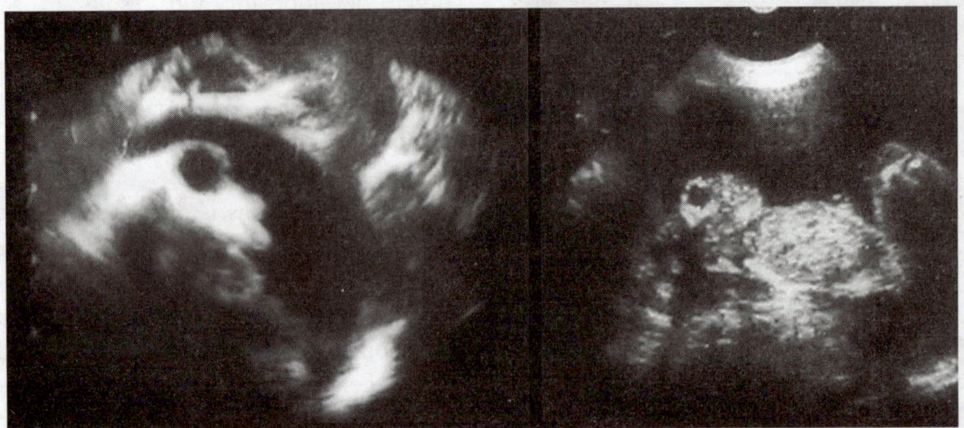

Figure 5.22: Anencephaly

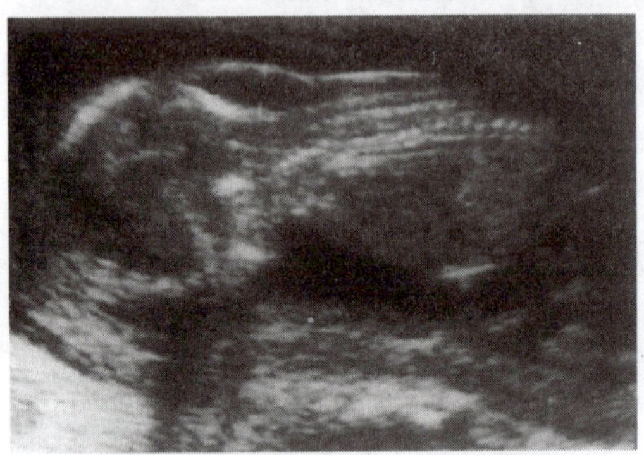

Figure 5.23: Nuchal translucency

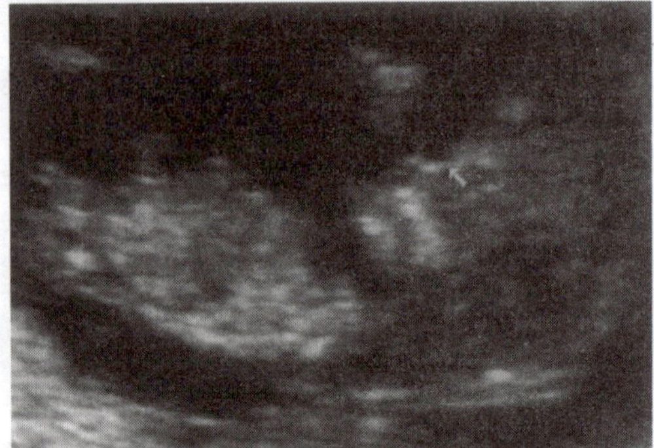

Figure 5.24: Absence of nasal bone

sonography, it appears as a bifid-looking embryo (Maggio et al 1985).

- *Acardiac twins*: The sonographic diagnosis of acardiac twins can be confirmed as early as at 11 weeks. Diffuse edema, cystic hygroma and absent cardiac pulsations are usually noted in the acardiac twin (van Allen et al 1983).
- *Hydrocephalus*: The presence of CSF up to 7 mm is normal, 7–10 mm is borderline and > 10 mm is indicative of ventriculomegaly (Fig. 5.21).

Detection of nuchal translucency: Abnormally thick nuchal translucency often signifies an increased risk of aneuploidy or abnormal karyotype (Taipale et al 1997) (Fig. 5.23). Even in fetuses with normal karyotype, as many as 27% demonstrate congenital malformations (van Vugt et al 1998). Hence, evaluation of posterior nuchal translucency is an essential part of first trimester sonogram. An anteroposterior measurement of more than 3 mm, measured from the membrane to skin surface, is considered abnormal.

- *Nasal bone*: Absence of nasal bone in scans done during 11–14 weeks suggests chromosomal abnormality, especially trisomy 21 (Fig. 5.24).
- *Ductus venosus flow*: In the scan at 11–14 weeks, if the ductus venosus shows reversal

of flow below the baseline, a chromosomal anomaly or major cardiac defect should be suspected (Colour plate 3).

Conclusion: Ultrasonography provides a simple, safe and effective method of diagnosing early pregnancy. With the availability of high-frequency and three-dimensional ultrasound technology, the human embryo can be better visualised, providing us further insights into human embryology and helping early detection of congenital anomalies.

References

Benoit B, T Hafner, A Kurjak, S Kupesic, I Banovic and T Bozele. 2002. Three-dimensional sonoembryology. *J Perinat Med* 30(1):63–73.

Bourne G. 1960. The microscopic anatomy of the human amnion and chorion. *Am J Obstet Gynecol* 79:1070–1073.

Bradley WG, CE Fiske and RA Filly. 1982. The double sac sign of early intrauterine pregnancy: Use in exclusion of ectopic pregnancy. *Radiology* 143:223–226.

Bronshtein M and Z Wiener. 1991. Early transvaginal sonographic diagnosis of alobar holoprosencephaly. *Prenat Diagn* 11:459.

Coppens M, P Loquet, M Kollen et al. 1996. Longitudinal evaluation of uteroplacental and umbilical blood flow changes in normal early pregnancy. *Ultrasound Obstet Gynecol* 7:114–121.

Coulam CHB, S Britten and DM Soenken. 1996. Early ultrasonographic measurements in normal pregnancies. *Hum Reprod* 11:1771–1774.

Daya S. 1993. Accuracy of gestational age estimation by means of the fetal crown rump length measurement. *Am J Obstet Gynecol* 168:903–908.

Filly RA, DH Chinn and PW Callen. 1984. Alobar holoprosencephaly: Ultrasonographic prenatal diagnosis. *Radiology* 151: 455.

Goldstein SR and R Wolfson. 1994. Transvaginal ultrasonographic measurement of early embryonic size as a means of assessing gestational age. *J Ultrasound Med* 13:27–31.

Horrow MM. 1992. Enlarged amniotic cavity: A new sonographic sign of early embryonic death. *Am J Roentgenol* 158:359–362.

Jauniaux E. 1996. Intervillous circulation in first trimester: The phantom of color Doppler Obstetric opera. *Ultrasound Obstet Gynecol* 8:73–76.

Johnson SP, NJU Sebine, RJ Snijders et al. 1997. Ultrasound screening for anencephaly at 10–14 weeks gestation. *Ultrasound Obstet Gynecol* 9:14.

Kurjak A, S Kupesic, I Banovic, T Hafner and M Kos. 1999. The study of morphology and circulation of early embryo by three dimensional ultasound and power Doppler. *J Perinat Med* 27(3):145–157.

Lasser PM, DB Peisner, J Vollebergh and I Timor-Tritsch. 1993. First trimester fetal biometry using transvaginal sonography. *Ultrasound Obstet Gynecol* 3:104–108.

Levi S, EA Lyons and DJ Lindsay. 1988. Early diagnosis of non-viable pregnancy with transvaginal US. *Radiology* 167:383–385.

Lorber J. 1971. The prognosis of occipital encephalocele. *Dev Med Child Neurol* 13:279.

Maggio M, NA Callan, KA Hamod et al. 1985. The first trimester ultrasonographic diagnosis of conjoined twins. *Am J Obstet Gynecol* 152:833.

Merz E, F Bahlmann and G Weber. 1995. Volume scanning in the evaluation of fetal malformations:

A new dimension in prenatal diagnosis. *Ultrasound Obstet Gynecol* 5:222.

Montenegro N, C Ramos, A Matias and H Barros. 1998. Variation of embryonic/fetal heart rate at 6–13 weeks gestation. *Ultrasound Obstet Gynecol* 11:274–276.

Moore KL and TVN Persaud. 1998. Organogenic period: The fourth to eighth weeks. In *The developing human: Clinically oriented embryology*, 6th ed, eds KL Moore and TVN Persaud, 85–100. Philadelphia: WB Saunders.

Nyberg DA, LA Mack, FC Laing and RM Patten. 1987. Distinguishing normal from abnormal gestational sac growth in early pregnancy. *J Ultrasound Med* 6:23–27.

Schats R, CAM Jansen and JW Wladiminoff. 1990. Embryonic heart activity: Appearance and development in early human pregnancy. *Br J Obstet Gynaecol* 97:989–994.

Seahore JH. 1978. Congenital abdominal wall defects. *Clin Perinatol* 5:61.

Stampone C, M Nicotra, C Muttinelli and EV Cosmi. 1996. Transvaginal sonography of the yolk sac in normal and abnormal pregnancy. *J Clin Ultrasound* 24:3–9.

Sterner H, A Stardach, O Spitzer et al. 1994. Three-dimensional ultrasound in obstetrics and gynecology: Technique, possibilities and limitations. *Hum Reprod* 9:1773.

Taipale P, V Niilesmaa, R Salonen and P Ylostalo. 1997. Increased nuchal translucency as a marker for fetal chromosomal defects. *N Engl J Med* 337:1654–1658.

Timor-Tritsch IE, D Farine and MG Rosen. 1988. A close look at early embryonic development with the high frequency transvaginal transducer. *Am J Obstet Gynecol* 159:676–681.

van Allen MI, DW Smith and TH Shepard. 1983. Twin reversed arterial perfusion (TRAP) sequence: A study of 14 twin pregnancies with acardius. *Semin Perinatol* 7(4):285.

van Vugt JMG, BWS Tinnemamma and RM van Zalen-Sprock. 1998. Outcome and early childhood follow up of chromosomally normal fetuses with increases nuchal translucency at 10–14 weeks gestation. *Ultrasound Obstet Gynecol* 11:407–409.

van Zalen-Sprock RM, JM Vugt and HP van Geijen. 1997. First trimester sonography of physiological midgut herniation and early diagnosis of omphalocele. *Prenat Diagn* 17: 511–518.

Yeh HC and JG Rabinowitz. 1988. Amniotic sac development: Ultrasound features of early pregnancy—the double bleb sign. *Radiology* 166:97–103.

6

Antenatal Fetal Surveillance

Gowri Ramanathan | Sabaratnam Arulkumaran

Introduction

Fetal surveillance is the assessment and monitoring of fetal behaviour and well-being. Antenatal fetal surveillance is traditionally offered to fetuses at risk of adverse perinatal outcome, with the aim of detecting early signs of uteroplacental insufficiency and hypoxia, so that timely intervention may prevent possible intrauterine death.

Certain factors have been shown to increase the risk of perinatal morbidity and/or mortality, for which there is evidence that antenatal fetal surveillance is beneficial. Although, with improved technology and skill, it is now possible to better monitor high-risk pregnancies, a large study has demonstrated that the perinatal mortality rate is now higher in the apparent 'low-risk' pregnancy than in the 'high-risk' pregnancy (Sim et al 1993). Further, the findings of the fourth annual report of the Confidential Enquiry into Stillbirths and Deaths in Infancy (CESDI 1997) have identified unexplained antepartum stillbirths as the largest area for improvements in perinatal mortality. Hence, the role of antenatal fetal surveillance is important, not only in high-risk pregnancies, but in all pregnancies in general.

Indications for Antenatal Fetal Surveillance

Fetal surveillance antenatally is usually initiated either in the event of a non-reassuring fetal sign (for example, reduced fetal movement or small for date fetus), or when indicated by either maternal or fetal risk factors. There are many medical and obstetric conditions than can endanger fetal well-being. Conditions associated with increased perinatal morbidity and/or mortality for which antenatal fetal testing may have an impact and includes small for gestational age (SGA) fetus (Soothill et al 1993), decreased fetal movement (Sadovsky et al 1977), post-date pregnancies (over 294 days) (McClure-Brown 1963; Phelan et al 1984), pre-eclampsia/chronic hypertension (Torres et al 1995), pre-pregnancy diabetes (von Kries et al 1997), insulin requiring gestational diabetes (Girz et al 1992), preterm prelabour rupture of membranes (PPROM) (Vintzileos 1996) and chronic (stable) abruption (Sholl 1987). Table 6.1 provides a non-exhaustive list of conditions that warrant close antenatal fetal surveillance; the timing of initiation of the testing is dictated by individual circumstances.

METHODS OF ANTENATAL FETAL ASSESSMENT

The ideal antenatal test would be one that is inexpensive, easy to perform and carries little, if any, risk to the mother and the fetus. The results of the test should be highly sensitive, specific, valid, reliable and reproducible. Unfortunately, there is no one test that meets all these requirements, hence the need to integrate some or all of the available tests for a more accurate depiction of fetal physiology. We discuss current methods of antenatal fetal surveillance used, namely ultrasound assessment of fetal weight, fetal activity or movement monitoring, the non-stress test (NST), contraction stress test (CST), ultrasound assessment of amniotic fluid volume, biophysical profile and Doppler evaluation of the fetoplacental or uteroplacental circulation.

Ultrasound Assessment of Fetal Weight (Fetal Growth Surveillance)

An SGA fetus, or a fetus that has failed to achieve a specific weight threshold which is generally defined as the tenth percentile (Chang et al 1992) is at greater risk of adverse perinatal outcome including stillbirth, birth hypoxia, neonatal complications (Cnattingius et al 1998; McIntire et al 1999) and impaired neurodevelopment (Roth et al 1999). Fetuses with growth compromise, when subjected to labour, are at increased risk of acidosis due to either uteroplacental insufficiency, lower metabolic reserves due to intrauterine malnutrition or pre-existing hypoxia, or umbilical cord compressions due to a reduction in amniotic fluid volume. This is however a heterogeneous group—approximately 50–70% of fetuses with birth weight below the tenth percentile for gestational age are constitutionally small (Ott 1988; Wilcox 1983). Once SGA is diagnosed, it is important to distinguish between the small, but normally grown, fetus and the growth restricted fetus at risk of adverse outcome.

Clinical risk assessment, for example, maternal risk factors such as hypertension or smoking, reduced fetal movements, a previous SGA baby, should be considered, along with the possibility of a constitutionally small fetus because the parents are short. Maternal

Table 6.1: Maternal and pregnancy-related conditions associated with increased prenatal morbidity/mortality where antenatal fetal surveillance may have an impact (Steer et al 1999)

Maternal Conditions	*Pregnancy-related Conditions*
Antiphospholipid syndrome	Pregnancy-induced hypertension/Pre-eclampsia
Hypertensive disorders	Insulin requiring gestational diabetes
Hyperthyroidism (poorly controlled)	Decreased fetal movements
Hemoglobinopathies (hemoglobin SS,SC, or S-thalassemia)	Multiple gestation (with significant growth discrepancy)
Cyanotic heart disease	Intrauterine growth restriction (IUGR)/small for gestational age (SGA) fetus
Systemic lupus erythematosus	Post-term pregnancies (> 41/42 weeks)
Chronic renal disease	Isoimmunisation (moderate to severe)
Type 1 diabetes mellitus	Previous fetal demise (unexplained/recurrent)
	Preterm prelabour rupture of membranes (PPROM) with oligohydramnios
	Polyhydramnios
	Chronic abruption

perception of an active fetus, fetal Doppler and biophysical profile offer important clues to distinguish a pathologically SGA fetus from one resulting from physiological factors (Baschat and Weiner 2000).

Clinical assessment by the symphysis-fundal height (SFH) measurement alone is a poor method of detecting SGA fetuses. Physical examination of the abdomen by inspection and palpation detects as few as 30% of SGA fetuses (Rosenberg et al 1982). Low sensitivity, high false-positive rates and significant intra- and interobserver variation make this test unsuitable for antenatal surveillance when used in isolation (Bailey et al 1989).

Ultrasonographic measurement of abdominal circumference (AC) and estimated fetal weight (EFW) are the most accurate diagnostic measurements to predict SGA (Chang et al 1992). Customised birth weight and ultrasound EFW charts that adjust for variables such as maternal weight, maternal height, ethnic group and parity have claimed better sensitivities for identifying SGA fetuses (Gardosi et al 1992). Similarly, the use of serial measurements of EFW looking at growth velocity of fetuses are superior to single estimates in predicting poor perinatal outcome (De Jong et al 1999); however, the use of fetal growth alone to diagnose growth restriction, especially when the time interval between the scan is less than two weeks, can lead to high numbers of false-positive results (Mongelli et al 1998). In recent years, the use of three-dimensional measurements has been shown to improve the accuracy of fetal size calculations (Schild et al 2000). Similarly, measurements of fetal subcutaneous tissue and fat volumetric measurements are proving beneficial in the late third trimester (Schwartz et al 2003).

Fetal Activity or Movement Monitoring

Fetal movement count is the oldest and by far the simplest of all fetal assessment techniques. All fetuses between 30 and 39 weeks of gestation and 98% of fetuses at 24–27 weeks gestation move by the 75th minute of observation, so maternal perception of movement should occur within 1.5 hours (Patrick et al 1982). A decrease in maternal perception of fetal movement often, but not invariably, precedes fetal death, in some cases by several days (Pearson et al 1976). This observation provides the rationale for fetal movement assessment by the mother ('kick counts') as a means of antepartum fetal surveillance.

Many methods of counting fetal movements have been proposed, with most data suggesting an improvement in perinatal outcomes with the early identification of decreased fetal activity (Moore et al 1989; Sadofsky et al 1973; Pearson et al 1976; Neldam 1980). Neither the optimal number of movements nor the ideal duration for counting movements has been defined, and no one technique is deemed superior. Compliance among low-risk pregnant women is highest when the monitoring method is minimally time-consuming and relatively simple (Davis 1987). The number of fetal movements perceived is arbitrary, though some studies suggest that a perceived lack of fetal movement for two hours or more requires further evaluation (Connors et al 1988; Moore et al 1989; Wilailak et al 1992). Routine fetal movement counting compared with this practice in selected groups has not been shown to be beneficial (Grant et al 1989). However, once a decrease in fetal movement is perceived, further and prompt investigation is warranted, either by external fetal heart rate monitoring or by ultrasonography.

Cardiotocography (CTG): The Non-stress Test (NST)

The non-stress test has been an important tool in fetal surveillance for many years and is used in nearly all pregnancies when complications arise. The basis of the non-stress test is that the heart rate of a fetus that is not acidotic or neurologically depressed will accelerate intermittently with fetal movement, and a normal fetal autonomic system exhibits reactivity in the fetal heart rate. The absence of accelerations and loss of reactivity, if not due to a fetal sleep cycle, is hence indicative of some degree of central nervous system depression, which includes fetal acidosis.

A normal test is defined as a reactive trace which requires a minimum of two accelerations (rise in fetal heart rate of at least 15 beats per minute above the baseline and lasting 15 seconds) during a 20-minute trace (Bishop 1981). It may be necessary to continue the tracing for 40 minutes or longer to take into account the variations of the fetal sleep–wake cycle. Acoustic stimulation may be performed to reduce overall testing time.

Despite its widespread use, the predictive value of a non-reactive trace is poor. While a reactive trace lowers the risk of intervention of fetal distress tenfold (Paul et al 1995), only 20–30% of fetuses with non-reactive trace undergo operative intervention for fetal distress, yielding a specificity of less than 50% for the non-reactive NST and a high false-positive rate (Bochner et al 1987). Moreover, interpretation of the CTG in the preterm period is more difficult, due to the physiological changes in the parasympathetic nervous system which gradually drops the baseline heart rate with increasing fetal maturity. The CTG of a non-compromised preterm fetus in the antenatal period is frequently non-reactive—from 24 to 28 weeks of gestation, up to 50% of NSTs may not be reactive (Lavin et al 1984), and from 28 to 32 weeks of gestation, 15% of NSTs are not reactive (Druzin et al 1985; Meis et al 1986).

Variable decelerations may be observed in up to 50% of NSTs (Dawes et al 1991). If non-repetitive and brief (<30 seconds), they indicate neither fetal compromise nor the need for obstetric intervention (Manning 1995). Repetitive variable decelerations (at least three in 20 minutes), even if mild, have been associated with an increased risk of cesarean delivery for a non-reassuring intrapartum fetal heart rate pattern (Dayal et al 1999; Bocking 2003). Fetal heart rate decelerations during an NST that persist for one minute or longer are associated with a markedly increased risk of both cesarean delivery for a non-reassuring fetal heart rate pattern and fetal demise (Brans et al 1989; Chauhan et al 1999; De Wit et al 2003).

The use of computerised CTG in the antenatal period has been shown to increase the ability to diagnose fetal hypoxia by reduced short-term variability (Dawes et al 1991; 1992); however, no studies have compared computerised CTG with standard CTG in relation to fetal outcome.

Contraction Stress Test (CST)

Fetal heart rate response to the transient depletion of fetal oxygenation can be tested by inducing contractions, either by nipple stimulation or by intravenous administration of dilute oxytocin. An already compromised fetus will show evidence of hypoxia with minimal contractions. The presence or absence of late fetal heart rate decelerations (that is, decelerations that reach their nadir after the peak of the contraction, and usually persist beyond the end of the contraction) is used to categorise the test as either negative (no late or significant variable decelerations), positive (late decelerations following 50% or more of contractions even if the contraction frequency is fewer than 3 in 10 minutes), equivocal/suspicious (intermittent late decelerations or significant variable decelerations), equivocal/hyperstimulatory (fetal heart rate decelerations that occur in the presence of contractions, more frequent than every two minutes or lasting longer than 90 seconds) or unsatisfactory (fewer than three contractions in 10 minutes or an uninterpretable tracing). Conditions associated with an increased risk of preterm labour and delivery, uterine rupture or uterine bleeding are contraindications to the CST, and these include preterm labour/patients at high risk of preterm labour, preterm prelabour rupture of membranes, history of extensive uterine surgery or classical cesarean delivery, and known placenta previa.

Ultrasound Assessment of Amniotic Fluid Volume

Amniotic fluid volume may be assessed qualitatively by clinical palpation; however, this is an inaccurate method. Ultrasonography permits subjective visual assessment or semi-quantitative assessment by enabling calculation of the amniotic fluid index (AFI) or deepest vertical pool; or quantitatively by invasive methods. It has been shown that abnormal amniotic fluid volume is associated with fetuses at risk of adverse outcomes. Oligohydramnios, defined as AFI of less than 5.0 cm (Phelan et al 1987), is linked with pulmonary hypoplasia, postural deformities, fetal distress and perinatal morbidity and mortality (Golan et al 1994). In the late second or third trimester, amniotic fluid volume reflects fetal urine production. Placental dysfunction may result in diminished fetal renal perfusion, leading to oligohydramnios. Amniotic fluid volume assessment can therefore be used to evaluate long-term uteroplacental function. The AFI is the summation of the deepest cord-free vertical pool in each of the four quadrants. The AFI has been shown to be a more accurate and reproducible method of determining abnormalities in amniotic fluid volume (ACOG 1993).

A meta-analysis of 18 studies with over 10,000 patients showed that an antepartum AFI of <5 cm was associated with increased risk of cesarean delivery for fetal distress (RR = 2.2; 95% CI 1.5–3.4) and a low Apgar score of less than 7 at five minutes (RR = 5.2; 95% CI 2.4–11.3) (Chauhan et al 1999). Other studies have shown that isolated oligohydramnios (AFI <5 cm) is associated with a fourfold risk of low birth weight and higher risk of admission to the Neonatal Intensive Care Unit (NICU), suggesting that pregnancies with isolated oligohydramnios require some form of fetal monitoring (Roberts et al 1998). Even a borderline AFI of more than 5 cm and less than 10 cm has been shown to be associated with increased risk of intrauterine growth restriction and overall adverse perinatal outcome (Banks et al 1999).

The modified biophysical profile (BPP) combines the NST (with the option of acoustic stimulation), as a short-term indicator of fetal acid–base status, with the AFI, as an indicator of long-term placental function. The modified BPP is considered normal if NST is reactive and AFI is more than 5, and abnormal if NST is non-reactive or AFI is 5 or less.

Biophysical Profile (BPP)

While the fetal heart rate assesses the short-term status of the fetus, the BPP is an indicator of long-term placental function and reserve. Manning described the BPP as NST together with four observations made by ultrasonography:

- Fetal breathing movements—one or more episodes of rhythmic fetal breathing movements of 30 seconds or more within 30 minutes
- Fetal movement—three or more discrete body or limb movements within 30 minutes
- Fetal tone—one or more episodes of extension of a fetal extremity with return to flexion, or opening or closing of a hand
- Determination of the amniotic fluid volume—a single vertical pocket of amniotic fluid exceeding 2 cm is considered evidence of adequate amniotic fluid (Manning 1995)

With scores of 2 (normal or present) or 0 (abnormal, absent or insufficient) for each of the five components, a composite score of 6 is considered equivocal, and a score of 4 or less is abnormal. The presence of oligohydramnios (largest vertical pocket of amniotic fluid volume less than 2 cm) warrants further evaluation, regardless of the composite score.

The value of this time-consuming test has not been evaluated in randomised controlled trials. However, in high-risk pregnancies, it has been shown to have a good negative predictive value for fetal death (Dayal et al 1999).

Doppler Evaluation of Fetoplacental and Uteroplacental Circulation

Umbilical artery Doppler flow velocimetry has been adapted for use as a technique of fetal surveillance, based on the observation that umbilical artery Doppler measures the resistance of the uteroplacental circulation, providing direct information on fetoplacental circulation, and identifies placental circulatory failure (Reuwer et al 1984). Histological examination has shown a strong correlation between the percentage of obliterated vessels and the resistance in umbilical artery blood flow as measured by the resistance index (Fok et al 1990).The Doppler ultrasound method for recording blood flow velocity waveforms in the fetal umbilical arteries is now a widely used indicator of fetal well-being.

There is compelling evidence that the use of umbilical artery Doppler to monitor high-risk fetuses reduces perinatal morbidity and mortality (Alfirevic et al 1995), and sigificantly reduces the number of antenatal admissions and inductions of labour. Westergaard (2001) showed that umbilical artery Doppler applied in high-risk pregnancies significantly lowered perinatal mortality by 34%, and the need for induction of delivery and emergency cesarean section rate by 22%.

Generally, placental resistance causes a reduction in fetal growth velocity first, followed by changes in fetal circulation (Bonnin et al 1993); fetal Doppler parameters provide the clearest evidence of deterioration in the fetal condition (Harrington et al 1999). A study comparing fetal heart-rate monitoring, biophysical profile and umbilical artery Doppler found that only umbilical artery Doppler had value in predicting poor perinatal outcomes in SGA fetuses (Soothill et al 1993; Baschat et al 2000). Absent or reversed end-diastolic flow in the umbilical artery is associated with increased perinatal mortality and morbidity (Karsdorp et al 1994), an 80% risk of hypoxia and a 46% risk of acidosis (Nicolaides et al 1988).

The fetal response to mild arterial hypoxemia includes redistribution of cardiac output to improve blood flow to the brain at the expense of the body (Richardson et al 1998). This process is identified by the demonstration of low-impedence Doppler waveforms from the middle cerebral artery (Vyas et al 1990). In growth-restricted fetuses, Doppler changes develop in a sequential manner. Early changes occur in the peripheral vessels (umbilical and middle cerebral arteries) and late changes include umbilical artery reverse flow, abnormal changes in the ductus venosus and aortic and pulmonary outflow tracts. It has been suggested that these late changes in vascular adaptation by the severely growth-restricted fetus are the best predictor of perinatal death (Ferrazzi et al 2002). The prognosis with time interval between early (15–16 days before delivery) and late changes (4–5 days before delivery) was significantly different. The shorter interval for the changes was associated with significantly greater perinatal death.

The investigation of uteroplacental circulation has added knowledge of how to identify at-risk patients for the future development of pre-eclampsia and fetal growth restriction during pregnancy by the identification of increased flow resistance and a 'notch' of the uterine artery waveform in the second trimester (Papageorghiou et al 2001; 2002). Abnormal uterine artery flow is considered to be a sign of placental maldevelopment in early pregnancy.

INTEGRATED FETAL SURVEILLANCE

The only effective therapy for fetuses at risk of adverse perinatal outcome secondary to uteroplacental insufficiency is delivery. With the risk of prematurity and its complications, particularly before 34 weeks gestation, precise antenatal fetal assessment is required to determine the timing of delivery, that is, when intrauterine risks exceed neonatal risks of adverse outcome.

It has been shown that in general, sequential changes occur in the tests of fetal well-being with progressive uteroplacental insufficiency. Once the diagnosis of fetal growth restriction has been made by fetal biometry, umbilical artery blood flow changes precede other cardiovascular responses. Evidence of brain-sparing subsequently develops with deterioration of placental function, followed by development of abnormal venous Doppler indices and abnormalities in biophysical parameters (Baschat 2003). The information gained through this concurrent evaluation offers the best prediction of fetal status and outcome.

Conclusion With increasing understanding of the mechanisms and manifestations of placental insufficiency as well as fetal adaptive responses, it has been recognised that no single antenatal fetal surveillance tool currently available can provide a complete assessment of fetal well-being. Usually, two or more of these methods may need to be integrated in the management of these at-risk pregnancies, with the surveillance plan aiming to maximise gestational age while minimising the risk of neonatal morbidity and mortality.

REFERENCES

Alfirevic Z and JP Neilson. 1995. Doppler ultrasonography in high-risk pregnancies: systematic review with meta-analysis. *Am J Obstet Gynecol* 172:1379–1387.

American College of Obstetricians and Gynecologists. 1993. Ultrasonography in pregnancy. *ACOG Technical Bulletin 187*. Washington, DC.

Bailey SM, P Sarmandal and JM Grant. 1989. A comparison of three methods of assessing inter-observer variation applied to measurement of the symphysis-fundal height. *Br J Obstet Gynaecol* 96:1266–1271.

Banks EH and DA Miller. 1999. Perinatal risks associated with borderline amniotic fluid index. *Am J Obstet Gynecol* 180:1461–1463.

Baschat AA and CP Weiner. 2000. Umbilical artery Doppler screening for detection of the small fetus in need of antepartum surveillance. *Am J Obstet Gynecol* 182:154–158.

Baschat AA. 2003. Integrated fetal testing in growth restriction: combining multivessel Doppler and biophysical parameters. *Ultrasound Obstet Gynecol* 21:1-8.

Bishop EH. 1981. Fetal acceleration test. *Am J Obstet Gynecol* 141:905–909.

Bochner CJ, AL Medearis, J Davis et al. 1987. Antepartum predictors of fetal distress in post-term pregnancy. *Am J Obstet Gynecol* 157:353–358.

Bocking AD. 2003. Assessment of fetal heart rate and fetal movements in detecting oxygen deprivation in-utero. *Eur J Obstet Gynecol Reprod Biol* 110:108–112.

Bonnin P, O Bailliart, W Kedra et al. 1993. Relationship between birth weight and umbilical Doppler blood flow velocity waveforms during the third trimester of pregnancy. *Eur J Med* 2:219–222.

Brans YW, DS Andrew, EB Dutton et al. 1989. Dilution kinetics of chemicals used for estimaton of water content of body compartments in perinatal medicine. *Pediatr Res* 25:377–382.

Chang TC, SC Robson, RJ Boys et al. 1992. Prediction of the small for gestational age infant: which ultrasonic measurement is best? *Obstet Gynecol* 80:1030–1038.

Chauhan SP, M Sanderson, NW Hendrix et al. 1999. Perinatal outcome and amniotic fluid index in antepartum and intrapertum periods: A meta-analysis. *Am J Obstet Gynecol* 181:1473–1478.

Cnattingius S, B Haglund and MS Kramer. 1998. Differences in late fetal death rates in association with determinants of small for gestational age fetuses: Population based cohort study. *BMJ* 316: 1483–1487.

Confidential Enquiry into Stillbirths and Deaths in Infancy. Fourth Annual Report. 1997. *Concentrating on Intrapartum Related Deaths 1994–5*. London: Maternal and Child Health Consortium.

Connors G, R Natale and C Nasello-Paterson. 1988. Maternally perceived fetal activity from twenty-four weeks' gestation to term in normal and at risk pregnancies. *Am J Obstet Gynecol* 158:294–299.

Davis L. 1987. Daily fetal movement counting. A valuable assessment tool. *J Nurse Midwifery* 32:11–19.

Dawes GS, M Moulden and CWG Redman. 1991. System 8000. Computerized antenatal FHR analysis. *J Perinat Med* 19:47–51.

Dawes GS, M Moulden and CWG Redman. 1992. Short-term fetal heart rate variation, decelerations, and umbilical flow velocity waveforms before labor. *Obstet Gynecol* 80:673–678.

Dayal AK, FA Manning, DJ Berck et al. 1999. Fetal death after normal biophysical profile score: An eighteen-year experience. *Am J Obstet Gynecol* 181:1231–1236.

De Jong CL, A Francis, HP Van Geijn et al. 1999. Fetal growth rate and adverse perinatal events. *Ultrasound Obstet Gynecol* 13:86–89.

De Wit AC and JG Nijhuis. 2003. Validity of the Hewlett-Packard actograph in detecting fetal movements. *Ultrasound Obstet Gynecol* 22:152–156.

Druzin ML, A Fox, E Kogut and C Carlson. 1985. The relationship of the nonstress test to gestational age. *Am J Obstet Gynecol* 153:386–389.

Ferrazzi E, M Bozzo, S Rigano et al. 2002. Temporal sequence of abnormal Doppler changes in the peripheral and central circulatory systems of the severely growth-restricted fetus. *Ultrasound Obstet Gynecol* 19:140–146.

Fok RY, Z Pavlova, K Benirschke et al. 1990. The correlation of arterial lesions with umbilical artery Doppler velocimetry in the placentas of small-for-dates pregnancies. *Obstet Gynecol* 75:578–583.

Gardosi J, A Chang, B Kalyan et al. 1992. Customised antenatal growth charts. *Lancet* 339:283–287.

Girz BA, MY Divon and IR Merkatz. 1992. Sudden fetal death in women with well-controlled, intensively monitored gestational diabetes. *J Perinat* 12:229–233.

Golan A, G Lin, S Evron et al. 1994. Oligohydramnios: maternal complications and fetal outcome in 145 cases. *Gynecol Obstet Invest* 37:91–95.

Grant A, D Elbourne, L Valentin and S Alexander. 1989. Routine formal fetal movement counting and risk of antepartum late death in normally formed singletons. *Lancet* 2 (8659): 345–349.

Harrington K, MO Thompson, RG Carpenter et al. 1999. Doppler fetal circulation in pregnancies complicated by pre-eclampsia or delivery of a small for gestational age baby: 2. Longitudinal analysis. *Br J Obstet Gynaecol* 106:453–466.

Karsdorp VH, JM van Vugt, HP Van Geijn et al. 1994. Clinical significance of absent or reversed end diastolic velocity waveforms in umbilical artery. *Lancet* 344:1664–1668.

Lavin JP Jr, M Miodovnik and TP Barden. 1984. Relationship of nonstress test reactivity and gestational age. *Obstet Gynecol* 63:338–344

Manning FA. 1995. Dynamic ultrasound-based fetal assessment: the fetal biophysical score. *Clin Obstet Gynecol* 38:26–44.

McClure-Browne JC.1963. Post-maturity. *Am J Obstet Gynecol* 85:573.

McIntire DD, SL Bloom, BM Casey et al. 1999. Birth weight in relation to morbidity and mortality among newborn infants. *N Engl J Med* 340:1234–1238.

Meis PJ, JR Ureda, M Swain, et al. 1986. Variable decelerations during nonstress tests are not a sign of fetal compromise. *Am J Obstet Gynecol* 154:586–590.

Mongelli M, S Ek and R Tambyraja. 1998. Screening for fetal growth restriction: a mathematical model of the effect of time interval and ultrasound error. *Obstet Gynecol* 92:908–912.

Moore TR and K Piacquadio. 1989. A prospective evaluation of fetal movement screening to reduce the incidence of antepartum fetal death. *Am J Obstet Gynecol* 160:1075–1080.

Neldam S. 1980. Fetal movememt as an indicator of fetal well-being. *Lancet* 1(8180):1222–1224.

Nicolaides KH, CM Bilardo, PW Soothill et al. 1988. Absence of end diastolic frequencies in umbilical artery. A sign of fetal hypoxia and acidosis. *Br Med J* 297:1026–1027.

Ott WJ. 1988. The diagnosis of altered fetal growth. *Obstet Gynecol Clin North Am* 15:237–263.

Papageorghiou AT, CKH Yu, R Bindra et al. 2001. Multicenter screening for preeclampsia and fetal growth restriction by transvaginal uterine artery Doppler at 23 weeks of gestation. *Ultrasound Obstet Gynecol* 18:441–449.

Papageorghiou AT, Yu CKH, Cicero S et al. 2002. Second-trimester uterine artery Doppler screening in unselected populations: A review. *J Maternal Fetal Neonatal Med* 12:78–88.

Patrick J, K Campbell, L Carmichael et al. 1982. Patterns of gross fetal body movements over 24 hour observation intervals during the last 10 weeks of pregnancy. *Am J Obstet Gynecol* 142:363–371.

Paul R and D Miller. 1995. Nonstress test. *Clin Obstet Gynecol* 38:3–10.

Pearson JF and JB Weaver. 1976. Fetal activity and fetal well-being: An evaluation. *BMJ* 1(6021): 1305–1307.

Phelan JP, CV Smith, P Broussard et al. 1987. Amniotic fluid assessment with the four-quadrant technique at 36-42 weeks gestation. *J Reprod Med* 32:540–542.

Phelan JP, LD Platt, S Yeh et al. 1984. Continuing role of the non-stress test in the management of postdates pregnancy. *Obstet Gynecol* 64:624–628.

Reuwer PJHM, HW Bruinse, P Stoutenbeek et al. 1984. Doppler assessment of the fetoplacental circulation in normal and growth retarded fetuses. *Eur J Obstet Gynecol Reprod Biol* 18:199–205.

Richardson BS and AD Bocking. 1998. Metabolic and circulatory adaptations to chronic hypoxia in the fetus. *Comp Biochem Physiol Mol Integr Physiol* 119:717–723.

Roberts D, EC Nwosu and SA Walkinshaw. 1998. The fetal outcome in pregnancies with isolated reduced amniotic fluid volume in the third trimester. *J Perinat Med* 26:390–395.

Rosenberg K, JM Grant and M Hepburn. 1982. Antenatal detection of growth retardation: actual practice in a large maternity hospital. *Br J Obstet Gynaecol* 89:12–15.

Roth S, TC Chang, S Robson et al. 1999. The neurodevelopmental outcome of term infants with different intrauterine growth characteristics. *Early Hum Dev* 55:39–50.

Sadovsky E and H Yaffe. 1973. Daily fetal movement recording and fetal prognosis. *Obstet Gynecol* 41:845–850.

Sadovsky E and WZ Polishuk. 1977. Fetal movement in utero: Nature, assessment, prognostic value, timing of delivery. *Obstet Gynecol* 50:49–55.

Schild RL, R Fimmers and M Hansmann. 2000. Fetal weight estimation by three-dimensional ultrasound. *Ultrasound Obstet Gynecol* 16:445–452.

Schwartz J and H Galan. 2003. Ultrasound in assessment of fetal growth disorders: is there a role for subcutaneous measurements? *Ultrasound Obstet Gynecol* 22:329–335.

Sholl JS. 1987. Abruptio placentae: Clinical management in nonacute cases. *Am J Obstet Gynecol* 156:40–51.

Sim D, RB Beattie and JC Dornan. 1993. Evaluation of biophysical fetal assessment in high risk pregnancy to assess ultrasound parameters suitable for screening in the low-risk population. *Ultrasound Obstet Gynecol* 3:11–17.

Soothill PW, RA Ajayi, S Campbell et al. 1993. Prediction of morbidity in small and normally grown fetuses by fetal heart rate variability, biophysical profile score and umbilical artery Doppler studies. *Br J Obstet Gynaecol* 100:742–745.

Steer PJ and P Danielian. 1999. Fetal distress in labour. In *High risk pregnancy: Management options,* 2nd ed, 1121–1149, ed DK James, PJ Steer, CP Wesner and B Gonik, Edinburgh: WB Saunders.

Torres PJ, E Gratacos and PL Alonso. 1995. Umbilical artery Doppler ultrasound predicts low birth weight and fetal death in hypertensive pregnancies. *Acta Obstet Gynecol Scandinavia* 74:352–355.

Vintzileos AM. 1996. Antepartum surveillance in preterm rupture of membranes. *J Perinat Med* 24:319–326.

von Kries R, R Kimmerle, JE Schmidt et al. 1997. Pregnancy outcomes in mothers with pregestational diabetes: A population-based study in North Rhine (Germany) from 1988 to 1993. *Eur J Ped* 156:963–967.

Vyas S, KH Nicolaides, S Bower et al. 1990. Middle cerebral artery flow velocity waveforms in fetal hypoxaemia. *Br J Obstet Gynaecol* 97:797–803.

Westergaard HB, J Langhoff-Roos, G Lingman et al. 2001. A critical appraisal of the use of umbilical artery Doppler ultrasound in high-risk pregnancies: Use of meta-analyses in evidence-based obstetrics. *Ultrasound Obstet Gynecol* 17:466–467.

Wilailak S, S Suthutvoravut, P Cherng-sa-ad et al. 1992. Assessment of fetal well-being: Fetal movement count versus non stress test. *Int J Gynecol Obstet* 39:23–27.

Wilcox AJ. 1983. Intrauterine growth retardation: Beyond birthweight criteria. *Early Hum Dev* 8: 189–193.

7

Anemia in Pregnancy

Asmita Muthal Rathore | Reva Tripathi

Anemia in pregnancy, though uncommon in the developed world, is the commonest medical disorder during pregnancy in developing countries. The prevalence of anemia complicating pregnancy in the developed world is reported to be about 18%, while in developing countries it varies from 35% to 75%. Nearly half of the total global numbers of anemic women live in the Indian subcontinent and the prevalence of anemia in pregnancy in India is 87.5% (WHO 1997). It is responsible for 40–60% of maternal deaths in non-industrialised countries (Bhatt 1997).

Hematological Changes in Normal Pregnancy

There are significant hematological changes during pregnancy. Plasma volume increases by about 50%. The increase starts early and is progressive throughout pregnancy, with a tendency to plateau in the last eight weeks. Similarly, there is an increase in red cell mass but the quantum of increase is debatable. The increase is influenced by iron intake even in women with normal hemoglobin, and is about 18% for women who do not receive iron supplement and about 30% for those who do (Letsky 2000).

The increase begins at the end of the first trimester and continues till the pregnancy reaches term. The increase in both plasma volume and red cell mass is related to fetal size and they are particularly big in women with a multiple pregnancy (Letsky 2002). Since the increase in plasma volume is more than that of red cells, there is a fall in hemoglobin, hematocrit and red cell count during pregnancy, but there is usually no change in red cell indices.

Changes at Labour and Puerperium

An increase in cardiac output is seen with each uterine contraction, magnifying the risk of cardiac failure—this is maximum in the second stage of labour. The blood loss during vaginal delivery is usually slightly more than 500 ml in singleton births and almost double in a twin delivery or a cesarean section. The abrupt decrease in blood volume during delivery is continued in puerperium due to postpartum diuresis. Similarly, the increments in red cell mass are lost acutely during delivery and then gradually as red cells reach the end of their lifespan. The hematocrit gradually increases and blood volume returns to non-pregnant levels around three weeks after delivery. Fluctuations in blood volume and hematocrit in the first few days following delivery depend on individual response to dehydration, pregnancy hypervolemia and the rapidity of blood loss. If increase in blood volume during pregnancy is appropriate, the loss of one litre of blood at delivery can be tolerated without causing a significant fall in hemoglobin concentration.

Definition of Anemia

Anemia is a condition of low circulating hemoglobin (Hb). The World Health Organization (1972) defines anemia in pregnancy as hemoglobin <11 g per cent and hematocrit of less than 33. It allows a fall of 0.5 g/dl and a cut-off value of 10.5 g/dl in the second trimester.

The Indian Council of Medical Research (Sharma 2003) classifies severity of anemia according to four grades:

Mild	10.0–10.9 g/dl
Moderate	7.0–9.9 g/dl
Severe	<7.0 g/dl
Very severe	<4.0 g/dl

Some experts consider Hb levels of 9–11 g/dl as mild anemia.

Etiological Classification of Anemia

Anemia can occur due to a variety of causes:

1. Nutritional
   Iron deficiency
   Folate deficiency
   Vitamin B_{12} deficiency
   Mixed deficiencies
2. Hemoglobinopathies
   Thalassemia
   Sickle cell anemia
3. Miscellaneous anemic disorders
   Aplastic anemia
   Autoimmune hemolytic anemia
   Anemia associated with chronic infections/disease

NUTRITIONAL ANEMIA

Nutritional deficiency is the most common cause of anemia in developing countries. As the name suggests, many factors are likely to be lacking in the diet, but frequently one of them predominates.

Iron Deficiency Anemia

About 80% of anemias in pregnancy are caused by iron deficiency. The pathophysiology is closely linked to iron metabolism. Iron is present in the body in three forms—heme iron (hemoglobin, myoglobin and iron-containing enzymes), transport (transferrin) and storage (ferritin). Most iron is contained in red blood cells.

A unique feature of iron balance in humans is that total body iron content is regulated mainly by variation in absorption and not by excretion. Thus, absorption is increased when iron stores are depleted. Heme iron of animal origin is more effectively absorbed than non-heme iron, putting vegetarians at a disadvantage—this is evident in the high prevalence of anemia in the Indian subcontinent. The combination of inadequate iron content in the average vegetarian diet and the lack of adequate reserves of iron in the majority of women during their reproductive years is further compounded by frequent pregnancies, worm infestation and malnutrition. The evolution of iron deficiency anemia occurs in three stages—initial depletion of iron stores, followed by reduction of serum iron levels and finally, frank development of anemia.

Iron requirements in pregnancy: The normal dietary intake may provide enough iron for daily requirements but not for the formation of iron stores; thus, more than 20% of women have depleted iron stores. The iron requirement of normal pregnancy is approximately 1000 mg, which includes maternal red cell expansion and fetoplacental needs. The gastrointestinal absorption of iron increases in the last two trimesters of pregnancy to about 1.0–3.0 mg/day. Absence of menstruation may contribute to conservation of about 240–480 mg of iron. Thus, a pregnant woman must have at least 500 mg of stored iron to fulfill the requirements of pregnancy without iron supplementation.

The daily adult iron requirement is about 2 mg/day; this increases during pregnancy to an average of about 4 mg/day, rising from 2.5 mg in the first trimester to 6.6 mg in the third trimester. Since less than 10% of total intake is absorbed, the diet must contain 40–60 mg of iron for a minimum of 4–6 mg of absorption. Since the iron content in the average daily diet is about 5–15 mg, supplements become mandatory.

Clinical features: These depend on the severity of anemia. Women with mild anemia may be asymptomatic and diagnosed as being anemic only on routine screening during pregnancy. Some may have symptoms of exertional dyspnea and easy fatigability which overlap with normal symptoms of pregnancy. In developing countries, it is not unusual to see moderate to severe anemia, especially in women who have inadequate antenatal care, poor nutrition and no iron supplementation during pregnancy.

Women with severe anemia may present with symptoms of breathlessness accompanied by gross pallor, general anasarca and congestive cardiac failure (CCF) due to a hyperdynamic circulation. Severe anemia may impair the oxygen carrying capacity but is usually well-compensated in chronic cases. Associated features such as stomatitis and signs of other vitamin deficiencies may be present.

Iron deficiency may affect the function of iron-dependent enzymes in the body resulting in impaired muscle function and exercise tolerance, epithelial changes and alteration in gastrointestinal function. These changes are the first to be corrected after initiating iron therapy and hence a subjective feeling of well-being is observed even before hemoglobin levels start to rise.

Maternal and fetal risks: Most women in the reproductive age group have a precarious iron balance which tends to deteriorate during pregnancy if treatment is not started early. Mild anemia may not affect pregnancy and labour, but the severity of anemia may increase in the later part of pregnancy or in subsequent pregnancies. Severe anemia may be associated with mortality or severe morbidity due to cardiac failure, pulmonary embolism or anoxic encephalopathy. The effects of iron deficiency on cellular function are believed to be associated with preterm labour. There is increased incidence of pre-eclampsia and sepsis. Intrapartum blood loss is also poorly tolerated.

The fetus derives its iron from maternal serum by active transport and there is reduction in fetal iron stores if the mother is iron deficient. However, except for low birth weight, adverse perinatal outcomes are infrequent even in severely anemic women (Levy et al 2005).

Diagnosis: Anemia can generally be diagnosed by simple and inexpensive laboratory tests. Table 7.1 compares various hematological investigations in different types of anemia.

- Hemoglobin concentration: Though reduction in Hb concentration is a late manifestation of iron deficiency, it is the simplest, most practical and cost-effective test for the diagnosis of anemia.
- Blood smear: Peripheral blood smear examination helps in differentiating various types of anemia (Fig. 7.1). In addition to

red cells, the appearance of other cells can contribute to a diagnosis.

- Red cell indices: Measurement of red cell indices, though not essential as first-line investigations, is useful in differentiating various types of anemia. Most modern analysers automatically report indices such as MCV, MCH, MCHC and red cell distribution width (RDW) which can be used as screening tests. RDW, an indicator of anisocytosis, is increased in most nutritional anemia but is normal in the beta-thalassemia trait.

Diagnosis: The following investigations may be used in some situations but requirement needs to be individualised:

- Serum iron and iron-binding capacity: It is an indicator of iron deficiency without overt signs of anemia. The iron binding capacity increases progressively with the severity of iron deficiency whereas the serum iron concentration decreases (Table 7.1). The normal transferrin saturation of 35–50% decreases to <15%.
- Ferritin: Depletion of iron stores is the first sign of iron deficiency, without overt anemia and can be detected by measuring ferritin levels.
- Free erythrocyte protoporphyrin: The normal level of protoporphyrin is 30 μg/dl of red cells which increases 2–3 times as there is not enough iron to convert all protoporphyrin to hemoglobin.
- Transferrin receptor: This appears to be a reliable indicator of cellular iron status but is not routinely available. It differentiates anemia of chronic inflammation from iron deficiency in combination with serum ferritin.
- Bone marrow examination: Depletion of iron stores without overt signs can be

Table 7.1: Comparison of commonly performed investigations in different types of anemia

Investigation	*Normal Pregnancy Values*	*Iron Deficiency Anemia*	*Megaloblastic Anemia*	*Thalassemia*
Hb (g/dl)	>10.5	<10.5 (vary with severity)	< 10.5	Normal or reduced
Blood smear	Normocytic normochromic	Microcytic hypochromic	Macrocytic	Microcytic hypochromic
Red cell indices				
MCV (fl)	70–96	Reduced	Increased	Very reduced
MCH (pg)	27–33	Reduced	Reduced	Very reduced
MCHC (g/dl)	30–35	Reduced	Reduced	Normal
Red cell width		High		Normal
Hb F (%)	<2	Normal	Normal	Raised
Hb A2 (%)	2–3%	Normal	Normal	Raised
Serum iron (μg/dl)	60–75	Reduced	Normal	Normal
Iron binding capacity (μg/dl)	350–400	Increased	Normal	Normal
Serum ferritin (μg/dl)	15–300	Reduced	Normal/reduced	Normal

detected by checking the iron content of the bone marrow. However, this method is invasive and is not routinely used.

- Investigations for contributory factors: Stool for ova and cyst, urine microscopy for asymptomatic bacteruria and peripheral smear for malarial parasite should be routinely performed. Renal function tests for chronic renal disease and chest x-ray for pulmonary tuberculosis are done if indicated by clinical suspicion.

Prevention: In developing countries, every pregnant woman needs iron supplementation which can be started as soon as nausea and vomiting of the early part of pregnancy is over. The WHO (1972) recommends that a supplement of 30–60 mg/day be given to

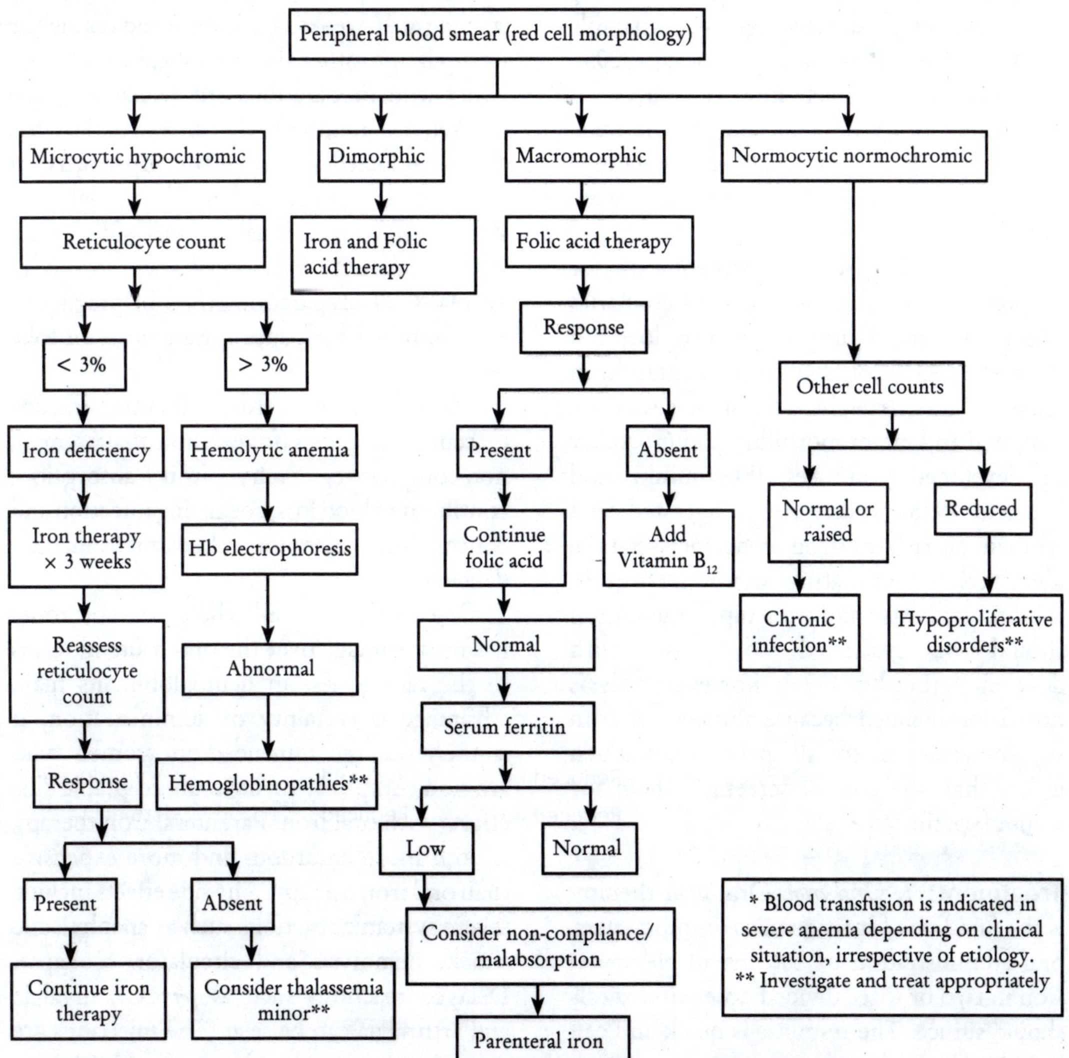

FIGURE 7.1: MANAGEMENT ALGORITHM FOR ANEMIA* (HB <10.5 G/DL)

women with adequate iron stores and 120–240 mg/day to those with none. The prophylaxis should continue throughout pregnancy and preferably for three months after delivery. For prophylaxis, the Government of India (CSSM Programme 1993) recommends 100 mg of elemental iron with 0.5 mg folic acid for at least 100 days in pregnancy. Poor compliance can be overcome by administration of two intramuscular (IM) injections containing iron (250 mg each) at a four-week interval along with tetanus toxoid, which gives comparable results (Bhatt 1997; Kumar et al 2005). Besides iron supplementation, measures for controlling other contributing factors such as worm infestations, malaria, unplanned pregnancies and inadequate antenatal care are important.

The need for iron supplementation for all pregnant women in developed countries is controversial. Current evidence does not show the benefit of iron supplementation in terms of birth weight, length of gestation, maternal and infant morbidity and mortality in developed countries (Hemminki and Starfield 1978). It has been suggested that women at risk of iron deficiency can be identified by estimating serum ferritin in the first trimester and iron supplementation should be restricted to those with deficiency (Letsky 1999); however, this is not recommended because the cost of iron supplementation to all pregnant women is less than the cost of screening them for serum ferritin.

Treatment: *1. Oral iron*: Oral iron therapy is the first line of management. In most cases, oral administration of 180 mg of elemental iron in two or three divided doses after meals should suffice. The response is quick and can be judged by both symptomatic improvement and significant increase in reticulocyte count, 5–10 days after therapy. Significant elevation in hemoglobin value can be expected after 2–3 weeks and the hemoglobin rises by 0.3–1.0 g per week irrespective of the route of administration and the compound used. The commonest problem with oral iron is gastrointestinal intolerance (nausea and diarrhea) experienced by about 10% of women undergoing treatment. Side effects of oral iron appear to be dose-related and can be minimised by using a daily dose of 100 mg, starting at 16 weeks of gestation and taking the iron pill *with* rather than *after* meals. Although many iron preparations are available in the market, no randomised controlled trial has been conducted to prove the superiority of one over the other and it is reasonable to start with conventional ferrous sulfate and ferrous fumarate because of their low cost. Virtually all preparations used in pregnancy are combined with appropriate doses of folic acid.

Causes of refractory anemia include inaccurate diagnosis (for example thalassemia), non-compliance, faulty iron absorption, continuing blood loss, coexisting infection and concomitant folate or other micronutrient deficiency.

2. Parenteral iron: While the parenteral route has no advantage over the oral route in terms of the rate of rise in hemoglobin, its main advantage is certainty of administration; it is therefore recommended in women who are non-compliant or have unacceptable side effects with oral iron. Parenteral iron therapy is both more hazardous and more expensive than oral iron therapy. The side effects include severe systemic reactions such as anaphylactic shock, hemolysis and circulatory collapse. Delayed reactions such as pyrexia, myalgia and arthralgia can be seen. The injections are painful and can cause skin staining but there is no risk of malignancy.

DOSE: The dose of parenteral iron is calculated using any one of the following two simple formulae:

a. Iron requirement in milligrams = Weight in pounds × 0.3 × Hb deficit in per cent
b. Iron requirement in milligrams = 250 mg of elemental iron × Hb deficit in g/dl

A further 50% should be added for replenishment of iron stores.

Parenteral iron is widely available as iron dextran and iron sorbitol citrate. Combinations of these along with folic acid and vitamin B_{12} are also available. Newer parenteral preparations (iron gluconate and iron sucrose complex) are associated with faster utilisation and lower incidence of anaphylactic reactions. Parenteral preparations can be given IM or IV. Since the maximum recommended dose of IM iron is 100 mg/day, several injections may be required. Oral iron should be stopped before giving iron sorbitol as it is associated with toxic reactions such as headache, nausea and vomiting if given simultaneously with oral iron.

Total dose intravenous infusion may occasionally be considered. In this, the total calculated dose of iron dextran is diluted in normal saline (1.5 g per 1000 ml) and administered initially at the rate of 1 ml in 30 minutes and if tolerated well, continued at the rate of 150 ml/hour. Drugs for treatment of anaphylactic shock should be immediately available.

BLOOD TRANSFUSION: If sufficient time is not available before delivery to achieve adequate hemoglobin levels before delivery, blood transfusion should be considered. In addition to its other (usual) hazards, blood transfusion during pregnancy increases the risk of precipitate labour and cardiac overload. The decision is easier in symptomatic women but there is no data that provides suitable guidelines for practice in asymptomatic women, though therapy is generally recommended if Hb is less than 6 g/dl after 36 weeks (WHO 2003). Packed cells are recommended for transfusion to avoid fluid overload, but the advantage of proteins in plasma should be considered in hypoproteinemic women. Diuretics (frusemide 40 mg IV) should be given prior to transfusion. Total or partial exchange transfusions are rarely required.

ROLE OF ERYTHROPOIETIN: Though effectively used in refractory anemia due to renal causes, its role in iron deficiency anemia is questionable. It has been tried with promising results, along with iron therapy, in severely anemic women who refuse blood transfusion on religious grounds. Recombinant erythropoietin is less immediately effective than blood transfusion, but considered safer in pregnancy, though its prohibitive cost restricts its use.

LABOUR MANAGEMENT: Anemia should ideally be corrected before labour. These women need careful monitoring during labour for fluid overload. Blood should be kept available at short notice and transfusion may be required in severely anemic women. The woman in labour should be propped up and appropriate analgesia given. The third stage of labour should be managed actively and even a minimal increase in blood loss should be treated aggressively as there is usually rapid deterioration. Prophylactic antibiotics should be considered.

Anemic women are at an increased risk of puerperal sepsis, lactation failure, subinvolution of uterus and thromboembolism, and should be carefully monitored. Oral iron therapy should be continued after the woman stabilises and she should be followed-up regularly. The woman should be strongly motivated to accept contraception for spacing of pregnancies. This would help the woman to regain her health.

Megaloblastic Anemia

The incidence of megaloblastic anemia varies from 0.2% to 5.0% (Letsky 2002); the majority of cases are due to folic acid deficiency and a very few due to vitamin B_{12} deficiency. Considerably greater number of women with normal peripheral smear have megaloblastic changes in the bone marrow.

Folate Deficiency

Folic acid should be taken along with iron during pregnancy. Dietary folate deficiency causing megaloblastic anemia probably occurs in about a third of all pregnant women (Letsky 1999).

Pathophysiology: Pregnancy causes a 20–30-fold increase in folate requirement (150–400 mg/day) to meet the needs of the fetus and the placenta, and to assist uterine hypertrophy and increase red cell mass. The placenta transports folate actively to the fetus even in the presence of deficiency in the mother; this causes plasma folate levels to decrease to roughly half the non-pregnant values by term. Plasma clearance of folate by kidneys is more than doubled. There is physiological increase in red cell size and this physiological macrocytosis may be masked by iron deficiency.

Predisposing factors: Usually folate deficiency is a part of overall malnutrition. Even though folate is found in nearly all natural foods it is easily destroyed by cooking. Women with multiple pregnancy, hemolytic or hereditary anemia and those on anticonvulsant therapy, especially phenytoin and phenobarbitone, are prone to megaloblastic anemia.

Clinical features: As in iron deficiency anemia, clinical features depend on the severity of the deficiency, but roughness of skin and glossitis are prominent features.

Maternal and fetal risks: Folic acid deficiency may be associated with abruption and pre-eclampsia, though this has not been established. Data supports an association between folic acid deficiency and neural tube defects, and peri-conceptional folic acid has been shown to reduce both first occurrence and recurrence of neural tube defects (MRC Vitamin Study Research Group 1991, Czeizel and Dudas 1992). Folate deficiency in the fetus is associated with low birth weight in the malnourished population. The risk of megaloblastic anemia in neonates is increased if the mother was folate deficient during pregnancy, especially if the delivery is preterm.

Diagnosis: It relies mainly on a macrocytic picture of peripheral blood film, though the hematological picture may indicate multiple deficiencies. Red cell indices show raised MCV. It should be suspected if the expected response to iron therapy is not achieved. Examination of suitably stained marrow aspirate will confirm diagnosis. Estimation of serum or red cell folate levels is not very helpful.

Prophylaxis: The WHO recommends that all women in the reproductive age group planning pregnancy should consume 400 mg of folic acid daily to prevent neural tube defects in the offspring; this should be continued during pregnancy. All epileptic women taking anticonvulsants should be given folate supplement in therapeutic doses.

Treatment: Once the diagnosis is made,

treatment should be started with oral folic acid, 5 mg daily. If there is no response to oral therapy for three weeks, parenteral folic acid should be given. Lactation provides an added folate stress and supplementation should be continued.

Vitamin B_{12} Deficiency

Anemia due to isolated Vitamin B_{12} deficiency is rare.

Pathophysiology: Pregnancy does not make a vast impact on maternal vitamin B_{12} levels. Vitamin B_{12} absorption is unaltered during pregnancy, but tissue uptake is increased causing a fall in serum B_{12}; this is more so in multiple pregnancies. It is preferentially transferred to the fetus at the expense of the mother. The recommended B_{12} intake during pregnancy is 3.0 mg/day which can be met by most non-vegetarian diets. Addisonian pernicious anemia, chronic tropical sprue and smoking, predispose to vitamin B_{12} deficiency.

Management: The diet of strict vegetarians may be deficient in B_{12}, so it should be supplemented. Most proprietary preparations of iron during pregnancy are combined with folic acid and Vitamin B_{12}. Treatment of established deficiency should be in the form of injectable vitamin B_{12} as gastrointestinal absorption is generally affected in these cases.

HEMOGLOBINOPATHIES

Hemoglobinopathies are autosomal recessive disorders of hemoglobin synthesis and are responsible for significant morbidity and mortality worldwide. In India, the distribution of specific disorders varies geographically and by community, and therefore, though common in certain areas, is seen rarely by obstetricians in other parts. The frequencies of beta-thalassemia minor ranges from 1% to 15%, sickle cell trait up to 40% and of alpha-thalassemia carriers reach >90% in some tribal communities (Mohanty et al 2002). The diagnosis of hemoglobinopathies early in pregnancy is particularly important, not only because of their clinical effects during pregnancy (they may complicate obstetric management), but also to help identify the fetus at risk of serious disease early, and plan relevant procedures accordingly.

Pathophysiology: There are three normal types of hemoglobin in adult humans—Hb A ($\alpha_2\beta_2$), Hb A_2 ($\alpha_2\delta_2$) and Hb F ($\alpha_2\gamma_2$). Since Hb A constitutes 95% of total circulating hemoglobin in adults, conditions affecting synthesis of Hb A alone are of clinical significance.

The hemoglobininopathies can result from:

- Impaired globin synthesis (thalassemia syndromes)
- Structural abnormality of globin (hemoglobin variants such as sickle cell syndromes)

The most important of these hemoglobinopathies are carrier states of beta-thalassemia and sickle cell hemoglobin (Hb S)—these are symptomless and have no direct effect on the length and quality of life. Homozygous disease is uncommon in obstetric practice and appropriate management by a multidisciplinary team can improve the outcome of pregnancy.

Thalassemia Syndromes

These are the commonest inherited disorders resulting in globin chain imbalance causing varying degrees of ineffective erythropoiesis and hemolysis in affected persons, thereby contributing to a wide range of clinical severity. These syndromes are divided into two main groups, alpha and beta, depending on the affected globin chain.

Beta-thalassemia

This is characterised by the formation of red cells with inadequate hemoglobin content due to the reduced rate of globin chain synthesis.

Beta-thalassemia major: This is a homozygous form and is rarely seen during pregnancy, as it is associated with significant morbidity and mortality in childhood. Life can be prolonged into the teens and early twenties only with regular blood transfusion, but puberty and growth are suboptimal and hence pregnancy is rare in the transfusion-dependent thalassemic girl. The greatest concern is that of chronic iron overload resulting in multiorgan dysfunction, anemia and intercurrent infection. Pregnancy is associated with marked anemia, increased transfusion requirement, concern about chelation therapy and high cesarean section rate. Organ function should be evaluated—extra folate will be required, but iron in any form is contraindicated. Erythropoietin, which stimulates hemoglobin F synthesis, may reduce transfusion requirements (Kovacs 2002). Women should be counselled, ideally before pregnancy, regarding the high risk of maternal and perinatal morbidity and mortality.

Beta-thalassemia minor: In the heterozygous state, life is normal except for mild anemia in some cases. In developing countries, the diagnosis is usually suspected when the woman being treated for anemia does not respond to oral iron therapy. Routine screening is suggested in many areas where prevalence is high.

Maternal and fetal risk: No significant maternal problems are expected in thalassemia minor, except for anemia, which may get aggravated during pregnancy. There are no fetal risks except for genetic transmission if both parents are affected.

Diagnosis: Anemia with abnormal red cell indices raises the suspicion which is confirmed on quantitative hemoglobin electrophoresis which shows raised concentration of Hb A2, with or without raised Hb F. Molecular techniques using DNA analysis can also be used.

Treatment: Women with thalassemia minor generally require oral iron and folate supplements in the prenatal period, but the dose should ideally be decided based on serum ferritin levels. Parenteral iron should not be given. However, to facilitate erythropoiesis, folic acid 5 mg daily is recommended.

Alpha-thalassemia

This occurs due to abnormalities in the synthesis of alpha globin chains. Alpha-thalassemia major in which there is no functional alpha chain is incompatible with life.

The disease burden of these syndromes and their public health importance have been largely neglected (Chui 2005). It is usually a gene deletion defect, and two forms of the trait result—alpha + and alpha 0 thalassemia, depending on whether three or two genes, respectively, are inherited instead of four. Alpha-thalassemia mutations are also common in Southeast Asia and they cause either Hb H disease (which is an intermediate form of thalassemia in which there is only one functional alpha gene) or Hb Barts hydrops fetalis (complete lack of the alpha globin gene).

Clinical features: Women may be anemic with severity of anemia and hematological changes more marked in alpha-thalassemia 0 than in alpha-thalassemia +. Women with Hb H disease will have chronic hemolytic anemia and 5–30% Hb H in their peripheral blood. They have normal life expectancy but may transmit alpha-thalassemia 0 or alpha-thalassemia + to their offspring.

Maternal and fetal risks: Women may become anemic during pregnancy when too much attention is paid to correcting the erythropoiesis. Presence of alpha-thalassemic hydropic fetus may be associated with life-threatening pre-eclampsia in the mother. Vaginal delivery may be associated with complications caused by a large fetus and bulky placenta.

Fetuses with the devastating Hb Barts hydrops fetalis may die in utero during the second or third trimesters or shortly after birth.

Diagnosis is based on hemoglobin estimation, red cell indices and DNA analysis, as Hb electrophoresis is not reliable. Management is the same as for beta-thalassemia minor.

Sickle Cell Syndromes

Out of about 250 hemoglobin variants known, Hb S is the most common. The sickling disorders include heterozygous state sickle cell trait (Hb AS), which is the most common, homozygous state sickle cell disease (Hb SS), compound variants such as sickle cell/Hb C disease and sickle cell/beta-thalassemia.

Pathophysiology: This is a variant of the beta globin chain where valine residue at the sixth position is replaced by glutamine. The average lifespan of RBCs in sickle cell patients is 17 days compared to the normal duration of 120 days (Oteng Ntim et al 2003). Hb S has the unique physical property of distorting red cells to sickle shapes, which block blood vessels, resulting in consequences like painful crises and infarction. The sickling phenomenon occurs particularly in conditions of lowered oxygen tension, acidosis, dehydration and cooling which cause stasis in small blood vessels.

Sickle Cell Disease: With advances in management, men and women with sickle cell disease now enjoy an improved quality of life well into adulthood (Hassell 2005) when they may elect to plan a family.

Clinical features: Most women with sickle cell disease will enter pregnancy with known diagnosis. The major problems associated with sickle cell disease are chronic hemolytic anemia and intravascular thrombosis leading to crises. The characteristic features are periods of health punctuated by acute episodes of painful crisis, due to intravascular sickling resulting in infarction. Clinical manifestations will depend on the organ involved. Renal complications are frequent. Aplastic crisis is the most common hematological crisis during pregnancy. Acute chest syndrome arising due to sickling in the lungs may be life-threatening.

Maternal and fetal risks: Sickle cell disease with pregnancy is a high-risk condition associated with high maternal mortality and morbidity. The causes of maternal death include pulmonary infection, infarction and embolism. Pregnancy has been associated with exacerbation of sickle cell disease and places women at an additional risk of obstetric complications. Severe maternal morbidity in these women is due to increased frequency of painful crises, infections, cerebrovascular accidents, pre-eclampsia/eclampsia, preterm labour and placental abruption. The incidence of spontaneous abortions is higher in these women.

Perinatal mortality and morbidity is increased due to the high incidence of stillbirths, neonatal deaths and low birth weight babies.

DIAGNOSIS: History is usually suggestive. The blood film may show sickle-shaped cells. Various osmotic fragility tests may help screen or suggest an initial diagnosis, which is confirmed by Hb electrophoresis or DNA analysis.

MANAGEMENT: Women with known diagnosis should undertake pregnancy in optimised health. All women should receive iron and folic acid supplements. There is no effective long-term method of reducing the chances of red cells to sickle in vivo, but risk factors such as anoxia and dehydration should be avoided and infections treated promptly. In the event of crises, aggressive supportive therapy should be instituted. A tourniquet should not be used.

1. Blood transfusion: Women with severe anemia may need blood transfusion if they are near term. Transfusion is also indicated in women with life-threatening illness and when crises do not respond to conservative management. The role of prophylactic transfusions to reduce the incidence of complications due to sickling is controversial. Regular transfusion to keep Hb at 9–12 g/dl with 60–70% Hb A is a common practice, but complications may exceed benefit and large trials are needed before guidelines can be suggested. Exchange transfusion has been successfully used in emergencies. Transfusion in women with Hb SS may require special care because atypical red cell antibodies may develop.

2. Erythropoietin: Stimulating hemoglobin F synthesis with recombinant erythropoietin appears a promising therapy for sickle cell disease (Czeizel and Dudas 1992) as the γ chain of fetal hemoglobin inhibits polymerisation of Hb S and thus sickling.

Antenatal care should aim for early detection of urinary tract infections, pre-eclampsia, renal and hepatic dysfunction and pathological fetal growth.

Labour: Adequate hydration should be ensured and hypoxia avoided. The role of additional oxygen and prophylactic antibiotics is doubtful. Careful maternal and fetal surveillance is necessary.

Postnatal care: Good hydration and oxygenation should be maintained, especially for the first 24 hours, as the risk of thromboembolism and crises are increased. Thromboprophylaxis should be considered. Contraceptive counselling should be provided.

Sickle Cell Trait: It is the most common sickle cell syndrome encountered during pregnancy. It offers some protection against falciparum malaria and is more commonly seen in endemic areas.

CLINICAL FEATURES: Women may have mild anemia or may be asymptomatic and are diagnosed on routine screening.

MATERNAL AND FETAL RISKS: In women with sickle cell trait there are no clinical implications, except for the slightly increased risk for crisis which occurs only in situations of extreme anoxia, acidosis and dehydration.

DIAGNOSIS: Anemia, if present, will be mild; Hb electrophoresis confirms the diagnosis.

MANAGEMENT: Management is routine—

extreme situations that may precipitate crises should be avoided. Oral iron and folic acid supplements should be given as usual.

Compound Variants: Hb SC is a milder variant with normal or near-normal levels of hemoglobin and may remain undiagnosed. Clinical manifestations of sickle cell beta-thalassemia are similar to Hb SS and will depend on the severity of the disease. There is increased risk of crisis in pregnancy, sometimes causing a delay in appropriate management; this could occasionally be fatal.

Prevention of hemoglobinopathies: Screening programmes to identify carriers and prevent the birth of homozygous children by prenatal diagnosis is seen as an important preventive measure to reduce the burden of disease. The screening strategies will have to vary according to the need. Screening tests suggested include red cell indices, osmotic fragility tests, solubility tests and high performance liquid chromatography (HPLC); confirmation is by Hb electrophoresis or newer molecular techniques. In women who are found to be carriers, the partner should be screened and if positive, genetic counselling and prenatal diagnosis offered. Molecular genetic techniques using DNA isolated from the amniotic fluid, chorionic villi or fetal blood are used for prenatal diagnosis. Pre-implantation genetic diagnosis (PGD) and IVF can be tried in some severe cases.

MISCELLANEOUS ANEMIC DISORDERS

Autoimmune Hemolytic Anemia: It is rarely encountered in pregnancy. Women with hemolytic anemia will have features of hemolysis such as jaundice, hepatosplenomegaly, decrease in Hb, presence of breakdown products like methemoglobin, abnormalities of red cell morphology and reticulocytosis that are hallmarks of hemolytic anemia. The rare combination of autoimmune hemolytic anemia and pregnancy carries a great risk to both mother and fetus. Very careful supervision and adjustment of steroid therapy is required.

Aplastic Anemia associated with Pregnancy

Pregnancy-associated aplastic anemia is a rare condition and the association is not well-explained. The main supportive measure is blood transfusions. Favourable maternal and neonatal outcome with transfusion support alone for this condition has been reported in the literature (Choudhury et al 2002; Kwon et al 2006). Pregnancy should be continued as long as the health of the mother is not impaired. Spontaneous remission can occur in 25–30% of patients. Rapid deterioration may necessitate termination of pregnancy.

Pregnancy following Bone Marrow Transplantation

There are reports of successful pregnancies in women with hematological malignancies after either autologous or allogeneic bone marrow transplantation (BMT). Holoweicka et al (2005) have reported six cases of uncomplicated pregnancies in five women treated with high-dose chemotherapy, radiotherapy and autologous BMT for acute lymphoblastic leukemia. All conceived between 15 and 52 months after transplantation. Relapse of leukemia during pregnancy was not noticed in this study.

Anemia associated with Chronic Infections/Disease

Anemia secondary to chronic infections is common in developing countries and will not respond to hematinics unless the primary pathology is treated.

Worm infestations are also common in developing countries and a direct relationship exists between the intensity of hookworm infection and blood loss. This can be diagnosed with simple tests such as stool examination and treated easily with albendazole or mebendazole. In highly endemic areas, routine antihelminthic treatment within prenatal care programmes should be considered. The importance of malaria as a major cause of anemia in pregnancy in endemic areas is well-recognised. Malaria prophylaxis in areas of high endemicity is an important strategy for controlling anemia in the community, including in pregnant women.

Urinary tract infection and asymptomatic bacteruria in pregnancy is associated with refractory anemia. It is important to screen patients and treat the infection appropriately. Chronic renal disorders lead to refractory anemia which will most likely respond to erythropoietin therapy.

References

Bhatt R. 1997. Maternal mortality in India–FOGSI-WHO study. *J Obstet Gynaecol Ind* 47:207–214.

Bhatt RV. 1997. Poor iron compliance and way out. *J Obstet Gynaecol Ind* **47:185–190.**

Chui DH. 2005. Alpha-thalassemia and population health in Southeast Asia. *Ann Hum Biol* 32(2): 123–130.

Czeizel AE and I Dudas. 1992. Prevention of first occurrence of neural tube defects by periconceptional vitamin supplementation. *New Engl J Med* 327:1832–1835.

Government of India. 1993. *Child Survival Safe Motherhood Programme*. Government of India.

Hassell K. 2005. Pregnancy and sickle cell disease. *Hematol Oncol Clin North Am* 19(5):903–916, vii-viii.

Hemminki E and B Starfield. 1978. Routine administration of iron and vitamins during pregnancy: and review of controlled clinical trials. *Br J Obstet Gynaecol* 85:404–410.

Holoweicka A, M Zielinska, W Rozmus, S Krzemien and J Holoweicki. 2005. Pregnancy outcome in five women after autologous bone marrow transplantation for acute lymphoblastic leukaemia. *Ginekol Pol* 76(10):799–805.

Kovacs BW. 2002. Anemia in pregnancy. In *Management of Common Problems in Obstetrics and Gynaecology,* 4th ed, ed DR Mishell Jr, TM Goodwin, PF Brenner, 22–25. Oxford: Blackwell Publishing.

Kumar A, S Jain, NP Singh and T Singh. 2005. Oral versus high dose parenteral iron supplementation in pregnancy. *Int J Gynecol Obstet* 89:7–13.

Kwon JY, Y Lee, JC Shin, JW Lee, JG Rha and SP Kim. 2006. Supportive management of pregnancy-associated aplastic anemia. *Int J Gynaecol Obstet* 95(2):115–120.

Letsky E. 1999. Anemia. In *High risk pregnancy—management options*, 2nd ed, eds DK James, PJ Steer, CP Weiner and B Gonik, 729–748. Edinburgh: WB Saunders.

Letsky E. 2000. Hematologic disorders. In *Medical disorders during pregnancy,* 3rd ed, eds William Barron, Marshall Lindheimer and John Davison, 267–315. St Louis: Mosby.

Letsky E. 2002. Blood volume, hematinics, anemia. In *Medical Disorders in Obstetric Practice,* 4th ed, ed Michael De Swiet, 29–60. Oxford: Blackwell Publishing.

Levy A, D Fraser, M Katz, M Mazor and E Sheiner. 2005. Maternal anemia during pregnancy is an independent risk factor for low birth weight and preterm delivery. *Eur J Obstet Gynecol Reprod Biol* 122(2):182–186.

Mohanty D, RB Colah, AC Gorakshakar, AH Nadkarni, SP Phanasgaonkar, S Shetty, K Ghosh and MB Mukherjee. 2002. Genetic disorders in hematological practice in India. *Community Genet* 5(3):197–200.

MRC Vitamin Study Research Group. 1991. Prevention of neural tube defects: results of medical research council vitamin study. *Lancet* 338:131–137.

Oteng Ntim E, M Lupton, S Mensah, EN Anionwu and P Steer. 2003. Sickle cell disease and pregnancy. In *Progress in Obstetrics and Gynaecology, ed* John Studd, Vol.16, 73–82. London: Churchill Livingstone.

Sharma JB. 2003. Nutritional anemia during pregnancy in nonindustralised countries. In *Progress in Obstetrics and Gynaecology,* ed John Studd. Vol.15, 103–122. London: Churchill Livingstone.

World Health Organization. 1972. Report of a WHO group of experts on nutritional anemias. Technical report series number 503. Geneva: WHO.

World Health Organization. 1997. WHO Global Database. Geneva: WHO.

World Health Organization. 2003. In *Handbook on Clinical Use of Blood,* 123–131. Geneva: WHO.

8

Current Trends in the Management of Diabetic Pregnancies

Muralidhar V Pai

Diabetes mellitus, a clinical syndrome characterised by deficiency of or insensitivity to insulin and exposure of organs to chronic hyperglycemia, is the most common medical complication of pregnancy.

DEFINITIONS AND CLASSIFICATION

Detection

The International Diabetes Center (Donald 2001) made the following recommendations regarding the practice guidelines for gestational diabetes:

Screening

Screen between 24 and 28 gestational weeks; with any risk factor, consider screening at first prenatal visit.

Screen with 50 g glucose challenge test: 1 hour plasma glucose >140 mg/dl positive; >120 mg/dl suspected.

Risk factors

The following factors are considered risk factors for diabetes in pregnancy.

- Body mass index >25 kg/m^2 (especially waist-to-hip ratio >1)
- Family history of type 2 diabetes (especially first-degree relatives)
- Age older than 25 years
- Multiparity
- Previous gestational diabetes: Macrosomic or large-for-gestational age infant (for example, >9 lb or 4000 g)
- Previous impaired fasting glucose with fasting plasma glucose 110–125 mg/dl
- Previous impaired glucose tolerance with oral glucose tolerance test two-hour glucose value 140–199 mg/dl
- American Indian or Alaska Native, African American, Asian, Hispanic, Pacific Islander

The ACOG recommends that all pregnant patients be screened for GDM. In the absence of known risk factors for GDM, a personal history may be sufficient (Expert Committee 2003).

Diagnosis

In the 100 g oral glucose tolerance test, the woman is asked to have a normal diet for three days prior to the test and asked to come overnight fasting (for at least 8 hours) on the day of the test. The fasting plasma glucose level is determined and then 100 g of oral glucose is administered. Three blood samples are drawn at hourly intervals. The recommended criteria for interpretation of this test are shown in Table 8.2.

GDM is diagnosed when fasting value is abnormal or any two values are met or exceeded, or if any single value is more than 200 mg/dl. If one value is abnormal, the International Diabetes Center recommends self-monitored blood glucose for seven days—if the average fasting blood glucose >95 mg/dl or the average two-hour post-meal >120 mg/dl, re-evaluate for gestational diabetes mellitus.

The WHO (1985) recommends the 75 gram two-hour oral glucose tolerance test; this approach is commonly used in Europe. The normal (non-diabetic) blood values are given in Table 8.4.

Levels between 140 and 200 mg/dl indicate

Table 8.1: Classification of diabetes during pregnancy (ACOG 1986)

Class	*Onset*	*Fasting Plasma Glucose*	*2 h PP Glucose*	*Therapy*
A1	Gestational	<105 mg/dl	<120 mg/dl	Diet
A2	Gestational	>105 mg/dl	>120 mg/dl	Insulin
Class	*Age of Onset*	*Duration (years)*	*Vascular Disease*	*Therapy*
B	Over 20	<10	None	Insulin
C	10–19	10–19	None	Insulin
D	Before 10	>20	Benign retinopathy	Insulin
F	Any	Any	Nephropathy	Insulin
R	Any	Any	Proliferative retinopathy	Insulin
H	Any	Any	Heart	Insulin

Table 8.2: ACOG (1994) criteria for diagnosis of GDM using 100 g oral glucose (plasma glucose values)

Time	*NDDG criteria (1979)*	*Carpenter and Coustan criteria (1982)*
Fasting	105 mg/dl (5.8 mmol/l)	95 mg/dl (5.3 mmol/l)
1 hour	190 mg/dl (10.5 mmol/l)	180 mg/dl (10 mmol/l)
2 hour	165 mg/dl (9.1 mmol/l)	155 mg/dl (8.6 mmol/l)
3 hour	145 mg/dl (8 mmol/l)	140 mg/dl (7.8 mmol/l)

Table 8.3: Indications for 100 g diagnostic oral glucose tolerance test

- Family history of diabetes
- Obese woman
- Unexplained maternal weight loss
- Previous history of GDM
- Previous history of congenital anomalies in the fetus
- Previous history of large infants
- Previous history of recurrent abortions or
- Previous history of unexplained fetal loss
- Persistent glycosuria
- Fasting plasma glucose >126 mg/dl or random plasma glucose > 200 mg/dl
- Positive 50 g oral glucose screening test

impaired glucose tolerance. This group is at increased risk of developing diabetes. Values greater than 200 mg/dl are diagnostic of diabetes mellitus.

Management

The general goal of therapeutic interventions of diabetes in pregnancy is to achieve and maintain blood glucose levels as near to normal as possible in order to reduce morbidity and mortality in the mother and the fetus.

PRECONCEPTION CARE FOR WOMEN WITH DIABETES

Care by an interdisciplinary diabetes healthcare (DHC) team (consisting of diabetes nurse educators, registered dietitians, obstetricians and endocrinologists/ internists), prior to conception and during pregnancy has been shown to minimise maternal and fetal risks in women with diabetes mellitus (Franz et al 1994). When such care results in optimal glycemic control, the risks of spontaneous abortion, congenital malformations, pre-eclampsia and progression of retinopathy are reduced (Glueck et al 2002). Women with type 1 or type 2 diabetes should strive to optimise glycemic control (Table 8.5). While an increasing number of women with type 2 diabetes are being managed in pregnancy clinics, they are often referred post-conception, while still using oral anti-hyperglycemic agents and with poor metabolic control. Whenever possible, women with type 2 diabetes who are planning pregnancy should be referred to the DHC team.

Use of oral hypoglycemic agents has always been debated. Based on the data currently available, it appears that glyburide could be safely and effectively utilised in the management of GDM. However, more intensive investigations regarding the safety and feasibility of oral agents in pregnancies complicated by type 2 diabetes are necessary. It is important to emphasise that it is the level of metabolic control achieved and not the mode of therapy that is crucial to improving outcome in these pregnancies (Homko et al 2004).

Women with poorly controlled diabetes have a two to threefold increased risk of offspring with congenital anomalies, including a 1% risk of neural tube defects. Folic acid supplement of 1–4 mg/day, from preconception until 13 weeks gestation, may reduce this risk (Glueck et al 2002).

APPROACH TO A PATIENT WITH TYPE I DIABETES

If the patient was not seen pre-conceptionally, initial evaluation must include an ophthalmological examination for evidence of retinopathy, a 24-hour urine test for creatinine clearance and total protein and albumin. Clinically detectable nephropathy in type 1 disease begins with microalbuminuria at 30–300 mg/24 hours of albumin. This may manifest as early as five years after the onset of diabetes (Nathan 1993). An ECG should be done for patients with a disease duration of more than five years or those who are above

Table 8.4: WHO (1985) criteria for diagnosis of GDM using 75 g oral glucose

Time	*Blood Glucose (mg/dl)*	*Plasma Glucose (mmol/l)*
Fasting	<110	<6.1
1 hour	<200	<11.1
2 hour	<140	<7.8

TABLE 8.5: RECOMMENDED GLYCEMIC TARGETS PRECONCEPTION AND DURING PREGNANCY

Pre-pregnancy
A_{1C} (%) = 7.0 (6.0, if possible)

Once pregnant
FPG and preprandial PG: 3.8–5.2 mmol/l (70–95 mg/dl)
1-hour postprandial PG: 5.5–7.7 mmol/l (100–140 mg/dl)
or
2-hour postprandial PG: 5.0–6.6 mmol/l (80–120 mg/dl)
Pre-bedtime snack PG: 4.0–5.9 mmol/l (70–105 mg/dl)
A_{1C} (%) = 6.0 (normal)

A_{1C}	glycosylated hemoglobin
FPG	fasting plasma glucose
PG	plasma glucose

the age of 30. All patients should have a triple test at 16–18 weeks and a detailed ultrasound examination with fetal echocardiography at 18–20 weeks, to rule out congenital anomalies.

Fetal surveillance is increased at 32 weeks of gestation, if vascular disease is present. Serial ultrasound is done to assess the fetal growth and amniotic fluid index. Polyhydramnios (AFI ≥20) or increased AC should alert the practitioner to less-than-ideal glucose control. If glucose values remain labile despite all attempts at management, it is best to deliver the fetus as soon as lung maturity is established by L:S ratio and prostaglandin by amniocentesis at 37 weeks.

Care of patients with insulin-dependent diabetes should be intensive. If not seen preconceptionally, prenatal vitamins should be started and additional folate given, 0.5 mg twice daily, because of the interaction of hyperglycemia with folate receptors. Prevention of hyperglycemia and ketoacidosis through rigorous control of blood glucose is mandatory.

Insulin therapy remains the mainstay of treatment for type 1 diabetes mellitus. Patients must receive initial and ongoing education that includes comprehensive information on care for and use of insulin, recognition and treatment of hypoglycemia, management of sick days, adjustments for food intake and physical activity and self-monitoring of blood glucose (SMBG).

INSULIN REGIMENS

A variety of insulin regimens have been used and studied. These should be adapted to the individual's treatment goals, lifestyle, diet, age, general health, motivation, capacity for hypoglycemia awareness and self-management, and social and financial circumstances. After an initial 'honeymoon period,' during which insulin requirements may decrease, the requirements will increase with time because of progressive beta cell destruction in both children and adults with type 1 diabetes.

The most successful protocols for type 1 diabetes rely on basal–bolus regimens with intermediate- or long-acting insulin, or extended long-acting insulin analogue once or twice daily as the basal insulin, and fast-acting insulin or rapid-acting insulin analogue as the bolus insulin for food intake at each meal (intensive therapy).

Optimal glucose levels before and during pregnancy are fasting levels of

70–90 mg/dl and one-hour postprandial values of 100–130 mg/dl or two-hour postprandial values of 90–120 mg/dl. This is best accomplished by pre-conceptual analysis and counselling, achievement of normal levels of glycosylated hemoglobin before pregnancy, frequent glucose monitoring, thoughtful control of diet and stabilisation of exercise. Counselling of the diabetic woman must include the family and the lifestyle changes necessary to attain the goals of normalisation of glucose levels.

Drug-induced hypoglycemia is a major obstacle for individuals with type 1 diabetes who are trying to achieve glycemic targets. Hypoglycemia can be severe and result in confusion, coma or seizure, requiring the assistance of other individuals. Significant risk of hypoglycemia often necessitates less stringent glycemic goals. The negative social and emotional impact of hypoglycemia may make patients reluctant to agree to intensifying therapy.

MANAGEMENT OF GESTATIONAL DIABETES MELLITUS

Therapeutic Considerations

All women with gestational diabetes mellitus (GDM) should receive nutritional counselling by a registered dietitian when possible. Individualisation of medical nutrition therapy (MNT) depending on maternal weight and height is recommended—it should include the provision of adequate calories and nutrients to meet the needs of pregnancy and should be consistent with the maternal blood glucose goals that have been established. Non-caloric sweeteners may be used in moderation.

For obese women (BMI >30 kg/m²), a 30–33% calorie restriction (to ≤25 kcal/kg actual weight per day) has been shown to reduce hyperglycemia and plasma triglycerides with no increase in ketonuria (International Diabetes Center 2003). Restriction of carbohydrates to 35–40% of calories has been shown to decrease maternal glucose levels and improve maternal and fetal outcomes (Langer et al 2000).

Insulin is the only pharmacological therapy that has most consistently been shown to reduce fetal morbidities when added to MNT. Selection of pregnancies for insulin therapy can be based on measures of maternal glycemia with or without assessment of fetal growth characteristics. When maternal glucose levels are used, insulin therapy is recommended when MNT fails to maintain self-monitored glucose at one of the following levels:

- Fasting whole blood glucose ≤95 mg/dl (5.3 mmol/l); fasting plasma glucose ≤105 mg/dl (5.8 mmol/l)
- one hour postprandial whole blood glucose ≤140 mg/dl (7.8 mmol/l); one hour postprandial plasma glucose ≤155 mg/dl (8.6 mmol/l)
- two hour postprandial whole blood glucose ≤120 mg/dl (6.7 mmol/l); two hour postprandial plasma glucose ≤130 mg/dl (7.2 mmol/l)

Measurement of the fetal abdominal circumference, early in the third trimester, can help identify a large subset of infants with no excess risk of macrosomia in the absence of maternal insulin therapy. This approach has been tested primarily in pregnancies with maternal fasting serum glucose levels < 105 mg/dl (5.8 mmol/l).

Human insulin should be used when insulin is prescribed, and SMBG should guide the dose and timing of the insulin regimen. The suggested starting dose is 0.7 U/kg of body weight. The total daily dose of insulin in the first trimester (weeks 5–12) is 0.7 U/kg/day; in the second trimester 0.8 U/g/day; in the third trimester (weeks 26–36) 0.9 U/kg/day and at term (weeks 36–40) 1.0

U/kg/day. The dose and timing of the insulin regimen should thereafter be guided by the SBGM levels, paying particular attention to insulin adjustment in the second and third trimesters. In fact, from Weeks 20 and 32 of gestation, there is a physiological progressive increase in insulin requirement of up to 50% of the initial dose (Langer et al 2000). The use of insulin analogues has not been adequately tested in GDM.

The most effective insulin regimen for insulin therapy during pregnancy consists of four injections per day. When multiple insulin injections are used to provide the basal need, NPH insulin is preferred because it has a more predictable absorption pattern than lente or ultralente insulin. Also, the recently developed long-acting insulin analogues have not yet been proven to be safe or efficacious in pregnancy.

Preferred use of NPH is to give a sixth of the total daily dose of insulin (I) as morning, dinner and bedtime injections. The other half of the total daily insulin dose should be short-acting insulin, given before each meal, to control postprandial glycemia. Many centres follow a convenient three-times-a-day regimen (pre-breakfast, pre-lunch and pre-dinner). Compensatory doses to adjust for high or low glucose levels are calculated as 3% of the total daily insulin requirement.

Continuous subcutaneous insulin infusion (CSII) therapy, through the utilisation of insulin pumps, could represent an optimal means to improve metabolic control with a reduction in the risk of hypoglycemia in diabetic pregnant women. Hospitalisation is not an elective choice for pregnant women with diabetes but it should be considered in cases of severe complications such as ketoacidosis, hypoglycemic coma or pre-eclampsia.

Oral glucose-lowering agents have generally not been recommended during pregnancy. However, one randomised, non-blind clinical trial compared the use of insulin and glyburide in women with GDM who were not able to meet glycemic goals on MNT (Langer 1998). Treatment with either agent resulted in similar perinatal outcomes. All patients were beyond the first trimester of pregnancy at the initiation of therapy.

Some studies have shown that the use of glyburide or metformin during pregnancy does not appear to be associated with an increase in congenital anomalies independent of glycemic control. However, the evidence is inadequate to warrant recommendation of their use in pregnancy (Diabetes Control and Complications Group 1996; Major et al 1998; McElvy et al 2000). Glyburide is not approved by the Food and Drug Administration (FDA) for the treatment of GDM and further studies are needed in a larger patient population to establish its safety.

Programmes of moderate physical exercise have been shown to lower maternal glucose concentrations in women with GDM. Although the impact of exercise on neonatal complications awaits rigorous clinical trials, the beneficial glucose-lowering effects warrant a recommendation that women without medical or obstetric contraindications be encouraged to start or continue a programme of moderate exercise as a part of treatment for GDM.

In itself, GDM is not an indication for cesarean delivery or for delivery before 38 completed weeks of gestation. Cesarean sections are recommended in the following cases—pre-eclampsia, fetal malformations, abnormal fetal presentations, advanced age of mother and previous cesarean sections. Prolongation of gestation beyond 38 weeks increases the risk of fetal macrosomia without reducing cesarean rates; hence, delivery in the 38th week is recommended, unless obstetric considerations dictate otherwise.

The main objective during labour is to maintain normal glycemic values, adequate hydration and caloric intake. If women are only on diet therapy, it is suggested that they avoid breakfast on the morning when delivery is planned. During delivery, an intravenous infusion of 5% glucose solution at the rate of 100–150 ml/hour and regular glucose monitoring is advised.

In the case of women on insulin treatment, during labour there is a reduction in the need for insulin and an increase in the demand for calories. The day before labour, women should follow their usual insulin and diet regimen with an injection at bedtime of intermediate insulin, adjusted to produce a satisfactory fasting blood glucose level. On the morning of the delivery, the woman should not receive either breakfast or a rapid acting insulin bolus. An intravenous insulin infusion of 1-2 U of short-acting insulin/hour together with a 5% glucose solution at 100–150 ml/hour is recommended. Blood glucose should be evaluated every hour or once in two hours and insulin infusion should be adjusted to obtain a glycemic target between 70 mg/dl and 130 mg/dl (3.8–7.2 mmol/l). During delivery, insulin infusion should be suspended while glucose infusion and glucose monitoring should be continued.

In the case of an elective cesarean section, the morning dose of insulin is withheld. A dextrose infusion with 1–2 U of short-acting insulin/hour is started and blood glucose is monitored every hour.

The neonates of mothers with GDM or with pregestational diabetes are at the same risk for complications, particularly those infants born macrosomic (birth weight > 4000 g). A pediatrician experienced in resuscitation of the newborn should be present, whether the delivery is vaginal or by cesarean section.

Breastfeeding, as always, should be encouraged in women with GDM.

Long-term Therapeutic Considerations

Reclassification of maternal glycemic status should be performed at least six weeks after delivery and according to the guidelines of the Report of the Expert Committee on the Diagnosis and Classification of Diabetes Mellitus (van Allen et al 2002) (Table 8.6).

If glucose levels are normal after delivery, glycemia should be reassessed at a minimum of three-year intervals. Women with IFG or IGT in the postpartum period should be tested for diabetes annually; these patients should receive intensive MNT and be placed on an individualised exercise programme because of their very high risk of developing diabetes. All patients with prior GDM should be educated regarding lifestyle modifications

Table 8.6: Criteria for the diagnosis of diabetes mellitus

Normoglycemia	*IFG and IGT*	*Diabetes Mellitus*
FPG <110 mg/dl	FPG ≥110 mg/dl and <126 mg/dl (IFG)	FPG ≥126 mg/dl
2-h PG† <140 mg/dl	2-h PG† ≥140 mg/dl and <200 mg/dl (IGT)	2-h PG† ≥200 mg/dl
—	—	Symptoms of DM and casual plasma glucose concentration ≥200 mg/dl

† PG = plasma glucose

that lessen insulin resistance, including maintenance of normal body weight through MNT and physical activity.

Medication that worsens insulin resistance (for example, glucocorticoids, nicotinic acid) should be avoided if possible. Patients should be advised to seek medical attention if they develop symptoms suggestive of hyperglycemia. Education should also include the need for family planning to ensure optimal glycemic regulation from the start of any subsequent pregnancy. Low-dose estrogen–progestogen oral contraceptives may be used in women with prior histories of GDM, as long as no medical contraindications exist.

References

American College of Obstetricians and Gynecologists. 1986. Management of diabetes in pregnancy. *Technical Bulletin No.92.* American College of Obstetricians and Gynecologists.

Donald R. 2001. ACOG clinical guidelines for management of gestational diabetes. *Obstet Gynecol* 98:525–538.

Expert Committee on the Diagnosis and Classification of Diabetes Mellitus. 2003. Report of the Expert Committee on the Diagnosis and Classification of Diabetes Mellitus. *Diabetes Care* 26 (Suppl. 1):S5–S20.

Franz MJ, ES Horton, JP Bantle, CA Beebe, JD Brunzell, AM Coulston, RR Henry, BJ Glueck CJ, P Wang, N Goldenberg et al. 2002. Pregnancy outcomes among women with polycystic ovary syndrome treated with metformin. *Hum Reprod* 17:2858–2864.

Glueck CJ, P Wang, S Kobayashi et al. 2002. Metformin therapy throughout pregnancy reduces the development of gestational diabetes in women with polycystic ovary syndrome. *Fertil Steril* 77: 520–525.

Homko CJ, E Sivan and AE Reece. 2004. Is there a role for oral antihyperglycemics in gestational diabetes and type 2 diabetes during pregnancy? *Treat Endocrinol* 3(3):133–139.

Hoogwerf and PW Stacpoole. 1994. Nutrition principles for the management of diabetes and related complications (Technical Review). *Diabetes Care* 17:490–518.

International Diabetes Center. 2003. Gestational diabetes practice guidelines. Minneapolis: International Diabetes Center.

Langer L, Dl Conway, MD Berkus, EM-J Xenakis, O Gonzales. 2000. A comparison of glyburide and insulin in women with gestational diabetes mellitus. *N Engl J Med* 343:1134–1138.

Langer O. 1998. Maternal glycemic criteria for insulin therapy in GDM, *Diabetic Care* 21 (Suppl 2): B91–B98.

Major CA, MJ Henry, M De Veciana, MA Morgan. 1998. The effects of carbohydrate restriction in patients with diet-controlled gestational diabetes. *Obstet Gynecol* 91:600–604.

McElvy SS, M Miodovnik, B Rosenn et al. 2000. A focused pre-conceptional and early pregnancy program in women with type 1 diabetes reduces perinatal mortality and malformation rates to general population levels. *J Matern Fetal Med* 9:14–20.

Nathan DM. 1993. Long-term complications of diabetes mellitus. *N Engl J Med* 328:1676.

The Diabetes Control and Complications Trial Research Group. 1996. Pregnancy outcomes in the Diabetes Control and Complications Trial. *Am J Obstet Gynecol* 174:1343–1353.

van Allen MI, C McCourt and NS Lee. 2002. Preconception health: Folic acid for the primary prevention of neural tube defects. A resource document for health professionals. Ottawa: Minister of Public Works and Government Services, Publication H39-607/2002E.

World Health Organization. 1985. Diabetes Mellitus Report of a WHO study group. *Technical Report series No.727.* Geneva:WHO.

9

Thyroid Diseases in Pregnancy

Sathisha Nayak | Sujatha Janakiraman

Introduction

Thyroid diseases are one of the common endocrine complications affecting pregnant women. Hypothyroidism (2.5%) is commonly encountered during pregnancy followed by hyperthyroidism (0.2%) and postpartum thyroiditis (ACOG Technical Bulletin 1993). Physiological changes associated with pregnancy may mimic thyroid disease in pregnancy and so, thyroid function evaluation must take this into consideration. Uncontrolled hyper or hypothyroidism may lead to serious maternal complications such as thyroid storm, heart failure or myxedema during pregnancy. The maternal thyroid function has a significant effect on the developing fetus because the supply of maternal thyroxin to the fetus is critical in early pregnancy for its central nervous system development, before fetal thyroid hormone secretion starts (Amino et al 1982). Evidence suggests that low level of thyroxin (T4) in the mother during pregnancy is associated with poor motor and cognitive development in the child later (Brander and Kivisaari 1984; Ballabio et al 1991; Amino et al 1999). Hence, maternal thyroid function screening during pregnancy seems logical but the cost-effectiveness of such an approach is under evaluation. Pre-pregnancy counselling for women with thyroid disease who are planning a pregnancy could help prevent most of the complications during pregnancy. Neonatal screening for babies delivered to mothers with thyroid disease should be part of the management plan as the disease process, complication or anti-thyroid medication could adversely affect the baby.

Physiological Changes in Thyroid Function during Pregnancy

Pregnancy induces both morphological and functional changes in the thyroid. Anatomically, there will be a slight diffuse enlargement of the thyroid which may be visible in about 10–15% of women during pregnancy (Brent 1997). Goitorous or nodular thyroids are pathological and need to be evaluated. Functionally, there would be an increase in serum levels of total thyroxin (T4), tri-iodothyronine (T3) and thyroid binding globulin (TBG), starting from the second month of pregnancy, which peaks at 18–20 weeks (Cooper et al 1983; Campbell et al 1992). Serum levels of free T4, free T3 and thyroid stimulating hormone (TSH) remain in the normal range as in non-pregnant women (Brent 1997). During pregnancy, the plasma iodine level falls due to increased iodine uptake by the fetus as well as increased renal clearance (Davis et al 1989; Brent 1997). WHO recommends 200 μg of iodine intake per day for pregnant women and 150 μg for non-pregnant women.

Thyroxin (T4) crosses the placenta and umbilical cord. T4 levels up to 50% of normal maternal serum levels have been detected in cases of congenital fetal hypothyroidism (Davis et al 1988). Thyrotropin–releasing hormone (TRH), thyroid stimulating antibodies, propylthiouracil and methimazole can all cross the placenta, but not TSH. TBG and iodine are actively transferred across the placenta, especially after 12 weeks of pregnancy. The endocrinal dynamics of pregnancy may mimic thyroid dysfunction and hence, careful clinical and laboratory evaluation are necessary in such cases (Ecker and Musci 1997; Dussault and Fisher 1999).

HYPOTHYROIDISM IN PREGNANCY

Hypothyroidism occurs in about 2.5% of all pregnancies including both clinical and subclinical cases (ACOG 1993).About 0.05% of all pregnant women have overt hypothyroidism (Ecker and Musci 2000). Subclinical hypothyroidism was reported in 2% of screened clinically euthyroid pregnant women (Freely 1979; Gerestein 1993). Interestingly, more than two-thirds of such cases were attributed to the transient hypothyroid state of early pregnancy (Gerestein 1990). Up to 20% of biochemically hypothyroid pregnant women could be clinically euthyroid (Gharib and Goellner 1993). Iodine deficiency is the largest single cause of hypothyroidism around the world and one billion people are at risk of developing the condition (Gibson and Tulchinsky 1980). Hence, iodine deficiency is the most common cause of hypothyroidism during pregnancy, particularly in areas at risk. Iodine deficiency before pregnancy and in the first half of the pregnancy can lead to significant fetal neurodevelopmental problems. Other rare causes of maternal hypothyroidism include idiopathic myxedema, Hashimoto's thyroiditis, thyroid surgery and radio-ablation.

Clinical Features: Clinical features of mild hypothyroidism include tiredness, lethargy, cold intolerance, weight gain and eyelid edema. In severe cases, dry skin, hair loss, hoarseness, constipation and goitre may be found.

Hypothyroidism is associated with increased risk of pre-eclampsia, preterm labour, stillbirth, fetal distress during labour, cardiac failure and PPH (Glinoer et al 1990; Gharib and Goellner 1993). There is no increased risk of congenital anomalies in the fetus (Glinoer et al 2000; Glinoer 2001). Subclinical autoimmune hypothyroidism in the mother may be associated with transient hypothyroidism in neonates (Glinoer et al 1994). Thyroid hormone replacement therapy does not cause fetal thyrotoxicosis as the placenta metabolises most of it, and therefore it is safe to breastfeed while on thyroid hormone replacement therapy. Children born to mothers with uncontrolled hypothyroidism during pregnancy are prone to significantly poor psychomotor development at 19 months (Ballabio et al 1991) and lower IQ at age 4 and 7 years.

Diagnosis: Diagnosis is quite often obvious in patients with pre-existing hypothyroidism but should be confirmed by low serum levels of free T4, free thyroxin index and increased TSH levels. A high degree of suspicion is warranted in those who have been exposed to thyroidectomy, Graves' disease or radio-ablation of the thyroid gland. Anti-thyroglobulin antibodies may be raised in up to 50% of cases of hypothyroidism caused by autoimmune thyroiditis and are almost always associated with raised antiperoxidase antibodies (Gibson and Tulchinsky 1980).

Management: Thyroid replacement with levothyroxin (0.1–0.2 mg per day) is the treatment of choice, and it should be started at the earliest. The clinical response and levels of TSH and free thyroxin should guide the dosage. The TSH and free T4 level should be monitored every eight weeks. The objective of the thyroid replacement therapy should be to keep TSH below 5 IU/ml. The requirements of thyroxin may increase by up to 50–100% as pregnancy advances (Haddow et al 1999). Inadequate pre-pregnancy dosage has been blamed for increased thyroxin requirements during pregnancy (Harris et al 1989). Thyroxin absorption is interrupted by ferrous preparations and antacids, hence they must be avoided at least four hours after a dose of thyroxin (Heyerdahl 1991; Kamjo et al 1998).

Myxedema coma is a rare complication, which has a mortality rate of about 20%. It can occur in poorly controlled hypothyroid pregnant women, often precipitated by pre-eclampsia or infection. Prompt diagnosis and management are essential. Management includes hospitalisation, thyroxin replacement and close monitoring.

Effect on Pregnancy: Labour is usually uneventful in optimally treated cases of hypothyroidism and hence, no special management is necessary. In the postnatal period, the neonate should be evaluated for evidence of thyroid dysfunction including TSH levels. Postpartum exacerbation is known to occur and so, long-term, regular follow-up is necessary for these patients, particularly those with thyroid autoantibodies. Even in well-controlled hypothyroidism, about 25% of pregnant women develop postpartum thyroiditis during the postnatal period (Klein et al 1991).

About 10–20% of subclinical cases progress to overt hypothyroidism within 1–4 years (Girling and de Sweit 1992). Hence screening and detection of sub-clinical patients is recommended.

HYPERTHYROIDISM IN PREGNANCY

Hyperthyroidism affects about one in 2000 pregnancies. About 90–95% of all cases are caused by Graves' disease (Lazarus et al 1997; Lazarus and Premawardhana 2005). Other causes include nodular goitre or solitary toxic nodule, gestational trophoblastic disease. A transient hyperthyroid state in pregnancy is described in cases of hyperemesis gravidarum and gestational transient thyrotoxicity. In hyperemesis gravidarum cases, high titres of hCG hormones result in thyroid stimulation, high levels of T4 and suppression of TSH. Anti-thyroid medications are rarely indicated and as the hCG level decreases, patients will be symptom-free. In gestational transient thyrotoxicity, which occurs in the first trimester, symptoms follow the levels of hCG and medication is rarely indicated.

Clinical Features: Clinical features of hyperthyroidism during pregnancy include tachycardia, nervousness, weight loss and tremors. Physiological changes of pregnancy can be differentiated from hyperthyroidism by checking the serum levels of free T4 and the FT4 index, which are raised, and TSH, which will be below normal in the latter.

Graves' Disease in Pregnancy

Graves' disease is the commonest cause of hyperthyroidism in pregnancy. It is caused by the presence of thyroid stimulating antibodies which act on TSH receptors and lead to hyperactivity of the thyroid gland. Proptosis, pretibial edema and external ocular muscle paresis are hallmarks of thyrotoxicosis. Interestingly, pregnancy seems to have a moderating effect on Graves' disease, explained by generalised immune system suppression and the presence of circulating thyroid stimulating hormone-blocking antibodies which inhibit thyroid stimulation (Lejeune et al 1992; Lei et al 1994). Thyroid-stimulating antibodies cross the placenta and may result in fetal thyrotoxicosis.

Effect of Pregnancy on Graves' Disease: Graves' disease often improves during the second and third trimesters but may get exacerbated in the first trimester due to hCG stimulation of thyroid receptors (Leung et al 1993). Recurrences are common 1–4 months following delivery, hence close follow-up is necessary in the postnatal period.

Effect of Graves' Disease on Pregnancy: Ideally, hyperthyroidism should be diagnosed and cured before pregnancy to prevent fetal and maternal complications. Uncontrolled, severe hyperthyroidism is associated with an increased risk of abortion, IUGR, preterm delivery (11–25%), pre-eclampsia, stillbirth (8–15%) and heart failure (Matuura et al 1997; Lucas et al 2000). Neonatal thyrotoxicosis can result in about 1% of babies born to mothers with Graves' disease due to transplacental passage of thyroid stimulating antibodies (Matuura et al 1997). Fetal thyrotoxicosis may result in craniosynastosis, heart failure and hepatosplenomegaly. High levels of such antibodies in the cord blood are suggestive of fetal or neonatal thyrotoxicosis. Hence, maternal serum thyroid stimulating antibody levels should be checked in all cases of thyrotoxicosis during pregnancy at term. Pregnant women with Graves' disease also develop thyroid stimulating hormone binding inhibitory antibodies or blocking antibodies which may cross the placenta and cause neonatal hypothyroidism (Mckenzie and Zakarijam 1978).

Commonly used anti-thyroid drugs can also cross the placenta and may give rise to fetal hypothyroidism. An ultrasound scan can be done to check for features of fetal hypothyroidism like fetal goitre or IUGR. The thyroid status of the fetus during pregnancy can be checked by either cordocentesis or amniocentesis.

The goal of the treatment should be to keep the patient asymptomatic and to achieve serum free T4 levels in the upper normal range. Anti-thyroid medication is the mainstay of treatment. Both propylthiouracil (PTU) and methimazole are safe and effective during pregnancy (Molitch 1995)—both belong to the thiamide group of drugs, which inhibit iodination of thyroglobulin and thyrogobulin synthesis by competing with iodine for the enzyme peroxidase. PTU also blocks peripheral conversion of T4 to T3 (ACOG Technical Bulletin 1993), a starting dose of 300–600 mg of PTU during pregnancy (100–150 mg every 8 hours) is recommended. Patients are reviewed at the end of the week and dosage can be adjusted according to the patient response. It may take up to 1–2 months for significant clinical response.

Free T4 levels are monitored monthly. The side effects of PTU include drug rash, pruritis, hepatitis, drug fever and bronchospasm. Agranulocytosis, which is a life-threatening complication, may occur in about 0.2% of all patients, particularly in the older age group and those on high doses of thiamide therapy (Montoro 1997). In such cases, immediate cessation of therapy is warranted and an improvement can be seen in days or weeks. Leucopenia can occur in about 10% of patients but does not warrant stopping the therapy. Breastfeeding is not contraindicated while the patient is on thiamide drugs, but these drugs must be taken just before or at least 3–4 hours after breastfeeding to decrease the level in breast milk.

Methimazole is blamed for anomalies in the fetus such as aplasia cutis, facial abnormalities and tracheo-esophageal fistula, but studies have not shown any such association (Montoro 1997). Propylthiouracil and methimazole carry the same risk of major anomalies when used in pregnancy (3% with PTU and 2.7% with methimazole) (Moosa and Mazzaferri 1997).

If a patient cannot tolerate the drug or develops serious complications following the thiamide drug, beta-blockers can be given to control symptoms which can also block conversion of T4 to T3. Propranolol, at a starting dose of 20–40 mg twice or thrice daily, is the drug of choice.

Due to the high vascularity of the thyroid gland during pregnancy, surgery is not recommended. However, when the patient is unable to tolerate anti-thyroid drugs or is unresponsive to medical treatment, surgical options may be considered. Radioiodine is contraindicated in pregnancy as it results in active fetal thyroid uptake, permanent fetal thyroid gland damage and neonatal hypothyroidism.

Thyroid Storm

Thyroid storm may complicate 1–10% of cases of hyperthyroidism complicating pregnancy. It is an emergency and the maternal mortality rate in such cases may be as high as 25% (Motaro et al 1981). The condition usually occurs in uncontrolled, severe cases of hyperthyroidism, and is often precipitated by infection, anemia, hypertension, labour or surgery. The clinical features include fever, nausea, diarrhea, dehydration, convulsions and cardiac arrhythmia. The condition is associated with a high risk of cardiac failure. Prompt diagnosis is essential even when the laboratory report on thyroid function tests is not available, as delay may lead to shock, stupor and coma.

Adequate fluid replacement, thermo-regulation and prompt treatment of the precipitating condition is the key to the management of thyroid storm (Davis et al 1989; Lazarus et al 1997). These patients are managed in the ICU with close monitoring of both mother and fetus. Invasive central monitoring and continuous cardiac monitoring may be indicated. General measures include correction of dehydration with intravenous fluids, electrolyte replacement, oxygen, antipyretics and cool blankets. PTU, beta-blockers, dexamethasone and iodides are given to rapidly control the symptoms of thyroid hyperactivity. Up to1 g of PTU can be given orally as a loading dose, followed by 200 mg every six hours. Potassium iodide is given as oral drops (5 drops every 8 hours). If the patient cannot take the medication orally, rectal suppositories of methimazole may be given. Phenobarbital can be given to control aggressive patients. Delivery is only indicated if the fetal condition warrants it.

POSTPARTUM THYROIDITIS

A common but underestimated condition characterised by thyroid dysfunction in the postpartum period occurs in about 5% of postnatal women worldwide (Nelson-Piercy 1997) and usually occurs within 1–8 months postpartum. About 70% of patients with anti-microsomal antibodies in early pregnancy and 25% of women with type 1 diabetes mellitus develop this condition (Othman et al 1990). A family history of autoimmune disorders may also be present in some cases (Pop et al 1999). Postpartum thyroiditis usually presents in two phases—the initial hyperthyroid state for 6 weeks to 6 months postpartum, and later the hypothyroid state up to one year following delivery.

Only about 25% display classical presentation, whereas about one-third of each present as either hyper or hypothyroidism alone. The underlying cause could be reactivation of the maternal immune system with autoantibodies against thyroid, which results in destructive transient lymphocytic thyroiditis. The hyperthyroid state is due to release of already accumulated thyroid hormones and not due to excessive production as in Graves' disease.

The clinical features are usually vague and non-specific like fatigue, palpitations and diffuse goitre. About 40% present with features suggestive of hyperthyroidism in the initial phase and another 40% with those of hypothyroidism. The hyperthyroid state usually last about 2 months (Pop et al 1991). Postpartum thyroiditis is associated with postnatal depression (often thyroid autoantibodies may be seen) (Singer et al 1995; Toft 1994).

Diagnosis is based on assessment of serum TSH, free T4 and anti-thyroid antibodies. Abnormal levels of TSH or T4 in the absence of thyroid stimulating antibodies during the first year postpartum is most likely to be due to postpartum thyroiditis. Postpartum recurrence of Graves' disease can be determined by checking for thyroid stimulating antibodies and iodine uptake—these will be raised in Graves' disease.

The majority of patients in the hyperthyroid state do not need any treatment and if symptoms are severe, beta-blockers may be given for symptomatic relief. Anti-thyroid medication has no role in the management. The hypothyroid state usually needs thyroxin replacement and must be guided by TSH levels and clinical response.

About 23% of women who recover from postpartum thyroiditis develop permanent hypothyroidism within five years (van Dijke et al 1987). A patient with thyroid antiperoxidase antibodies and one with very high levels of TSH are at a higher risk of developing permanent hypothyroidism (Vander Spuy and Jacobs 1984). Routine screening is not recommended but those at risk need be scanned at 3 and 6 months postpartum (Wasserstrum and Anania. 1995). About 70% develop recurrent postpartum thyroiditis (Weetman 2000).

THYROID NODULE DURING PREGNANCY

Evaluation: Nodularity of the thyroid gland during pregnancy calls for evaluation, as normal changes of pregnancy induce only diffuse thyroid enlargement. About 5–30% of these nodular goitres are likely to be malignant. Ultrasound evaluation can differentiate between solid and cystic mass, and should be the investigation of choice. Fine needle aspiration of the thyroid nodule is safe during pregnancy—it offers good sensitivity and specificity. If the nodule is growing, is associated with lymphadenopathy or is more than 4 cm in size (or more than 2 cm of solid mass), biopsy is indicated. Cystic lesions are usually benign (Wing et al 1994). The radioiodine uptake test is contraindicated during pregnancy as fetal uptake may result in fetal thyroid ablation. Most thyroid malignancies are well differentiated and so, do not spread or metastasise rapidly. Delaying thyroid surgery until after delivery does not alter the prognosis (Wing et al 1994). However, surgery may be contemplated, in case a thyroid malignancy is diagnosed before 24 weeks of pregnancy.

References

ACOG Technical Bulletin Number 181. 1993. Thyroid disease in pregnancy. *Int J Gynecol Obstet* 43:82–88.

Amino TN, H Tada, Y Hikada, LM Crapo, A Stagnaro-Green. 1999. Therapeutic controversy screening for postpartum thyroiditis. *J Clin Endocrinol Metab* 84:1813–1921.

Amino TN, O Tanizawa, H Mori et al. 1982. Aggravation of thyrotoxicosis in early pregnancy and after delivery in Graves' disease. *J Clin Endcrinol Metab* 55:108–112.

Ballabio M, M Posychinda, RP Ekins. 1991. Pregnancy induced changes in thyroid function: Role of human chorionic gonodotrophin as putative regulator of maternal thyroid. *J Clin Endocrinol Metab* 73:824–831.

Brander A and L Kivisaari. 1984. Ultrasonography of the thyroid during pregnancy. *J Clin Ultrasound* 17:403.

Brent GA. 1997. Maternal thyroid function tests in pregnancy. *Clin Obstet Gynecol* 40:3–15.

Campbell NRC, BB Hasinoff, H Stalts et al. 1992. Ferrous sulfate reduces thyroxin efficacy in patients with hypothyroidism. *Ann Intern Med* 117:1010–1013.

Cooper DS, D Goldminz, AD Levin et al. 1983. Agranulocytosis associated with antithyroid drugs. *Ann Intern Med* 98:26–29.

Davis LE, KJ Leveno and FG Cunningham. 1988. Hypothyroidism complicating pregnancy *Obstet Gynecol* 72:18–112.

Davis LE, MJ Lucas, GDV Hankins FG Cunningham. 1989. Thyrotoxicosis complicating pregnancy. *Am J Obstet Gynecol* 160:63–70.

Dussault JH and DA Fisher. 1999. Thyroid function in mother of hypothyroid newborns. *Obstet Gynecol* 93:15–20.

Ecker JL and TJ Musci. 1997. Treatment of thyroid disease in pregnancy. *Prescribing in Pregnancy* 24:575–589.

Ecker JL and TJ Musci. 2000. Thyroid function and disease in pregnancy. *Curr Prob Obstet Gynecol Fertil* 23:109–122.

Freely J. 1979. Physiology of thyroid function in pregnancy. *Postgrad Med* 55:336–339.

Gerestein HC. 1990. How common is postpartum thyroiditis?: a methodologic overview of the literature. *Arch Intern Med* 150:1397–1400.

Gerestein HC. 1993. Incidence of postpartum thyroid dysfunction in patients with type I diabetes mellitus. *Ann Intern Med* 118:419–423.

Gharib H and JR Goellner. 1993. Fine needle aspiration biopsy of the thyroid: An appraisal. *Ann Intern Med* 118:282–289.

Gibson M and D Tulchinsky. 1980. The maternal thyroid. In *Maternal-fetal endocrinology,* eds D Tulchinsky, J Ryan, 115–128. Philadelphia: WB Saunders.

Girling JC and M de Sweit. 1992. Thyroxin dosage during pregnancy in women with primary hypothyroidism. *Br J Obstet Gynecol* 99:368–370.

Glinoer D and F Derange. 2000. The potential repercussions of maternal, fetal, and neonatal hypothyroxinemia on the progeny. *Thyroid* 10:871–887.

Glinoer D, M Riahi, JP Grun et al. 1994. Risk of sub-clinical hypothyroidism in pregnant women with asymptomatic autoimmune thyroid disorders. 79:197.

Glinoer D, PT de Nayer, P Bourdeoux et al. 1990. Regulation of maternal thyroid during pregnancy. *J Clin Endocrinol Metab* 71:276–287.

Glinoer D. 2001. Pregnancy and iodine. *Thyroid* 11:471–481.

Haddow JE, GE Palomaki, WC Allan et al. 1999. Maternal thyroid deficiency during pregnancy and subsequent neuropsychological development of the child. *N Engl J Med* 341:549–555.

Harris B, M Fong, S Johns et al. 1989. Transient postpartum thyroid dysfunction and postnatal depression. *J Affect Disord* 17:243.

Heyerdahl S. 1991. Intellectual development in children with congenital hypothyroidism in relation to T4 replacement. *J Pediatr* 118:850–855.

Kamjo K, T Saito, M Sato et al. 1998. Transient sub-clinical hypothyroidism in early pregnancy. *Endocrinol Japan* 37:397–403.

Klein RZ, JE Haddow, JD Fax et al. 1991. Prevalence of thyroid deficiency in pregnant women. *Clin Endocrinol* 35:41–46.

Lazarus JH and LD Premawardhana. 2005. Screening for thyroid disease in pregnancy. *J Clin Pathol* 58(5):449–452.

Lazarus JH, F Ammari, R Oretti, AB Parkes, CJ Richards and B Harris. 1997. Clinical aspects of recurrent postpartum thyroiditis. *Br J Gen Pract* 47:305–308.

Lei Y, AD Sperber and S Shany. 1994. Non-specific intestinal absorption of levothyroxin by aluminum hydroxide. *Ann J Med* 97:363–365.

Lejeune B, M Lemone, J Kinthaer et al. 1992. The epidemiology of autoimmune and functional thyroid disorders in pregnancy. *J Endocrinol Invest* 15(Suppl 2):77.

Leung AS, LK Millar, PP Koonings et al. 1993. Perinatal outcomes in hypothyroid pregnancies. *Obstet Gynecol* 81:349–353.

Lucas A, E Pizaro, ML Granada et al. 2000. Postpartum thyroiditis: Epidemiology and clinical evolution in a non-selected population. *Thyroid*; 10:71–77.

Matuura N, S Harada, Y Ohyama et al. 1997. The mechanism of transient hypothyroidism in infants born to mothers with Graves' disease. *Paediatr Res* 42:214–218.

Mckenzie JM and M Zakarijam. 1978. Pathogenesis of maternal Graves' disease. *J Endocrinol Invest* 2:182.

Molitch ME. 1995. Pituitary, thyroid, adrenal, and parathyroid disorders. In *Medical disorders during pregnancy* WM Barron, MD Lindheimer (eds). Missouri: Mosby Year Book, 99–109.

Montoro MN. 1997. Management of hypothyroidism during pregnancy. *Clin Obstet Gynecol* 40:65–80.

Moosa M and EL Mazzaferri. 1997. Outcome of differentiated thyroid cancer diagnosed in pregnant women. *J Clin Endocrinol Metab* 82:2862.

Motaro M, JV Collea, SD Fraiser and JH Mestman. 1981. Successful outcome of pregnancy in women with hypothyroidism. *Ann Intern Med* 94:31–34.

Nelson-Piercy C. 1997. Thyroid and parathyroid disease In *Handbook of Obstetric Medicine*. Oxford: ISIS Medical Media, 80–94.

Othman S, DI Phillips, AB Parkes et al. 1990. A long-term follow-up of postpartum thyroiditis. *Clin Endocrinol* 32:559–564.

Pop VJ, JL Kujjpens, van Baar et al. 1999. Low maternal free thyroxin concentration during early pregnancy is associated with impaired psychomotor development in infancy. *Clin Endocrinol* 50:149–155.

Pop VSM, H de Rooy, HL Vader et al. 1991. Postpartum thyroid dysfunction and depression in an unselected population. *N Engl J Med* 324:1815–1816.

Singer PA, DS Cooper, EG Levy et al. 1995. Treatment guidelines for patients with hyperthyroidism and hypothyroidism. *JAMA* 273:808.

Toft AD. 1994. Thyroxin therapy. *N Engl J Med* 331:174–180.

van Dijke UP, Heydendael RJ, De Kleine MJ et al. 1987. Methimazole, carbimazole and congenital skin defects. *Ann Intern Med* 106:60–61.

Vander Spuy ZM and HS Jacobs. 1984. Management of endocrine disorders in pregnancy Part 1- Thyroid parathyroid disease. *Postgrad Med J* 60:245–252.

Wasserstrum N and CA Anania. 1995. Perinatal consequences of maternal hypothyroidism in early pregnancy and inadequate replacement. *Clin Endocrinol* 42:353–358.

Weetman AP. 2000. Graves' disease. *New Eng J Med* 343:1236–1248.

Wing DA, LK Millar, PP Koonings et al. 1994. A comparison of propylthiouracil versus methimazole in the treatment of hyperthyroidism in pregnancy. *Am J Obstet Gynecol* 170:90–95.

10

Heart Disease in Pregnancy

Parvathi Bhat

Heart disease as a complication is seen in 1% of pregnant women. In the past, rheumatic heart disease accounted for the majority of the cases; but now, over the past three decades, it has almost disappeared in developed countries. Meyer et al (1994) described pregnancies that were complicated by cardiac disease based on data collected over 10 years; they found that only a few were caused by rheumatic fever.

Tan and de Swiet (1998) in a study of the prevalence of heart disease diagnosed de novo in a West London population found that this was an uncommon problem with low prevalence and more common in the immigrant population.With better medical and surgical management, women with congenital heart disease can now attempt to have a baby under supervision. The other types of heart diseases are less common. Maternal mortality due to heart disease has decreased remarkably over the past fifty years; however, it still contributes significantly in certain parts of the world.

The healthy heart is able to cope with the marked hemodynamic changes stimulated by pregnancy, but this has a profound effect on underlying heart disease in pregnant women. A working knowledge of the normal physiology of pregnancy is often helpful in the management of patients with heart disease.

Normal Physiological Changes during Pregnancy

Profound hemodynamic alterations occur during pregnancy, labour and delivery and in the postpartum period.

Most pregnant women have peripheral edema and regular venous distension. They also have audible physiological systolic murmurs, created by augmented blood flow. Often a physiological, third heart sound (S3), reflecting the volume overloaded state, can be appreciated.

Whenever possible, women with pre-existing cardiac lesions should receive preconception counselling, including a discussion about contraception, maternal and fetal risk during pregnancy and the potential long-term maternal morbidity and mortality.

The New York Heart Association (NYHA) functional class is often used as a predictor for outcome.

Class I Uncompromised: These are patients with cardiac disease and no limitation of physical activity. They do not have symptoms of cardiac insufficiency, nor do they experience anginal pain.

Class II Slightly compromised: These are patients with cardiac disease and slight limitation of physical activity. These women

Table 10.1: Normal hemodynamic changes during pregnancy (Maroo and Raymond 2003)

Hemodynamic Parameter	*Change during Normal Pregnancy*	*Change during Labour and Delivery*	*Change during Postpartum Period*
Blood volume	↑ 40–50%	↑	↓
Heart rate	10–15 beats/minute	↑	↓
Cardiac output	↑ 30–50% above base line	↑ Additional 50%	↑ Initially within preload, then with diuresis
Blood pressure	↓ 110 mm of Hg	↑	Returns to base line
Stroke volume	↑ 1st and 2nd trimester, slight ↓ in 3rd trimester	↑ 300–500 cc per contraction	↓
Systemic Vascular resistance	↓	↑	Returns to base line

are comfortable at rest, but if ordinary physical activity is undertaken, discomfort results in excessive fatigue, palpitation, dyspnea or anginal pain.

Class III Markedly compromised: These are patients with cardiac disease and marked limitation of physical activity. They are comfortable at rest, but less than ordinary activity causes discomfort due to excessive fatigue, palpitation, dyspnea or anginal pain.

Class IV Severely compromised: These are patients with cardiac disease and the inability to perform any physical activity without discomfort. Symptoms of cardiac insufficiency or angina may develop at rest and if any physical activity is undertaken, discomfort increases.

Women graded as NYHA Class III or Class IV face a mortality rate of as much as 7% and a morbidity rate of 50%. These women should be strongly counselled against pregnancy.

Five factors have been found to be predictive of maternal cardiac complications. These factors are listed in Table 10.2.

Cardiac lesions can be congenital or acquired. In addition, these patients can be further classified as low risk, intermediate risk or high risk pregnancies.

Low Risk

1) Atrial septal defect
2) Ventricular septal defect
3) Patent ductus arteriosus
4) Asymptomatic with low mean gradient (<50 mm Hg) and normal left ventricle (LV) function (ejection fraction [EF] >50%)
5) Aortic regurgitation (AR) with normal LV function and NYHA class I or II
6) Mitral valve prolapse (MVP) isolated or with mild/moderate MR and normal LV function
7) MR with normal LV function and NYHA class 1 or II
8) Mild/Moderate mitral stenosis (MS), mitral valve area (MVA) >1.5 cm^2 mean gradient <5 mm Hg) without severe pulmonary hypertension
9) Mild/Moderate pulmonary stenosis (PS)

TABLE: 10.2: PREDICTORS OF MATERNAL RISK OF CARDIAC COMPLICATIONS (MAROO AND RAYMOND 2003)

1. Prior cardiac event (heart failure, transient ischemic heart attack, stroke prior to pregnancy)
2. Prior arrhythmia (symptomatic sustained tachyarrhythmia or bradyarrhythmia requiring treatment)
3. NYHA functional class >2 or cyanosis
4. Valvular and outflow tract obstruction (aortic valve area <1.5cm^2, mitral valves <2cm^2 or left ventricular outflow tract gradient >30mm Hg)
5. Myocardial dysfunction (LVEF* <40%) or restrictive cardiomyopathy or hypertrophic cardiomyopathy

** - LVEF = Left ventricular ejection fraction*

10) Repaired acyonotic congenital heart disease without residual cardiac dysfunction

INTERMEDIATE RISK

1) Large left-to-right shunt
2) Coarctation of the aorta
3) Marfan's syndrome with a normal aortic root
4) Moderate/Severe MS
5) Mild/Moderate aortic stenosis (AS)
6) Severe PS
7) History of prior peripartum cardiomyopathy with no residual ventricular dysfunction

HIGH RISK

1) Eisenmenger's syndrome
2) Severe pulmonary hypertension
3) Complex cyanotic heart disease (tetralogy of Fallot [TOF], Ebstein's anomaly, truncus arteriosis [TA], transposition of the great arteries [TGA], tricuspid atresia)
4) Marfan's syndrome with aortic root or valve involvement
5) Severe AS with or without symptoms
6) Aortic and/or mitral valve disease with moderate/severe LV dysfunction (EF <40%)
7) NYHA class III to IV symptoms associated with any valvular disease or with cardiomyopathy of any etiology
8) History of peripartum cardiomyopathy with persistant LV dysfunction (Banow et al 1998)

Causes of Heart Disease

Rheumatic heart disease: This is on the decline but still exists in certain regions.

Congenital heart disease: Better medical management along with newer surgical techniques has enabled more girls with congenital heart disease to reach childbearing age (Morgan and Howitt 1965, Brickner et al 2000). Congenital heart disease now constitutes about half of all cases of heart disease encountered during pregnancy (Bitsch et al 1989, McFaul et al 1998).

Hypertensive heart disease: This is frequently complicated by heart disease of obesity and has become a relatively common cause of peripartum heart failure at Parkland Hospital (Cunningham et al 1986).

Other varieties are even less common and include:

- Coronary
- Thyroid
- Syphilitic
- Kyphoscoliotic
- Idiopathic cardiomyopathy
- Cor pulmonale

- Constrictive pericarditis
- Various forms of heart blocks
- Isolated myocarditis

Diagnosing Heart Disease in Pregnancy

Sometimes, heart disease can be diagnosed early in life, before a woman can embark on pregnancy; however, in some women it may have become apparent only during pregnancy.

Many of the physiological changes of normal pregnancy tend to make the diagnosis of heart disease more difficult. The common symptoms and clinical findings discussed below should lead to suspicion of cardiac problems.

Maternal mortality Although sporadic fatalities will be seen in all forms of heart disease in pregnancy, maternal mortality is highest in conditions that lead to obstruction of blood flow, especially pulmonary blood flow. For example, Eisenmenger's syndrome, where maternal mortality is 30–50% (Morgan and Howitt 1965).

An elevation in pulmonary vascular resistance is seen in primary pulmonary hypertension associated with a maternal mortality of 40–50% (Morgan and Howitt 1965). In contrast, in women with Fallot's tetralogy, in which pulmonary vascular resistance is normal, the reported maternal mortality rate varies between 4% and 20%.

Fetal outcome The fetal outcome among mothers who have rheumatic heart disease during pregnancy is usually good, and there is very little difference between these mothers and those who do not suffer from the disease (Brickner et al 2000).

However, the babies are likely to be lighter at birth by about 200 g. In mothers with cyanotic congenital heart disease, the fetuses are generally growth restricted and fetal loss including abortion may be as high as 45%. The prevalence of congenital heart disease in infants whose mothers have congenital heart disease varies between 3% and 14% (Nora 1978 Whittemore et al 1982).

Management The most important factor in management is history taking. As far as possible, pregnant women with heart disease should be managed in a combined Obstetric/Cardiac clinic. As with all forms of medicine, history is the most important single factor in the assessment of a patient who may have heart disease.

The most common symptom of heart disease in pregnancy is breathlessness (Morley and Lim 1995). Some pregnant women do experience slight breathlessness during pregnancy which may not be due to a cardiac problem. It is therefore important to consider whether the woman suffered from breathlessness before she became pregnant. Syncope occurs in severe aortic stenosis, hypertrophic cardiomyopathy, Fallot's tetralogy and Eisenmenger's syndrome. It is also a feature of normal pregnancy. Chest pain may occur in severe aortic stenosis or, more commonly, in pregnancy with hypertrophic cardiomyopathy.

Physical signs Systolic murmur is common in pregnancy and problems may occur when they are present. The significant murmurs are:

- Pansystolic murmurs of ventricular septal defect, mitral regurgitation or tricuspid regurgitation
- Late systolic murmurs of mitral regurgitation, mitral valve prolapse or hypertrophic cardiomyopathy
- Ejection systolic murmur louder than grade 3/6 of aortic stenosis

- Ejection systolic murmurs that vary with respiration in pulmonary stenosis

Investigations Most diagnostic cardiovascular studies are non-invasive and can be conducted safely in pregnant women.

Common investigations

1) Chest radiography: It is not helpful in diagnosis of minor degrees of heart disease but will show typical changes in hemodynamically significant cardiac pathology. The benefit of diagnosing serious and potentially fatal cardiac disease far outweighs possible radiation risk.
2) Electrocardiography: T wave inversion in lead III, S–T segment changes and Q waves which are usually considered pathological, occur during normal pregnancy. Hence, electrocardiography helps in the diagnosis of dysrhythmias rather than structural abnormalities of the heart.
3) Echocardiograph: The majority of structural cardiac abnormalities can be detected by echocardiography. This is the investigation of choice in pregnancies as there is no radiation hazard and detailed information is available.
4) If indicated, right heart catheterisation can be performed with limited x-ray fluoroscopy. On rare occasions, it may be necessary to perform left heart catheterisation. Technetium^{99}-labelled albumin or red cells are used to evaluate ventricular function.

Preconceptional counselling is very important and a woman with significant heart disease may benefit from it before making the decision to become pregnant (Table 10.3). The American College of Obstetricians and Gynecologists (1992) has adopted the three-tiered classification according to risks for death during pregnancy. These risks may be used to help counsel women about conception.

General Management: Although a number of generalisations regarding management may be made, few women actually fit any regular pattern of cardiac disease. Thus, individualisation is essential for achieving optimum outcome.

It is preferable to provide management for a pregnant woman with a cardiac disease as a team, with a cardiologist and an anesthesiologist. Four concepts that affect management are emphasised by the American College of Obstetricians and Gynecologist (1992):

i) The 50% increase in blood volume and cardiac output by the early third trimester
ii) Further fluctuations in volume and cardiac output in the peripartum period
iii) A decline in systemic vascular resistance, reaching a nadir in the second trimester and then rising to 20% below normal by the late stages
iv) Hypercoagulability of special importance in women requiring anticoagulation in the non-pregnant state with coumarin derivatives

Labour and Delivery: In general, delivery should be accomplished vaginally unless there are obstetrical indications for a cesarean delivery. The impact of the hemodynamic adaptations of pregnancy on an ailing heart must be reduced and this can be done by the following measures.

- The pregnant cardiac patient in labour should be in the left lateral position and preferably even during delivery or shifted to the dorsal position at the time of delivery, thus reducing hemodynamic impairment.

Table 10.3: Risks for maternal mortality caused by various heart diseases (Cunningham et al 2001)

Cardiac Disorder	*Percentage*
Group 1 – Minimal Risk	0–1
Atrial septal defect	
Ventricular septal defect	
Patent ductus arteriosis	
Pulmonic or tricuspid disease	
Fallot's tetrology, corrected	
Bioprosthetic valve	
Mitral stenosis, NYHA Classification I & II	
Group 2 – Moderate Risk 2A	5–15
Mitral stenosis, NYHA Classification III & IV	
Aortic stenosis	
Aortic coarctation without valvular involvement	
Fallot's tetralogy uncorrected	
Previous myocardial infarction	
Marfan's syndrome, normal aorta	
Moderate Risk 2 B:	
Mitral stenosis with atrial fibrillation	
Artificial valve	
Group 3 – Major Risk	25–50
Pulmonary hypertension	
Aortic coarctation with valvular involvement	
Marfan's syndrome with aortic involvement	

- She should be provided with effective pain relief. During early labour, morphine 2–4 mg may be used; later if the patient is not on anticoagulants, an epidural analgesic can be administered by an experienced obstetric anesthesiologist. Many pregnant cardiac patients benefit from a double catheter epidural anesthesia technique. This method limits the extent of sympathetic blockade and its effect on intravascular volume pooling and blood pressure. Epidural narcotics, for example, morphine and fentanyl are preferred to epidural anesthetics when there is some degree of contraindication to epidural administration of local anesthetics—for example, in aortic stenosis, mitral stenosis, aortic coarctation, Marfan's syndrome with dilated aortic root or hypertrophic subaortic stenosis.
- Cardiac patients in labour should be monitored with pulse oximetry. Mild degrees of desaturation in labour need not be corrected. Pulmonary edema and an inability to tolerate labour may develop. The most important aspect of intrapartum care in a pregnant woman with cardiac disease is the control of the rate of intravenous fluid administration. Patients with congenital or acquired heart disease and with artificial prosthetic valves should have antibiotic prophylaxis to avoid subacute bacterial endocarditis.

The Antibiotic Treatment Recommended by the American Heart Association is as follows:

Antibiotic dosage: Aqueous crystalline

Penicillin G (2–4 million IM or IV) or ampicillin (1.0 g IM or IV) plus gentamycin (1.5 mg/kg, not to exceed 80 mg IM or IV) or streptomycin (1.0 g IM) as an initial dose to be given 30 minutes to an hour before the procedure. If gentamycin is used, administer a similar dose of gentamycin and penicillin (or ampicillin) every 8 hours for two additional doses. If streptomycin is used, administer a similar dose of streptomycin and penicillin (or ampicillin) every 12 hours for two additional dosages.

For women who are allergic to penicillin, vancomycin (1.0 g IV given over 30 minutes to 1 hour) plus streptomycin (1.0 g IM) at a single dose of these antibiotics given over 30 minutes to 1 hour before the procedure is probably sufficient but the same dose may be repeated after 12 hours. For patients with significantly compromised renal functions, it may be necessary to modify the dosage of antibiotics used. During prolonged procedures or in delayed healing, it may be necessary to provide additional doses of antibiotics.

Pregnant cardiac patients who are not on anticoagulants tend to develop thromboembolisation in the postpartum period. Relative immobilisation, pooling of blood in the lower extremities and alteration in coagulation and fibrinolysis that occur in peripartum combine to produce an environment that favours thrombus formation in the lower extremities. The risk of thromboembolisation is approximately 2% for patients with rheumatic heart disease. To prevent this serious complication, early ambulation should be initated shortly after delivery, pneumatic compression of the lower extremities should be performed or a prophylatic low dose heparin should be given during labour, delivery and the immediate postpartum period. Immediately after delivery, the uterus decreases markedly in size and ceases to obstruct the return circulation to the heart. Most of the blood contained in the uterine vessels is suddenly infused into systemic circulation. These two phenomena combine to increase the preload and, in a cardiac patient, may exceed the pumping ability of the heart, resulting in acute pulmonary edema. Patients with mild mitral stenosis and fixed cardiac output are at risk of this complication. To avoid this, the patient should be placed in a sitting position after delivery. This will increase venous pooling in the lower extremities and decrease the venous return to the heart. Normally, after delivery, oxytocin is given to make the uterus contract. In a patient with cardiac disease, oxytocin should not be administered as a bolus as it may cause a sudden drop in peripheral vascular resistance and produce hypotension. In addition, ergot alkaloids should not be used in cardiac patients as they cause significant vasoconstriction and elevation of blood pressure.

Vital signs should be taken frequently between contractions. Increase in pulse rate above 100 per minute or a respiratory rate above 24 breaths, particularly when associated with dyspnea, may suggest impending ventricular failure. With any evidence of cardiac decompensation, intensive medical management must be instituted immediately.

Valvular Heart Disease

Rheumatic fever is becoming rare in parts of the country, but is still encountered very often in other areas. During epidemics of streptococcal pharyngitis, as many as 3% of untreated young adults may develop rheumatic fever.

Mitral Stenosis Rheumatic endocarditis causes three-fourths of the cases of mitral stenosis. As a result, blood flow from the left atrium to the ventricle is impeded. If mitral stenosis is tight, dilatation of the left atrium may be seen and the left atrial pressure is clinically elevated. This could result in significant passive pulmonary hypertension and fixed cardiac output leading to ventricular failure and pulmonary edema. About 25% of women have cardiac failure for the first time during pregnancy (Caulin-Glaser and Setaro 1999). The surface area of the normal mitral valve is 4.0 cm^2. Due to stenosis, there is narrowing of this valve and, if this progresses to less than 2.5 cm^2, the patient may become symptomatic and present with dyspnea due to pulmonary venous hypertension and pulmonary edema. The patient may also complain of fatigue, palpitation, cough and hemoptysis.

Management

i) Limited physical activity
ii) If symptoms of pulmonary congestion develop, dietary sodium should be restricted and the patient started on diuretics
iii) Beta blocker can be given to slow the heart rate in response to activity and anxiety
iv) In cases of atrial fibrillation, IV Verampil 5–10 mg should be given or the electrocardio version must be admnistered. For chronic fibrillation, digoxin, a beta blocker or a calcium channel blocker can be given to slow ventricular response. Anticoagulants such as heparin can also be given.

Mitral Valve Prolapse: This is caused by the presence of a pathological connective tissue disorder termed myxomatus degeneration, which involves the mitral valve leaflets, the annulus or the chordae tendinae.

Women with mitral valve prolapse are usually asymptomatic and are diagnosed by routine physical examination or echocardiography. The few who are symptomatic complain of palpitation, dyspnea, atypical chest pain, anxiety and syncope. Pregnant women with mitral valve prolapse rarely have cardiac complications. Pregnancy-induced hypervolemia may improve the alignment of the mitral valve (Rayburn et al 1987) when symptomatic beta blockers are used; but when mitral valve prolapse is associated with regurgitation, it is considered a significant risk factor for the development of bacterial endocarditis, and antibiotic prophylaxis must be administered.

Mitral Insufficiency: This develops when improper coaptation of mitral valve leaflets during systole leads to left ventricular dilatation and hypertrophy.

Etiology

Rheumatic fever, mitral valve prolapse, left ventricular dilatation of any etiology such as dilated cardiomyopathy, mitral valve vegetation—known as Libman-Sacks endocarditis, which is common in women with antiphosphospholipid antibodies—coexisting with systemic lupus erythematosus (Roldan et al 1996) may cause mitral insufficiency. Mitral regurgitation is well tolerated during pregnancy due to decreased systemic vascular resistance. Prophylaxis against bacterial endocarditis is required in labour.

Aortic Stenosis: Aortic valve stenosis is a disease of ageing and if present at a younger age, is usually congenital. It is caused by bicuspid valve stenosis, resulting in a systolic pressure gradient between the left ventricle and the systemic arterial outflow tract.

First, left ventricular hypertrophy occurs and the end diastolic pressure becomes elevated. A decline in ejection fraction and reduced cardiac output is observed, after which heart failure and sudden death occur. Mild-to-moderate stenosis is well tolerated in pregnancy, while severe aortic stenosis is extremely dangerous. For asymptomatic patients, close observation is advocated while in severe conditions, valve replacement or valvotomy using cardio pulmonary bypass should be considered.

During labour, these patients should be monitored preferably with pulmonary artery catheterisation; patients with aortic stenosis are dependent on adequate end diastolic ventricular filling pressure to maintain cardiac output and systemic perfusion. Sudden decrease in end diastolic volume may result in hypotension, syncope, myocardial infarction and sudden death. Hence, for these women, maintaining adequate intravascular volume is important during labour. The labour analgesic of choice is a narcotic epidural analgesic, which helps to avoid hazardous hypotension. Bacterial endocarditis prophylaxis is given at delivery and prophylactic forceps are used.

Aortic Insufficiency: Aortic regurgitation is the diastolic flow of blood from the aorta into the left ventricle.

Etiology

Rheumatic fever, connective tissue abnormalities and congenitally acquired lesions are some of the probable causes of the condition. In Marfan's syndrome, the aortic root is dilated resulting in insufficiency. Aortic and mitral valve insufficiency have been linked to appetite suppressants fenfluramine and dexfenfluramine (Gardin et al 2000). Symptoms require treatment for heart failure which includes bed rest, sodium restriction and use of diuretics. Epidural analgesia is preferred for vaginal or cesarean delivery and bacterial endocarditis prophylaxis is given.

Congenital Heart Disease: Most babies born with congenital heart disease require cardiac catheterisation or surgery. Otherwise, they invariably die within the first year. The remaining require surgery in childhood and 85% survive to adulthood (Moodie 1994).

According to Nugent et al (1990), the more common lesions at birth are ventricular septal defect (28%), pulmonary stenosis (10%), patent ductus arteriosis (8%), arterial septal defect (7%), aortic stenosis (4%) and coarctation of the aorta (4%).

Mendelson and Lang (1995) have divided the congential heart lesions complicating pregnancy into three groups:

i) Volume overload or left-to-right shunts: Arterial septal defects, ventricular septal defects
ii) Pressure overload: Aortic and pulmonary stenosis, coarctation of the aorta, hypertrophic subaortic stenosis
iii) Cyanotic lesions or right-to-left shunts: Fallot's tetralogy, Eisenmenger'a syndrome.

Other Cardiovascular Conditions

1) Pulmonary hypertension and high pulmonary blood pressure may be secondary to cardiac or pulmonary disease. Primary pulmonary hypertension can be idiopathic or caused by antiphospholipid antibodies. Maternal mortality is high whether pulmonary hypertension is primary or secondary in severe cases but the mild-to-moderate types tolerate pregnancy, labour and delivery (Weiss et al 1998).
2) Peripartum cardiomyopathy: This is a diagnosis of exclusion and is similar to dilated cardiomyopathy occurring in non-pregnant adults. The review panel from the National Heart, Lung and Blood Institute concluded that the

disease is an acute condition rather than a pre-existing one preceding pregnancy. Chronic hypertension with superimposed pre-eclampsia is a common cause of heart failure during pregnancy.

Women with cardiomyopathy present with the signs and symptoms of congestive heart failure—dyspnea, orthopnea, cough, palpitation and chest pain. Cardiomegaly may be present; echocardiographic and Doppler studies show increased end diastolic dimensions, an ejection fraction <45% and/or fractional shortening of <30% (Hibbard et al 1996). Management consists of treatment for heart failure, restriction of sodium intake and use of diuretics to reduce preload. Afterload is accomplished with hydralazine or other vasodilators. Digoxin is given unless complex arrhythmias are observed. Low dose heparin is recommended to prevent pulmonary embolism.

Surgeries for Heart Disease in Pregnancy

Valvular heart disease is the most common indication for cardiovascular surgery during pregnancy (Parry and Westaby 1966, Brady and Duff 1989; Weiss et al 1998, Mahli et al 2000). Cardiac surgery can be performed during pregnancy with relative safety for the mother, with a maternal mortality rate of 3%–6% and a fetal mortality rate of 20%–30%. Maternal deaths were reported in 9% of valvular surgical procedures and in 22% of aortic dissection repairs and pulmonary embolectomies. The current recommendation for open heart surgery during pregnancy includes:

- Avoidance of open heart surgery, if possible, during the first trimester. The risk of teratogenesis due to drug administration, and possible cardiopulmonary bypass during the first trimester of pregnancy is always present
- Use of high flow, high pressure, normothermic bypass during the procedure
- Fetal heart and uterine monitoring to allow adjustments to blood flow and pharmacological manipulation to ensure adequate placental perfusion
- If the fetus is >28 weeks of gestational age, to opt for cesarean section concurrently prior to cardiac operation

References

Banow RO, B Carabello, AC de Leon Jr et al. 1998. Guidelines for the management of patients with valvular heart disease. Executive Summary – A report of the American College of Cardiology American Heart Association Task Force on Practice Guidelines (Committee on management of patients with valvular heart disease) *Circulation* 98:1949–84.

Bitsch M, C Johansen, A Wennevold and M Osler. 1989. Maternal heart disease. A survey of a decade in a Danish university hospital. *Acta Obstet Gynecol Scand* 68:119.

Brady K amd P Duffy. 1989. Rheumatic heart disease in pregnancy. *Clin Obstet Gynecol* 32: 21–40.

Brickner ME, LD Hillis and RA Lange. 2000. Congenital heart disease in adults Part I. *N Eng J Med* 342:256.

Caulin-Glaser T and JF Setaro. 1999. Pregnancy and cardiovascular disease. In *Medical complications during pregnancy*, 5th ed, 111, eds Burrow GN and Duffy P. Philadelphia: Saunders.

Cunningham FG, JA Pritchard, GDV Hankins, PL Anderson, MK Lucas and KF Amstrong. 1986. Idiopathic cardiomyopathy or compounding cardiovascular events. *Obstet Gynecol* 67:157.

Cunningham GF, NF Gant, KJ Leveno et al. 2001. Cardiovascular disease, *Williams Obstetrics*. 21st ed; 182.

Gardin J, D Schumacher, G Constantine, KD David, C Leung and CL Reid. 2000. Valvular abnormalities and cardiovascular status following exposure to dexfenfluramine or phenteramine/ fenfluramine. *JAMA* 283:1703.

Hibbard JU, M Lindheimer and RM Lang. 1996. A modified definition for peripartum cardiomyopathy and prognosis based on echocardiography. *Obstet Gynecol* 94:311.

Mahli A, S Izdes and D Coskun. 2000. Cardiac operations during pregnancy: review of factors influencing fetal outcome. *Ann Thorac Surg* 69:1622–1626.

Maroo A and R Raymond. 2003. *Pregnancy and heart disease*. The Cleveland Clinic Foundation.

Mendelson MA and RH Lang. 1995. Pregnancy and Heart disease. In *Medical disorder during pregnancy*, 2nd ed, 129, eds Barnes WM and MD Lindhermer. St.Louis: Mosby Yearbook.

Meyer NL, B Mercer, A Khoury and B Sibai. 1994. Pregnancy complicated by cardiac disease: maternal and perinatal outcome. *J Mat Fetal Med* 3:31.

Moodie D. 1994. Adult congenital heart disease. *Curr Opin Cardiol* 9:137.

Morgan Jones A and G Howitt. 1965. EisenMenger Syndrome in Pregnancy. *Br Med J* I:1627–1631.

Morley CA and BA Lim. 1995. The risk of delay in diagnosis of breathlessness in pregnancy. *Br Med J* 311:1083–1084.

Nora JJ. 1978. The evolution of specific genetic and environmental counselling in congenital heart disease. *Circulation* 57:205–213.

Nugent EW, WH Planter, JE Edwards and WH William. 1990. The pathology, abnormal physiology, clinical recognition and medical and surgical treatment of congenital heart disease. In *The Heart*, 7th ed, 655, eds Hurst JW, RC Schland, CE Rackley, EH Sonnenblick and NK Wenger. New York: McGraw Hill.

Parry AJ and S Westaby. 1966. Cardiopulmonary bypass during pregnancy. *Ann Thorac Surg* 61: 1865–1869.

Pearson GD, JC Veille, S Rahimtoola, J Hsia, CM Oakley, JD Hosenpud, A Ansari and KL Baughman. 2000. Peripartum Cardiomyopathy. National Heart, Lung and Blood Institute and Office of Rare Diseases (National Institute of Health Workshop Recommendations and Review) *JAMA* 283:1183.

Rayburn WF, MS LeMire, JL Bird and AJ Buda. 1987. Mitral valve prolapse: echocardiographic changes during pregnancy. *J Reprod Med* 32:185.

Roldan CA, BK Shively and MH Crawford. 1996. An echocardiographic study of valvular heart disease associated with systemic lupus erythematosus. *N Engl J Med* 335:1424.

Tan J and M de Swiet. 1998. Prevalance of heart disease diagnosed de novo in pregnancy in a West London population. *Br J Obstet Gynaecol* 105:1185.

Weiss BM, L Zemp, B Seifert, OM Hess. 1998. Outcome of pulmonary vascular disease in pregnancy: a systemic overview from 1978 through 1996. *J Am Coll Cardiol* 31:1650.

Weiss BM, LK von Segesser, E Alon, B Seifert and MI Turna. 1998. Outcome of cardiovascular surgery and pregnancy: a systematic review of the period 1984–1966. *Am J Obstet Gynecol* 179: 1643–1653.

Whittemore R, JC Hobbins and MA Engle. 1982. Pregnancy and its outcome in women with and without surgical treatment of congenital heart disease. *Am J Cardiol* 50:641.

11

Liver Disease in Pregnancy

Narayanan R

Pregnancy does not change the size of the liver. In the third trimester, the enlarging uterus displaces the liver superiorly and posteriorly. Therefore, a palpable liver suggests significant hepatomegaly and underlying liver disease. Hepatosplenomegaly should be absent in a normal pregnancy, but because examination of the abdomen may be difficult when the uterus is gravid, the condition may be difficult to detect. Some peripheral edema is also common during pregnancy, as are some findings that usually connote chronic liver disease, such as telangiectasia, particularly on the chest, back and face, and palmar erythema, which occurs in up to 60% of normal pregnant women but disappears after delivery. These findings are signs of high circulating estrogen levels. Liver biopsies performed during uncomplicated pregnancies reveal no pathological changes.

The anatomical and physiological changes that accompany pregnancy alter physical findings and liver biochemistry. Yet, normal pregnancy does not significantly affect liver metabolism or function. The pregnant state is usually mildly cholestatic because of the increase in endogenous estrogens.

In an uncomplicated pregnancy, many laboratory test results may appear abnormal according to standards derived from a non-pregnant population. Pregnancy does not alter the expected values for serum bilirubin, aminotransferases, glutamyl transpeptidase, nucleotidase or prothrombin time. During pregnancy, the liver's metabolic, synthetic and excretory functions are affected by the increased serum estrogen and progesterone. Serum albumin concentration decreases during pregnancy and reaches its nadir towards the end of pregnancy, secondary to an increase in plasma volume. Alkaline phosphatase activity is increased during the third trimester, both because of leakage of placental alkaline phosphatase into the maternal circulation and because of increased maternal bone turnover. Because of this lack of specificity, alkaline phosphatase activity is a poor test for the diagnosis of cholestasis during the third trimester of pregnancy. Serum transaminase levels are within normal values during pregnancy. Increase in transaminase levels was found during labour and is, most probably, secondary to leakage from the contracting uterine muscle. Serum levels of Upsilon-glutamyl-transferase (UpsilonGT) and 5' nucleotidase are normally unchanged. Total and free bilirubin serum levels are lower in pregnancy because of hemodilution and low albumin concentration (albumin being the protein that transports bilirubin).

Liver disease is a rare complication of pregnancy, but when it occurs, it may do so in a dramatic and tragic fashion for both mother and infant. Diseases such as acute fatty liver of pregnancy (AFLP) may begin innocuously with mild symptoms and liver enzyme abnormalities, but, if left untreated, can progress to jaundice, liver failure and even death. Liver diseases occurring during pregnancy can be divided into three categories:

- liver diseases unique to pregnancy
- acute liver disease coincident with pregnancy
- pregnancy occurring in a patient with established chronic liver disease.

LIVER DISEASES UNIQUE TO PREGNANCY

Hyperemesis Gravidarum

Hyperemesis gravidarum is characterised by nausea and vomiting; in severe cases, it may lead to dehydration and malnutrition. It generally occurs during the first trimester of pregnancy, although it may also appear as late as the 20th week. Abnormal liver enzyme values have been reported in up to 50% of women hospitalised for hyperemesis. Mild hyperbilirubinemia (a bilirubin value of less than 4 mg/dl) with elevations in both direct and indirect fractions have been found in half the women hospitalised for this condition. Alkaline phosphatase may be elevated to twice the normal value, and aminotransferase values can rise to as much as 200 U/l. On biopsy, the liver tissue either appears normal or has fatty changes. The mechanism of hyperbilirubinemia is unknown, but the condition is probably related to malnutrition and impaired excretion of bilirubin, because laboratory test results show that the values return to normal within days after resumption of adequate nutrition and restoration of fluid balance. Genetic predisposition and high circulating levels of estrogens are thought to be causative factors. The mean birth weight of babies born to women with severe hyperemesis gravidarum (defined as a loss of more than 5% of body weight) is significantly lower than that of the offspring of women with mild hyperemesis gravidarum.

Pregnancy Toxemias and the HELLP Syndrome

In severe pre-eclampsia or eclampsia, liver involvement can be detected by abdominal tenderness and abnormal liver biochemistry. Jaundice is uncommon. Hepatocellular necrosis can occur from endothelial damage and platelet and fibrin deposition in the sinusoids. The characteristic epigastric or substernal pain called pre-eclamptic angina is attributed to hepatic subcapsular stretching. Subcapsular hematoma and hepatic rupture rarely develop.

The HELLP syndrome (hemolysis, elevated liver enzymes, low platelets) is usually associated with 5–10% of pre-eclampsia; occasionally, it may arise in the absence of either hypertension or proteinuria. The precise cause remains unclear, but vascular endothelial damage plays a pivotal role. Liver complications are similar to those in pre-eclampsia. Aspartate amino transferase (serum glutamic oxalocetic transaminase or AST (SGOT)) above 50 IU/l and lactic dehydrogenase above 180 IU/l with a low platelet count and hemolysis confirm the diagnosis of HELLP. Differentiation of AFLP from the HELLP syndrome may be clinically difficult, but the treatment—prompt delivery and supportive care—is identical for both. Maternal mortality may be as high as 25%, occurring as a result of cerebral hemorrhage, cardiopulmonary arrest, disseminated intravascular coagulation (DIC), adult respiratory distress syndrome, pulmonary edema, renal failure, sepsis, hepatic hemorrhage or encephalopathy.

Intrahepatic Cholestasis of Pregnancy

Intrahepatic cholestasis of pregnancy accounts for 20–25% of cases of jaundice during pregnancy. The cause is unknown. There is a clear genetic predisposition, which is likely to show autosomal dominance. The non-childbearing women affected by this condition may develop pruritis while taking the oral contraceptive pill, or cyclical pruritis related to menstruation. The cholestasis (failure of bile formation) represents an exaggerated response of the liver to the normal increase in endogenous estrogens during pregnancy.

Clinical Features: Presentation is typically in the third trimester with insidious onset of pruritus. In half of these patients, jaundice follows. Other cholestatic features include dark urine and, occasionally, pale stool. Otherwise, women generally feel well, without nausea, vomiting or abdominal pain. Serum alkaline phosphatase and cholesterol may rise, but aminotransferases are likely to be only modestly elevated. Ultrasound and cholangiography are normal. The evaluation of a pregnant woman with cholestasis involves excluding other causes of jaundice and pruritus including viral hepatitis, primary biliary cirrhosis and biliary tract disease by appropriate laboratory and ultrasound investigations. Liver biopsy, which shows only cholestasis without inflammation, may be necessary in some atypical cases.

Management: Although a benign condition for the mother (other than the inexorable pruritus), intrahepatic cholestasis may decrease fetal survival and increase the risk of prematurity. Treatment is supportive with bile salt-binding agents such as cholestyramine. Ursodeoxycholic acid therapy improves bile formation, perhaps washing out 'toxic' bile acids and pruritogenic agents. S-adenosylmethionine, which alters membrane fluidity, and rifampin, which increases the excretion of pruritogenic agents, also work. Treatment for cholestasis and pruritus is, however, generally unsatisfactory. Delivery should occur as soon as fetal lung maturity is documented, to prevent the increased risk of stillbirth. Parenteral vitamin K may be needed to correct a prothrombin deficiency. Early delivery by 37–38 weeks has been shown to reduce fetal mortality.

Symptoms usually abate within two weeks of delivery. There is a significant risk of recurrence with subsequent pregnancies and with the use of oral contraceptives or other estrogens.

Acute Fatty Liver of Pregnancy

Acute fatty liver of pregnancy is characterised by fatty infiltration of the liver. It may rapidly progress to hepatic failure and death. Acute fatty liver may be uncommon (one in 13,000 deliveries), but should be given due importance, being associated with a maternal mortality rate of 18% and fetal mortality rate of 23%. The cause is unknown, but the microvesicular fat that accumulates in hepatocytes probably represents disordered intermediary fat metabolism, perhaps related to mitochondrial injury.

Clinical Features: Acute fatty liver of pregnancy almost invariably presents in the third trimester, with a peak frequency around 36–37 weeks of gestation. Occasionally, it will become apparent only after delivery. Association with nulliparity, twin gestations, male fetus and pre-eclampsia or eclampsia has also been observed. Presentation can vary from nonspecific symptoms to fulminant hepatic failure. Nausea and vomiting, with or without abdominal pain, are common. Examination may reveal a tender liver. Pruritus is uncommon and would suggest the possibility of a different liver problem such as intrahepatic cholestasis of pregnancy. Progressive hepatic failure then rapidly supervenes, with the development of jaundice, generalised bleeding from coagulopathy, hypoglycemia, hepatic encephalopathy and renal failure. Such severe cases have an inexorable downhill course unless the fetus is delivered; even so, deterioration may continue for a further 48–72 hours.

Laboratory features include a moderately elevated aminotransferase, which is usually around 300 IU/l but may range from normal (N = 5 – 60 IU/l) to 1000 IU/l. The amenotransferases are normally present in low concentration, usually less than 40 IU/l. Plasma levels up to 300 IU/l are non-specific and may be seen in a number of hepatic diseases. Alkaline phosphatase and serum bilirubin are elevated. Liver biopsy reveals tiny droplets of fat (microvesicular fat) inside the hepatocytes.

Diagnosis: Diagnosis requires a high degree of suspicion, as the presentation is often nonspecific. Acute fatty liver of pregnancy should be considered whenever marked nausea and vomiting develop in the third trimester of pregnancy. Suspicion increases with a twin pregnancy, nulliparity or signs of toxemia. Ultrasound or CT scan may detect the presence of increased fat in the liver and help exclude complications such as a subcapsular hematoma or some other entity such as choledocholithiasis. Liver biopsy is diagnostic. Biopsy, even through the transvenous route (necessary when a coagulopathy makes percutaneous liver biopsy hazardous), should be done if the results will alter management. For example, differentiation of acute viral hepatitis from acute fatty liver is important to determine whether rapid delivery is indicated. Delivery can be lifesaving in acute fatty liver.

Management: Management involves aggressive supportive care. The only definitive treatment for the condition is prompt delivery. The risk of acute fatty liver of pregnancy is not increased in subsequent pregnancies.

LIVER DISEASE INCIDENTAL TO PREGNANCY

Viral Hepatitis

a) Hepatitis A: The incidence of acute hepatitis A (HAV) during pregnancy is no different from that of the acute infection in the specific geographic area.

The clinical presentation, disease course, treatment and sequela are similar to those of non-pregnant patients except that pruritus is more common due to the high estrogen state. Perinatal transmission is most probably secondary to horizontal transmission at the time of delivery. Both the inactivated vaccine against HAV and the postexposure immunoglobulin prophylaxis are safe in pregnancy.

b) Hepatitis B: Hepatitis B (HBV) is a double-stranded, enveloped, DNA virus, which is highly infectious and transmitted parenterally by percutaneous or mucosal exposure, sexually, and from the mother to the infant. The clinical presentation and course of the disease are similar to that of non-pregnant infected individuals. Diagnosis of acute HBV infection is made by detecting the HBV surface antigen (HBsAg) in the serum, and confirmed by the presence of IgM antibodies to HBV core antigen (HBcAg). Hepatitis e (envelope) antigen is present in almost all acute infections and represents high infectivity. As long as HBsAg is present, the individual is infectious. As the anti-HBe antibody develops, infectivity decreases. Acute HBV complicates about 1–2 of every 1000 pregnancies.

If acute maternal infection occurs in the first trimester and resolves, the risk of neonatal infection is minimal. In contrast, an infection during the second and third trimesters poses a threat of 10% and 90%, respectively, for vertical transmission. Most perinatal transmission occurs intrapartum (95%). Intrauterine infection is rare. The risk factors for intrauterine transmission are maternal serum HBeAg positivity, history of threatened preterm labour and presence of HBV in the placenta. A child born to an HBeAg-positive mother has a 70%–90% chance of being infected. A child infected with HbeAg at birth has a 90% chance of progressing to chronic infection, while an infection between 7 and 12 months progresses to chronicity in 40% of cases. Only 10–20% of cases of the infection occurred between 1 and 3 years of age. The presence of HBsAg in pregnant women does not pose an additional risk for the pregnancy and its outcome. Since 1991, a recommendation to vaccinate individuals in high-risk groups, such as children born to HBsAg-negative mothers (with an addition of immunoprophylaxis with HBV immunoglobulin for children of HBsAg-positive mothers) has been followed. The vaccine is safe to use in pregnancy. Passive and active immunisations, given together, are very effective in preventing neonatal transmission and in reducing the carrier state of infants born to HBeAg/HBsAg-positive-women from 70–90% to almost 0%.

With proper immunoprophylaxis, breastfeeding of infants by chronic HBV carrier women poses no additional risk factor for the transmission of the HBV virus.

c) Hepatitis C: Hepatitis C (HCV) is an enveloped, single-stranded RNA virus. It is less common than HBV, but HCV infection becomes chronic in a larger proportion of cases (80%). Percutaneous transmission accounts for at least 60% of cases; others may have no identifiable risk factors. To date, childhood acquisition of HCV infection through maternal–infant transmission has become the most important mode of spread. The prevalence of detectable HCV antibodies in pregnant women is 1% overall (range 0.1–2.4%), which is not very different from that in the general age-matched population. Approximately two-thirds may be expected to have an active infection with detectable serum HCV RNA. Different studies have drawn different conclusions regarding the effect of pregnancy on chronic infection with HCV. The data from these studies is inconsistent and currently no definitive conclusion can be drawn. To date, HCV is not considered a contraindication for pregnancy. Since HCV RNA levels fluctuate during pregnancy, they should be measured in the third trimester. This is because the first trimester levels may not be representative or predictive of HCV RNA concentrations at the time of delivery. Chronic infection with HCV does not have an adverse effect on the pregnancy and its outcome. Since passive transmission of IgG antibodies to HCV takes place through the placenta, the presence of detectable anti-HCV antibodies in the newborn does not mean that a perinatal infection has occurred. Detectable anti-HCV antibodies in infants more than 18 months old or detectable HCV RNA in infants 3–6 months old can indicate mother-to-infant transmission of the infection. If the mother is viremic with detectable HCV RNA, the transmission rate reaches 4.3%. The higher the viral load, the greater the likelihood of transmission. Co-infection with HIV significantly increases the risk of HCV transmission, which is 19.4% in co-infected mothers, when compared to a much lower risk of transmission in mothers with HCV alone. Antiretroviral treatment for HIV during pregnancy results in a decrease in the rate of HCV transmission, to the levels of women who are not co-infected with HIV. The HCV genotype has no effect on transmission. Amniocentesis or fetal blood monitoring through the scalp vein catheter is considered a relative contraindication during pregnancies of mothers with HCV infection. The type of delivery (cesarean versus vaginal) does not seem to influence the rate of mother-to-infant transmission. Although the HCV virus can be detected in breast milk and the colostrum, breastfeeding is not considered a risk factor for HCV transmission. Treatment of HCV infection with alpha-interferon and ribavirin is contraindicated during pregnancy. Alpha-interferon is contraindicated in children under the age of two years because of severe neurotoxicity and ribavirin is teratogenic. Screening of all prospective mothers is still not indicated. However, screening of high-risk groups such as HIV-positive women, women with previous or current use of injection drugs or current or previous sex partners known to use injection drugs, women who received blood transfusions and those from certain geographic areas may be advantageous. The outcome of perinatally infected children is still not clear. Several studies have demonstrated spontaneous clearance of HCV within 6–24 months of age. It is still to be investigated whether HCV acquired through mother-to-infant transmission is different from transfusion-related HCV and adult onset HCV.

d) Hepatitis D: Hepatitis D (HDV) is a single-stranded, circular RNA virus, which depends on the presence of the HBV virus for its replication. One of the main routes of transmission is from the mother to the infant. Co-infection with HBV and HDV causes a more severe disease, with a much higher chronicity rate (70%–80% of infected patients will develop cirrhosis), and a much more rapid course of disease. The measures used to prevent HBV infection are also effective against HDV.

e) Hepatitis E: Hepatitis E (HEV) is a non-enveloped, single-stranded RNA virus. It is endemic in developing countries and is associated with the same route of transmission, risk factors and chronicity rate as HAV. During pregnancy, HEV can cause fulminant hepatitis indistinguishable from AFLP. There is a significant mortality rate of 16% in pregnant women with acute HEV infection. Transmission occurs intrapartum and peripartum through close contact between the mother and the neonate. Evidence suggests significant vertical transmission rates among HEV RNA–positive mothers of up to 50%. Among women with symptomatic infection, the rate of transmission is up to 100%, with significant perinatal morbidity and mortality.

PREGNANCY IN WOMEN WITH PRE-EXISTING LIVER DISEASE

Effect of Pregnancy on Pre-existing Liver Disease

Pregnancy is unusual in patients with chronic liver disease. Fertility becomes nearly normal when cirrhosis is well compensated or the active liver disease improves with appropriate therapy (as in autoimmune hepatitis on steroids). The degree of hepatic impairment determines the risk for the mother during pregnancy. Hemorrhage from esophageal varices is the most significant complication of cirrhosis in pregnancy. The increased blood volume and flow through the azygous system that are a part of any normal pregnancy raise the pressure in the esophageal veins; in established cirrhosis, this increases variceal size and the likelihood of bleeding.

Pre-existing chronic liver disease requires careful monitoring of the patient for worsening disease, as well as monitoring of the developing fetus. Most often, women with pre-existing liver disease are able to carry the fetus safely to term.

Autoimmune Chronic Active Hepatitis

Flare-up of chronic active liver disease (CALD) has been reported during pregnancy. However, it is not clear whether the flare-ups of CALD have actually been induced by pregnancy, since autoimmune hepatitis is a disorder characterised by exacerbations and remissions. The drugs used to treat CALD—for example, prednisone and azathioprine—may be used during pregnancy without adverse effects on the fetus. However, pregnant women who have CALD (with or without therapy) have a higher incidence of both stillbirths and delivery of premature infants.

Chronic Viral Hepatitis

There is little evidence that pregnancy influences the clinical course of either chronic active or chronic persistent viral hepatitis. Sometimes, worsening of chronic hepatitis B and hepatitis C has been reported.

Primary Biliary Cirrhosis (PBC)

Pregnancy often leads to an increase in the biochemical parameters of cholestasis in women with primary biliary cirrhosis. After delivery, these abnormalities return to their pre-pregnant values. Clinically, PBC does not exhibit an accelerated course during pregnancy. Since PBC tends to occur in older women, PBC and pregnancy are not often seen as concomitant problems in the same patient.

Cirrhosis

Cirrhotic women may sustain a normal pregnancy without any worsening of hepatic function. However, women with cirrhosis are less fertile and have higher rates of both stillbirths and premature infants. In addition, cases of worsening hepatic function, jaundice and hepatic failure have been reported in pregnant women with cirrhosis. Although intravascular blood volume may increase and esophageal varices may develop during pregnancy (even in normal women), it is not clear that the risk of variceal hemorrhage is increased during pregnancy in cirrhotic women. A history of variceal hemorrhage in one gestation does not indicate the same for subsequent pregnancies. The preferred modality for treating bleeding esophageal varices during pregnancy is endoscopic ligation or sclerotherapy.

Cholestatic Disorders

Patients with the Dubin–Johnson syndrome commonly demonstrate an elevation in conjugated bilirubin during pregnancy. On the other hand, patients with the Gilbert syndrome do not develop an increase in unconjugated bilirubin. Patients with the rare syndrome of benign recurrent intrahepatic cholestasis (BRIC) usually develop jaundice during pregnancy. In addition, unaffected relatives of patients with BRIC may develop cholestasis during pregnancy.

Wilson's Disease

Wilson's disease is a rare genetically transmitted disturbance in copper metabolism that leads to copper toxicity and death, usually before the age of 30. Women with this disorder should be maintained on 0.75–1 g/day of penicillamine during gestation. This dosage has not been associated with any untoward side effects in the newborn. Discontinuation of medication during pregnancy has been associated with worsening of the hepatic disease.

Hepatic Adenoma or Focal Nodular Hyperplasia

Both hepatic adenoma and focal nodular hyperplasia are common benign hepatic tumours. Although lesions have been reported to enlarge or rupture, this seems to be an extremely rare event.

References

Benjaminov FS and J Heathcote. 2004. Liver disease in pregnancy. *Amer J Gastro Enterol* 99:12, 2479–2485.

Berg B, G Helm, L Petersohn et al. 1986. Cholestasis in Pregnancy. *Acta Obst Gynecol Scand* 65: 107–113.

Cahill KM. 1962. Hepatitis in Pregnancy. *Surg Gynecol Obstet* 114:545–552.

Everson GT. 1998. Ob-Gyn interactive case challenge—liver disease in the third trimester of pregnancy. *Medscape Women Health* J 3(2).

Hilsden RJ and EA Shaffer. 1997. Liver disease in pregnancy. *First Principles of Gastroenterology* 14(17):552–570.

Hunt MD, M Christine, MD Sharare, I Ala. 1999. Liver disease in pregnancy. *Amer Fam Phys* 59:212–225.

Knox TA and LB Olans. 1996. Liver disease in pregnancy. *N Engl J Med* 335:569–576.

Lee WM. 1992. Pregnancy in patients with chronic liver disease. *Clin North Am* 21:889–903.

Riely CA. 1994. Hepatic disease in pregnancy. *Amer J Med* 9)1A):185–225.

Rinaldo P WR TReem, CA Riely et al. 1997. Liver disease in pregnancy. *N Engl J Med* 336:377–379.

12

Tropical Diseases in Pregnancy

Vanita Suri

Diseases that are prevalent in the hot and humid climate of the tropics and subtropics are called tropical diseases. These include a wide variety of infections which can be bacterial (for example, typhoid) or parasitic (for example, malaria). Most of these infections are endemic in India, which is a tropical country. Pregnancy leads to alteration in immunity, thus increasing the mother's susceptibility to infection. The choice of drugs available to treat these diseases is also limited due to fear of teratogenicity. Only those diseases that are commonly encountered during pregnancy and have an important bearing on maternal and fetal outcome are discussed in this chapter.

MALARIA

Malaria is the most important of the parasitic diseases of humans. It affects more than one billion people annually with 1–3 million deaths each year. Though it has been almost eradicated from North America, Europe and Russia, it is still a major problem in the tropics. About 90% of cases are reported each year in sub-Saharan Africa. In India, after the initial drop in incidence, the epidemiological situation has reached a plateau. Infants, young children and pregnant women have been identified as high-risk groups. Malaria is quite prevalent in the north-eastern states of India mainly because the topography and climatic conditions are favourable for malaria transmission. Among these states, Assam reports the maximum number of malaria cases followed by Arunachal Pradesh, Tripura and Meghalaya (Park 2002).

Etiology

Malaria is a protozoan infection caused by four species of Plasmodium, namely, *Plasmodium falciparum, Plasmodium vivax, Plasmodium malariae* and *Plasmodium ovale*. It is transmitted in humans by the bite of a certain species of infected female Anopheles mosquito. Malaria can also be acquired through blood transfusion, organ transplantation, use of contaminated needles or during parturition.

The saliva of the mosquito contains sporozoites, which immediately enter the hepatocytes where they change into exoerythrocytic forms. After a silent stage of approximately one week, merozoites are released from the liver, which invade red cells and then through further replication, lead to rupture of red blood cells. The merozoites of *Plasmodium falciparum* invade all red cells, leading to a higher degree of parasitemia, while the merozoites of *Plasmodium vivax* invade only young red cells and those of *Plasmodium malariae* only senescent red cells. The clinical features of malaria result from the damage to the red blood cells. The exoerythrocytic forms of

Plasmodium vivax and *Plasmodium ovale* can remain dormant in the liver for extended periods and thus cause relapse after many months.

Clinical Features

The clinical features of malaria manifest in three stages—cold, hot and sweating. The severity depends on the species of *Plasmodium*, the patient's state of immunity, intensity of infection (degree of parasitemia) and concomitant conditions like malnutrition or pregnancy. The symptoms begin with a flu-like prodrome followed by paroxysmal fever, rigor, abdominal pain, headache and bodyache. Fever may be continuous in *Plasmodium falciparum* infection. Other signs include intravenous hemolysis, anemia, thrombocytopenia, hepatomegaly and spleenomegaly. *Plasmodium falciparum* can also cause cerebral malaria, kidney failure, coma and death. During pregnancy, the blood flow in the placenta may be disrupted due to sequestration of red blood cells (Duffy 2003).

Effect of Pregnancy on Disease

Knowledge about malaria in pregnancy is derived from studies carried out in tropical Africa. Systematic studies from malaria endemic regions in India are few and have been carried out in Chandigarh (Sholapurker et al 1988), Surat, Gujarat (Nair et al 1993) and Jabalpur, Madhya Pradesh (Singh et al 1999). Prevalence of malaria in pregnancy is higher than in the normal groups (Singh et al 1999). The incidence increases three to fourfold during the second and third trimesters of pregnancy and in the immediate postpartum period (Diagne et al 2000). The parasite density is highest in the third trimester for both vivax and falciparum types (Sholapurker et al 1988).

Pregnancy increases susceptibility to malaria as well as its severity (Robier et al 1999). HIV infection can predispose the pregnant woman to higher incidence of malaria and increase its severity, thus affecting the fetus and the newborn (Whitty et al 2005). In endemic countries, this disease is more common in primigravidas, who also have a higher degree of parasitemia than the non-pregnant and multigravidas (Luzzi et al 1993). Malaria may mimic other disorders in pregnancy, thus delaying diagnosis and increasing maternal and fetal morbidity and mortality (Prien-Larsen et al 1993). Cerebral malaria is a common complication of severe *P. falciparum* infection with high mortality during pregnancy (Singh et al 1999). The increased prevalence and severity of malaria in pregnancy may be due to changes in cell-mediated immunity and antibody response during pregnancy (Mvondo et al 1992).

Effect of Disease on Pregnancy

In pregnant women, malaria affects the decidual vessels and placenta (Ismail et al 2000). It leads to increased incidence of abortion and preterm labour (Menendez et al 2000). Maternal malaria infection is the most important infectious cause of low birth weight in tropical Africa (Taha et al 1993) and similar results have been shown in the study conducted by Singh et al. It has been seen that pregnant women with falciparum malaria are more anemic than non-infected pregnant controls or infected non-pregnant women. Whether as a cause or a result, anemia is a definite contributor to low birth weight in newborns. The other cause is cytotrophoblastic thickening due to the malarial parasite. Many workers have shown that malaria leads to a decrease in maternal transfer of antibodies to the fetus, such as respiratory syncytial virus, *S. pneumoniae*, *H. influenzae* and tetanus (Brair et al 1994; Wesumperuna et al 1999).

Neonatal infection is less common. The incidence varies from 0.1% to 42%. Congenital malaria can occur in symptomatic as well as asymptomatic women. The incidence is low in immune mothers due to spontaneous clearing of infection by the transfer of IgG antibodies, but the incidence can be as high as 10% in non-immune mothers (Subramanian et al 1992). The neonates become symptomatic after 2–8 weeks of birth or symptoms may appear within a few hours of birth, simulating neonatal sepsis (Subramanian et al 1992). According to Hulbert's review (1992), neonates manifest with fever, anemia, hepatomegaly and spleenomegaly. Since it mimics other congenital infections, high index of suspicion is necessary for establishing diagnosis.

Diagnosis

Suspicion of malaria is aroused by epidemiological and clinical evidence. Blood smears help in making the diagnosis—thick smears optimise the chance of detection of parasite but cannot help identify the species; thin smears help in identifying the species and estimating the magnitude of infection. Since the malarial parasite localises in the placenta, placental blood smears can also demonstrate presence of the parasite and can assist in diagnosing congenital malaria.

The malarial fluorescent antibody test, which becomes positive after two weeks of primary infection is of great value in epidemiological studies. Antigen capture assay (dipstick) is the latest and one of the simplest diagnostic techniques used for the detection of *Plasmodium falciparum* (WHO 1986).

Treatment

Malaria needs to be treated immediately and intensively according to the National Malaria Eradication Programme (NMEP). The National Antimalaria Programme has recommended that any fever in endemic areas during transmission season without any other obvious cause may be considered as malaria and investigated and treated accordingly.

Chloroquine is the drug of choice during pregnancy for treatment of *P. vivax, P. malariae and P. ovale* infections; treatment varies according to the endemicity of the area (Park 2002). In high-risk areas, presumptive treatment is started on day 1 with chloroquine (600 mg) followed by the same dose on day 2 and half the dose on day 3. After confirmation of diagnosis, primaquine should be given for radical treatment in *P. vivax* infection. As primaquine is contraindicated during pregnancy, it should be reserved till after delivery. In chloroquine-resistant *P. falciparum* infection, single dose pyrimethamine/sulfadoxine combination is given if the patient is not near term, or oral quinine may be prescribed. Clindamycin is given if *P. falciparum* malaria was acquired in Southeast Asia because of the multidrug resistance of these strains (Panisko et al 1990). Mefloquine is a new drug that is active against chloroquine-resistant and multi-drug-resistant strains of *P. falciparum*. It has been safely used in pregnancy (Briggs et al 1998). In low-risk areas, presumptive treatment is started on day 1 with 600 mg of chloroquine and the same dose is repeated after 24 hours on confirmation of diagnosis. Primaquine, which should be given for radical cure, is contraindicated during pregnancy.

For severe and complicated malaria, the patient should be hospitalised. Parenteral quinine should be given. In the US, quinidine is given in place of quinine as the latter is not available (CDC). Though the drugs belong to classes C and D, respectively, the benefits to the mother and fetus outweigh the risk. In some Asian countries, Chinese drugs derived from artemisinin are being used as first line drugs for severe malaria. No reports are available regarding their safety during pregnancy. Exchange transfusion should be considered if parasitic load is very high (Wong et al 1992). Determining the safety and effectiveness of new antimalarials in pregnancy is required (Duffy et al 2005).

Chemoprophylaxis

Chemoprophylaxis appears to be of limited value in areas of endemic malaria, but still desirable in pregnant women living in high-risk areas to reduce maternal mortality from life-threatening complications of malaria and to decrease the incidence of low birth weight babies. WHO (1996) has recommended the use of effective and safe anti-malarial drugs during pregnancy to prevent the adverse effects of malaria on the mother, fetus and newborn, but NMEP in India does not endorse it. The Ministry of Health has permitted the treatment of febrile episodes only.

Chemoprophylaxis is recommended in pregnant women before travel to endemic areas. Chloroquine (300 mg) is given orally once a week, started 1–2 weeks before entering and continued till four weeks after leaving the endemic area (Bradley et al 1995). Pregnant women should be discouraged from traveling to areas known to have many cases of multi-drug-resistant *P. falciparum* infection (Briggs 1998). If it cannot be avoided, measures should be taken against mosquito bites in the form of protective clothing, mosquito nets and repellents. Mefloquine prophylaxis should be given after the first trimester (Nosten et al 1995).

A number of vaccines are under evaluation. A synthetic 'cocktail' vaccine for *Plasmodium falciparum* called SPF 66, developed by Dr M Patarroyo in Colombia has been field-tested and found to be effective (Olliaro et al 1996). Another vaccine PFS 25 has been clinically tried in the USA and in Africa.

AMEBIASIS

Amebiasis is an intestinal infection caused by the protozoan *Entamoeba histolytica.*

Its incidence is high in tropical countries such as Mexico and India and in tropical Asia and Africa. Infection is acquired by ingestion of cysts from contaminated water and food. Less common modes of transmission include oral and anal sexual practices. About 90% of patients remain asymptomatic; symptoms develop 2–6 weeks after ingestion of the cyst. Patients may manifest with abdominal pain and diarrhea or full-blown dysentery. Amebiasis may take a fulminent course during pregnancy with severe abdominal pain, high fever and profuse diarrhea. Prognosis is worse if liver abscess develops. Constantine et al have reported acute rupture of hepatic abscess during pregnancy. Routine stool identification of amebae cannot differentiate between *Entamoeba histolytica* and *Entamoeba dispar,* which is non-pathogenic. An antigen test can be used to distinguish *E. histolytica* from *E. dispar* where the clinical picture does not suggest invasive amebiasis and the stool specimen shows trophozoites of Entamoeba (Tanyuksel et al 2003).

Treatment

Metronidazole is the drug of choice. Large observational studies of women exposed to metronidazole during pregnancy and meta-analysis indicate that metronidazole does not increase the rate of birth defects (Burtin et al 1995). Tinidazole is another alternative in FDA Category C. A review in 1985 (Rao) indicated that tinidazole was similar to metronidazole in having low potential risk of teratogenicity. The safest approach would be to avoid the use of both metronidazole and tinidazole in the first trimester of pregnancy as far as possible. Paromomycin, though less effective, can be prescribed with reasonable safety during the first trimester (*Med Letter* 2004).

GIARDIASIS

Giardiasis is a common intestinal parasitic infection caused by *Giardia lamblia*. The transmission of *G. lamblia* occurs through contaminated water or food. It may be present in asymptomatic carriers or cause acute or chronic illness. The alteration in the immunological and gastric state may predispose the pregnant woman to symptomatic infection. It is associated with prolonged diarrhea which is more severe in pregnancy (Karen et al 1981). The drugs for treatment include metronidazole, tinidazole, quinacrine, paromomycin and nitazoxanide. Metronidazole and tinidazole should be avoided during the first trimester (Jones et al 2005). Paromomycin is recommended in such situations though it is less effective (Karen et al 1981).

COMMON HELMINTHIC DISEASES

Worm infestations are very common in tropical countries. These are closely related to the unavailability of potable water, inadequate disposal of human waste and warm and humid climate. These infections can lead to nutritional deficiency and thus cause anemia in pregnant women. If left untreated they can often lead to low birth weight babies (Christian et al 2005). Commonly isolated parasites during a study conducted in India among anemic pregnant women were *Ankylostoma duodenale*, *Ascaris lumbricoides*, *Taenia solium*, *Trichuris trichura* and *Entrobius vermicularis*. Other organisms were *E. histolytica* and *G. lamblia*.

Hookworm Disease

Infestation with *A. duodenale* or *Necater americanus*, known as hookworm disease, is commonly seen in a warm, moist climate in tropical and subtropical regions. Hookworm infection is widely prevalent in India. *N. americanas* is predominant in south India and *A. duodenale* in north India. The prevalence of hook worm infection in pregnant women in the rural plains of Nepal was found to be 78.8% (Navitsky et al 1998).

The hookworm enters the body (usually through the feet) by penetrating the skin. Ankylostoma can also be acquired by the oral route by direct ingestion of infective larvae through contaminated fruits and vegetables. This infection causes chronic blood loss leading to iron deficiency anemia. The worm lives in the jejunum where it attaches itself to the mucus membrane to feed and secrete an anticoagulant causing bleeding. It causes increased maternal morbidity, low birth weight babies, abortion, stillbirths and impaired lactation (Santiso 1997).

The prevention and control of hookworm infection includes sanitary disposal of feces, chemotherapy, correction of anemia and health education. Different drugs that can be used against this infection include albendazole, mebendazole, levamisole, pyrantel pamoate and bephenium hydroxy naphthoate. A single 500 mg dose of mebendazole combined with weekly iron doses is recommended in pregnancy for population coverage (Santiso 1997). As a rule, all drugs should be avoided during the first trimester.

Ascariasis

Ascariasis is the most common helminthic infestation. It is the infection of the small intestine caused by the roundworm *Ascaris lumbricoides* transmitted by the ingestion of food or drink contaminated with soil containing infective eggs. The infection may be asymptomatic or may manifest with nausea and/or abdominal pain. It is an important cause of nutritional deficiency and anemia in pregnancy. The larvae can migrate to the lungs causing pulmonary manifestations. Diagnosis is established by examination of stool. Treatment should be given in pregnancy only for symptomatic infection and intestinal obstruction by worms. Albendazole, mebendazole or pyrantel pamoate are the recommended drugs (Med Letter 2004). Albendazole and mebendazole are Class C drugs (FDA). As a rule, they should not be used in pregnancy. However, a few studies conducted in Sierra Leone and Sri Lanka have shown these drugs to be safe (De Silva et al 1999). The WHO has made the recommendation of giving a single dose oral anthelminthic to pregnant and lactating women. However, no drug should be given in the first trimester. The effect of pyrantel pamoate, which is used in ascariasis, has not been adequately studied in pregnancy.

Typhoid Fever

Typhoid fever is a systemic infection caused by a Gram-negative bacillus, *Salmonella typhi*. It occurs in all parts of the world where sanitation is substandard. Typhoid fever is now uncommon in developed countries but continues unabated in the developing countries of Africa, Asia and Latin America. Typhoid fever is endemic in India.

Typhoid fever is transmitted through the feco-oral route, urine-oral route, from respiratory secretions, vomitus or other body fluids. Following ingestion, the organisms penetrate the gastrointestinal tract in the duodenum and enter the bloodstream. From the liver, the organisms reach the bile where they multiply rapidly and re-enter the intestinal tract. The gall bladder is always infected and may be the source of infection in those who become typhoid carriers. Hemorrhage from ileal blood vessels and perforation may occur. Diarrhea is also associated. Fever is due to tissue endotoxin. It is remittent and is associated with headache, malaise and anorexia (Sadan et al 1986). Splenomegaly, relative bradycardia, stepwise fever and leukopenia are some of the important signs. Clinical suspicion of typhoid is confirmed by culturing blood for *Salmonella typhi* and performing the Widal test.

Typhoid fever poses a special risk to the pregnant mother and fetus. *S typhi* can cross the placenta thus affecting the fetus and causing fetal loss (Amster et al 1985). The incidence of typhoid fever in pregnancy was 1.28–2. 8% in the past. There has been a steady decline in its incidence because of the availability of effective antibiotics. Reports about this condition in pregnancy are scarce. Pregnancy generally does not alter the clinical picture or the laboratory findings of a patient with typhoid fever. In a study by Seoud et al (1988), relative bradycardia, which is often seen in patients, was absent in pregnant patients and the patients who received antipyretics had a hypothermic response, which is not seen commonly in non-pregnant patients. This sudden hypothermia can be dangerous for the fetus.

Early reports published before the development of effective chemotherapy indicated increased maternal mortality rates and increased incidence of premature labour and spontaneous abortions in patients with typhoid fever (Amster et al 1985). Currently, it is believed that with early diagnosis and prompt treatment there is no increase in maternal mortality and fetal morbidity.

The proposed treatment for typhoid fever in pregnancy is use of ampicillin or amoxicillin for 2–3 weeks. Ciprofloxacin has been used in multi-drug–resistant enteric fever in seven patients by Koul et al (1995) without any effect on the neonates.

Leishmaniasis

The term Leishmaniasis refers to various clinical syndromes caused by the protozoa of the genus Leishmania. It is endemic in the tropics, subtropics and southern Europe. Visceral leishmeniasis (kala azar) is commonly seen in Bihar and northeastern India. The causative species is *L. donovani*, and is transmitted by sandflies. It can also be transmitted parenterally and congenitally. In spite of the increasing incidence of kala azar in India, pregnancy in infected women is quite uncommon. Either the disease is responsible for infertility or it leads to abortion. There are only sporadic case reports regarding kala azar during pregnancy (Thakur et al 1993).

It is difficult to treat kala azar in pregnancy because the commonly used drugs, stibogluconate and pentamiadine, have been found to be unsafe in pregnancy (WHO 1990). However, if the disease is not treated, it may cause an increase in maternal morbidity and lead to congenital leishmaniasis in the neonate. Two cases of congenital leishmaniasis have been reported by Eltoun et al (1992). Amphotericin B may be used as an alternative in treating leishmaniasis in pregnancy, though long-term results about its safety are not yet known. Thakur et al have reported five pregnant patients with visceral leishmaniasis who were treated with Amphotericin B. All the patients were cured of the disease and the fetuses suffered no untoward effects. However, as the safety of the drugs used for treatment of kala azar is not proven, it is better to defer the treatment until after delivery, if possible.

References

Amster R, JB Lessing, AJ Jaffa and MR Peeyser. 1985. Typhoid fever complicating pregnancy. *Acta Obstet Gynecol Scand* 64(8):685–686.

Bradley DJ and DC Warhurst. 1995. Malaria prophylaxis. Guidelines for travelers from Britain. *BMJ* 310:709.

Brair ME, BJ Brabin, P Milligan et al. 1994. Reduced transfer of tetanus antibodies with placental malaria. *Lancet* 343:208.

Briggs GG, RK Freeman, and SJ Yaffe (eds). 1998. *Drugs in Pregnancy and Lactation*, 5th ed. Baltimore: Williams and Wilkins.

Burtin P, A Taddio, O Ariburno, TR Einarson and G Korean. 1995. Safety of metronidazole in pregnancy: a metaanalysis. *Am J Obstet Gynecol* 172:525–529.

Christian P, SK Khatry and KP West Jr. 2005. Antenatal anthelminthic treatment, birthweight and infant survival in rural Nepal. *Lancet* 366:95.

De Silva NR, JLGJ Sivisena, DPS Gunasekera, MN Ismail and HJ De Silva. 1999. Effects of mebendazole therapy during pregnancy and birth outcome. *Lancet* 353: 1145–1149.

Diagne N, C Rogier, CS Sokhna, A Tall, D Fontinelle, C Roussilhon, A Spiegel and J-F Trape. 2000. Increased susceptibility to malaria during the early postpartum period. *N Engl J Med* 343:598.

Duffy PE and M Fried. 2005. Malaria in the pregnant woman. *Curr Top Microbiol Immunol* 295:169–200.

Duffy PE. 2003. Maternal immunization and malaria in pregnancy. *Vaccine* 21:3358.

Eltoun IA, EE Zijlsta, MS Ali, HW Galib, MMH Sati, B Eltoum et al. 1992. Congenital leismaniasis and leishmaniasis in the placenta. *Am J Trop Med Hyg* 46:57–62.

Hulbert TV. 1992. Congenital malaria in the United States: Report of a case and review. *Clin Infect Dis* 14:922.

Ismail MR, J Ordi, C Menendez, PJ Ventura, JJ Aponte, E Kahigwa, R Hirt, A Cardesa and PL Alonso. 2000. Placental pathology in malaria: A histological, immunohistochemical and quantitative study. *Hum Pathol* 31:85.

Jones JL, J Schulkin and JH Maguire. 2005. Therapy for common parasitic diseases in pregnancy in the United States: A review and a survey of obstetrician/gynecologists' level of knowledge about these diseases. *Obstet Gynecol Surv* 60(6):386–393.

Karen A, VE Delbene and MS Amstey. 1981. Giardiasis in pregnancy. *Am J Obstet Gynecol* 140:895.

Koul PA, JI Wani and A Wahid. 1995. Ciprofloxacin for multiresistant enteric fever in pregnancy. *Lancet* 346(8970):307–308.

Luzzi GA and TE Peto. 1993. Risk factors of malaria infection during pregnancy in Burkina Faso: Suggestion of a genetic influence. *Am J Trop Med Hyg* 48:358.

Med Letter. 2004. Drugs for parasitic infections. *Med Lett Drugs Ther* 1189:1–12.

Menendez C, PL Alonso, J Ordi, MR Ismail, PJ Ventura, JJ Aponte, E Kahigwa and F Font. 2000. The impact of placental malaria on gestational age and birthweight. *J Infect Dis*181:1740.

Mvondo JL, MA James and CC Cambell. 1992. Malaria and pregnancy in Cameroonian women. Effect of pregnancy on Plasmodium falciparum parasitemia and the response to chloroquine. *Trop Med Parasitol* 43:1–5.

Nair LS and AS Nair. 1993. effects of malaria infection on pregnancy. *Ind J Malariol* 30:207–214.

Navitsky RC, ML Dreyfuss, J Shrestha, SK Khatry, RJ Stoltzfus and Albonico. 1998. Ancylostoma duodenale is responsible for hookworm infections among pregnant women in the rural plains of Nepal. *J Parasitol* 84(3):647–651.

Nosten F and RN Price. 1995. New antimalarials: a risk benefit analysis. *Drug Safety* 12:264.

Olliaro P, J Cattani and D Wirth. 1996. Malaria, the submerged disease. *JAMA* 275:230.

Panisko DM and JS Keystone. 1990. Treatment of malaria. *Drugs* 39:160.

Park K. 2002. Epiemiology of communicable diseases. In *Park's Textbook of Preventive and Social Medicine*, ed K Park,192–201. New Delhi: Banarsidas Banot.

Prien-Larsen JC and M Stjernquist. 1993. Malaria in pregnancy: A master of masquerade. *Acta Obstet Gynecol Scand* 72:496.

Rao FJC. 1985. Safety of nitroimidazoles. *Sczend J Infect Dis* 46(suppl):72–81.

Robier C, A Tall, N Diagne, D Fontenille, A Spiegel and JF Trape. 1999. Plasmodium falciparum clinical malaria: lessons from longitudinal studies in Senegal. *Parasitologia* 41:255.

Sadan O, LH Mathews, AB Koller and RG White. 1986. Typhoid fever in pregnancy. Case report and review of the literature. *Acta Obstet Gynecol Scand* 65(7):807–809.

Santiso R. 1997. Effects of chronic parasitosis on women's health. *Int J Gynaecol Obstet* 58:129–136.

Seoud M, G Saade, M Uwaydah and R Azoury. 1988. Typhoid fever in pregnancy. *Obstet Gynecol* 71(5) :711–714

Sholapurker SL, AN Gupta and RC Mahajan. 1988. Clinical course of malaria in pregnancy: a prospective controlled study from India. Transactions of the *Royal Society of Tropical Medicine and Hygiene* 82:376–379.

Singh N, MM Shukla and VP Sharma. 1999. Epidemiology of Malaria in Pregnancy in Central India. *Bull WHO* 77(7):567–572.

Subramanian D, KJ Moise and AC White. 1992. Imported malaria in pregnancy: Report of four casec and review of management. *Clin Infect Dis* 15:408.

Taha T, RH Gray and AA Mohamedani. 1993. Malaria and low birth weight in central Sudan. *Am J Epidemiol* 138:318.

Tanyuksel M andWA Petri Jr. 2003. Laboratory diagnosis of amoebiasis. *Clin Microbiol Rev* 16: 1713–1729.

Thakur CP, GP Sinha, V Sharma and D Barat. 1993. The treatment of kala azar during pregnancy. *Natl Med J India* 6(6):263–265.

Whitty CJ, S Edmonds and TK Mutabingwa. 2005. Malaria in pregnancy. *BJOG*. 112(9):1189–1195.

WHO. 1986. The clinical management of acute malaria. *SEARO* No. 9. New Delhi: World Health Organization.

WHO. 1990. WHO model prescribing information, drugs used in parasitic diseases. Geneva: World Health Organization, 14–22.

WHO. 1996. The World Health Report of the Director-General: Fighting disease Fostering development. Geneva: World Health Organization.

Wong RD, AR Murthy, GE Mathisen et al. 1992. Treatment of severe falciparum malaria during pregnancy with quinidine and exchange transfusion. *Am J Med* 92:561.

13

Viral Infections in Pregnancy

K Uma Devi

Even though technological advancements have proved useful for the dignosis, management and prevention of viral infections, many viruses are yet to be identified. During pregnancy, viral infections pose a more perplexing and difficult problem because the degree of fetal damage caused cannot be predicted with certainty.

DIAGNOSTIC AND THERAPEUTIC DILEMMAS

- Mild or subclinical infections may adversely affect the fetus and the newborn.
- Specific laboratory tests may not enable accurate diagnosis of infectivity.
- Ethical dilemmas about maternal treatment of infections to prevent maternal–fetal transmission (for example, HIV) may be encountered.
- Specific treatment is not available for most infections.

Prevalence and Epidemiology

The prevalence and epidemiology of viral infections in pregnancy have changed in the past five decades, with the emergence of new viral infections and mutations to existing viruses, causing considerable therapeutic anxieties.

Effect of Viral Infections on Pregnancy

Cell-mediated immune responses may be suppressed during pregnancy by placental hormones, fetal and serum products and cytokines. These responses would revert to normal in the postpartum period. Thus, genital warts that may increase during pregnancy regress markedly in the puerperium. However, interferon, which is produced by the placenta, may protect the fetus.

Viral infections can occur in utero (that is, congenital infection), at birth or in the neonatal period, with very different outcomes (Table 13.1). The spectrum of fetal involvement ranges from asymptomatic infection to long-term sequelae and intrauterine fetal demise. The presentation in the fetus is heterogenous and depends on the infecting organism, gestational period and immune status of the mother.

Pathogenesis of Fetal Infection

Maternal viral infections can affect the fetus, either directly or indirectly, through the systemic effects of maternal illnesses such as high fever or associated metabolic derangements as in variola, varicella and measles. The routes of infection can be ascending (herpes simplex), hematogenous or iatrogenic (cytomegalovirus after intrauterine blood transfusion), or may result from the use of fetal scalp monitors (HSV and HIV).

Viral Teratology

In the human fetus, teratogenesis occurs during the embryonic period (maximum) and fetal period (beginning at the end of the eighth week). The sensitivity to teratogenesis decreases as differentiation progresses.

Pathophysiology of Viral Teratogens: The mechanisms postulated for developmental defects are placental dysfunction, chromosomal injury, cellular necrosis and antigen-antibody complex formation.

Teratogenic Viruses: The known teratogenic viruses are rubella, cytomegalovirus, herpes simplex virus, Venezuelan equine encephalitis virus and varicella. Other suspected teratogenic viruses are coxsackie virus, mumps, western equine encephalitis virus, rubella, echovirus, influenza, vaccinia and the hepatitis viruses.

Clinical and Laboratory Diagnosis of Viral Infections in Pregnancy

The laboratory diagnosis of viral infections is based on demonstrating the presence of one or both of the following:

- The virus (particles, antigens or by culture)
- Antibody to the virus (host immune response)

The specimens to be collected from the pregnant women and the neonates consist of serum (single/paired) urine, throat swab, lesion scrape/swab, vesicle fluid, nasopharyngeal aspirate and cerebrospinal fluid according to the suspected viral infection. This should then be transported at 4°C on wet ice. Prenatal diagnosis of viral infections by amniocentesis

Table 13.1: Possible outcomes of viral infections in the fetus or neonate

Congenital Infection	*Perinatal Infection*
Resorption of embryo	Acute illness resulting in either complete recovery or long-term sequelae
Abortion	Death
Stillbirth	Persistent infection, clinical or subclinical with late sequelae
Prematurity	Delayed manifestation
Intrauterine growth restriction	
Clinical disease at birth	
Congenital malformation or defect	
Death in infancy	
Symptomatic infection	
Late onset congenital disease or defect/Normal infant	

(Source: Marie LL. 2000. Viral infections in medical complications during pregnancy, ed Burrow GN and Duffy TP, 5th edition; 337-362, WB Saunders Company, Harcourt Asia PTE Ltd.)

and chorion villus biopsy is still not a routine diagnostic option. Table 13.2 lists the viruses that may adversely affect the fetus or newborn.

Viral infections in pregnancy can be studied under the following categories:

1. Infections that may be unduly severe in pregnancy

a. Influenza
b. Herpes virus
c. Hepatitis viruses
d. Poliomyelitis
e. Blood-borne viral infections
f. Japanese encephalitis

2. Infections that may damage the fetus if acquired early in pregnancy

a. Rubella
b. Cytomegalovirus
c. Varicella
d. Human parvovirus B19

3. Infections acquired in later pregnancy and intrapartum

a. Varicella
b. Herpes simplex virus Types 1 and 2
c. Newly described human herpes viruses (Types 6, 7 and 8)
d. Enteroviruses
e. Human papillomaviruses
f. Hepatitis B viruses
g. Hepatitis C virus
h. Human T cell lymphototrophic viruses (HTL I)

4. Sexually transmitted viral infections

a. Hepatitis B
b. HIV
c. Herpes simplex
d. Human papilloma virus
e. CMV

Table 13.2: Viruses that may infect or damage the fetus/neonate

Virus Infection	*Birth Defects*	*Persistent Infection*	*Fetal Death*
Rubella	Yes	Yes	Yes
Cytomegalosis	Yes	Yes	Yes
Varicella	Yes	Occasional	Yes
HSV I and II	Rare	No	Neonate
HPV B19	No	Yes	Yes
HIV I and II	No	Yes	Yes
Hepatitis B	No	Yes	No
Hepatitis C	No	Yes	Unknown
Hepatitis E	No	Insufficient data	Yes
Polyomyelitis	No	No	Yes
Coxsackie B virus	No	No	Yes
Japanese B encephalitis	Unknown	Unknown	Yes
Lassa fever	No	No	Yes
HTLV I	No	Yes	No
HTLV II	No	?	No

(Source: Basic Science in Obstetrics & Gynaecology. A textbook for MRCOG Part I, 3rd ed, ed de Swiet M Chamberlain & Bewett P Churchill Livingstone, Edinburg 2002: 126-127)

5. Intrauterine central nervous system infections

a. Rubella
b. Cytomegalovirus
c. Herpes simplex virus Type 2
d. Varicella zoster virus
e. Lymphocytic choriomeningitis virus
f. Western equine encephalitis virus

Some of these viruses are discussed in detail.

VIRAL INFECTIONS CAUSING FETAL DAMAGE IN EARLY PREGNANCY

RUBELLA

Epidemiology: Rubella (also known as German measles, three-day measles or the third disease) is caused by a single-stranded RNA togavirus and spread by nasopharyngeal droplets, with an incubation period of 14–21 days. This virus travels from the upper respiratory tract to the cervical lymph nodes and is then disseminated hematogenously throughout the body. A disease prodrome of malaise, fever, headache, conjunctivitis and pharyngitis, lasting 1–5 days, precedes the classic manifestations of widespread pink/red maculopapular rash and generalised lymphadenopathy. The duration of the rash is approximately three days, beginning in the face (forehead) and migrating distally. Infection is greatest in the prodromal and rash period. Therefore, the patient may be contagious for a period of 7–10 days (ACOG 1992).

With the licensure of an effective vaccine in 1969, the frequency of rubella has declined by almost 99%. Antibodies against rubella do not normally appear in the serum until after the rash has developed. Acquired immunity to rubella usually lasts for life. Second infections have occurred after natural infections and vaccination, but recurrent infections are generally not associated with serious illness, viremia or congenital infection. About 25–50% of infections may be asymptomatic. Sometimes, thrombocytopenic purpura, encephalitis and Guillain-Barre syndrome have been reported in adults (Yaginuma et al 1996).

Effect of Maternal Infection on the Fetus and Newborn: FETAL INFECTION: Fetal infection follows maternal viremia and decidual infection, and a state of chronic infection occurs. This is caused by the inhibition of multiplying fetal cells and delayed and deranged organogenesis due to destruction of clones of cells early in fetal life or vascular insufficiency as a result of endothelial infection. Fetal infection depends on the mother's immune status and may occur at any time during the pregnancy, but the greatest risk is in the first trimester and rises again near term (Miller 1982; Mellinger et al 1995).

CONGENITAL RUBELLA SYNDROME (CRS)

In the first ten weeks of gestation, CRS occurs in about 90% of those who are infected. This figure drops to 50% at 11–12 weeks and to 33% at 13–16 weeks. After the twelfth week, deafness is usually the sole manifestation, and after 17–18 weeks, defects attributable to rubella are rare. The risk of congenital malformations again rises to 60% at 31–36 weeks. At this stage, the infants may become infected but are not necessarily adversely affected. Although fetal loss can occur (20%) very early in gestation, most pregnancies are carried to term. Differences in the clinical manifestations of CRS may be attributed to strain differences (Uda et al 1983). Preconceptional rubella in the mother does not result in fetal infection, provided the illness occurs earlier than 12 days after the last menstrual period (Enders et al 1988). In utero exposure to the rubella infection has been hypothesised to increase the liability to schizophrenia in adulthood by adversely affecting the maturation of critical structural and functional components in the brain (Brown et al 2002).

CRS includes a triad of malformations consisting of cataract, sensorineural hearing loss and congenital heart disease, and its expanded version includes a constellation of defects with associated manifestations that are thought to result from chronic viremia. These manifestations could be transient, permanent or late onset (Table 13.3). Transient manifestations appear within a few days after birth and result from abnormalities in cellular immune function. Most of them are benign and self limiting.

Permanent manifestations are physical or functional abnormalities detected within the first year of life and may result from injury to the tissues by the virus. Late onset or developmental manifestations are seen in children who are apparently normal at birth, but show clinically recognisable features later in childhood.

Effects of Infection on Pregnant Women: Pregnancy does not alter the severity of the illness in the mother. Infection with other viruses (enterovirus, parvovirus B19 and arbovirus) may present with very similar clinical features. If the clinician caring for the pregnant woman suspects rubella, the illness should be investigated virologically and diagnosed as 'rubella' until proven otherwise.

Rubella Re-infection: Re-infection is seen less frequently after natural immunity than when compared to vaccine-induced immunity. Present estimates place the risk to the fetus after rubella re-infection at around one-tenth of the risk associated with primary rubella (Cradlock-Watson, 1985; Morgan et al, 1991).

TABLE 13.3: MANIFESTATIONS OF CONGENITAL RUBELLA SYNDROME

Frequency	*Type*	*Manifestations*
Common	Transient	IUGR, hepatosplenomegaly, thrombocytopenic purpura, meningoencephalitis, lymphadenopathy, acute interstitial pneumonia, blueberry muffin lesions, bony or EEG abnormalities
	Permanent	IUGR, postnatal growth restriction, patent ductus arteriosus, pulmonary hypoplasia, cataract, microophthalmia, retinopathy, microcephaly, mental and motor retardation
	Late onset	Deafness, motor and mental handicap, language defect and IDDM
Uncommon	Transient	Hemolytic anemia, leucopenia, hepatitis, large anterior fontanelle, prematurity, myocarditis, myositis, nephritis, interstitial pneumonitis, cloudy cornea
	Permanent	ASD/VSD, glaucoma, intracranial calcification, renal artery stenosis, thymic hypoplasia, tooth defect, tracheoesophageal fistula, cleft palate, hand abnormalities, biliary atresia
	Delayed	Coarctation of aorta, chronic progressive encephalitis, thyroiditis, GH deficiency, subretinal vascularisation, keratoconus, lens absorption

Risks from Inadvertent Rubella Immunisation during Pregnancy: Although in 2% of instances, the vaccine virus has crossed the placenta to cause fetal infection, this is not associated with the congenital rubella syndrome (CDC 1987; Best et al 1994). The maximum theoretic risk of congenital damage has been calculated to be 1.4% (Bart et al 1985). Therefore, inadvertent vaccination during pregnancy is not by itself an indication for termination of pregnancy. However, pregnancy should be avoided for three months after vaccination.

Laboratory Diagnosis: Screening for rubella immune status should be a routine part of the first antenatal examination in every pregnancy. Evidence of fetal infection later in the pregnancy can be confirmed by identifying rubella-specific RNA using reverse transcriptase polymerase chain reaction (RT-PCR) in blood obtained by fetal blood sampling (Daffos et al 1984; Bosma et al 1995).

Management: Since history is unreliable, laboratory tests should be done to confirm the diagnosis. Laboratory investigations and interpretations of results are based on the following:

- The incubation period of rubella is 13–20 days. Thus, any rubella antibody that is detected within the first two weeks after exposure is almost certainly due to previous immunity. Hence, if infection has occurred, it will be detected only five weeks after exposure, at the latest.
- Rubella-specific IgM antibodies and/or a significant rise in antibody titre between paired sera are indicative of recent stimulus from primary or re-infection.

If infection is documented serologically, the risk to the baby should be discussed with the parents and they should be counselled about the decision to continue or terminate the pregnancy. Assessment of the risk is a statistical one and the fate of a particular fetus cannot be predicted with certainly. Direct evidence of fetal damage is conclusive. Tests such as cordocentesis and amniocentesis predict only fetal infection, which anyway occurs in the majority of cases; hence, these prenatal diagnostic techniques help to document fetal infection rather than fetal damage and are therefore of limited value. Figure 13.1 shows an algorithm of the management of rubella infection in pregnancy.

Prevention:

- Immunisation of all adult women contemplating pregnancy by evaluating their serostatus.
- Identification and vaccination of unimmunised women immediately after childbirth or abortion.
- Education of parents about the dangers of rubella infection.
- Vaccination of all susceptible hospital personnel.
- Vaccination of all susceptible women working in school, collegiate and health services and identification of serostatus and vaccination of women who visit family planning and infertility clinics.

Rubella Infection—Summary:

- Rubella is caused by the RNA togavirus.
- The incubation period is 2–3 weeks and the communicable period is one week before to four days after the appearance of rash.
- Virologic diagnosis is based on serology.
- Rising antibody titres (fourfold) signify recent infection.

- Rubella-specific IgG3 is present in all primary infections but not in re-infections.
- Since infections in the first trimester carry an 80% risk of fetal infection and congenital malformation, termination of pregnancy should be offered. The risk decreases to 25% in the second trimester.
- Human IgG decreases disease symptoms but not teratogenicity.
- Rubella re-infection carries negligible risk to the fetus.
- Only preventive and opportunistic vaccination can curb this devastating fetal disease.
- Rubella vaccine is contraindicated in pregnancy. However, inadvertent vaccination has not been found to cause fetal damage.
- In utero exposure could increase the fetus's susceptibility to schizophrenia since brain maturation could be affected.
- Prenatal diagnostic methods can only confirm fetal infection and not fetal damage.
- Detailed ultrasound evaluation can identify some, but not all, malformations.

Cytomegalovirus (CMV)

CMV is a double-stranded DNA herpes virus. Humans are the only known hosts of this virus. After the initial infection, it remains latent in the host cells (monocytes, bone marrow and the kidneys) like other herpes simplex viruses. Recurrent infections are usually caused by reactivation of the endogenous latent virus rather than re-infection with a new strain of the virus. Reactivation is common in immunosuppressed hosts.

Epidemiology: By adulthood, 40–100% of the population is infected with CMV. The virus can be transmitted by droplet infection and direct contact through infected saliva and urine (from congenitally infected babies), and sexually through infected cervical secretions and semen. It can also be transmitted vertically from mother to child, either in utero or perinatally through the infected maternal genital secretions or breast milk and iatrogenically through blood transfusions and transplantation of infected organs.

CMV produces three disease syndromes that are clinically important:

- Heterophine negative mononucleosis
- Intrauterine and congenital infection
- Infection in the immunocompromised patient

The Guillain–Barre syndrome is a well-known complication of CMV disease, and its hematological manifestations (leucopenia, thrombocytopenia and anemia), have been reported in pregnant women with CMV disease. The potential complications in immunocompromised individuals include pneumonia, hepatitis, gastroenteritis, retinitis and meningoencephalitis.

Effect of Infection on Pregnant Women: The risk of primary infection during pregnancy is approximately 1% and pregnancy does not seem to increase the severity of the disease.

Effect of Maternal Infection on the Fetus and Newborn: In early pregnancy, spontaneous abortion has been associated with placentitis (Altshuler 1974). CMV-induced anomalies occur over a wider gestational age than in rubella, wherein severe damage is restricted to the first 16 weeks of pregnancy. Fortunately, congenital infections resulting from recurrent infections are less often associated with clinically apparent sequelae than those from primary infections (Fig. 13.2). Early fetal infection causes brain anomalies, whereas late fetal infection results

Figure 13.1: Management of rubella in pregnancy

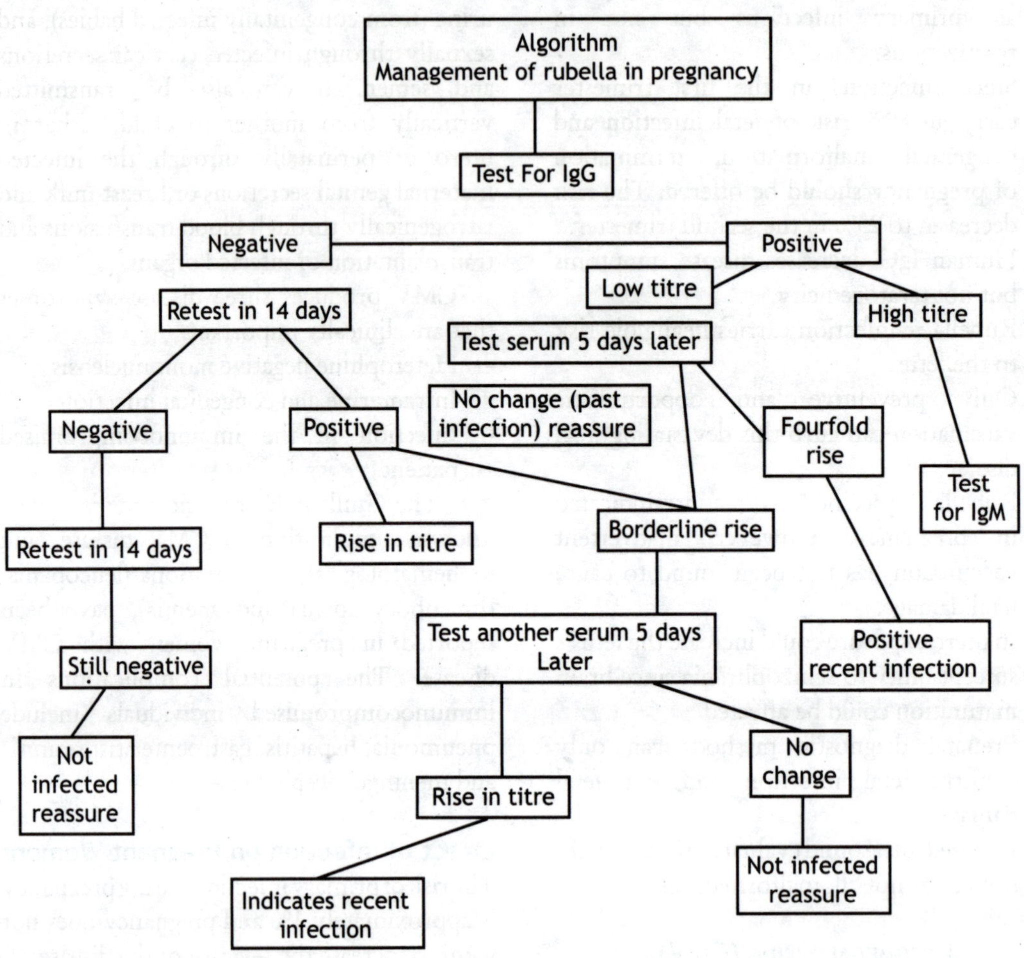

(Modified from *Medical Disorders in Pregnancy,* ed William M Barrow)

in hepatitis and thrombocytopenia.

Most CMV-infected neonates show no apparent signs of CMV infection at birth. Approximately 10% of infected newborns display systemic signs, which consist of jaundice, hepatomegaly, splenomegaly, petechial or purpuric rash, intrauterine growth restriction or respiratory distress. Neurological signs of intrauterine CMV infection include microcephaly, chorioretinitis, seizures, sensorineural hearing loss and hypotonia or hypertonia. Unfortunately, maternal immunity to CMV does not prevent recurrence, reactivation or exogenous re-infection or congenital infection. The risk of seroconversion among susceptible women during pregnancy is 1–4%.

Primary CMV infection is transmitted to the fetus in 40% of cases, and transmission is more likely in the first half of pregnancy. Only 5–7% of congenital infections are symptomatic at birth. A further 10–15% of cases could have hearing defects or psychomotor retardation. Natural immunity results in 70% reduction of congenital CMV infection in future pregnancies. Re-infection can take place with a different strain of virus that can cause fetal infection and symptomatic congenital disease. Re-infection from recurrent maternal infection reactivation is less often associated with clinical sequelae.

Transplacental transmission of the virus and fetal damage may be due to a specific CMV-induced defect in maternal cell immunity or high viral load. A high CMV DNA load in amniotic fluid is a good indicator of symptomatic congenital infection. Amniocentesis is the method of choice for fetal sampling in possible congenital infections, but should be delayed until six weeks after maternal CMV seroconversion (Grade A). Hyperechogenic bowel may be the earliest manifestation in ultrasound.

The commonest abnormality in congenital CMV is sensorineural deafness; this being a more frequent cause of deafness than bacterial meningitis, congenitally acquired rubella and genetic factors put together (Griffiths 2000). After Down syndrome, congenitally acquired CMV is the second most common known cause of motor retardation. At birth, symptomatic infants typically present with intrauterine growth restriction, jaundice, hepatosplenomegaly, petechital or thrombocytopenic rash, chorioretinitis and encephalopathy. Microcephaly may also be present at birth or develop during the early months of life. Areas of periventricular calcification may be seen radiologically.

Intrapartum and Postpartum Infection If acquired intrapartum or through breastfeeding, rather than damaging the infant, acquisition of CMV may be beneficial because it may immunise the infant naturally.

Late sequelae: The common sequelae appear as a result of central nervous system infection. About 25% of cases experience auditory deficiency. Mental retardation affects 93% of newborns with severe infection and 20% of those who are symptomatic at birth. Visual difficulties affect 25% of newborns with symptomatic infection and include chorioretinitis, optic neuritis, optic atrophy, cataracts and microophthalmia.

Primary Infection: This is best diagnosed if seroconversion of CMV-specific IgG is demonstrated in paired acute and convolescent sera that is assayed simultaneously. There is no absolute IgG titre that can clearly differentiate acute from

Figure 13.2: Effect of maternal infection

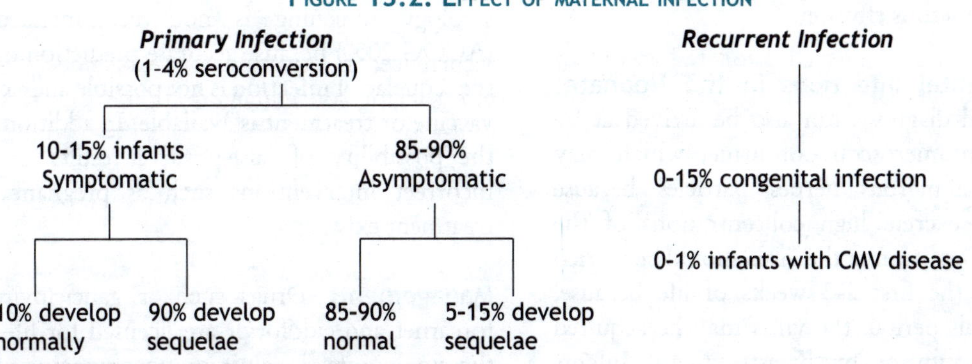

(Adapted from *Stagno and Whiteley*)

recurrent infection. A fourfold or greater change in the IgG titre is consistent with recent acute infection. In the acute phase of infection, virus-specific IgM antibodies are seen in the serum.

Diagnosis of CMV Disease: Identification of the virus in amniotic fluid by combined culture and quantitative PCR leads to the diagnosis of CMV in around 80% of fetal infections, but repeated sampling (on at least two occasions) is required to achieve maximal sensitivity (Liesnard C et al 2000) (Level II). Cordocentesis is not justified in these cases, because fetal blood culture and CMV-specific IgM antibodies are frequently negative in umbilical blood sampling (Griffiths et al 1995). Amniocentesis is the method of choice for diagnosing congenital infections but must be delayed until six weeks after maternal CMV (Grade A). However, isolation of the virus in amniotic fluid or fetal blood does not delineate the severity of fetal injury. Ultrasound detects a large proportion of affected fetuses and, though not specific for CMV, is invaluable in providing information about the severity of fetal impairment. These include microcephaly, ventriculomegaly, intracerebral calcification, hydrops, growth restriction, oligohydramnios, fetal heart block, echogenic bowel, renal dysplasia and isolated serous effusion.

Congenital Infections in the Neonate: A rapid diagnosis can also be arrived at by electron microscopy of urine, which may show numerous herpes particles because infants excrete high concentrations of the virus. Detection of the virus should be carried out in the first 2–3 weeks of life because, after this period, the virus may be acquired intrapartum or by breastfeeding. Infants infected congenitally by CMV may excrete the virus for up to 5–7 years. A positive IgM result may indicate a more serious prognosis. Maternal IgG masks seroconversion in the baby, but IgG in the infected infant persists beyond the 6–12 months expected for transplacentally acquired antibodies. Sensitivity of PCR does not exceed that of shell vial assay of urine culture, which is the gold standard for diagnosing congenital infections.

Postnatal Diagnosis of Sequelae: Neuroimaging studies provide useful information regarding the effects of CMV infection on the developing brain and the likelihood of neurodevelopmental sequelae. Approximately 50% of infants with intrauterine CMV infection have periventricular calcification—a hallmark of intrauterine infection—and infants with calcification have higher rates of permanent neuro developmental disabilities (Boppana et al 1999; Noyala et al 2001). Because CT detects small calcifications more effectively than MRI, the former should be the initial imaging study. After two years, MRI could be used to detect other disorders of neuronal migration. Figure 13.3 shows an algorithm for the evaluation of suspected maternal CMV infection.

Maternal Screening for CMV: Maternal serology screening is not recommended (ACOG 2000) because accurate prediction of the sequelae of infection is not possible and no vaccine or treatment is available. In addition, the possibility of false-positive results and incorrect interventions such as pregnancy treatment exist.

Management: Drugs such as ganciclovir, forcarnet and cidoforvir are licensed for life-threateninginfectionsinimmunocompromised patients. Ganciclovir is available only for intravenous administration and has significant hematological toxicity (neutropenia). Neonates with congenital CMV infection and CNS signs at birth should be treated with ganciclovir according to the recent protocol from the collaborative antiviral study group (Grade A). Acyclovir is not useful because the virus does not induce its own thymidinekinase. Figure 13.4 shows the management of CMV-infected pregnant women.

About 95% of congenital infections in infants have no apparent sequelae and no absolute indication for termination of pregnancy on the grounds of risk to the fetus exist. However, parents may find it difficult to accept the risk of hearing and intellectual defects that occur in 5% of babies born to mothers with primary CMV infection.

Prevention: Recombinant glycoprotein B vaccines are currently being studied; however, at present, neither CMV vaccines nor an effective mode of passive prophylaxis is available. Hence, prevention of maternal primary infection, especially in early pregnancy, by basic measures such as good hygiene is of the utmost importance. Data on the efficacy of any strategy to prevent sexual transmission of the infection is as yet unavailable.

Summary:

- Infection is usually asymptomatic, except for a mild infectious mononucleosis-like syndrome in immunocompetent patients.
- Congenital defects may follow infection at any stage in pregnancy, and deafness and subtle intellectual defects may become apparent only much later. The incidence of congenital infection varies between 0.3% and 3%, and 5% will be symptomatic at birth.
- Routine serological or virological screening for CMV is not justified.
- About 95% of infected children have no apparent sequelae. Hence, there is no indication for termination of pregnancy if only infection is documented.
- Since no vaccine is available as of date, prevention by following universal precautions and handwashing is the only strategy.
- Ultrasound helps to identify infants with sequelae.
- Long-term survivors experience neurodevelopmental delays in up to 90% and hearing loss in 60%.

Varicella Zoster Virus (VZV)

The VZ virus is a DNA herpes virus that can cause varicella or zoster infection. The virus remains in the dorsal root ganglia after primary infection and gets reactivated years later to produce shingles (herpes zoster). Varicella (chickenpox) is the acute primary disease and herpes zoster is the recurrent form of the infection. In the temperate zones, more than 95% of individuals are infected in childhood and most adults, even without a history of varicella, are immune when tested. About 5–15% of childbearing women are susceptible. Primary varicella virus infection in pregnancy is uncommon, affecting approximately three in 1000 pregnancies. Patients are infective during prodromal febrile illness, 2–3 days before the rash appears, and communicability lasts up to five days after the rash manifests, till the crusts dry up.

Maternal zoster is usually not associated with risk to the fetus because there is little or no viremia and infection is associated with a rapid varicella zoster IgG booster response. A small number of infants with

FIGURE 13.3: AN ALGORITHM FOR THE EVALUATION OF SUSPECTED MATERNAL CMV INFECTION

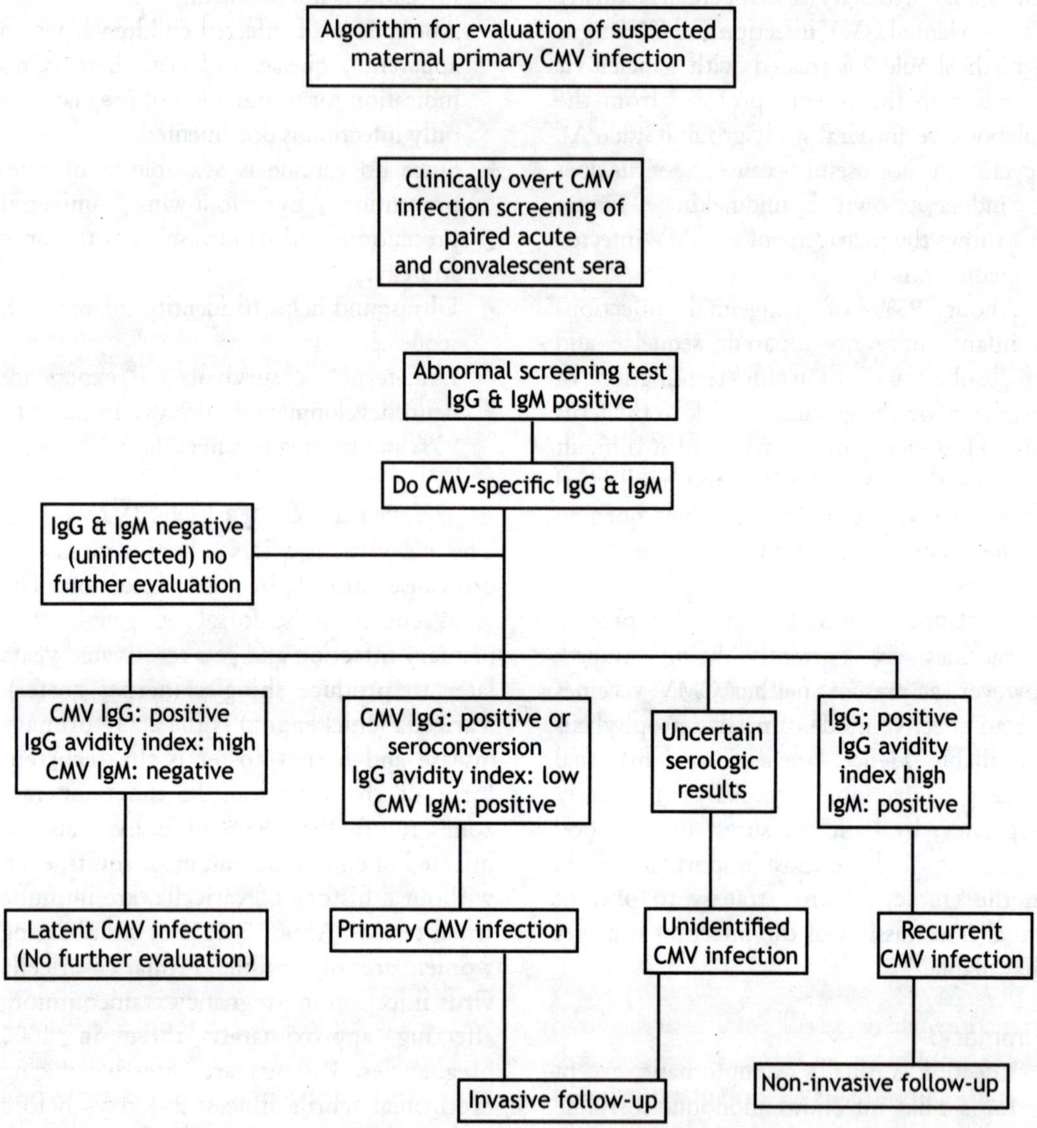

Algorithm for evaluation of suspected maternal primary CMV infection

→ Clinically overt CMV infection screening of paired acute and convalescent sera

→ Abnormal screening test IgG & IgM positive

→ Do CMV-specific IgG & IgM

- IgG & IgM negative (uninfected) no further evaluation
- CMV IgG: positive; IgG avidity index: high; CMV IgM: negative → Latent CMV infection (No further evaluation)
- CMV IgG: positive or seroconversion; IgG avidity index: low; CMV IgM: positive → Primary CMV infection → Invasive follow-up
- Uncertain serologic results → Unidentified CMV infection → Invasive follow-up
- IgG; positive; IgG avidity index high; IgM: positive → Recurrent CMV infection → Non-invasive follow-up

(Adapted from Williams Obstetrics, ed Gary F Cunningham et al. McGraw-Hill 2001. Chapter 58: Infections)

malformations following maternal zoster have been described; these malformations comprise microcephaly, microophthalmia, cataracts and talipes equinovarus (Webster 1977).

Primary varicella infection in pregnancy can be associated with an adverse outcome in three ways:

- Maternal VZ infection
- Congenital varicella syndrome

- Varicella infection of the newborn

Maternal varicella zoster infection

Effect of Infection on Pregnant Women: Generally, varicella is more severe in adults than in children. The age-specific death/case ratio increases from 1/100,000 in children to 31/100,000 in adults. A review of the literature reveals 118 reported cases in pregnancy, with 24 developing varicella pneumonia and 11 fatalities (Enders et al 1994).

This increase in severity could be due to a bias towards reporting more severe cases. There is no evidence that the course of herpes zoster in pregnant women is different from that of nonpregnant women. Pulmonary involvement (pneumonia) occurs in about 10% of pregnant women with varicella, which is not more frequent than in non-pregnant adults. Death may occur as a result of pulmonary insufficiency, bacterial superinfection or progressive pulmonary fibrosis. Onset during the third trimester is a risk factor for fetal outcome (Smego et al 1991). Mechanical ventilation may be required and mortality rates up to 6% have been reported.

Effect of Maternal Infection on the Fetus and the Newborn: Congenital varicella syndrome, varicella infection of the newborn, spontaneous abortion, stillbirth and premature delivery are the effects of maternal infection on the fetus and the newborn. Overall, approximately 1% of infants exposed to VZV early in pregnancy develop congenital varicella, with a range of 0–0.9%. Varicella embryopathy followed maternal infection in the first 20 weeks of gestation in 2% of babies, and infection later in pregnancy may result in neonatal herpes zoster. Fetal exposure later in pregnancy is associated with only congenital varicella lesions. It has been hypothesised that recurrent zoster infection in utero (and not varicella) could cause cutaneous and limb abnormalities, whereas acute varicella is responsible for neurological lesions. Less than half the babies born with the fetal varicella syndrome survive to their second birthday.

High-resolution ultrasonography, when carried out five weeks after the primary infection, may demonstrate some of the structural malformations (Table 13.4).

Perinatal Varicella (Varicella in the Newborn): Up to 50% of fetuses are infected when maternal infection occurs 1–4 weeks before delivery, and one-third of these babies develop clinical varicella despite high titres of passively acquired maternal antibodies. This infection can be lethal in 20–30% of infants if the maternal infection occurs four days before delivery and up to two days postpartum. Congenital varicella infection has been reported in 17% of term infants born to mothers who had varicella infection within 4–5 days of delivery, and the fatality rate was 31% (De Nicola et al 1979). Babies with no clinical evidence of varicella infection

Figure 13.4: Management and counselling of women with CMV infection in pregnancy

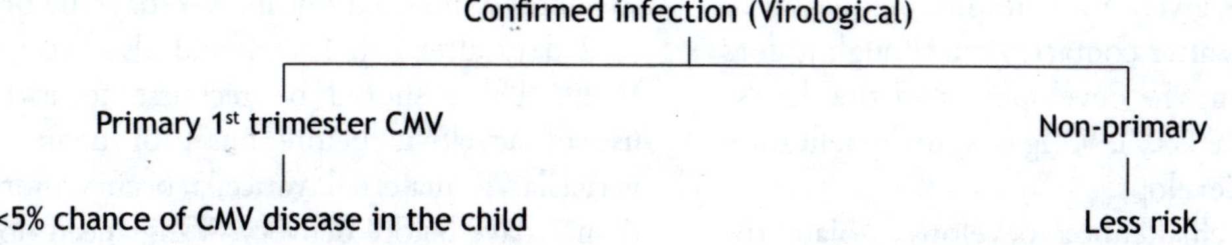

at birth can develop herpes zoster in infancy, consistent with primary infection in utero.

Table 13.5 describes the consequences of contracting varicella infection in late pregnancy while Table 13.6 shows the correlation between the onset of the infection and the mortality rate.

Neonatal varicella is characterised by pneumonitis, hepatitis and disseminated intravascular coagulation. The severity of the neonatal infection is directly related to the presence of maternal antibodies in the circulation of the newborn. The mother starts to produce and transfer protective antibodies to the fetus approximately five days after onset of the disease. Thus, babies born five days or more after the beginning of the maternal disease will be protected. Babies that develop neonatal varicella between birth and five days of age will also be protected. In contrast, mortality will be elevated if the neonatal rash appears between Days 5 and 10. Neonatal infection after Day 10 is usually mild and is likely to have been acquired postnatally.The fetus too may develop in utero varicella that heals by the time of birth. These babies are carriers of the virus and will develop herpes zoster during childhood.

Maternal Management of Varicella in Pregnancy: If a non-immune pregnant woman has contact with VZV, her VZV antibody status should be investigated within 24–48 hours, either using a fresh serum sample or a sample obtained at the time of booking the visit. If she is not immune to VZV, she should be given VZV immunoglobulin up to 10 days after contact, even though it does not prevent the development of the disease (Byrne et al 2007). VZIg is of no benefit once varicella develops.

Once chickenpox develops, isolate the patient from all other pregnant women and neonates. If they present with rash within 24 hours and the gestation period is over 20 weeks, oral acyclovir can be prescribed (UK Advisory Group on Chickenpox). The patient should be carefully monitored, and hospitalisation may be required if any respiratory symptoms occur. The lesions are dense and hemorrhagic, new lesions continue to develop six days after onset, clinical deterioration occurs or the gestation is over 36 weeks (Byrne et al 2007). Varicella pneumonia, and particularly severe episodes of adult varicella, should be treated with acyclovir 10 mg/kg, 8 hourly intravenously for seven days. No teratogenic effects of acyclovir have yet been documented. Another antiviral drug that can be used is vidarabin in doses of 10 ml/kg over a two-hour period, every day for five days.

Routine use of acyclovir may be justified since the alternative can be much more severe. In severe cases of varicella pneumonia, assisted ventilation may be necessary. Illness during the third trimester is more likely to result in maternal fatality, and regular or recent smokers are more likely to have lung complications. Tocolytics can be used to delay delivery for at least five days. Since the vaccine virus is not secreted in breast milk, postpartum vaccination should not be delayed because of breastfeeding.

The neonates should also receive VZIZ if the mother receives VZIg prophylaxis in the five days before delivery because it is unlikely that sufficient antibodies would have crossed the placenta in this period. Neonates born to mothers infected within 5–7 days before to 2 days after delivery should also receive VZIg. There should be recourse to early use of acyclovir before onset of neonatal varicella. If maternal varicella occurs more than 7 days before delivery, VZIg need not be administered to the baby. The following

Table 13.4: Varicella embryopathy

Varicella Embryopathy
Intrauterine growth restriction
Dermatological: skin loss or scarring
Skeletal: hypoplasia of bone and muscle, often with rudimentary digits
CNS: cortical and cerebellar atrophy, microcephaly, mental retardation, dysfunction of bowel and bladder sphincters
Ophthalmic: microophthalmia, chorioretinitis, optic atrophy, cataracts
Gastrointestinal and genitourinary malformation
Ultrasound findings: polyhydramnios, hydrops fetalis, hypoechogenic foci within the liver

Table 13.4 summarises the management of varicella in pregnancy.

Prevention: *Prevention of varicella among susceptible exposed pregnant women*

There is no evidence that VZIg given within 24 hours of contact prevents intrauterine infection (Level II). Although VZIg prevents and/or ameliorates maternal disease, it is unclear if such passive immunisation prevents fetal infection. The recommended dose of VZIg is 125 units per 10 kg of body weight up to a maximum of 625 units intramuscularly. Figure 13.5 shows the options available for the prevention of varicella in pregnant women.

Nonpregnant exposed women: Attenuated virus vaccine (varivax) is administered the patient is advised to avoid pregnancy for one month. Inadvertent vaccination within one month or during pregnancy should lead to counselling. No cases of congenital varicella were reported by the Varicella Pregnancy Registry. Risk from vaccine virus is less than that from the wild virus.

Human Parvovirus

The human parvovirus, B19, is a single-stranded DNA virus. This is the causative agent for both erythema infectiosum (slapped cheek disease or fifth disease) and transient aplastic crisis (TAC), in patients with chronic hemolytic anemia. It replicates in rapidly proliferating cells such as erythroblast precursors, and only individuals with the erythrocyte membrane P antigen are susceptible. The receptor (the P antigen) has been identified in various cells (mature human erythrocytes, erythroid progenitor cells, fetal cardiac myocytes, placenta, endothelial cells and megakaryocytes).

In 1975, B19 was discovered when blood donor serum number B19, used as a negative control in an assay for the hepatitis B virus, gave a false-positive reaction and parvovirions were visualised in the serum subsequently. In 1984, the adverse effects of parvovirus B19 on the human fetus were first reported. This includes miscarriage, stillbirth and hydrops fetalis. The association between hydrops fetalis and B19 infection was first recognised in a patient undergoing an evaluation for elevated maternal serum alphafetoprotein (MSAF).

Erythema Infectiosum (EI): EI is a mild, exanthematous, self-limiting illness that usually occurs in childhood. It is worldwide in distribution, with its highest incidence in late spring and early summer. The incubation period is 4–14 days. The differential diagnosis for EI includes rubella, roseola, rubeola and scarlet fever. Transmission occurs through respiratory secretions, close contact between hand and mouth, fomites and by droplets, rather than aerosols. Although the risk is low, transmission can also occur though blood products, especially pooled coagulation factor concentrates.

The parvovirous B19 infection has two phases. The first phase is characterised by viral replication in the bone marrow, viremia and viral shedding in the throat. The second phase, associated with rash and arthalgia, is coincident with immune response and the presence of antigen-antibody complexes. The rash initially appears in the face giving a 'slapped cheek' appearance before spreading to the trunk and limbs but sparing the palms. The rash is lacy or reticular in pattern, persists for several days and occasionally recurs. Non-classic distribution of the rash on the palms and soles, sparing the face, can also occur. After contact with the virus, the respiratory secretions become positive 5–10 days later and the rash appears 17–18 days later. Transmissibility is maximum before the rash appears. Infection is often subclinically associated with nonspecific flu-like symptoms. In adults, the rash may be morbilliform and indistinguishable from the rash of rubella or may even be purpuric, resembling Henoch-Schönlein purpura. The pattern of joint involvement resembles rheumatoid arthritis and can be mistaken for Lyme disease or systemic lupus erythematosus (SLE). Simultaneous presentation of acute parvovirous and SLE has also been described (Cope, 1992). In industrialised countries, about 50% of women are immune, with an annual seroconversion rate of about 1.5%.

Transient Aplastic Crises (TAC): A second major clinical presentation, TAC occurs primarily in individuals with underlying hemoglobinopathy and results from viral infections of the bone marrow, which cause reticulocytopenia and hypoplastic erythroid series in the bone marrow and red cell aplasia. The crisis resulting from the parvovirus infection generally lasts approximately 7–10 days and may necessitate transfusions during this period. Abnormalities in the number of white blood cells and platelets have also been noted but are not usually clinically relevant. TAC patients are infectious. Spontaneous recovery occurs in 2–4 weeks, but in immune-deficient patients, chronic severe anemia and autoimmune disorders may be

TABLE 13.5: CONSEQUENCES OF VARICELLA INFECTION IN LATE PREGNANCY

Onset of Rash in Mother	*Babies with Varicella*	*Mortality*
4 days antepartum to 2 days postpartum	16%	31%
>5 days antepartum	32%	0%

(Based on data from Meyers JD, J Infect Dis 129:215-217 1974)

TABLE 13.6: CORRELATION BETWEEN PERIOD OF ONSET AND MORTALITY

Day of Onset of Rash in Neonate	*Neonatal Deaths*	*Neonatal Cases*	*Mortality (%)*
0-4	0	22	0
5-10	4	19	21

present. In addition to patients with chronic hemolytic anemia and immunodeficiency, pregnant woman represent a third group at increased risk as a consequence of the fetal effects of B19.

Maternal Parvovirous B19 Infection: The estimated incidence of human parvovirus B19 infection in the United Kingdom is 1 in 400 pregnancies. Infection in pregnant women is about as severe as in non-pregnant adults. Based on the virological findings in aborted fetuses, the risk of transplacental infection has been estimated to be 33–51%. Infection in the first 20 weeks of gestation is estimated to cause fetal loss in 9% of pregnancies and hydrops fetalis in 3% of patients. There are isolated reports of infections as late as Week 39, causing stillbirth (Hellman 1991). Thus, fetal infection can be severe and sometimes fatal (Table 13.8).

Fetal and Neonatal Effects: In non-immune, pregnant individuals (50% of the population), the presence of an acute infection carries at least 1 in 5 risk of transplacental transmission (Level II). In apporoximately 30% of maternal infection, the virus is transmitted to the fetus and intrauterine infection usually terminates uneventfully, when the maternal antibody crosses the placenta. However, spontaneous abortion may occur in the first half of the pregnancy and hydrops fetalis in the second half. The overall risk to the fetus from maternal B19 infection is estimated at 1–6.5% with fetal demise usually occurring 3–6 weeks after maternal infection (Gratacos et al 1995; Levy et al 1997), suggesting that damage is due to fetal infection rather than the indirect effects of maternal infection. No developmental abnormalities were observed in children monitored for late sequelae up to 10 years of age (Miller 1998).

Fetal Effects subsequent to Organogenesis: Although parvoviruses are known animal teratogens, only a single case report has described the teratogenic effect of a B19 infection in a first trimester abortion. Multiorgan involvement with

TABLE 13.7: SUMMARY OF MANAGEMENT OF VZV INFECTION IN PREGNANCY

Clinical Scenario	*Risk*	*Action*
VZI early pregnancy	Minimal risk to fetus	Discuss with parents, no indication for recommending termination of pregnancy
VZI 5-20 days antipartum	Risk of neonatal varicella Prognosis good Baby potentially infected	No VZIg Acyclovir for severe neonatal illness Nursed in isolation and early discharge from hospital
VZI <5-7 days antepartum and <2 days postpartum	Risk of neonatal varicella 5% fatality risk Baby potentially infectious	VZIg to neonate Treat neonate with acyclovir Separate neonate from mother Nurse in isolation ?Acyclovir for the mother
Neonate exposed to postnatal varicella (nonmaternal)	Severe disease uncommon	VZIg to prevent neonatal infection if mother seronegative

microophthalmia, lens abnormalities, skeletal muscle degeneration and vascular endothelial damage in the fetus and placenta was observed. Spontaneous abortion and intrauterine fetal death occur in the second or third trimester. Alfafetoprotein has been reported to be elevated in two cases of intrauterine B19 infection prior to the development of hydrops.

FIGURE 13.5: ALGORITHM OF THE OPTIONS AVAILABLE FOR THE PREVENTION OF VARICELLA IN PREGNANT WOMEN

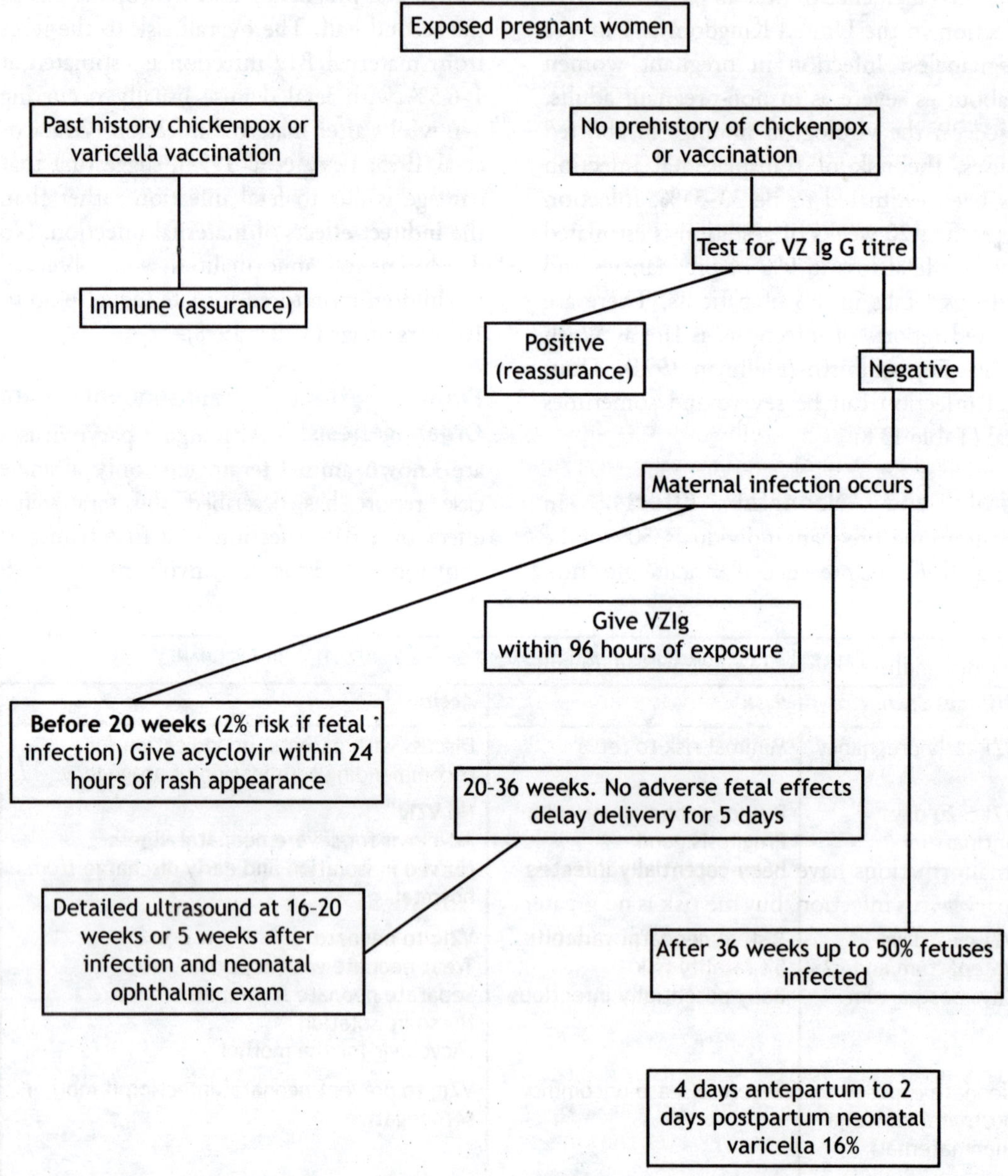

Whether this is a consequence of increased fetal hepatic production or transplacental leakage, or some other process, is unknown. Fetal hydrops is the most ominous manifestation of congenital parvovirus infection and occurs in 3% of pregnancies, between 9 weeks and 20 weeks. Neonatal anemia has been shown in infants infected during the third trimester.

Non-immune Hydrops Fetalis (Pathophysiology): The pathophysiology is probably similar to isoimmunisation with the combination of shortened red cell lifespan (45–70 days), increased hematopoiesis and decreased hepatic function. The fetal red cell mass increases about 34-fold between the third and sixth months of gestation. This setting is conducive for intracellular viral replication in rapidly dividing cells, causing red cell maturation arrest and leading to aplastic crises with resultant severe anemia and cardiac failure. Non-immune hydrops fetalis and isolated ascites with significantly increased middle cerebral artery Doppler velocity indices are indicative of fetal anemia. Reticulocytosis (>20%) indicates recovering erythropoiesis. A combination of high output cardiac failure, hypoalbuminemia aggravated by direct, viral-induced myocarditis and hepatitis could be responsible for the hydropic changes in the fetus.

Congenital Defects: Congenital malformations have been reported following parvovirus infection, but the risk is no greater than the base line risk in the general population (Katz 1996; Tiessen 1994). Persistent neurological morbidity and abnormalities including hypotonia, arthrogryposis, motor developmental delay, infantile spasms, intracranial calcification and ventriculomegaly have been reported. However, even the longest epidemiological survey had only a 30% power to detect a doubling of the frequency of developmental delay, from 7.5–1.5% (Rodis 1998; Conry 1993).

Diagnosis: A pregnant woman with an unexplained morbiliform or purpuric rash, or a patient with chronic hemolytic anemia and aplastic crises, should be evaluated for parvovirus infection, especially when there is an outbreak.

Diagnosis of Maternal Infection: Antibody assay is the recommended method since viral DNA is present only for a transitory period. Both rubella and B19 antibodies should be measured. Radioimmunoassay and enzyme-linked immunosorbent assays detect B19 IgM in approximately 90% of cases by the third day after the onset of symptoms. Titres start to decline 30–60 days after onset of the illness. A patient who is seronegative should be tested again 2–3 weeks later, depending on the timing of the exposure. HPV B19 IgG is usually present by the seventh day of illness and persists for life. If maternal infection is confirmed, the fetus should be visualised by serial ultrasound scans to enable early detection of fetal hydrops.

Diagnosis of Fetal Infection: Fetal complications can occur two or more months after maternal infection. If fetal hydrops is documented by ultrasound, cordocentesis could be performed to detect B19-specific IgM or IgA in fetal blood, although such investigations are relatively insensitive. In infants with persistent congenital infection, the virus does not circulate in the blood but is present in low levels in the bone marrow and can be detected by PCR.

Management of Human Parvovirus B19 Infection in Pregnancy: Pregnant women with acute infection should be treated symptomatically. Early recognition and transfusion, when necessary, can reduce the overall risk of 0.5% mortality to about 0.15%. Women exposed to parvovirus early in pregnancy must be reassured that the risk is low, and investigated virologically if they develop any signs or symptoms of infection. They should then be followed up by serial ultrasound evaluation to detect hydrops fetalis.

If mild hydrops is detected, a conservative approach is recommended. For worsening hydrops, diagnostic cordocentesis and intrauterine red blood cell transfusion should be considered at tertiary fetal medicine centres. If intravascular transfusion is impossible because of gestational age, intraperitoneal transfusion may be feasible. Because the fetus can recover without treatment in 34% of cases and intrauterine blood transfusion can cause fetal death, further study is needed to better define the risks and benefits of this treatment. The role of digitalisation of the fetus is unclear. Figure 13.6 shows the algorithm for early pregnancy exposure to parvovirus B19.

Prevention: Prevention of the parvovirus B19 infection is difficult since no vaccine is currently available. There is no evidence that antiviral treatments prevent maternal fetal infection. Pregnant healthcare workers should avoid caring for patients with TAC or confirmed hosts with chronic infection who are highly contagious. However, they do not need to avoid infected children because infection is greatest before any clinical illness.

Conclusion: Routine screening for parvovirus B19 infections in pregnancy does not seem to produce significant benefits, and maternal infection does not warrant therapeutic termination of pregnancy. Information about this infection should be provided to all women working in close contact with young children, not only in antenatal clinics but also in preconception and family planning clinics. All cases of non-immune hydrops fetalis with serology showing potential for early infection with parvovirus B19 should be managed in fetal medicine centres (Brown et al 1984). All pregnant women with nonvesicular rash should be investigated for rubella and parvovirus B19 infection.

INFECTIONS ACQUIRED IN LATER PREGNANCY, INTRAPARTUM AND POSTPARTUM

Herpes Simplex Virus (HSV)

HSV belongs to the Herpes viridae family of double-stranded DNA viruses. This family includes CMV, VZV, Epstein–Barr virus (EBV) and the recently described human herpes virus 6 (HHV-6) that infects B lymphocytes

Table 13.8: Outcome of human parvovirus B19 infection

Risk of acquiring infection	*1 in 400*
Transplacental infection	33-51.5%
Excess fetal loss	9%
Risk of hydrops fetals	3 %
Third trimester intrauterine fetal death	7.5 %
Number congenitally infected	20% (Persistent salivary IgG)
Outcome of survivors	No abnormalities

and is associated with lymphoproliferative disorders. In adults, typical lesions are vesicular or ulcerative, involving only the skin and mucus membranes. Widespread infection involving the central nervous system occurs only in people with debilitating disease. On the other hand, the newborn is subject to systemic, and frequently lethal diseases because of an incompletely developed immune system.

Herpes simplex virus infections once contracted are lifelong and the virus persists in the sensory root ganglia, most frequently in the trigeminal (HSV I) or sacral (HSV II) ganglia. HSV Type I is most commonly associated with herpes labialis and HSV Type II with genital herpes. In reality, however, a lot of overlap between these subtypes is seen (Whitley et al 2001). Approximately 70–90% of oral and 75% of genital herpes infections are asymptomatic. In the affluent groups, HSV I infection is delayed until adulthood in 50–70% of cases.

The issues with HSV in pregnancy are that it presents particular management difficulties and periodic recrudescences. The two types (HSV I and II) possess similar tissue tropism and perinatal impact, although Type I recurs less frequently than Type II in the genital area.

The level of virus present in non-visible lesions is likely to be 100–1000 times lower than in overt lesions. Around 20% of pregnant women have serological evidence of past HSV II infections, although only a quarter of these women are aware that they have had genital herpes. A history of genital herpes ('Do you have or have you ever had genital herpes?') has a positive predictive value of 92% and negative predictive value of 67% in identifying pregnant women who are HSV II seropositive. History of HSV I is also important because previous HSV I infection can influence the outcome of the subsequent genital HSV II experience. The disease is transmitted by intimate mucocutaneous contact or infected body secretions coming into contact with mucosal surfaces. The virus can also enter directly through breaches in the skin, such as may occur in contact sports or through the needle puncture site on the scalp of a baby when fetal monitors are attached during delivery. No firm clinical evidence that transmission occurs through contact with toilet seats, towels or hot tubs has been found. Rare cases of acquisition of the disease from truly asymptomatic individuals have been reported. The herpes virus has been isolated from the genitalia of 0.02–1% of adult females. Positive cultures of 0.6% were found in asymptomatic pregnant women. Asymptomatic shedding in pregnancy is 10% after a primary episode and 0.5% after recurrent episodes.

Herpetic Syndromes: Clinically, there are three herpetic syndromes in adults—first episode (primary and non-primary) and recurrent genital herpes.

First episode genital herpes: A first episode (or 'initial') infection is the first clinically overt infection at a particular site, irrespective of prior serological status.

First episode primary: A first episode primary is the clinical presentation of herpes without antibodies to either HSV I or HSV II.

First episode non-primary infection comprises an initial clinical episode, with either HSV I or HSV II, in patients with antibodies to the other viral serotypes. It is similar in presentation to recurrent episodes. As many as two-thirds of women with HSV II antibodies acquired the infection asymptomatically.

Recurrent genital herpes: Recurrent or secondary infections are milder, with a shorter viral shedding (3–5 days), in which a patient provides the previous history of lesions at the same site. These usually follow reactivation of the virus from latency, although re-infection cannot be initially excluded.

From a purely clinical standpoint, it is possible to diagnose only the first episode and recurrent infection. Serological information is required to differentiate primary from non-primary first episode infections.

Infections with one type confer some protection from subsequent first episode non-primary infections by the other type. Hence, primary infections are usually more severe than non-primary first episode infections, which in turn are more severe than recurrent infections. Since about half the childbearing-aged population is already HSV I seropositive, true primary infections with HSV during pregnancy are uncommon.

Fetal Transmission: Primary genital herpes (2%) in pregnancy has been associated with a more severe course, an increase in miscarriage in first trimester infections and premature delivery in third trimester infections in some studies. The risk of transmission to the fetus is greatest when primary genital herpes occurs at term and has a range of 30–50% for infants delivered vaginally. Recurrent HSV is much more common than primary infection during pregnancy, and in these cases, the fetus has only a 3–5% chance of being infected because of lower virus titres and the protective effect of transplacental maternal antibodies. Transmission is much more likely if a lesion is present in a recurrent infection site, and asymptomatic shedding is associated with an extremely low risk of transmission to the fetus. Factors affecting the transmission of HSV to the fetus include high virus titres, lack of transplacental antibodies, ruptured membranes of more than 6 hours and trauma to fetal skin. Recent acquisition of genital HSV, whether primary or non-primary first episode, is associated with a high rate of perinatal infection. Asymptomatically infected patients can give birth to seriously infected neonates, and these mothers constitute about 70% of cases. Among infants with disseminated herpes, the risk of death or serious sequelae is about 50%.

Effect of Infection on Pregnant Women: The incubation period for herpes infection is 2–14 days (median 4–6 days). The episode starts with local pain, itching or tingling, followed by focal vesicular lesions. These lesions progress to crusted lesions and this sequence can last between 6 and 30 days before healing is complete. HSV may involve the oral mucosa, eyes (conjunctivitis or keratitis), fingers (herpetic whitlow), central nervous system (encephalitis, meningitis) or genital mucosa (genital herpes).

Primary genital herpes may vary in intensity in pregnancy but is usually associated with fever, headache, myalgia and malaise as well as genital lesions. These may be extensive and bilateral and involve the vulva, cervix and urethra with discharge, dysuria and sometimes urine retention (10–15%). Rectal or perineal lesions may be seen, usually with a history of rectal intercourse. Over 9% of first episode genital herpes present with atypical features including nonspecific vulvar erythema, fissure, furuncles or excoriation and would not be recognised unless virological tests are done.

HSV II can cause mild aseptic meningitis and HSV I encephalopathy and the meningitis is self-limited. A more severe but rare complication of primary or genital (or oral) herpes in pregnancy is widespread dissemination of the virus, leading to necrotising hepatitis with or without thrombocytopenia, leucopenia, coagulopathy and encephalitis. Left untreated,

Figure 13.6: An algorithm for early pregnancy exposure to parvovirus B19

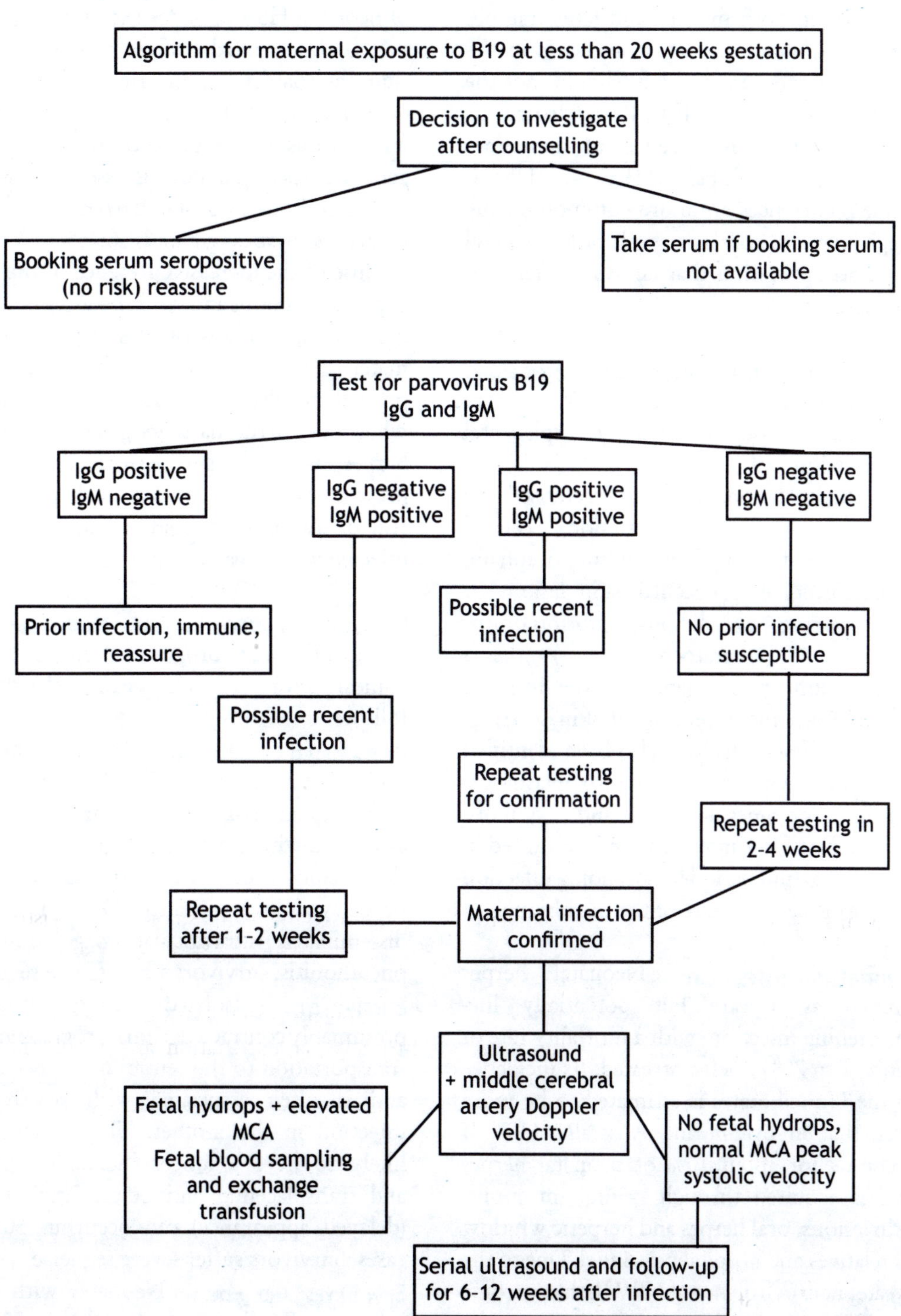

these manifestations have a mortality rate of over 50% in both mother and fetus. Herpes hepatitis is a rare disease that occurs in the third trimester and which should not be confused with the HELLP syndrome or acute fatty liver. Recurrences are ten times more frequent with HSV II than with HSV I. These recurrences are more common during pregnancy, possibly as a result of the general immunosuppression that allows the fetus to be tolerated.

Congenital and Neonatal Infection: Congenital infection with HSV is rare and usually associated with transplacental transmission of primary genital herpes early in gestation. It is characterised by intrauterine growth restriction, central nervous system involvement (microcephaly, hydranencephaly), vesicular skin lesions or skin scarring, eye lesions (chorioretinitis, microphthalmia, keratoconjuctivitis) and, in a smaller number, enlargement of the liver and spleen. With the exception of skin scarring, these manifestations have also been identified in infants with congenital toxoplasmosis, rubella, cytomegalovirus and syphilis. Intrauterine HSV infection can be acquired in the intrapartum period by ascending infection after prolonged rupture of the membrane.

Neonatal Infection: Neonatal herpes simplex is a rare but potentially life-threatening infection, with a mortality rate of more than 70% if left untreated. Its incidence in the United States is estimated to be more than that in Britain and Australia. HSV II accounts for about 10% of neonatal herpes and is acquired through genital infections, skin lesions, oral herpes and herpetic whitlow of relatives and hospital personnel. Due to the greater neurovirulence of HSV II, the outcome for HSV I-infected neonates appears to be better than for HSV II. The portal of entry of neonatal HSV includes the umbilical cord, eye, oral and nasal orifices and traumatised skin. Internal fetal monitoring in the presence of active genital herpes has been associated with serious neonatal infections. First episode genital herpes near term is associated with a higher risk of neonatal herpes (41%) than recurrent herpes genitalis (2–5%). This is because of the increased presence of the virus in primary lesions and virus shedding of longer duration, and a lack of passively transferred maternal antibodies to protect the fetus. The practice of culturing the virus before delivery, when one of the partners gives a history of herpes, is no longer performed since the presence of the virus does not help predict the risk of transmission, and infants can still be infected with negative cultures.

Clinical Picture in the Neonate: For therapeutic and prognostic purposes, the clinical picture of neonates can be classified as follows:

Disseminated infection: Involvement of multiple organs, especially the brain, liver, lungs and adrenal glands is characteristic and associated with the worst prognosis. Vesicular skin lesions occur in 80% of cases but may be delayed in appearance. Death is due to disseminated intravascular coagulation and pneumonitis; survivors suffer severe sequelae.

Encephalitis: Isolated encephalitis is presumably contracted from retrograde axonal transportation to the central nervous system, and is often associated with reactivation infection in the mother. These infants are likely to have a longer incubation period and transplacental antibodies. Skin vesicles (delayed appearance) can occur in 60% of cases. Survivors suffer severe sequelae.

Skin, eyes and mouth: Neonates with HSV infection localised to the skin, eyes or mouth have the most favourable prognosis. Nevertheless, approximately 10% will have long-term neurological sequelae. Disseminated infections commonly present at 9–10 days of age, encephalitis at 16–17 days of age and localised skin, eye or mouth infections at 10–11 days may be seen. Consequently, neonates do not usually become ill until after they are discharged from the hospital.

Diagnosis: Electron microscopy of vesicular fluid, aspirated into a 1-ml syringe with a 26-G needle, can demonstrate the presence of the herpes virus within minutes by negative contrast. Culture by shell vial assay of scrapings or swabs from the base of the ulcer can establish diagnosis within 24 hours.

The gold standard diagnostic test of viral culture has a recognised false-negative rate. Rapid tests, including a monoclonal antibody test and ELISA are available, but their use is optimal only in high prevalence populations. PCR is more sensitive than standard culture techniques and is becoming more widely available. Tzanck smears are neither sensitive nor specific to HSV and are not encouraged. A sensitive and specific test for HSV with rapid results obtained at the onset of labour is required but is not yet available. Thus, clinical management at delivery is solely dependent on careful examination of the mother's genital tract for lesions.

Surveillance culture of the mouth, nasopharynx, eyes, urine, stool or rectum and cerebrospinal fluid should be obtained in exposed infants, 24–48 hours after birth. Restriction endonuclease mapping of isolates have helped to trace the source of some neonatal infections.

Management of Herpes in Pregnancy

General: This is a recurrent, unpleasant disease with no permanent cure. It may lead to relationship and psychosexual problems and counselling should form an essential part of its management. Abstinence should be advised when infective lesions are present. Intravenous acyclovir is the most effective treatment (Level II) and secondary bacterial and fungal infections should be treated. Hospitalisation may be required for retention of urine or painful micturition for catheterisation and administration of intravenous acyclovir.

The obstetrician has the responsibility of managing episodes during gestation and preventing any hazard to the baby during delivery. Treatment consists of supportive measures such as analgesics, topical anesthetics and good hygiene. Frequent bathing followed by thorough drying of the affected areas with a hair dryer provides temporary relief. Use of suppressive acyclovir produces significant reduction in maternal infection at vaginal delivery and cesarean section (Reiff-Eldridge et al 2000; Brocklehurst et al 1998). Valacyclovir (prodrug of acyclovir) and famicyclovir (metabolised to penicillin) also work against HSV, but currently no data is available about the safety of these drugs for use in pregnancy.

Antepartum: The history of the patient should be documented and the appropriate mode of delivery discussed. Antepartum maternal viral cultures are not required since they do not help in predicting the risk of exposure to the fetus at the time of delivery (Arvin et al 1986). Due to the suppression of the immune system during pregnancy, early recourse to intravenous acyclovir is recommended and no fetal teratogenicity or toxicity has been reported. The genitourinary physician should be involved in the management of the patient. Primary genital herpes should be treated in the last four weeks of gestation with daily suppressive acyclovir to prevent recurrence at term, thereby reducing the need for delivery by cesarean section.

Intrapartum: If herpetic lesions are present on the vulva or cervix, or if the first episode occurs within 6 weeks of the due date, delivery should be by cesarean section and done electively in the latter case (Level II).

For recurrent HSV, if herpetic lesions are visible, cesarean section is recommended; however, there is no consensus on routine cesarean section. Frequent, symptomatic recurrences during pregnancy should be treated with acyclovir from 36 weeks and vaginal delivery is not contraindicated (Level IV). Fetal scalp monitoring should also be avoided.

Postpartum: Breastfeeding is recommended if there are no lesions around the nipples. Close contact with the baby should be avoided if orofacial lesions are present. Use of acyclovir does not proscribe breastfeeding, since it does not harm the baby (Table 13.9).

Newly Described Human Herpes Viruses (Types 6, 7 and 8): HHV-6 infection can occur in utero but there is little information about the role of these viruses in causing congenital infections. HHV-8 transmission occurs within families, but not during delivery or by breastfeeding. These studies were conducted at French Guiana, which has a prevalence rate of 15% for persons aged 15–40 years.

Human Papilloma Virus (HPV)

HPV is a virus that causes warts (Condyloma acuminata), and about 100 genotypes have been identified. They are found on the skin, genital tract, oral cavity and respiratory tract. Condyloma acuminata, often called genital warts, are sexually transmitted. The risk factors associated with HPV infection include early onset of sexual activity, multiple sex partners, cigarette smoking and long-term use of oral contraception. Between 500,000 and 1 million new cases of HPV occur annually in the United States. Spontaneous regression within two years is common as a result of cell-mediated immunity. Conditions associated with depression of T cell function such as pregnancy, transplantation, HIV infection and immunosuppressive drugs have been linked to an increase in the prevalence, size and number of warts.

Genital Warts: Genital warts predominantly affect the young, and prevalence is highest among the 16–25 year age group. The risk of acquiring the virus by sexual contact with an infected partner is high (65%) and the incubation period ranges from 3 weeks to 8 months with an average of 2.8 months. More than 35 HPV types infect the genital tract. Types 6 and 11 cause exophytic condylomas. Types 6 and 16 are low oncogenic risk groups and Types 16 and 18 are high-risk categories.

Genital Warts in Pregnancy: Condyloma acuminata can grow more rapidly during pregnancy and are located over the genital tract and the perianal regions. They can grow so large as to cause dystocia and severe hemorrhage when disruption occurs during vaginal delivery. They also provide foci for secondary bacterial infection, which can adversely affect the fetus (chorioamnionitis, intrapartum fetal infection). Transmission can occur during birth through the infected birth canal, or occasionally, in utero.

Respiratory Papilloma Virus

This virus is associated with a long period of latency before the lesions are visualised. Laryngeal papillomas or respiratory papillomatosis, transmitted by the aspiration of HPV-infected secretions during delivery, are caused by virus Types 6 and 11. Voice change and abnormal cries can occur, and lesions appear in the larynx, trachea, nose, lips and oral cavity. The highest risk is in children younger than five years. Conjunctival papillomatosis in infants has also been reported. These complications are rare, despite the frequency of genital HPV.

Diagnosis: Warts are diagnosed by clinical examination and, when in doubt, histological examination can be conducted. Papanicolau smears can be used to detect characteristic koilocytes. Subclinical lesions require colposcopic examination and staining with 3% acetic acid or iodine for visualisation of affected areas. DNA probes are available to distinguish common high- and low-risk HPV types. However, treatment is based on clinical diagnosis.

Management: Management of these lesions in pregnancy poses a few problems. Excision of the lesions by cautery or use of cryosurgery seems to be the best approach to treatment during pregnancy. Often, multiple applications and modalities may be required. Trichloracetic acid, electrocautery and laser therapy could also be used. Podophyllin, podofilox and imiquimod should not be used during pregnancy. Genital warts by themselves are not an indication for cesarean section, provided they are detected and adequately managed. The risk of respiratory papillomatosis in a baby born to a mother with genital warts is very low (1 in 1000) and does not by itself justify cesarean section (CDC, 2002a). Cesarean section may be indicated when genital warts obstruct the birth canal or lead to excessive bleeding. Laryngeal papillomatosis poses a difficult problem. Limited but transient success has been achieved with interferon. Surgery remains the mainstay when papillomas compromise the airway. Surgery may be needed every year and scarring may occur.

Prevention: Condoms provide some protection. Both, prophylactic vaccines to prevent infection and therapeutic vaccines to destroy HPV-infected cancer cells, are under development.

Polyomaviruses

Infection by the polyomaviruses JC and BK are common, and 50–80% of the population is infected by adulthood. Reactivations occur in 25% of women during pregnancy with viruria documented in 3–7%. Virus reactivation does not produce any obvious disease in the mother. Seventeen children with a range of congenital abnormalities (prematurity, hyperbilitubinemia, seizures, cerebral defects) were found to have an IgM antibody to the BK virus early in life (3–90 days old), and the virus was isolated from the urine of one child (Rziha et al 1978). Unequivocal evidence of congenital infection has not yet been documented.

Viral Hepatitis in Pregnancy (see Chapter 11)

The viruses that cause hepatitis are hepatitis viruses (A–E), Epstein–Barr virus, cytomegalovirus and yellow fever virus.

Lymphocytic Choriomeningitis (LCM) Virus

LCM, first identified as a cause of human infection in the 1930s, infects the feral mouse and hamsters. The infected animals chronically excrete the virus in urine, feces and respiratory secretions, and human infection results from inhalation of infected aerosols, direct contact with infected animals or ingestion of material contaminated by infected excreta. Intrauterine LCM infection is a rare condition but no surveillance studies have been performed to establish the incidence of the disorder.

Clinical Features: The clinical features of congenital LCM virus infection mimic those of intrauterine cytomegalovirus disease and congenital toxoplasmosis. Among 26 reported cases reviewed by Wright and colleagues in 1997, 88% had chorioretinopathy, 43% had macrocephaly at birth and 13% were microcephalic. Occasionally, infants with vesicular or bullous skin lesions were seen. Approximately 50% of mothers who gave birth to infants with congenital LCM virus infection recalled influenza-like symptoms during pregnancy, and one-fourth reported contact with rodents, usually mice, during their pregnancies.

Diagnosis: The diagnosis of congenital LCM virus infection is established by serological studies of the mother and newborn. Detection of LCM virus–specific IgM in the serum strongly supports diagnosis. Imaging studies in infants may show hydrocephalus, intracranial calcification and cortical dysplasia.

Prevention, Treatment and Prognosis: Currently, no vaccine exists for prevention but pregnant women can reduce their risk by avoiding mice-infested areas and pet hamsters. Effective postnatal antiviral therapy of the LCM virus has not been described.

Approximately 35% of infants die from complications of congenital LCM virus infection (Wright 1997). Most surviving infants have neurodevelopmental sequelae and can develop progressive hydrocephalus.

Venezuelan Equine Encephalitis (VEE)

Intrauterine infection with VEE, a pathogen endemic to Latin America, causes severe fetal disease with stillbirth and hydranencephaly. VEE is a togavirus found predominantly in Central and South America. Humans are infected by a mosquito vector and the illness is usually mild. VEE produces an influenza-like illness during which some patients develop signs of encephalitis. VEE infection in pregnancy has been associated with increased spontaneous abortion rate and destruction of the cerebral cortex of the fetus to produce cystic changes (hydranencephaly, microophthalmia and joint anomalies).

Japanese Encephalitis

Japanese encephalitis is a mosquito-borne infection caused by a flavivirus and found in the Far East and Southeast Asia, in areas where paddy fields and pig farming coexist. Usually asymptomatic infection may be associated with encephalitis in 1 in 200 cases, carrying a mortality rate of 30–40% and permanent neurological sequelae in a high proportion of survivors. High maternal and fetal mortality rates have been reported in pregnancy. The Japanese encephalitis virus has been shown to cross the placenta.

Three doses of vaccines have been recommended for people staying in endemic countries for longer than a month, during or after the rainy season. Local and allergic reactions have been reported with the vaccine. The risk associated with disturbing an unstable pregnancy must be weighed against the risk of acquiring infection. Since allergic reactions can occur as late as 10 days after the vaccination, patients are advised to avoid long-haul flights until 10 days have elapsed. Appropriate clothing and insect repellants are also emphasised for preventing infection.

Enteroviruses

The enteroviruses comprise a genus of the Picornaviridae family that includes the poliovirus (3 types), Group A coxsackie virus (types), Group B coxsackie virus (six types), echovirus (31 types), enterovirus (Types 68–71) and the hepatitis virus.

Enteroviruses are named after their propensity to replicate in the enteric tract but they can also cause widespread maternal, fetal and neonatal infections. The manifestations of non-polio enterovirus infections are protean, and range from subclinical infections and undifferentiated fevers with or without a rash (rubelliform, vesicular) to respiratory infections, aseptic meningitis, myocarditis, conjunctivitis, herpangina and hand, foot and mouth disease.

Echoviruses

They may cause a rubelliform rash and may be mistaken for rubella.

Poliovirus

Due to the immunisation policy of the WHO, poliomyelitis has been eradicated throughout the world, except in parts of Central Africa and the Indian subcontinent. Polio in pregnancy causes more severe infection than that in the non-pregnant population, with a higher incidence of paralytic complications. The severity of paralytic disease increases with gestational age (Siegel et al 1955). Transplacental transmission of the poliovirus and coxsackie virus after maternal infection early in pregnancy have been reported. Neonatal poliomyelitis carries a 25% mortality risk. Inactivated subcutaneous poliovaccine is recommended for susceptible pregnant women who wish to travel to endemic areas. However, the live polio vaccine has been used for mass vaccination during pregnancy without harmful fetal effects (Harjulehto 1989). Other enteroviral infections are not thought to bc more severe than in non-pregnant women, although atypical complications (for example, disseminated peritoneal infection and uterine atony after cesarean section) have been reported with coxsackie B2 virus infection.

Table 13.9: Dosage Of Acyclovir Treatment In Pregnancy (Category B)

Indication	*Route*	*Dosage**
Mild herpetic lesions	Oral	
Severe genital lesions	Oral/Intravenous	200 mg, five times daily/400 mg, three times daily for five days.
Suppressive therapy (genital herpes late in pregnancy)	Oral	400 mg, three times daily from 36 weeks to term
Herpes encephalitis	Intravenous	10 mg/kg, slow infusion over one hour, then 8 hourly for 14-21 days
Severe herpes zoster	Oral	800 mg, five times daily for 7 days
Severe varicella or varicella pneumonia	Oral or intravenous depending on severity	800 mg, four times daily or 10 mg/kg by slow infusion over one hour, repeated 8 hourly for 5 days

* Dosage should be reduced in renal impairment

(Modified from Medical Disorders in Pregnancy, edited by William M Barrow et al.)

Table 13.10: Management of Genital herpes infection at various stages of pregnancy

Clinical Category	Management
Overt genital herpes at labour	Cesarean section
Overt genital herpes earlier in pregnancy	Treat with acyclovir and monitor. If primary give daily suppressive acyclovir from 36 weeks to term to prevent recurrence
First episode at first or second trimester and no recurrence	Treat with acyclovir. Vaginal delivery
First episode within 6 weeks of the due date	Cesarean section
Past history of genital herpes but no clinical episode during the current pregnancy	Inspect genitalia including cervix during labour. If there are no lesions vaginal delivery, and cesarean section if lesions are present.

Transmission and Pathogenesis: Enteroviruses are transmitted postnatally, predominantly by the feco–oral route, but respiratory transmission is also possible. The incubation period is usually 3–6 days. A viremia seeds target organs and the virus is shed from the throat, urine, stool and cervix.

Transmission to the fetus or newborn may occur transplacentally, but the majority of infections are probably acquired either during the birth process or after birth (Modlin 1986). Ascending infection may also occur, presumably from an infected cervix (Reyes 1986). Enteroviruses have been recovered from amniotic fluid associated with chorioamnitis and fetal demise (Neilsen 1988).

Congenital Infections: Even though a number of case reports have implicated non-polioenteroviruses as a cause of spontaneous abortion, stillbirth and fetal loss in the second and third trimesters, population-based studies have not proved the same. The rates of congenital abnormalities were not increased in large studies, except one study which showed cardiovascular and gastrointestinal tract anomalies with coxsackie viruses (Brown 1971). The polio and echoviruses were not associated with any congenital abnormalities. The estimated risk of congenital abnormalities in coxsackie virus infection is too small to justify termination of pregnancy.

Perinatal Infections: Transplacental transfer can occur late in gestation and neonatal enterovirus infections have been documented following cesarean section (Nagington 1978; Modlin 1986; Spector 1983). Infections contracted in utero during maximal maternal viremia, with delivery before maternal antibody development, tend to be the most severe. Postnatal transmission resuts in milder illness. Infections are acquired from the birth canal during delivery or postnatally from exposure to maternal blood, feces or oropharyngeal secretions.

Most newborns are asymptomatic but severe hepatitis in echovirus infections and myocarditis in coxsackie B virus infections can occur. Nosocomial infections in hospital nurseries have also been documented. Low birth weight and prematurity are risk factors for the disease.

Diagnosis: Virological diagnosis of enterovirus infections can be made by the isolation of the virus from stools, throat swabs and other organs and body fluids.

Treatment and Prevention: There is no specific antiviral therapy for enterovirus infections. Immunoglobulins have been used to treat infections, but its value remains untested. Careful attention to handwashing and restricting visitors during enterovirus epidemics are also recommended.

MOLLUSCUM CONTAGIOSUM

Molluscum contagiosum is caused by a poxvirus, molluscum contagiosum, and humans are the only hosts. People of all ages can be affected and transmission is through personal contact or fomites. It can be a marker for sexually transmitted infections, especially AIDS.

It is usually found all over the body in children, and over the genital area, perianal region and upper thighs in adults. They may last a few weeks or some years and are found as crops of popular skin lesions 2 mm to 1 cm in size, with an expressible core of degenerating epidermal cells and keratin.

Molluscum does not pose any additional problem during pregnancy. The characteristic skin lesions and the molluscum bodies in histopathological examination confirm the diagnosis. Treatment is by curettage and cryotherapy.

WEST NILE VIRUS

This is a mosquito-borne flavivirus and a human pathogen. It is transmitted by mosquito bites, typically in late summer. The incubation period is 3–14 days. The infection is usually mild or asymptomatic and less than 1% of adults develop meningoencephalitis.

The presenting symptoms are fever, mental status changes, muscular weakness and coma. Fetal infection has been described at 27 weeks with chorioretinitis and cystic changes in the temporal lobe. Breastfeeding is not prescribed. There is no effective antiviral treatment available and supportive treatment is the only way of management.

RESPIRATORY VIRUSES

The common cold and respiratory tract infections are caused by more than 200 antigenically distinct respiratory viruses, and the commonest viruses are rhinovirus, coronavirus and adenovirus. Adenovirus infections can cause pneumonia.

Fetal Effects: Conflicting reports of fetal neural tube defects (anencephaly) have been attributed to maternal cold infections, fetal myocarditis, non-immune hydrops fetalis and adenovirus infections. Childhood myocarditis has also been linked to adenovirus infections.

SEVERE ACUTE RESPIRATORY SYNDROME (SARS)

SARS is caused by a coronavirus, and since 2002, several outbreaks of community-acquired pneumonia have been reported in Asia and North America. Travel to an endemic area increases the likelihood of diagnosis.

SARS progresses in a triphasic pattern—with fever and myalgia in the first week, recurrent fever, diarrhea and hypoxemia in the second week and acute respiratory distress requiring ventilatory support in the third phase (seen in 20% of patients). The mortality rate is related to acute lung injury.

The CT changes in the lungs include ground-glass opacities to unilateral and bilateral consolidation. Lymphopenia, thrombocytopenia and elevated lactate dehydrogenase have also been reported.

Fetal Illness and Maternal Outcome: SARS generally has a poor outcome in pregnancy. No fetal transmission has been reported, except small bowel perforation in two preterm neonates.

Management: In pregnancy, clarithromycin 500 mg twice daily, with augmentin (amoxicillin with clavulinate 375 mg) three times daily, is recommended. Severe illness is treated with ribavarin and corticosteroids.

Epstein-Barr Virus (EBV)

EBV is a herpes virus that causes infectitious mononucleosis, commonly called glandular fever, which is a disease of adolescents and young adults. Hence, most adults are seropositive and infections are uncommon in pregnancy. EBV is also the etiological agent for Burkitt's lymphoma and nasopharyngeal carcinoma.

The patient presents with fever, malaise, sore throat, petechial rash in the soft palate and a macular rash, hepatitis, cervical lymphadenopathy, hepatosplenomegaly and, sometimes, meningitis. Presence of specific IgM antibodies and positive monospot tests and the Paul-Bunnell test signify presence of the infection.

About 3-4% of pregnant women are susceptible to EBV. A few studies have shown congenital malformations, namely, congenital heart disease, central nervous system malformations, cataracts, biliary atresia, microphthlmia, metaphysitis and low birth weight associated with serological and virological evidence of EBV infection (Goldberg et al 1981). However, there is no convincing evidence that primary EBV infection in pregnancy causes congenital defects. Even though several positive cases of possible vertical transmissions were identified, the outcome of the affected infants was not reported (Meyohas et al 1996).

Usually, symptomatic treatment and administration of corticosteroids for neurological complications is recommended.

Hantavirus

These are RNA viruses and members of the family Bunyaviridae. They are associated with a rodent reservoir. An outbreak due to infection with Sin Nombre virus in Western United States in 1993 was characterised by severe non-cardiogenic pulmonary edema and a fatality rate of 45%. Transplacental transmission can cause fetal demise and preterm birth. It has been associated with hemorrhagic fever and renal symptoms. Prevention is by lowering exposure to infected rodents.

Viral Hemorrhagic Fevers

Viral hemorrhagic fevers can be caused by arenaviruses infections (Lassa fever, Bolivian hemorrhagic fever), filoviruses (Marburg and Ebola), yellow fever (flavivirus) and dengue in severe cases. Maternal and fetal mortality is highest if infection is acquired in the last trimester and a fourfold increase in seen in women who underwent evacuation after spontaneous abortion.

Lassa fever occurs in rural areas in West Africa, and humans are infected by exposure to the secretions and excretions of the rodent, Mastomys natalensis. Ribaverin is given for both, prophylaxis and for treatment, and is effective if given early in the course of infection.

Measles

The measles (rubeola, red measles, first disease) virus is a single-stranded, RNA paramyxovirus, closely related to the canine distemper virus. It causes a highly contagious, febrile infection of childhood, characterised by cough, coryza and conjunctivitis, followed by an erythematous maculopapular rash and pathognomonic Koplik's spots on the oral buccal epithelium. Malnutrition and vitamin A deficiency greatly increase the associated morbidity and mortality. Pneumonitis is the usual cause of death in adults. In elderly patients, hepatitis, encephalomyelitis and sclerosing panencephalitis can occur. Nearly 90% of adults acquire immunity in childhood.

Measles in Pregnancy: Increased risk of measles pneumonitis in the third trimester of pregnancy and increased mortality from heart failure and pulmonary edema has been established (Kamaci et al 1996; Eberhart et al 1993; Gershon et al 1995). Increased risk of spontaneous abortion, premature labour and low birth weight baby has also been observed. There is no difference in the incidence of congenital malformations. Since the incubation period of measles is 13–14 days, measles occurring in the newborn in the first 10 days of life is regarded as resulting from intrauterine transmission, and after 14 days is due to postnatal transmission. One report suggests that measles virus infection in utero may be a risk factor for Crohn's disease (Ekbom et al 1996).

Postnatal infection in the newborn is more severe than childhood infection. One-third of babies exposed to the virus in utero develops the disease, and fatality is higher in babies born prematurely (56%) than at term (20%). Measles is not a case for termination of pregnancy.

Management: Human gamma globulin should be given as soon as possible within 72 hours of exposure up to 7 days. Aerosolised ribavirin may be tried in life-threatening infections. Even though ribavirin has a theoretic potential for teratogenicity, it should not be withheld from a severely ill patient with measles pneumonia. Measles vaccination is contraindicated in pregnancy since it is a live vaccine.

Mumps

The mumps virus is an RNA virus and a member of the paramyxovirus family. It is an acute, generalised, non-exanthematous infection with a predilection for the parotid and salivary glands. It may also affect the brain, pancreas and gonads. It is transmitted by saliva and droplet contamination and the incubation period is 14–18 days. Parotitis occurs within 24 hours of onset of prodrome of fever, malaise, myalgia and anorexia. Although the disease is usually self-limited and complication free, it can be associated with aseptic meningitis, pancreatitis, mastitis, thyroiditis, myocarditis, nephritis, arthritis and orchitis (in postpubertal manes). By the age of 20 years, about 75% of the population would be infected.

Mumps in Pregnancy: Mumps infection does not pose any serious problems for the mother but transplacental transmission may occur, and in the first trimester, it is associated with double the fetal loss than in controls (Siegel et al 1966; Kurtz et al 1982).

There are no convincing reports that gestational mumps is associated with endocardial fibroelastosis (Gersony 1966). Perinatal mumps does not present a significant clinical problem. Laboratory diagnosis is made serologically by the complement fixation test.

Management: Symptomatic treatment with analgesics, bed rest and application of cold or heat to the parotids has been recommended.

Prevention: The live attenuated mumps vaccine is contraindicated in pregnancy. When given with the rubella vaccine, pregnancy should be avoided for the next three months. When monovalent mumps vaccine is given, pregnancy should be avoided for one month. However, inadvertent vaccination during pregnancy should not be considered as an indication for termination of pregnancy.

Influenza

The influenza A and B viruses are RNA viruses of the family Orthomyxoviridae. Influenza A is more serious than influenza B and it usually develops during winter. Symptoms include fever and cough, and the infection can be confirmed with rapid enzyme immunoassay and immunofluorescence assay. Influenza is usually a self-limiting illness, except in those with underlying debility and respiratory and cardiac illnesses. The risk of serious medical complications increases during pregnancy, especially in the third trimester, due to the effect of pregnancy on the cardiovascular and respiratory systems.

Fetal Effects: No firm evidence that influenza A causes congenital malformations such as fetal neural tube defects exists, even though they have been reported in some studies. There is controversial evidence that fetal exposure to influenza A may predispose the child to schizophrenia later (Kunugi et al 1995).

Prevention: Since serious medical complications can occur during pregnancy, the Advisory Committee in Immunisation Practices of the United States recommends that women who are beyond the first trimester of pregnancy during the influenza season be vaccinated. Even though the vaccine is an inactivated agent and should be safe for administration at any time during pregnancy, the CDC recommends deferring vaccination of pregnant women until beyond the first trimester (CDC, 2004). However, if there is a high-risk medical disorder such as diabetes, heart disease, asthma and HIV infection, delay is not warranted. There is no evidence of teratogenicity, and clinical illness is prevented in 70–90% of healthy adults. The cold-adapted, live, attenuated vaccine administered intranasally is not recommended for pregnant women.

Management: Chemoprophylaxis with amantadine and vimantadine has been effective against the influenza A virus (ineffective against influenza B) in 70–90% of healthy adults. Neuraminidase inhibitors such as oseltamivir and zananivir have also been used to reduce the duration of complicated illness by about one day. Since these drugs are FDA category C drugs, they should be used when the potential benefits outweigh the risks. Unfortunately, these drugs do not prevent serious complications such as pneumonia.

Infected pregnant women should be advised to remain and rest at home. They should maintain hydration and use acetaminophen/paracetamol (650 mg orally every 4–6 hours, maximum 4 g/24 hours), as needed, to lower their temperature and reduce discomfort from headache and myalgias. They should be evaluated for pneumonia and preterm labour. They should also be treated with either zanamivir 10 mg or oseltamivir 75–150 mg orally twice daily for five days.

Conditions that Mimic Congenital Virus Infections: Several non-infectious disorders produce clinical features that can resemble intrauterine infections. Aicardi syndrome, Warburg syndrome, incontinentia pigmenti and neonatal Graves' disease are among the non-infectious disorders that may occasionally be confused with an intrauterine infection.

Immunisation during Pregnancy:

- Do not give live virus vaccines during pregnancy, unless the health of the mother is at serious risk, and only after discussing the risks with the patient.
- Inactivated vaccine alternatives are available for poliomyelitis.
- Inadvertent rubella vaccination has not been associated with fetal damage.
- Even though it is not contraindicated, inactivated vaccines are better given before or after pregnancy.
- The TC-83 vaccine for VEE and the vaccine for small pox are known to cause fetal damage.
- Gamma globulins are not hazardous to pregnant women.
- Efforts should be made to immunise all unimmunised mothers in the postpartum period.
- The rabies (diploid cell) and Hepatitis B vaccines are safe in pregnancy.
- Influenza vaccination is recommended after the first trimester of pregnancy and women with underlying medical conditions should be vaccinated regardless of the stage of pregnancy.
- Live attenuated viral vaccines (polio, measles, rubella and mumps) are best avoided in pregnancy, but inadvertent vaccination has not caused fetal damage, and hence is not reason for termination of pregnancy. Since viremia has been documented after oral polio vaccination, it should be avoided. Inactivated polio vaccine is a preferable alternative.
- Yellow fever vaccination is also not associated with fetal damage, However, it is advisable to give the vaccine as late in the pregnancy as possible.
- Vaccines that are reactogenic may cause fever and result in miscarriage.
- Vaccination of children of pregnant mothers need not be postponed because they only shed the viruses and do not transmit them. If the pregnant mother or any member in the family has not been immunised against polio, after the vaccination of the children, the secondary contacts may become infected with a mutated virulent virus. Hence, in such circumstances, the pregnant mother should receive killed polio vaccine while her children receive the live oral version.

Conclusion Tremendous progress has been made towards understanding and treating specific viral infections during pregnancy but much remains to be accomplished. Viral hemorrhagic fevers can be fatal to the fetus and the mother. Advances in diagnosis and therapeutics have decreased the risk of vertical transmission. Yet, the large economical divide between the developed and developing nations has resulted in limitations in administering appropriate therapy. Hence, the risk of vertical transmission is a continuing problem in these nations. The long-term effects of many antiviral agents on children are yet to be discovered.

References

Altshuler G. 1974. Immunologic competence of the immature human fetus: Morphologic evidence from intrauterine cytomegalovirus infection. *Obstet Gynaecol* 43:811–816.

American College of Obstetricians and Gynecologists. 2003. Immunisation during pregnancy. Committee opinion No.282.

Arvin AM, PA Hendsleigh, CG Prober et al. 1986. Failure of antepartum maternal cultures to predict the infant's risk of exposure to herpes simplex virus at delivery. *N Engl J Med* 315:796–800.

Bart SW, HC Stellan, SR Preblind et al. 1985. Fetal risk associated with rubella vaccine: An update. *Rev Infection Dis* 7:595.

Basic Science in Obstetrics & Gynaecology. 2002. A textbook for MRCOG Part I, 3rd ed. ed de Swiet M Chamberlain and P Bewett Churchill Livingstone: Edinburg, p 126–127.

Blanc WA. 1981. Pathology of the placenta, membranes and umbilical cord in bacterial, fungal and viral infections in man. In *Perinatal disease* ed RL Naeye, JM Kissana, N Kaufmam, Baltimore: Williams and Wilkins:67.

Boppana SB, KB Fowler, Y Vaid et al. 1999. Neuroradiographic findings iin the newborn and long term outcome in children with symptomatic congenital cytomegalovirus infection, *Pediatrics* 99.

Bosma TJ, KM Corbett, S O'Shea et al. 1995. PCR for detection of rubella virus RNA in clinical samples. *J Clin Microbiol* 33:1075–1079.

Brocklehurst P, G Kinghan, O Carney et al. 1998. A randomized placebo controlled trial of suppressive acyclovir in late pregnancy in women with recurrent genital herpes infection. *Br J Obslet Gynaecol* 105:275.

Brown AS and ES Susser. 2002. In utero infection and adult schizophrenia. *Ment Retard Dev Disabil Res Rev* 8 (1):51–57.

Brown GC and RS Karunas. 1971. Relationship of congenital anomalies and maternal infection with selected enteroviruses. *Am J Epidemiol* 95:207.

Brown T, A Anand and LD Ritchie. 1984. Intrauterine parvovirus associated with hydrops fetalis. *Lancet* 2:1033–1034.

Byrne BMP, PA Crowley and D Carrington. 2007. Chicken pox in pregnancy. Royal College of Obstetricians and Gynaecologists. Clinical 'Green Top' Guidelines. London: RCOG.

Conry JA, T Torok and I Andres. 1993. Perinatal encephalopathy secondary to in utero human parvovirous B 19 (PV infection). *Neurology* 43:A346.

Cope AP, A Jones and M Brozonic et al. 1992. Possible induction of systemic lupus erythematosus by human parvovirus. *Ann Rheum Dis* 51:803 Centers for Disease Control and Prevention:2004

Cradock-Watson JE, MKS Ridehalgh, MJ Anderson et al. 1985. Rubella, re infection and the fetus, *Lancet* 1:1039, 1985.

De Nicola LK and JB Hauston. 1979. Congenital and neonatal varicella (editorial). *J Pediatr;* 94:175.

Eberhart JE, Phillips JE, PD Frederick, RC Baron et al. 1993. Measles in pregnancy. A descriptive study of 58 cases. *Obstet Gynecol* 82.

Ekhbom A, P Daszak, W Kraas et al. 1996. Crohn's Disease after in utero measles virus exposure. *Lancet* 348:515.

Enders G, E Miller, J Cradock-Watson et al. 1994. Consequences of varicella and herpes zoster in pregnancy, prospective study of 1739 cases. *Lancet* 343: 1548–1550.

Enders G, U Wickerl Packer, E Miller et al. 1988. Outcome of confirmed periconceptional maternal rubella. *Lancet* I: 1447–1114.

Feldman RG, J Bryant, KN Ives et al. 1987. A novel presentation of coxsackie B2 virus infection during pregnancy. *J Infect* 15:73–76.

Fox H. 1981. Placental involvement in maternal systemic infection. In: Rosemberg HS, Bernstein J. ed., *Perspectives in Pediatric Pathology*. Vol. 6 New York: Masson: 63.

Gershon AA. 1995. Chickenpox, measles and mumps. In *Infections diseases of the fetus and newborn infant* 4th ed. JS Remington and JO Klein, 565–618 Philadelphia: WB Saunders.

Gersony WM, SL Katz, AS Nadas. 1966. Endocardial fibroelastosis and the mumps virus. *Pediatrics* 37:430.

Goldberg GN et al. 1981. Association with African Burkitts lymphoma and hairy leukoplakia in patients with AIDS and Hodgkins lymphoma. *JAMA* 240:15,79.

Goldberg GN et al. 1981.Association with African Burkitts lymphoma and hairy leukoplakia in patients with AIDS and Hodgkins lymphoma. *JAMA* 240:15,7.

Gratracos E, PJ Torres, J Vidal et al. 1995. The incidence of human parvovirus B19 infection during pregnancy and its impact on perinatal outcome. *J Infect Dis* 171:1360.

Griffiths PD. 1995. Cytomegalovirus. In *Principles and practice of clinical virology*, 3rd ed. ed. Zuckerman AJ, JE Banavala, JR Pattison, Chichester: John Viley and Sons 69.

Griffiths PD. 2000. Cytomegalo virus In *Principles and practice of clinical Virology* 4th ed. ed. Zuckerman AJ, JE Banavala, JR Pattison, Chichester: John Wiley and Sons 79–116.

Harjulehto F, T Aro, T Hovi et al. 1989. Congenital malformation and oral poliovirus vaccination during pregnancy. *Lancet* 1:771.

Hehlmann R. 1991. Human Retroviruses In *Textbook of human virology* 2nd ed. ed RB Belshe, 274–306. St Louis: Mosby Year Book.

Kamaci M, CG Zorlin and A Belhar. 1996. Measles in pregnancy. *Acta Obstetr Gynecol Scand* 75:3.

Katz V1, MC McCoy, JA Kuller and WF Hausan. 1996. An association between fetal parvovirus B19 infection and fetal anomalies: A report of few cases. *Am J perinatal* 13:43.

Kunugi H and S Nauko.1995. Schizophrenia following in utero exposure to the 1957 influenza epidemics in Japan. *Am J Psychiatry* 152:450.

Kurtz JB, AH Tonulinson and J Pearson. 1982. Mumps virus isolated from a fetus.*BMJ;* 284:47.

Le CT, S Chang, MH Lipson. 1983. Epstein-Barr virus infections during pregnancy. *Am J Dis Child* 137:466.

Levy R, A Weissman, G Blomberg et al. 1997. Infection by parvovirus B 19 during pregnancy: A review. *Obstet Gynecol Surv* 52:254.

Low-Beer NM and JR Smith. 2002. Management of genital herpes in pregnancy. Royal College of Obstetricians and Gynaecologists. Clinical 'Green Top' Guidelines. London: RCOG.

Marie LL. 2000. *Viral infections in medical complications during pregnancy*, ed Burrow GN and Duffy TP, 5th ed. 337–362, WB Saunders Company, Harcourt Asia PTE Ltd..

Mellinger AK, JD Cragon.,WL Atkinson, et al. 1995. High incidence of congenital rubella syndrome after a rubella outbreak. *Pediatr Infect Dis J* 14(7):573–578.

Meyohas MC, V Marechal, N Desire et al. 1996. Study of mother to child Epstein-Barr virus transmission by means of nested PCRs. *J Virol* 70:6816.

Miller E, CK Fairley, BJ Cohen et al. 1998. Immediate and long term effect of human parvovirous B19 infection in pregnancy. *J Obstet Gynaecol* 105:174–175.

Miller E, JE Cradock-Watson and TM Pallock. 1982. Consequences of confirmed maternal rubella at successive stages of pregnancy. *Lancet* 2(8302):781–784.

Modlin JF. 1986. Perinatal echovirus infection. Insights from a literature review of 61 cases of serious infection and 16 outbreaks in nurseries. *Rev Infect Dis* 8:918.

Modlin JF. 1988. Perinatal echovirus and Group B coxsackie infections. *Clin Perinatal* 15:233.

Morgan-Capner P, E Miller, JE Vurdien et al. 1991. Outcome of pregnancy after maternal re infection with rubella. *Communicable Disease Report* 1:R57–59.

Nagington J, TG Wreghitt, G Gandy et al. 1978. Fatal echovirus 11 infections in outbreak in special-care baby unit. *Lancet* ii 725.

Neilsen JL, GK Berryman and GDV Hankins. 1988. Intrauterine fetal death and the isolation of echovirus 27 from amniotic fluid. *J Infect Dis* 158:501.

Plotkin SA. 1988. Mechanisms and pathways of congenital infections. *Clin Perinatal* 15:163.

Reiff-Eldridge RA, CR Heffner, SA Ephron et al. 2000. Monitoring pregnancy outcomes after prenatal drug exposure through prospective pregnancy register: A pharmaceutical company communication. *Am J Obstet Gynecol* 182:159.

Reyes MP, D Zalenski, F Smith et al. 1986. Coxsackie virus positive cervices in women with febrile illness during the third trimester of pregnancy. *Am J Obstet Gynecol* 155:159.

Rodis JF, C Rodner, AA Hansen et al. 1998. Long term outcome of children following maternal human parvovirus B19 infection. *Obstet Gynaecol* 91:125, 1.

Rziha HJ, BH Belohradsky, U Schneider et al: 1978. BK virus II: Serologic studies in children with congenital disease and parents with malignant tumours and immunodeficiencies. *Med Microbiol Immunol* 165:83–92.

Seigel M and M Greenberg. 1955. Incidence of poliomyelitis in pregnancy, its relation to maternal age, parity and gestational period. *N Engl J Med* 243:841–847.

Siegel M and HT Fuerst. 1966. Low birth weight and maternal virus diseases: A prospective study of rubella, mumps, chicken pox and hepatitis. *JAMA* 197:86–92.

Smego RA and MO Asperilla. 1991. Use of acyclovir for varicella pneumonia during pregnancy. *Obstet Gynecol* 78:1112.

Spector SA, RC Straube. 1983. Protean manifestations of perinatal enterovirus infections. *West J Med* 138:847.

Tiessen RZG, AMV Van Elsacker-Niele, CHR Vermey-Keers et al. 1994. A fetus with a parvovirus B19 infection and congenital anomalies. *Prenatal* 14:173.

Webster MH, CS Smith. 1977. Congenital abnormalities and maternal herpes zoster. *K Med J* 2;1193

Whitley RJ and B Roizman. 2001. Herpes simplex virus infections. *Lancet* 357:1513–1518.

Wright R, D Johnson, M Neumann et al. 1997. Congenital lymphocytic choriomeningitis virus syndrome: A disease that mimics congenital toxoplasmosis or cytomegalovirus infection. *Pediatrics* 100: E9.

Yaginuma Y, M Kawamura, M Ishikawa et al 1996. Guillian–Barre syndrome in pregnancy. *J Obstet Gynaecol* 22:47–49.

14

HIV in Pregnancy

Rashmi Bagga

When an HIV-infected woman is planning a pregnancy or is diagnosed with HIV during pregnancy, there are two major concerns. The first is about the management of her HIV disease, and the second about perinatal transmission and the methods to reduce this. The risk of perinatal transmission is 15–20% in non-breastfeeding populations in Europe and 25–40% in the breastfeeding population in Africa. The risk of perinatal transmission is higher in developing countries, possibly because of infant feeding practices such as breastfeeding, longer duration of breastfeeding and the universality of this practice in these areas (Working Group on Mother-to-Child Transmission of HIV 1995). Perinatal transmission can be reduced to less than 2% with suitable measures such as anti-retroviral therapy (ART), delivery by elective cesarean section and avoidance of breastfeeding. However, some of these interventions may not be easy to follow in resource-poor countries like India. WHO has modified some of these interventions for resource-constrained countries so that they are less costly but still provide the benefit of reducing perinatal transmission (World Health Organization 2004). However, no intervention guarantees a zero transmission rate of HIV infection to the baby.

THE HIV EPIDEMIC

Today HIV/AIDS has assumed epidemic proportions and increasingly affects women and children. Globally, just under half of all people living with HIV are women. This is primarily because of heterosexual transmission, and the fastest increase in the proportion of women with HIV infection is in Asia, Eastern Europe and Latin America. In 2004, an estimated 39.4 million people in the world were HIV-positive, of which 37.2 million were adults, 17.6 million were women and 2.2 million were children below 15 years (UNAIDS/WHO 2004). Up to July 2006, 38.6 million people were estimated to be living with HIV/AIDS, and 27 million have died since the beginning of the epidemic. About 4.9 million people became infected with HIV in 2005, including 700,000 children, most of whom were infected by perinatal transmission. Of these children, 70% were born in sub-Saharan Africa, 25% in southeast Asia and 5% in Latin America and the Caribbean (UNAIDS 2006). Each day, 14,000 people become infected with HIV, with increasing numbers of young adults, women and children. Fifteen hundred children are infected daily by perinatal transmission, despite the knowledge that ART administered at the time of delivery and to the infant after birth may largely prevent this. Unfortunately, ART prophylaxis that can prevent perinatal or mother-to-child transmission (MTCT) reaches only 10% of affected mothers (Schwartlander et al 2006). MTCT is the most important cause of HIV infection in children in developing countries, though its incidence has been significantly reduced in developed countries. In 2003, less than 1000 children were estimated to have acquired the infection in North America and western Europe, and less than 100 in Australia and New Zealand (World Health Organization 2004).

The Prevention of Parent-to-Child Transmission of HIV/AIDS (PPTCT) programme was started in India in 2002 by the National AIDS Control Organisation (NACO). Based on HIV prevalence rates in the adult population, estimated from the National Sentinel Surveillance Round conducted during 2003, India's states and union territories were divided into three groups—those with a high prevalence of HIV infection of >1% among antenatal women (Maharashtra, Tamilnadu, Karnataka, Andhra Pradesh, Manipur and Nagaland), those with a moderate prevalence of <1% among antenatal women and >5% among high-risk groups (Gujarat, Goa and Pondicherry), and those with a low prevalence of <1% among antenatal women and <5% among high-risk groups (Manual for Management of HIV/AIDS in Children, NACO, IAP, WHO, UNICEF 2004). Currently, there are more than 4000 Integrated Counselling and Testing Centres (ICTCs) in government hospitals in India. These offer PPTCT services to pregnant women. Of these, 502 are located in Obstetrics and Gynecology departments and in maternity homes where the patients are predominantly pregnant women. The Joint Technical Mission on PPTCT (2006) estimated that out of 27 million annual pregnancies in India, 189,000 occur in HIV-positive women. In the absence of any intervention, an estimated 56,700 infected babies will be born annually. The PPTCT programme entails counselling and testing of pregnant women in ICTCs. Pregnant women who are found to be HIV-positive are given a single dose of nevirapine at the time of labour; their newborns also get a dose of nevirapine immediately after birth to prevent transmission of HIV from the mother. The PPTCT services cover only about 10% of pregnancies in the country. In 2006, 2.1 million pregnant women accessed this service and 16,500 of them were found to be HIV-positive. To provide universal access to PPTCT services, further scale-up is planned up to the level of Community Health Centres and the Primary Health Centres, as well as in the private sector by forging public-private partnerships. NACO hopes to reduce the proportion of infants infected with HIV/AIDS by 50% by 2010 (NACO, India 2007).

Pathogenesis

HIV-1 and HIV-2 are DNA retroviruses that cause acquired immunodeficiency syndrome (AIDS). HIV-1 causes the most infections worldwide, including in India, whereas the HIV-2 virus is endemic in West Africa. Transmission routes are chiefly sexual (homosexual or heterosexual), through blood or body fluids and from an HIV-infected mother to the fetus/infant. Retroviruses have the unique ability to make DNA copies of their own genome within the host cells by transcription from RNA with the help of the reverse transcriptase enzyme. The HIV virus attacks the host cells that have the CD4 antigen. These are chiefly T lymphocytes, some monocyte macrophages and microglial brain cells. After the virus attaches itself to the host cells with the help of CD4 receptors, it gains entry into the host cells, where it uses the reverse transcriptase enzyme to transcribe its genomic DNA. Viral DNA is incorporated into cellular DNA and after cell death, many virions are released into the bloodstream and these attack more T cells. Cell life is shortened by this infection and thus, the number of T lymphocytes falls gradually, insidiously and profoundly, leading to immunosuppression. Viremia can be detected and quantified by using viral-RNA assays. The initial infection is similar to that of any acute viral syndrome and lasts for a few days. This is followed by a long latency period (5–10 years) during which the HIV-infected individual is asymptomatic. Ultimately, with profound immunosuppression, the clinical symptoms and signs of AIDS manifest. HIV antibodies in blood are detected 3–6 months after the initial infection.

HIV Testing in Women Planning a Pregnancy or During Pregnancy Ideally, all women planning a pregnancy should undergo HIV testing so that if they are found to be HIV-positive their disease status can be assessed. If they are found to have an advanced stage of the disease which needs ART, the viral levels should be reduced (undetectable or less than 500–1000 copies per ml) to minimise perinatal transmission. However, this is rarely the scenario in India. The next best opportunity for screening for HIV infection is during early pregnancy. NACO recommends routine, voluntary HIV screening of all pregnant women after counselling and obtaining informed consent, so that appropriate measures can be taken to ensure a favourable outcome for the mother and the baby. If a woman declines testing, she should be counselled again at subsequent visits and the benefits of HIV screening must be explained. Screening only high-risk women may not help detect all HIV-infected women because, in India, the chief mode of transmission is heterosexual, and HIV-infected women do not belong to any well-defined risk group. Most such women may be unsuspecting victims of a legal monogamous relationship in which they acquire infection from their partner who may have contracted the infection from elsewhere. Currently, NACO has established Integrated Counselling Testing Centres (ICTC) in hospitals all over India. These provide free HIV screening and ART to pregnant women, their partners, children and anyone else who desires HIV screening.

Pregnancy and HIV Disease Progression

It is thought that pregnancy, because of its associated hormonal changes or suppression of cellular immunity, may lead to HIV disease progression. However, data from the United States and Europe has not substantiated this (Burns et al 1998; Saada et al 2000). Normally, the CD4 count falls during pregnancy and then returns to the pre-pregnancy levels in the postpartum period; and there is no increased risk of accelerated immunosuppression during pregnancy. A French cohort study of 365 women with a known date of HIV sero-conversion reported the relative risk of disease progression associated with pregnancy as 0.7 (Saada et al 2000). Some studies from developing countries suggest that the disease may progress with pregnancy but the results are not easy to interpret because of small sample size and selection bias related to indications for testing (Watts 2002). An observational study of 140 HIV-seropositive asymptomatic women of childbearing age in Haiti (1984–1992), in which 44 women were pregnant or became pregnant during the study period, showed that there was a trend towards earlier manifestation of HIV-related symptoms among the pregnant cohort, but no significant difference was observed in the rate of progression to AIDS or death between pregnant and non-pregnant women (Deschamps et al 1993). Another study among 71 tribal women with AIDS in Manipur, India (1992–1996) to assess the impact of pregnancy on maternal AIDS showed that pregnancy in women with AIDS had a detrimental effect on maternal as well as obstetric outcome and accelerated disease progression (Kumar et al 1997). A meta-analysis suggested that pregnancy in HIV-positive women may be associated with a small increase in the risk of adverse maternal outcome, but further large-scale observational studies of pregnant and non-pregnant HIV-infected women with long-term follow-up are required (French and Brocklehurst 1998).

Effect of HIV Disease on Pregnancy Outcome HIV infection, especially when advanced, may adversely affect pregnancy, with increased risk of spontaneous abortion, fetal growth restriction, low birth weight and preterm birth but no increase in congenital malformations (Brocklehurst and French 1998). Higher rates of adverse outcomes are reported with more advanced HIV infection (Watts 2002; Brocklehurst and French 1998). In addition, such women have increased susceptibility to certain infections and alteration in their natural course/treatment. These include vulvovaginal candidiasis, bacterial vaginosis, genital herpes, syphilis, human papilloma virus infection, cytomegalovirus infection, toxoplasmosis and hepatitis B and C (Anderson 2001). Dual infection with HIV and malaria produces additional detrimental effects on maternal and infant survival (Ticconi et al 2003).

HIV Infection and Perinatal Transmission

Timing of perinatal transmission Perinatal transmission can occur during pregnancy, labour or delivery, or while breastfeeding. According to the Pediatric Virology Committee of the AIDS Clinical Trials Group in the United States, a child with a positive DNA-PCR (polymerase chain reaction) within 48 hours of birth is likely to have been affected in utero during the antenatal period, while a positive PCR within 7–90 days of birth indicates an intrapartum infection (Rouzioux et al 1995). Some proportion of transmissions (25–35%) occurs during the antenatal period as the HIV virus has been shown to cross the placental barrier early in pregnancy; most of these transmissions occur in the late third trimester (after 36 weeks) (Lewis et al 1990). Most transmissions (65–75%) take place during the intrapartum period. The postulated mechanisms are materno-fetal microtransfusions during uterine contractions and exposure of the baby's mucocutaneous surfaces to maternal blood and cervico-vaginal secretions during delivery. Breastfeeding is associated with a twofold increase in transmission and it results in an excess transmission rate of 12–16%. The risk is maximal during the first six months of life (NACO India 2004).

Factors influencing vertical transmission of HIV (Anderson 2001, Kapoor et al 2004) HIV-related factors: The risk is reduced when the plasma HIV RNA levels are undetectable, in case of infections with HIV-2, the viral phenotype is T cell tropic (more risk with macrophage tropic virus phenotype) and high CD4 levels are seen. The risk is reduced by the use of antenatal and neonatal ART.

Maternal factors The risk of perinatal transmission is increased in the presence of advanced HIV disease, AIDS-related symptoms, substance abuse, Vitamin A deficiency, smoking, co-existing sexually transmitted infections (STIs) and unprotected sexual intercourse. A trial with Vitamin A supplementation did not lower the overall MTCT rate but reduced the number of preterm births, and among preterm babies, reduced HIV transmission (Coutsoudis et al 1999). A randomised trial in Tanzania showed that multivitamin supplementation, but not Vitamin A, during pregnancy was associated with significant increase in CD4, CD8 and CD3 counts. The clinical relevance of multivitamin supplementation for vertical transmission of HIV and the progression of disease was not known, but such supplementation appeared to be a low-cost means of substantially decreasing adverse pregnancy outcomes and increasing T cell counts in HIV-infected women. The beneficial effects of multivitamins on birth outcome may have been mediated through improved maternal immune status (Fawzi et al 1998).

Obstetric factors: The risk is increased with prolonged labour, ruptured membranes (2% per hour of ruptured membranes), episiotomy, operative vaginal delivery, invasive fetal monitoring like scalp blood sampling, vaginal delivery, placental abruption and chorioamnionitis (Read 2000). Elective cesarean section performed prior to ruptured membranes or onset of labour (~38 weeks) reduces vertical transmission in all HIV-infected women except in those with HIV-RNA levels of <1000 copies/ml, as, in this situation, vertical transmission is already very low (<2%) and elective cesarean section does not reduce it further. Elective cesarean confers a higher benefit in reducing perinatal transmission in women with advanced disease and high viral loads, but at the cost of higher morbidity in the mother.

Fetal and neonatal factors: The risk is higher in preterm babies. It also increases with breastfeeding especially mixed feeding, breast infection or cracked nipples and oral candidiasis in the infant.

Pre-pregnancy Counselling and Contraception

All HIV-infected women should be counselled regarding planning or avoiding a pregnancy, according to their desire. If pregnancy is to be deferred, contraception is advised. Consistent and correct use of condoms (either male or female) at each sexual intercourse must be emphasised and hormonal contraception (combined oral pills or progestin-only contraceptives) may be offered in addition to condoms for better contraceptive efficacy. Though hormonal contraceptives can lead to increased virus shedding in the genital tract and increased cervical ectopy, given their effectiveness and overall safety, they remain an option for these women. Estradiol levels from oral contraceptives are reduced by nevirapine, ritonavir and nelfinavir; this may reduce contraceptive efficacy (MMWR 1998; Saada et al 2000). Interactions between medroxyprogesterone acetate and anti-retroviral drugs are being studied, but this agent is a reasonable choice. Intrauterine devices may be offered to HIV-infected women who have a low risk of STIs and do not have severe immune suppression. They should be used with caution because of increased risk of pelvic inflammatory disease and increased duration and volume of bleeding associated with their use. Spermicides such as nonoxynol-9 are to be avoided. Though nonoxynol-9 is HIV-cidal, this beneficial effect is negated by its effect on the vaginal mucosa. Local inflammation and vaginal mucosal injury caused by prolonged use of nonoxynol-9 further increases the transmission of STIs and HIV (Anderson 2001).

If an HIV-infected woman is planning a pregnancy, evaluation of her disease status including CD4 count and HIV-RNA levels should be done. If required, treatment with anti-retrovirals (ARV) may be initiated to optimise the disease status. STIs must be screened for and treated. Good general health and nutrition must be ensured and lifestyle modifications such as avoidance of substance abuse encouraged. Hepatitis B immunisation should be carried out.

Antenatal Management HIV-infected women are cared for by a team comprising an obstetrician, a physician conversant with HIV infection management, a pediatrician and a health counsellor who co-ordinates the patients' care. Management strategies are summarised as follows:

Assessment of HIV disease status and ARV: Clinical assessment and laboratory investigations are carried out to classify the pregnant woman as asymptomatic HIV-positive or having an advanced disease. Women with AIDS-defining illnesses or severe symptoms of HIV infection are started on ARV therapy irrespective of their CD4 count. Asymptomatic women with a CD4 count of <200/ml definitely need ARV and those with a CD4 count of 200–350/ml may also be offered ARV. Some clinicians initiate ARV if the CD4 count is >350/ml but plasma viral load is very high (>100,000 copies/ml) (http://aidsinfo.nih.gov 2004).

The highly active anti-retroviral therapy (HAART) regimen recommended by the WHO as first-line therapy comprises two nucleoside reverse transcriptase inhibitors (NRTIs) (zidovudine or ZDV and lamivudine or 3TC) and one non-nucleoside reverse transcriptase inhibitor (NNRTI) (nevirapine or NVP). Another NNRTI, efavirenz, is teratogenic in monkeys (causes anencephaly, anophthalmia or cleft palate) and is better avoided during pregnancy. ZDV and 3TC have not been shown to be teratogenic in animals in concentrations similar to those used in humans. The rates of birth defects among infants born to more than 400 women exposed to ZDV and 3TC during the first trimester were no higher than those of infants born to women exposed after the first trimester or infants in the Metropolitan Atlanta Congenital Defects Program of the Centers for Disease Control and Prevention (Antiretroviral Pregnancy Registry 2001). ZDV, 3TC and NVP cross the placenta and provide prophylaxis to the fetus, unlike protease inhibitors (PIs) which do not cross the placenta (WHO 2004). Didanosine and stavudine are two other NRTs that may be given in pregnancy, but not together, as cases of lactic acidosis, some fatal, have been reported in pregnant women who receive these two NRTs together. ZDV, 3TC and stavudine are FDA pregnancy category C drugs; NVP and didanosine belong to category B.

NRTIs bind to mitochondrial DNA polymerase gamma and may cause mitochondrial dysfunction. This manifests clinically as myopathy, cardiomyopathy, neuropathy, lactic acidosis, or fatty liver of pregnancy (Watts 2002). ZDV has hematologic toxicity (anemia, neutropenia and thrombocytopenia), 3TC is associated with mitochondrial dysfunction and NVP is linked to cutaneous rash and hepatotoxicity. NVP hepatotoxicity is 10 times higher when the CD4 count is >250/ml (Baylor and Johann-Liang 2004). Hepatitis develops in about 1% of those who receive NVP and may be fatal (Watts 2002). Carcinogenicity of ART drugs is another concern. An increase in the incidence of tumours of the liver, lungs, and reproductive system was reported in rodents exposed in utero to zidovudine at 30 times the dose used in humans, but no increase was found in a similar study using lower doses. Data from studies on humans does not suggest an increase in the incidence of tumours in children with prenatal exposure to ART. Among 727 children exposed to ZDV in utero and followed up for six years, no tumours or deaths from cancer occurred (Watts 2002; Hanson et al 1999).

Antenatal evaluation: At the initial visit, the obstetric details and medical history are noted. A physical examination including an obstetric examination is performed. In addition, a pelvic examination is carried out to collect a PAP smear used to screen for cervical dysplasia and to check for any STIs or vaginal infections which are then appropriately treated. The investigations include blood group, STS, hepatitis B surface antigen, anti-HCV, urine analysis, Mantoux test, complete hemogram, liver function tests, toxoplasma and cytomegalovirus screening. CD4 count, HIV-RNA levels, complete blood counts and liver function tests are repeated every 3–4 months. A screening test for gestational diabetes is done at 24–28 weeks. Ultrasound to screen for congenital fetal malformations is desirable. It is unclear whether invasive procedures such as amniocentesis and chorionic villous sampling for prenatal diagnosis increase the risk of perinatal HIV transmission. The use of amniocentesis among HIV-infected women is uncommon, and the use of chorionic villus sampling is rare (Watts 2002). The risk may be higher among untreated women and therefore such procedures should be avoided (Mandelbrot et al 1996).

Prevention of opportunistic infections: If CD4 count is <200/ml, a once-daily tablet of double strength trimethoprim-sulphamethoxazole should be given for prophylaxis of pneumocystis carinii pneumonia (PCP) and toxoplasmosis. Folate supplementation is even more important for women who receive this. In case of a positive Mantoux test of >5 mm, isoniazid 300 mg with pyridoxine 50 mg daily has been suggested for mycobacterium tuberculosis prophylaxis after excluding active tuberculosis (Anderson 2001). However, its routine use in endemic countries like India is not recommended as tuberculin positivity in the general population is high. Drug resistance to isoniazid is increasingly being encountered and chemoprophylaxis may not prevent re-infection. In India, approximately 50% of the adult population is tuberculin-positive and therefore this may not be taken as an indication for isoniazid prophylaxis. However, in the event of a documented recent tuberculin conversion and/or recent exposure or close contact with active tuberculosis, isoniazid prophylaxis may be considered (Khilnani 2004).

Immunisation Pneumococcal and influenza vaccines are recommended before the flu season begins. The hepatitis B vaccine must be given in anti-HBc–negative patients. The hepatitis A vaccine is administered to women with chronic hepatitis C. Vaccination should ideally be administered after HIV-RNA has been suppressed to undetectable levels with ARV, to prevent increase in the risk of transmission that theoretically accompanies the transient increase in HIV-RNA after immunisation.

Anti-retroviral therapy for prevention of perinatal transmission According to the US Public Health Service Task Force Recommendations, any pregnant woman who does not require HAART for her own disease status but who has a HIV RNA level of >1000 copies/ml is considered eligible for HAART; this is done to reduce MTCT. Women with RNA levels of <1000 copies/ml are eligible for the ACTG 076 (AIDS Clinical Trial Group) protocol in which ZDV (300 mg BD) is given throughout pregnancy, after the first trimester and intrapartum to the mother and for 6 weeks to the neonate (2 mg/kg weight given 6 hourly) (http://aidsinfo.nih.gov 2007). If the RNA level at 36 weeks is <1000 copies/ml, there is no further benefit from an elective cesarean as MTCT would already have been reduced to <2% with ARV. All other women may undergo elective cesarean at 38 weeks to further reduce MTCT. Breastfeeding is not recommended in these settings.

However, such optimal therapies may not be available and practical in resource-constrained countries such as India. The WHO has identified four regimens of abbreviated ARV for women in resource-limited settings who do not need ARV for their own health and stipulated that selection of the ARV drug regimen is to be made at the national level, based on issues of efficacy, safety, drug resistance, feasibility and acceptability. The most efficacious of these regimens is ZDV 300 mg BD antenatally from 28 weeks of gestation, 300 mg 3 hourly during labour; in addition, a single dose NEV 200 mg must be given to the mother at onset of labour and a single dose of NEV (2 mg/kg weight. given between 48 and 72 hours after birth) plus a week of ZDV (2 mg/kg weight given 6 hourly) to the infant. This has been adopted by Thailand and is associated with a vertical transmission rate of <2% even without the added benefit of elective cesarean (Coovadia 2004). The second and third WHO regimens involve the independent use of either of these drugs. NACO, India has adopted the single-dose NEV strategy to the mother and child; this is available free of cost in all ICTCs for pregnant women. The fourth regimen is ZDV and 3TC from 36 weeks of pregnancy and for one week postpartum, both to the mother and the baby.

Use of single-dose NVP at the onset of labour may lead to drug resistance in the mother later, as NVP has a long half-life. The US Public Health Service Task Force reports that studies in South Africa and Cote d'Ivoire have shown that giving a cover or tail of ZDV plus 3TC for 3–7 days postpartum to women who receive a single dose of NVP at the onset of labour may reduce this resistance (http://aidsinfo.nih.gov 2007).

Mode of Delivery and Intrapartum Management Elective cesarean at 38 weeks lowers the MTCT (OR 0.43) both in women who receive ZDV monotherapy and those who do not receive ARV but not in women on HAART with RNA levels of <1000 copies/ml (Watts 2002). However, the morbidity and mortality associated with cesarean delivery is 5–7 times that of vaginal delivery, a fact to be remembered while discussing its benefits and risks with the patient. Its benefit in reducing MTCT is more in women with high viral loads. The pregnant woman should be counselled regarding the mode of delivery and infant feeding practices during the antenatal period and supported in whatever decision she takes.

If a woman reports in labour that is freely progressing, vaginal delivery may be opted for. ARV is continued during labour, and if the woman has been taking ZDV (ACTG 076 or Thailand protocol), intrapartum ZDV orally 300 mg 3 hourly may be initiated if intravenous ZDV is not available. Single-dose NEV at onset of labour is administered to women who receive ZDV as per the Thailand protocol or do not receive any antenatal ARV. There is no advantage in adding single-dose NEV to women who are already on HAART or the ACTG 076 protocol, as it does not further reduce perinatal transmission. During labour, care is taken to minimise the duration of membrane rupture, avoid invasive monitoring (scalp electrodes, scalp blood sampling) and operative vaginal delivery including episiotomy. Artificial rupture of membranes is avoided, and the interval between rupture and delivery minimised by augmenting labour as needed after spontaneous rupture has occurred. Chlorhexidine (0.25%) vaginal lavage during labour has not proved beneficial, except when membranes were ruptured for >4 hours (Biggar et al 1996). The infant should be washed of all secretions and blood before any invasive procedure is performed. Universal precautions should be followed in all deliveries. Broadspectrum antibiotics should be given intrapartum to prevent maternal infection.

Postpartum Management Wound healing and uterine involution are assessed and broadspectrum antibiotics given for 3–7 days. Contraception (described earlier) and the need for life-long follow-up must be discussed.

Breastfeeding or Alternate Feeding? Breastfeeding is known to increase MTCT. There is a cumulative risk of HIV transmission with increased duration of breastfeeding—0.7% per month in the first 5 months, 0.6% at 6–11 months and 0.3% at 12–17 months (Miotti et al 1999). In developing countries where infant mortality is caused by malnutrition and infection than AIDS itself, the WHO recommends that a choice of exclusive breastfeeding with early and rapid weaning at 6 months be offered after proper counselling. The option of alternative feeding can be offered to the mother only if it is acceptable, feasible, affordable, sustainable and safe (AFASS criteria). Mixed feeding should never be allowed as such children are more likely to acquire HIV than exclusively breastfed children because of infection-related injuries to the gastrointestinal mucosa (WHO 2004).

Care of the HIV-exposed Infant The HIV DNA-PCR test is today used for the early diagnosis of HIV infection in newborns; it has a sensitivity of 93% in the first 14 days of life. Cord blood sample must not be taken because of chances of contamination with maternal blood. The neonate should be tested within 48 hours of birth, at 1–2 months of age and at 4–6 months of age. HIV can be excluded if two tests at age >1 month are negative, one of which is at age >4 months. All exposed infants must be given PCP prophylaxis beginning at 4–6 weeks till HIV infection is excluded (Anderson 2001). Finally, an HIV antibody assay by ELISA at 18 months of life confirms presence or absence of HIV infection in the baby. This cannot be done till 18 months of age as maternal HIV antibodies may persist in the baby till then and provoke a false-positive result.

REFERENCES

Anderson JR. 2001. HIV and reproduction in *A guide to the clinical care of women with HIV* ed JR Anderson 2001;. http://www.hab.hrsa.gov/

Baylor MS and R Johann-Liang. 2004. Hepatotoxicity associated with nevirapine use. *J Acquir Immune Defic Syndr* 35:538–539.

Biggar RJ, PG Miotti, TE Taha, L Mtimavalye, R Broadhead, A Justesen, F Yellin, G Liomba, W Miley, D Waters, JD Chiphangwi and JJ Goedert. 1996. Perinatal intervention trial in Africa: effect of a birth canal cleansing intervention to prevent HIV transmission. *Lancet* 347:1647–1650.

Brocklehurst P and R French. 1998. The association between maternal HIV infection and perinatal outcome: a systematic review of the literature and meta-analysis. *Br J Obstet Gynaecol* 105: 836–848.

Burns DN, S Landesman, H Minkoff, DJ Wright, D Waters, RM Mitchell, A Rubinstein, A Willoughby and JJ Goedert. 1998. The influence of pregnancy on human immunodeficiency virus type 1 infection: Antepartum and postpartum changes in human immunodeficiency virus type 1 viral load. *Am J Obstet Gynecol* 178:355–359.

Coovadia H. 2004.Antiretroviral agents: How best to protect infants from HIV and save their mothers from AIDS. *N Engl J Med* 351:289–292.

Coutsoudis A, K Pillay, E Spooner, L Kuhn and HM, Coovadia, for the South African Vitamin A Study Group. 1998. Randomized trial testing the effect of vitamin A supplementation on pregnancy outcomes and early mother-to-child HIV-1 transmission in Durban, South Africa. *AIDS* 13:1517–1524.

Deschamps MM, JW Pape, M Desvarieux, P Williams-Russo, S Madhavan, JL Ho and WD Johnson Jr. 1993. A prospective study of HIV-seropositive asymptomatic women of childbearing age in a developing country. *J Acquir Immune Defic Syndr* 6:446–551.

Fawzi WW, GI Msamanga, D Spiegelman, EJ Urassa, N McGrath, D Mwakagile, G Antelman, R Mbise, G Herrera, S Kapiga, W Willett, DJ Hunter. 1998. Randomised trial of effects of vitamin supplements on pregnancy outcomes and T cell counts in HIV-1-infected women in Tanzania. *Lancet* 351 (9114):1477–1482.

French R and P Brocklehurst. 1998. The effect of pregnancy on survival in women infected with HIV: A systematic review of the literature and meta-analysis. *Br J Obstet Gynaecol* 105: 827–835.

Guidelines for the use of antiretroviral agents in HIV-1 infected adults and adolescents. 2004. http://AIDSInfo.nih.gov

Guidelines on Care, Treatment and Support for Women Living with HIV/AIDS and their Children in Resource-constrained Settings. 2004. AIDS epidemic update. *Joint United Nations Programme on HIV/AIDS, UNAIDS/WHO*. www.unaids.org.

Hanson IC, TA Antonelli, RS Sperling, JM Oleske, E Cooper, M Culnane, MG Fowler, LA Kalish, SS Lee, G McSherry, L Mofenson and DE Shapiro. 1999. Lack of tumors in infants with perinatal HIV-1 exposure and fetal/neonatal exposure to zidovudine. *J Acquir Immune Defic Syndr Hum Retrovirol* 20:463–467.

Interim report: 1/1/89-1/31/01. May 2001. Wilmington, NC: Antiretroviral Pregnancy Registry.

Kapoor A, A Kapoor, SN Vani. 2004. Prevention of mother to child transmission of HIV. *Ind J Paediatr* 71:247–251.

Khilnani GC. 2004. Tuberculosis and Pregnancy. *Ind J Chest Dis Allied Sci* 46:105–111.

Kumar RM, SA Uduman, AK Khurrana. 1997. Impact of pregnancy on maternal AIDS. *J Reprod Med* 42:429–434.

Lewis SH, C Reynolds-Kohler, HE Fox, JA Nelson. 1990. HIV-1 in trophoblastic and villous Hofbauer cells, and haematologic precursors in eight-week fetuses. *Lancet* 335:565–568.

Mandelbrot L, MJ Mayaux, A Bongain, A Berrebi, Y Moudoub-Jeanpetit, JL Benifla, N Ciraru-Vigneron, J Le Chenadec, S Blanche and JF Delfraissy. 1996. Obstetric factors and mother-to-infant transmission of human immunodeficiency virus type 1: the French perinatal cohorts. *Am J Obstet Gynecol* 175:661–667.

Manual for management of HIV/AIDS in children. 2004. NACO, IAP, WHO, UNICEF.

Miotti PG, TE Taha, NI Kumwenda, R Broadhead, LA Mtimavalye, L Van der Hoeven, JD Chiphangwi, G Liomba and RJ Biggar. 1999. HIV Transmission through Breastfeeding: A Study in Malawi. *JAMA* 282: 744–749.

National AIDS Control Organisation (NACO), India. 2004. Guidelines for the Prevention of Mother to Child Transmission of HIV www.naco.nic.in.

PPTCT. National AIDS Control Organisation (NACO), India. 2007. www.naco.nic.in.

Public Health Service Task Force Recommendations for Use of Antiretroviral Drugs in Pregnant HIV-Infected Women for Maternal Health and Interventions to Reduce Perinatal HIV Transmission in the U.S. 2007. http://AIDSInfo.nih.gov

Read J, for the Intl Perinatal HIV Group. 2000. Duration of rupture of membranes and vertical transmission of HIV-1: A meta-analysis from fifteen prospective cohort studies. *7th Conf Retrovirus Opportunistic Infect* (Abst 659).

Report of the NIH panel to define principles of therapy of HIV infection and guidelines for the use of antiretroviral agents in HIV-infected adults and adolescents. 1998. *MMWR Morb Mortal Wkly Rep* 47:1–82.

Rouzioux C, D Costagliola, M Burgard, S Blanche, MJ Mayaux, C Griscelli and AJ Valleron. 1995. Estimated timing of mother-to-child human immunodeficiency virus type 1 transmission by use of a Markov model: the HIV Infection in Newborns French Collaborative Study Group. *Am J Epidemiol* 142:1330–1337.

Saada M, J Le Chenadec, A Berrebi, A Bongain, JF Delfraissy, MJ Mayaux and L Meyer. 2000. Pregnancy and progression to AIDS: results of the French prospective cohorts. *AIDS* 14:2355–2360.

Schwartlander B, I Grubb and J Perriens. 2006. The 10-year struggle to provide antretroviral treatment to people with HIV in the developing world. *Lancet* 368: 589.

Ticconi C, M Mapfumo, M Dorrucci, N Naha, E Tarira, A Pietropolli and G Rezza. 2003. Effect of maternal HIV and malaria infection on pregnancy and perinatal outcome in Zimbabwe. *J Acquir Immune Defic Syndr* 34:289–294.

UNAIDS. 2006. Report on the global HIV/AIDS Epidemic. 2006. Program on HIV/AIDS. Geneva: Joint United Nations

Watts DH. 2002. Management of human immunodeficiency virus infection in pregnancy. 2002. *N Engl J Med* 346:1879–1891.

Working Group on Mother-to-Child Transmission of HIV. 1995. Rates of mother-to-child transmission of HIV-1 in Africa, America and Europe: results from 13 perinatal studies. *J Acquir Immune Defic Synder Hum Retrovirol* 8:506–10.

World Health Organization Expert Consultation, Geneva. 2004. Antiretroviral drugs for treating pregnant women and preventing HIV infection in infants. Geneva: World Health Organization.

15

Autoimmune Diseases in Pregnancy

Gita Radhakrishnan

Autoimmune diseases, also referred to as connective tissue or collagen vascular disorders, most commonly occur in women of childbearing age (Beeson 1994). Although some conditions such as ankylosing spondylitis are more common in men, over 70% of individuals with autoimmune diseases are women. These diseases occur when, due to as yet unknown reasons, the immune system is stimulated to produce antibodies directed against self or normal tissues. These misdirected antibodies are called autoantibodies. The stimulus responsible for their production is known, but a variety of inciting reasons are suspected that include bacterial or viral injury to genetically susceptible tissues.

Autoantibodies may induce immune injury in connective tissues in two ways. First, they may react with antigens directly—this is the cytotoxic mechanism. Alternatively, they may combine with antigens to form immune complexes. When these complexes are fixed in tissues, they activate the complement cascade resulting in the release of several chemotactic factors. This leads to polymorphonuclear cell infiltration, immune complex phagocytosis and subsequent lysosomal enzyme release into tissues causing inflammation—this is the immune-complex mechanism.

The dramatic physiologic changes in hormones during pregnancy, including the increase in estrogen, certainly affect the course of autoimmune diseases. The state of enhanced humoral immunity (antibody response) and weakened cellular immunity suggested by some investigators leads to variable effects that are dependent on the specific disease process (Wegmann et al 1993). Cell-mediated autoimmune disorders, such as rheumatoid arthritis, tends to improve during pregnancy, whereas those characterised by excessive autoantibody production, such as systemic lupus erythematosus, often worsen (Luster et al 1984).

An intriguing phenomenon has been used to explain the predilection of autoimmune disorders for women. Fetal cells are present in maternal blood starting in the first trimester. There have been many observations on the role of 'fetal cell microchimerism' to explain immune mediated diseases (Adams et al 2004). By this mechanism, persistent fetal cells such as thymocytes became engrafted in maternal tissues, or immortal lymphocytes circulate in the maternal circulation and stimulate the production of autoantibodies. Lupus may therefore represent a chronic graft versus host response to transplacentally acquired fetal cells, as suggested for some thyroid diseases and systemic sclerosis (Srivatsa et al 2001; Jimenez and Arlett 2005).

Classification

Autoimmune diseases can be classified as follows:

Systemic diseases

- Systemic lupus erythematosus
- Antiphospholipid syndrome
- Rheumatoid arthritis
- Systemic sclerosis

Organ specific diseases

- ***Endocrine diseases***
  Graves hyperthyroidism
  Hashimoto's thyroiditis
  Juvenile diabetes mellitus (type I)
- ***Skin diseases***
  Psoriasis
  Vitiligo
- ***Neuromuscular diseases***
  Myasthenia gravis
  Fibromyalgia
- ***Blood and blood vessels***
  Pernicious anemia
  Hemolytic anemia
  Temporal arteritis
- ***GI system***
  Autoimmune hepatitis
  Crohn's disease
  Ulcerative colitis

Systemic autoimmune diseases have significant effects on maternal and perinatal outcome during pregnancy and will be discussed in this chapter, while the organ specific autoimmune diseases will be dealt with in other sections.

SYSTEMIC LUPUS ERYTHEMATOSUS (SLE)

Lupus is a heterogenous syndrome with a complex pathogenesis, and its genetic contribution is clustered on the 1q and 6p chromosomes. Immune system abnormalities include overactive B lymphocytes that are responsible for autoantibody production. These result in tissue and cellular damage, when autoantibodies or immune complexes are directed at one or more cellular nuclear components. Almost 90% of cases are women. The prevalence in women of childbearing age is about 1 in 500 (Lockshin 2000). The 10- and 20-year survival rates are 75% and 50%, respectively (Jacobsen et al 1999). Infection, lupus flares, end-organ failure, and cardiovascular disease account for most deaths.

Genetic influences are implicated by a higher concordance with monozygotic compared with dizygotic twins and a 10% frequency in patients with one affected family member. The relative risk of disease is increased threefold if HLA-DR2 or DR3 genes are found. Under the influence of multiple genes, often triggered by environmental stimuli and highly influenced by gender, a number of clinical syndromes may develop, fulfilling diagnostic criteria for lupus.

Clinical Findings

Lupus is notoriously variable in its presentation, course and outcome. Clinical manifestations may be confined initially to one organ system, with others becoming involved as the disease progresses (Table 15.1). Alternatively, the disease may initially manifest by multisystem involvement. Common findings are malaise, fever, arthritis, rash, pleuropericarditits, photosensitivity, anemia, and cognitive dysfunction. At lease half of these patients have renal involvement.

Laboratory Findings

Identification of antinuclear antibodies (ANA) is the best screening test, however, a positive test result is not specific for lupus. For example, low titres are found in normal individuals, other autoimmune diseases, acute viral infections, and chronic inflammatory processes. Several drugs can also cause a positive reaction. Antibodies to double-stranded DNA (dsDNA) and to Smith (Sm) antigens are relatively specific for lupus, whereas other antibodies are not.

Anemia is common, and there may be leukopenia and thrombocytopenia. Proteinuria and casts are found in that half of patients with glomerular lesions, and there may be renal insufficiency. Other laboratory findings include false-positive syphilis serology, prolonged partial thromboplastin time, and positive serum rheumatoid factor assay.

Diagnosis

Most often patients present to the obstetrician with SLE already diagnosed. Rarely, the clinical picture of pre-eclampsia with renal involvement may be the first presentation. The revised criteria of the American Rheumatism Association for diagnosis of systemic lupus are in Table 15.2. If any 4 or more of these 11 criteria are present, serially or simultaneously, the diagnosis of lupus is made.

Drug-induced Lupus: Numerous drugs have been reported to induce a lupus-like syndrome. These include procainamide, quinidine, hydralazine, α-methyldopa, phenytoin and phenobarbital. Drug-induced lupus is rarely associated with glomerulonephritis, and it usually regresses when the medication is discontinued. It is rare in pregnancy.

Lupus and Maternal Outcome: Important factors for pregnancy outcome include whether the disease is active at the beginning of pregnancy, age and parity, coexistence of other medical or obstetrical disorders, and whether there are antiphospholipid antibodies.

Several studies indicate that during pregnancy, lupus improved in about one-third patients, remained unchanged in a third and one-third patients worsened. In a

Table 15.1: Clinical manifestations of systemic lupus erythematosus (Hahn 2001)

Organ System or Process	Clinical Manifestations	Percentage of patients
Systemic	Fatigue, malaise, fever, weight loss	95
Musculoskeletal	Arthralgias, myalgias, polyarthritis, myopathy	95
Hematological	Anemia, hemolysis, leukopenia, thrombocytopenia, lupus anticoagulant	85
Cutaneous	Malar (butterfly) rash, discoid rash, photosensitivity, oral ulcers, alopecia, skin rashes	80
Neurological	Cognitive dysfunction, mood disorder, headache, seizures	60
Cardiopulmonary	Pleuritis, pericarditis, myocarditis, Libman-Sachs endocarditis	60
Renal	Proteinuria, casts, nephrotic syndrome, renal failure	60
Gastrointestinal	Anorexia, nausea, pain, diarrhea	45
Thrombosis	Venous (10%), arterial (5%)	15
Ocular	Conjunctivitis	15
Pregnancy	Recurrent abortion, early pre-eclampsia, stillbirth	30

given pregnancy, lupus may suddenly flare or worsen without warning biochemical or clinical parameters (Ruig Irastorza et al 1996; Kamashta et al 1997). In one well-controlled prospective study of 80 women who had SLE during pregnancy, only 13% had flares that clearly were due to SLE (Lockshin 1989). Another group of investigators noted a high rate (70%) of flares in 61 SLE pregnancies (Urowitz et al 1993); however, a cohort of age- and disease-matched controls had a similar rate of flares (80%). In contrast, a few other studies have reported increased flares in lupus pregnancies (Petri et al 1991; Wong et al 1991; Ruiz-Irastorza et al 1996).

Regardless of whether or not the rate of SLE flares increase during pregnancy, flares are common and may occur during any trimester or postpartum. The precise risk of flare postpartum is also controversial; older studies suggest a worsening of disease postpartum, while recent works suggest the opposite (Lockshin 1984; Petri 1991). One fact is certain, **Lupus can be life threatening to both the mother and her fetus-infant.** Petri in 1998 reported a 7% risk of major morbidity during pregnancy and estimated a one in 20 chances, of a life-threatening event. Generally, these are due to renal impairment, myocarditis or serositis.

Remission of SLE immediately before and at the time of conception (ideally for 6–12 months) probably decreases the chances for SLE exacerbations during pregnancy and postpartum (Petri et al 1991). It has been demonstrated that active disease at the time of conception, active nephritis, a systemic lupus erythematosus disease activity index score of 5 or more, and abruptly stopping hydroxychloroquine therapy are significant risk factors for lupus flares (Beeson 1994).

In general, pregnancy outcome is better if:

1. Lupus activity has been quiescent for at least six months before conception.
2. There is no active renal involvement manifest by proteinuria or renal dysfunction.

Table 15.2: The 1997 Revised Criteria of American Rheumatism Association for Systemic Lupus Erythematosus (Hochberg 1997)

Criteria	*Comments*
Malar rash	Malar erythema
Discoid rash	Erythematous patches, scaling, follicular plugging
Photosensitivity	Present
Oral ulcers	Usually painless
Arthritis	Noncrosive involving two or more peripheral joints
Serositis	Pleuritis or pericarditis
Renal disorder	Proteinuria greater than 0.5 g/day or <3+ dipstick; or cellular casts
Neurological disorders	Seizures or psychosis without other cause
Hematological disorders	Hemolytic anemia, leukopenia, lymphopenia or thrombocytpenia
Immunological disorders	Anti-dsDNA or anti-Sm antibodies, or false-positive VDRL, IgM or IgG anticardiolipin antibodies, or lupus anticoagulant
Antinuclear antibodies	Abnormal titre of ANAs

3. Superimposed pre-eclampsia does not develop.
4. There is no evidence of antiphospholipid antibody activity.

RENAL DISEASE

Approximately 50% of patients who have lupus will develop renal disease. Lupus nephritis is a result of immune complex deposition, complement activation, and inflammation in the kidney. Several reports have emphasised the potential for a permanent decrease in renal function and maternal mortality after pregnancy in women who have active lupus nephritis (Fine et al 1981; Burkett 1985). On the other hand, more recent series indicate excellent outcome for most women who have mild renal disease (Packham et al 1992). A review of several retrospective reports, including 242 pregnancies in 156 women who had lupus nephritis, demonstrated that 59% of patients had no change in their renal function, 30% experienced transient renal impairment, and 7% had permanent renal insufficiency (Burkett 1985). Two recent large series confirmed these findings (Bobrie et al 1987; Packham et al 1992).

It is clear that there is a strong correlation between the severity of the renal insufficiency before conception and the risk deterioration during pregnancy and postpartum. The general consensus is that women who have a serum creatinine level above 1.5 mg/dl have a significantly increased risk of deterioration in renal function (Jungers et al 1982; Burkett 1985). Conversely, patients who have serum creatinine levels below 1.5 mg/dl can be reassured that pregnancy will probably not increase the rate of deterioration of renal function. These effects appear to be independent of the specific type of nephritis as demonstrated by histologic studies.

Although most authorities recommend continuation of immunosuppressive therapy during pregnancy in women with nephritis, it is not clear whether the dosage should be increased peripartum. Although it is often stated that this is the time that activation or exacerbations are most likely to develop, conclusive evidence is not available.

PRE-ECLAMPSIA

Pre-eclampsia, a common complication in women who have SLE, occurs in approximately 30% of pregnancies (Lockshin 1994). Clinically apparent renal disease, underlying hypertension, and antiphospholipid antibodies, all increase the risk for pre-eclampsia. In one prospective series, pre-eclampsia occurred in 7 of 19 women who had lupus nephritis (37%), compared with 15 of 106 who did not (14%) (Lockshin 1994). The use of high-dose steroids also may predispose women to pre-eclampsia. The increased rate of pre-eclampsia in women who have SLE in the absence of known risk factors may be attributed to the unrecognised renal disease present in virtually all SLE patients.

In certain cases, it may be difficult to distinguish pre-eclampsia from a lupus flare or nephritis. Both disorders can be characterised by proteinuria, hypertension, fetal growth restriction, and multiorgan dysfunction. Often the two conditions coexist, and it may be difficult to make a definitive diagnosis. Ensuring the correct diagnosis is imperative, however, to determine clinical management. Table 15.3 outlines features that may prove helpful in the distinction between the two conditions. Renal biopsy may be used in those instances wherein certain diagnosis of lupus nephritis is required.

EFFECTS OF LUPUS ON THE FETUS AND NEONATE

Fetal growth restriction and perinatal mortality

and morbidity are increased significantly in pregnancies complicated by lupus (Table 15.4). Prognosis is worsened with a lupus flare, significant proteinuria, renal impairment and with associated hypertension, development of pre-eclampsia, or both (Aggarwal et al 1999; Carmona et al 1999; Scott 2002). The factors at least partially responsible for adverse fetal consequences include decidual vasculopathy with placental infarction and decreased perfusion.

Table 15.3: Characteristics that may be useful in distinguishing SDLE flare with lupus nephritis from preeclampsia (Warren 2004)

Test	*Pre-eclampsia*	*SLE*
Serologic		
Decreased complement	+	+++
Elevated Ba or Bb fragments with low CH50	±	++
Elevated anti-dsDNA	-	+++
Antithrombin III deficiency	++	±
Hematologic		
Microangiopathic hemolytic anemia	++	-
Coombs positive hemolytic anemia	-	++
Thrombocytopenia	++	++
Leukopenia	-	++
Renal		
Hematuria	+	+++
Cellular casts	-	+++
Elevated serum creatinine	±	++
Elevated ratio of serum blood urea nitrogen/creatinine	++	±
Hypocalciuria	++	±
Liver		
Serum transaminases	++	±

- not present, ± rarely present , + sometimes present, ++ often present, +++ almost always present

NEONATAL LUPUS ERYTHEMATOSUS

Neonatal lupus erythematosus (NLE) is a rare syndrome, occurring in approximately 1 in 20,000 live births (Lee 1993). It is most commonly characterised by fetal and neonatal congenital heart block (CHB), skin lesions, and less commonly, thrombocytopenia, anemia, and hepatitis (Lee 1993). Approximately half of infants who have NLE have CHB, half have skin disease, and 10% have both (Lee 1993; McCune et al 1987).

It now is clear that NLE is due to immune-mediated damage from maternal autoantibodies crossing the placenta, most commonly SSA (Ro). SSB (La) antibodies are found in 50% to 75% of these women in conjunction with SSA (Ro). An important point is that maternal SLE is not a prerequisite for NLE, and many cases occur in otherwise asymptomatic mothers who have circulating autoantibodies. Some of these individuals will, indeed, ultimately develop connective tissue disorders. However, autoantibodies alone are insufficient to cause NLE, as has been illustrated by reports of twins, discordantly affected, and a low recurrence rate of NLE (10–25%) (McCune 1987). In these instances, other contributing factors such as certain HLA types, especially DR3, may increased the risk (Watson et al 1984).

Clinical manifestations of NLE are variable. Cutaneous and hematological disorders do not cause permanent morbidity and resolve by an age of six months, consistent with the disappearance of maternal antibodies (Lee 1993). In contrast, cardiac complications can be fatal (Watson et al 1984; McCune et al 1987). Cutaneous lesions of NLE are red, scaling plaques present on the scalp and face with histologic characteristics consistent with cutaneous lesions in adults. Cardiac lesions associated with NLE are CHB and endocardial fibroelastosis. The anti-SSA binds to myocardial tissue and is associated with pancarditis, fibrosis, and calcifications replacing the atrial ventricular (AV) node and, occasionally, the sinoatrial (SA) node. The effect can be seen throughout the myocardium, resulting in diffuse fibroelastosis. CHB is usually detected in utero as fetal bradycardia, with a rate between 60 and 80 beats per minute. It is typically recognised between 16 and 25 weeks gestation. Fetal echocardiography demonstrates a structurally normal heart with AV dissociation. In some cases, CHB can cause fetal hydrops and fetal death in utero. These two events have prompted the use of antepartum steroid therapy or plasmapheresis (Bierman et al 1988) in an attempt to improve outcome. Some reports of improved cardiac function and resolution of CHB after steroid therapy are available (Copel et al 1995), but the use of steroids for prophylaxis in women who have SLE and anti-SSA is of unproven efficacy and is not recommended. Despite persistent bradycardia, some infants who have CHB have good cardiac function and do not require intervention. The remaining 36% to 86% of infants need pacemakers (Groves et al 1996). About 15–33% of neonates develop diffuse myocardial involvement and heart failure resulting in death during infancy (McCune et al 1987; Groves et al 1996). Among survivors, a substantial proportion will become symptomatic, need pacemakers or die (Groves et al 1996). Few data are available regarding long-term prognosis, and only a few cases of adult-onset connective tissue disease in patients who have NLE, have been reported.

Clinical Management of Systemic Lupus Erythematosus in Pregnancy

Medical and obstetric management: Management of SLE should include preconception counselling regarding medical and obstetric risks as discussed above. Patients

Table 15.4: Maternal and perinatal effects of systemic lupus erythematosus (Warren and Silver et al 2004)

Outcome	*Description*
Maternal	
Lupus flare	Overall a third flare during pregnancy Flare can be life-threatening (1 in 20 chance) Flares associated with worse perinatal outcomes Prognosis worse if antiphospholipid antibodies present Increased incidence common with nephritis
Preeclampsia	Controversial if incidence is increased
Preterm labour	Increased
Perinatal	
Preterm delivery	Increased with preeclampsia
Growth restriction	Increased
Stillbirth	Increased, especially with antiphospholipid antibodies
Neonatal lupus	About 10% incidence (transient except for heart block)

should undergo testing for renal function and hematological abnormalities. The panel of tests should include serum creatinine, 24-hour urine for protein and creatinine clearance, hematocrit and platelet count. In addition, patients should be tested for aPLs. Nonsteroidal antiinflammatory drugs (NSAIDs) and cytotoxic agents should be discontinued before conception. Finally, conception should ideally be delayed until the patient has been in remission for at least six months.

During pregnancy, patients should be co-managed by an obstetrician and a rheumatologist. Obstetric visits should be as frequent as every two weeks during the first two trimesters and weekly during the third trimester. Blood pressure, urine and symptoms of lupus flare should be assessed at each visit.

MANAGEMENT DURING PREGNANCY: This consists primarily of monitoring the clinical

TABLE 15.5: MANAGEMENT PROTOCOL FOR PATIENTS WHO HAVE SLE

Priorities

A. Avoid medication that is harmful to the fetus
B. Prompt detection of pre-eclampsia and uteroplacental insufficiency
C. Distinguish between lupus exacerbations and pre-eclampsia
D. Appropriate detection and treatment of lupus flares

Management

A. Pre-conception counselling
   1. Discuss potential pregnancy complications including pre-eclampsia, preterm labour, miscarriage, fetal death, fetal growth restriction, and neonatal lupus
   2. Clinically evaluate lupus activity; delay pregnancy until remission
   3. Evaluate patient for nephritis, hematologic abnormalities, and antiphospholipid antibodies
   4. Discontinue NSAIDs and cytotoxic agents
B. Antenatal care
   1. Frequent visits to assess SLE status and to screen for hypertension
   2. Serial ultrasounds to evaluate interval fetal growth
   3. Antenatal surveillance at 32 weeks or earlier if indicated
C. Treatment of SLE exacerbations
   1. Mild to moderate exacerbations
      a. If the patient is taking glucocorticoids, increase the dose to at least 20-30 mg/d
      b. If the patient is not taking glucocorticoids, start 15-20 mg/d of prednisone
   2. Severe exacerbations without renal or central nervous system manifestations
      a. Recommend rheumatology consultation and consider hospitalisation
      b. Glucocorticoid treatment 1.0-1.5 mg/kg; expect clinical improvement in 5-10 days
      c. Taper the glucocorticoids once the patient demonstrates clinical improvement
      d. If patient cannot be tapered off high doses of glucorticoids, consider starting cyclosporine, plaquinil or azathioprine
   3. Severe exacerbations with renal or central nervous system involvement
      a. Hospitalise and arrange rheumatology consultation
      b. Initiate intravenous glucocortioid treatment, 10-30 mg/kg/d of methylprednisolone for 3-6 days
      c. Maintain patient on 1.0-1.5 mg/kg of oral prednisone
      d. When the patient responds, taper the glucocorticoid
      e. For unresponsive patient, consider starting cyclophosphamide or plasmapheresis

conditions of both maternal and fetal patients and maternal laboratory values. Pregnancy-induced thrombocytopenia and proteinuria resemble lupus disease activity, and the identification of a lupus flare is confounded by the increase in facial and palmar erythema of normal pregnancy. Monitoring of lupus activity and identification of pending lupus flares by a variety of laboratory techniques has been recommended. The sedimentation rate cannot be interpreted because of pregnancy-induced hyperfibrigenemia. Although falling of low levels of complement components C_3, C_4 and CH_{50} are more likely to be associated with active disease, higher levels provide no insurance against disease activation. Buyon and colleagues (1999) recommended that hypocomplementemia should be attributed to disease activity in pregnant women in the following circumstances:

- when there is decreased C_3, C_4 or CH_{50} levels without evidence of a synthetic defect;
- when levels of C_3, C_4 or CH_{50} fall by 25% as pregnancy progresses; or
- when there are normal levels of C_3, C_4 or CH_{50} but other evidence of complement activation such as abnormal levels of C_{3a}.

Serial hematological studies may detect changes in disease activity. Hemolysis is characterised by a positive Coombs test, anemia, reticulocytosis and unconjugated hyperbilirubinemia. Thrombocytopenia, leukopenia or both may develop.

Serum transminase activity reflects hepatic involvement, as does a rise in serum bilirubin. Azathioprine therapy too may induce enzyme elevations. Urine is tested frequently to detect new-onset or worsening proteinuria. Overt proteinuria that persists is an ominous sign, even more so if accompanied by other evidence of the nephrotic syndrome or abnormal serum creatinine levels.

The fetus should be closely observed for adverse effects. Fetal growth is monitored closely and careful attention is given to the development of hypertension. Some recommend screening for anti-SS-A and anti-SS-B antibodies, and if found, fetal cardiac function should be evaluated. Antepartum fetal surveillance is done as for any high-risk pregnancy.

Unless hypertension develops, or there is evidence of fetal compromise or growth restriction, pregnancy is allowed to progress to term. Peripartum corticosteroids in 'stress doses' are given to women who are taking these drugs or who have recently done so.

Medication: The medical management of SLE includes four categories of drugs—NSAIDs, antimalarials, corticosteroids and cytotoxic agents (Table 15.6). NSAIDs and aspirin are the most common antiinflammatory agents used in the treatment of SLE. Unfortunately, their use during pregnancy is associated with significant fetal morbidity. For this reason, these agents should be avoided during pregnancy. Glucocorticoids are the most effective treatment for SLE, considered safe for routine use during pregnancy given their lack of teratogenic effects. Hydrocortisone, prednisone or prednisolone are preferred because these steroids largely are inactivated by 11-β-hydroxysteroid dehydrogenase in the plasma (Lee 2003). Less than 10% of active drug reaches the fetus, and the risk of fetal adrenal suppression is extremely low. Dexamethasone and β-methasone (fluorinated corticosteroids) should be avoided because they are inactivated to a much lesser degree by the placenta.

Potential maternal side effects of glucocorticoids include osteopenia, glucose intolerance, infection, sodium and water retention, hypertension, cataracts and avascular

TABLE 15.6: MEDICATIONS USED FOR PATIENTS WHO HAVE SLE (WARREN 2004)

Medication	*Pregnancy category*	*Recommendations*
NSAIDS	B	Avoid, especially in the third trimester
Hydroxychloroquine	C	Limited data available on use in pregnancy Teratogenicity based on studies of chloroquine Stopping hydroxychloroquine is associated with increased risk of SLE flares, therefore recommend continue medication if needed to control SLE
Glucocorticoids	B	Avoid fluorinated glucocorticoids as they cross placenta High doses are associated with significant maternal side effects and subsequent fetal side effects Avoid empiric treatment and minimise dose
Cyclosporin A	C	Extensive experience in pregnant renal transplant patients Not an animal teratogen Appears to be safe in humans Long-term follow-up studies are limited
Azathioprin	D	Teratogenic in animals Appears to be safe in humans
Cyclophosphamide	D	Associated with cleft palate and skeletal abnormalities Avoid if possible; may be needed in severe cases of proliferative nephritis
Methotrexate	X	Embryolethal and therefore should be avoided Also associated with multiple congenital abnormalities (aminopterin syndrome)

necrosis. These agents may also contribute to an increased risk for gestational diabetes, pre-eclampsia, preterm premature rupture of membranes (PPROM), and fetal growth restriction during pregnancy (Cowchock et al 1992). Despite these side effects, the benefits of steroids outweigh the risk in women who have SLE. The smallest effective dose of glucocorticoids should be used to effectively control symptoms. 'Stress doses' should be administered at the time of labour and delivery in patients who are receiving chronic steroids (for more than three weeks).

Due to concerns of untoward fetal effects, most other immunosuppressive drugs are reserved for refractory cases of SLE. Azathioprine has been associated with fetal growth impairment and neonatal immune suppression The cytotoxic agents cyclophosphamide and methorexate may be human teratogens and are best avoided. Antimalarial drugs can accumulate in melanin-containing tissues and have been associated with ear (Caruso 1993) and eye damage in case reports. However, normal fetal outcome after exposure to antimalarials has been reported (Wolfe and Cordeo 1985; Parke 1998), and the benefits may outweigh the risks in severe cases. In fact, a recent prospective study demonstrated that stopping hydroxychloroquine treatment during pregnancy was associated with a significant increase in the risk of lupus flares (Jungers et al 1982). Therefore, if a patient requires this medication to control her disease, stopping the drug is relatively contraindicated. In fact, hydroxychloroquine is rapidly gaining favour as a first-line therapy for the treatment of SLE, even during pregnancy.

Long-term prognosis and contraception:

In general, women with lupus and chronic vascular or renal disease should limit family size because of the morbidity associated with the disease as well as increased adverse perinatal outcomes. Tubal sterilisation may be advantageous. It is performed with greatest safety postpartum or whenever the disease is quiescent. Oral contraceptives must be used with caution in women with lupus because vascular disease is relatively common. Progestin-only implants and injections provide effective contraceptions with no known effects on lupus flares. Intrauterine devices should not be prescribed if the woman is receiving immunosuppressive therapy.

ANTIPHOSPHOLIPID SYNDROME

Antiphospholipid antibodies (aPL) are a heterogenous family of autoantibodies directed against phospholipid binding plasma proteins. Of this family of approximately 20 antibodies, the two most clinically significant are the lupus anticoagulant (LA) and the anticardiolipin antibodies (aCL). Although they may be found in normal persons, they too are associated with antiphospholipid syndrome.

The antiphospholipid syndrome (APS), as originally defined, refers to the association of persistently positive titres of LA or aCL with either arterial and venous thrombosis or recurrent miscarriages or thrombocytopenia (Hughes 1983). In the two decades since this description of APS, there has been an explosion of interest in the relationship between aPL and adverse pregnancy outcome at all gestational ages. The current obstetric criteria for the definition of the APS are as follows:

1. One or more unexplained deaths of a morphologically normal fetus, at or beyond the 10th week of gestation, with normal fetal morphology documented by ultrasonography or by direct examination of the fetus.
2. One or more premature births of a morphologically normal neonate, at or before the 34th week of gestation, because of severe pre-eclampsia or severe placental insufficiency.
3. Three or more unexplained consecutive spontaneous abortions before the 10th week of gestation, with maternal anatomical or hormonal abnormalities and paternal and maternal chromosomal causes excluded.

Approximately a third of patients who have SLE also have aPLs. Individuals who have SLE and APS are considered to have secondary APS, while those who have APS and no other connective tissue disorders have primary APS.

Obstetric Complications

The incidence of aPLs in general obstetric population is about 5%. The association between APS and pregnancy loss has been confirmed in numerous retrospective studies, with rates of pregnancy loss quoted as high as 90% (Branch 1992; Rai 1995). Prospective studies have since confirmed this association

(Cowchock 1992; Out 1992; Pattison 1993; Lynch 1994; Yasuda 1995).

An unusually large proportion of pregnancy losses associated with aPL are second- or third-trimester fetal deaths. Mid-trimester fetal deaths account for only a small percentage of all pregnancy losses in the general population. However, one cohort study of pregnancy losses in 76 women (333 pregnancies) with APS reported that 50% of the losses were fetal deaths (Oshiro 1996). Eighty per cent of these women suffered at least one fetal death.

Recurrent spontaneous abortion too is associated with aPL. Several case control studies have demonstrated a higher proportion of positive tests for LA and aCL in women who have recurrent pregnancy losses compared with controls (Out 1991; Parazzin 1991; Yetman 1996).

As opposed to recurrent pregnancy loss and fetal death, aPLs are rarely associated with sporadic early pregnancy loss—these are most commonly attributable to genetic abnormalities.

Pregnancies that result in live births are often complicated by fetal growth restriction, pre-eclampsia, uteroplacental insufficiency evidenced by abnormalities in antepartum surveillance, and preterm birth. Intrauterine growth restriction occurs in 15% to 30% of women who have APS (Kutteh 1996; Lima 1996). Abnormal fetal heart rate tracings prompting delivery has been reported in up to 50% of women who have APS. Half of all pregnancies in a large cohort study of women who had APS had abnormal fetal heart rate tracings, prompting iatrogenic preterm birth (Branch 1992). Placental insufficiency may be evident in fetal heart tracings as early as the second trimester (Druzin 1987). Pre-eclampsia in women who have APS is often severe and presents relatively early in gestation (second trimester). Several investigators reported aPL in women who have pre-eclampsia ranging from 11% to 17% (Branch 1989; Moddley 1995). In one series from the University of Utah, 16% of women with severe pre-eclampsia presenting before 34 weeks of gestation had clinically relevant levels of aPL. However, a recent study failed to demonstrate an association between aPL and pre-eclampsia (Lee 2003). Preterm birth is usually iatrogenic and due to pre-eclampsia, IUGR, or abnormal fetal testing, and occurs in one-third of women who have APS (Yasuda 1995; Kutteh 1996). Delivery before 34 weeks is most likely in women who meet clinical and laboratory criteria for APS.

Medical Complications

Perhaps the most serious medical complication associated with aPL is thrombosis (Sletnes et al 1992). Approximately 70% of thrombotic events are venous and occur in the lower extremities, but arterial thomboses and cerebrovascular accidents also are common (Khamashta et al 1988). Atypical thromboses in unusual sites should prompt suspicion of APS and further investigation. Antiphospholipids are present in approximately 2% of individuals who have unexplained thrombosis (Malm et al 1992) and in approximately 5% of patients who have thrombotic strokes who are less than 50 years of age (Brey et al 1990). Transient central nervous system manifestations of ischemia also are common in APS patients. Most thrombotic events in women who have APS occurred in association with estrogen-rich states, such as pregnancy or oral contraceptive use (Branch et al 1992; Silver et al 1994; Lima et al 1996). Oral contraceptives that contain estrogen should, therefore, be avoided. In addition, patients who have aPLs and a history of thrombosis are at increased risk for recurrence (33–69% without treatment).

Autoimmune thrombocytopenia also has been linked to aPL, occurring in up to 40% of patients who have primary APS (Harris 1985). The thrombocytopenia associated with APS is difficult to distinguish from ITP. Fortunately, they are treated in a similar fashion. Other medical complications include autoimmune hemolytic anemia, livedo reticularis, chorea gravidarum, cutaneous ulcers, renal insult, pulmonary hypertension and transverse myelitis. Postpartum complications include a severe illness characterised by fever and cardiopulmonary disorders that may be life-threatening.

Diagnosis of Antiphospholipid Antibody Syndrome

By international consensus, APS is diagnosed on the basis of clinical and laboratory criteria (Levine et al 2002). One of two clinical criteria that include vascular thrombosis or certain pregnancy morbidity must be present. In addition, at least two laboratory criteria that include LAC activity, or medium- to high-positive specific IgG or IgM-ACAs must be confirmed on two occasions, six weeks apart.

Indications to identify lupus anticoagulant and antiphospholipid antibodies:

- Unexplained second- or third-trimester loss
- Early-onset severe pre-eclampsia
- Venous or arterial thrombosis, unexplained fetal growth restriction
- Autoimmune or connective tissue disease
- False-positive serological test for syphilis
- Prolonged coagulation studies
- Positive autoantibody tests

Few areas of medicine have generated as much controversy and confusion as laboratory testing for aPL. Clinicians should recognise the limitations of available assays and test in a laboratory experienced in aPL testing.

Lupus anticoagulant: LA is a misnomer, as it is present in patients who do not have SLE and predisposes to clotting, not bleeding. It is detected in plasma by any one of several phospholipid-dependent clotting assays, such as the activated partial thromboplastin time, dilute Russell viper-venom time, plasma clotting time or kaolin clotting time. The sensitivity of these assays may be laboratory-dependent and is affected by the reagents and phospholipids used.

These assays use phospholipids as a template for the interaction of the enzymes and cofactors in the clotting cascade. LA binds to phospholipids or epitopes created by protein-phospholipid interactions, interfering with clotting factors and leading to a prolongation of clotting time. This observation prompted the term lupus anticoagulant.

Factors other than LA may cause prolonged clotting times. For this reason, a confirmatory test must be used to confirm the presence of LA (Fig. 15.1). The affected patient's plasma is mixed with normal plasma. If a clotting factor deficiency is responsible for the prolonged clotting time, the addition of normal plasma (and the deficient factor) will correct the clotting time. In contrast, if LA is present in the affected plasma, the clotting test will remain abnormal. A second confirmatory test involves the addition or removal of phospholipid, which would bind LA, and thus normalise the clotting time. For example, if LA is present, preincubation of plasma with phospholipid will bind LA and normalise the clotting time. LA is not quantified, but simply reported as present or absent.

Anticardiolipin antibody: ACL is detected by immunoassays using cardiolipin as the antigen. Results from assays use international standard sera to assign numeric values termed

Fig. 15.1: Detection of lupus anticoagulant phospholipid dependent clotting test

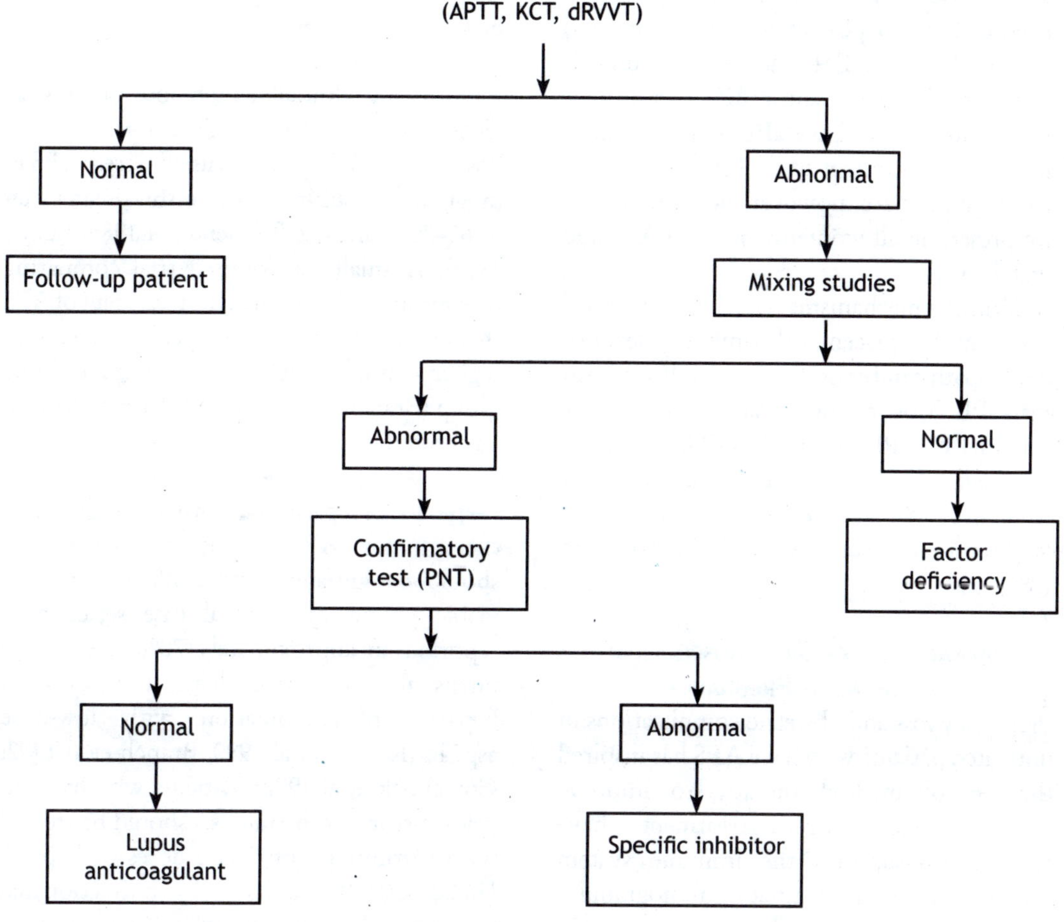

GPL (IgG aCL), MPL (IgM aCL), or aPL (IgA aCL) units. In turn, these units are semiquantitated and reported as negative and low-, medium-, or high-positive.

Low-positive aCL, isolated IgM aCL, and aPL are of questionable clinical significance. Medium-high-positive levels of aCL (as well as LA) correlate best with aPL-related disorders and thus form the diagnostic criterion for APS (Harris 1987; Alarcon et al 1992). Positive tests for aPL should be confirmed on two occasions, several weeks apart.

Many women who have LA have aCL, and those who have aCL have LA, but the correlation is imperfect. Regardless, both independently correlate with the clinical features of APS, and testing for both LA and aCL in patients suspected of having APS is recommended.

Pathogenesis of Antiphospholipid Syndrome

The obstetric complications of APS are all results of abnormal placental function. These observations, in conjunction with the association of APS with thrombosis, led to the hypothesis that thrombosis in the uteroplacental circulation is responsible for pregnancy loss in women who have APS. Decidual vasculopathy also has been proposed to contribute to placental insufficiency and fetal loss (Silver 1991). Evidence of thrombosis or infarction was present in 82% of placentas from women who have aPL and fetal death in a large case-control study (Out et al 1991). These findings are, however, nonspecific and not present in all women who have APS and fetal demise.

Multiple mechanisms have been proposed to explain the placental thrombosis, decidual vasculopathy and episodic vascular thrombosis with aPL. Most attention has focused on the potential for aPL (or anti-β_2-GP-I) to initiate a cascade of thrombogenic mediators after binding to damaged endothelium, platelets or gestational tissues (Walsh 1985; Lockshin 1996).

Management of Antiphospholipid Syndrome in Pregnancy

Pregnancy loss and obstetric complications in untreated patients who have APS has inspired the use of medical therapy to improve fetal outcome. Current treatments have three goals—suppress the immune system (prednisone and intravenous immunoglobulin [IVIG]), prevent thrombosis (heparin and aspirin), and improve placental blood flow by decreasing the thromboxane-to-prostacycline ratio (aspirin). A summary of the management of APS in pregnancy is depicted in Table 15.8.

Low dose aspirin: Low dose aspirin, 60–80 mg, given daily blocks the conversion of arachidonic acid to thromboxane A2, while sparing prostacyclin production. This results in reduced thromboxane A2, which aggregates platelets and causes vasoconstriction, while sparing prostacyclin which has the opposite effect. There appear to be no major side effects from low dose aspirin, other than the slight risk of small vessels bleeding during surgical procedures.

Prednisone: Initially, high-dose prednisone (at least 40 mg/d) in combination with low dose aspirin (80 mg/d) was used to treat APS in pregnancy, resulting in successful pregnancies in 60–70% of cases (Branch et al 1985; Lubbe 1983). A small, randomised trial comparing prednisone and heparin in the treatment of APS showed the two to be of similar efficacy, with higher complication rates in the prednisone group (Branch 1992). Since that time, heparin has been the treatment of choice.

Heparin: Heparin is considered first line therapy for APS during pregnancy and should be initiated after confirmation of a viable pregnancy. Several case series have reported an approximately 70% rate of live births after treatment with unfractionated heparin in combination with low-dose aspirin (Rosove et al 1990; Branch et al 1992; Cowchock et al 1992). Patients who have no prior history of thrombosis should be treated with thromboprophylactic doses of heparin (10,000–20,000 units of unfractionated heparin daily). Patients who have a history of thrombosis should receive a dose of heparin that will provide anticoagulation. The goal of therapy is to maintain the activated partial thromboplastin time at 1.5 to 2.5 times the normal value. Because LA causes a prolongation of the activated partial thromboplastin time, this test cannot be used to monitor anticoagulation in patients who test positive for the lupus anticoagulant. Rather, anti-factor Xa levels are followed. Anti-factor Xa levels should fall between 0.4 and 0.7 U/ml for full anticoagulation with unfractionated heparin.

Side effects of heparin include bleeding,

Management of patients who have APS

Goals of therapy

A. Embryonic and fetal survival
B. Prompt detection of uteroplacental insufficiency and pre-eclampsia
C. Prevention of thrombosis

Management

A. Pre-conception counselling
   1. Review pregnancy risks, such as miscarriage, fetal death, pre-eclampsia, fetal growth restriction, uteroplacental insufficiency, and preterm birth
   2. Evaluate the accuracy of the diagnosis; confirm the presence of antiphospholipid antibodies, if necessary

B. Antenatal care
   1. When a live embryo is detected, start subcutaneous unfractionated heparin 10,000–20,000 units/d in divided doses or the equivalent doses of low molecular weight heparin; full anticoagulant doses should be used in patients who had prior thrombosis
   2. Calcium supplementation and axial skeleton weight-bearing exercise
   3. Frequent assessment for the development of pre-eclampsia
   4. Serial ultrasounds to evaluate interval fetal growth
   5. Fetal surveillance starting at 32 weeks or earlier if there is evidence of placental insufficiency
   6. If a patient has a history of a thromboembolic event, or suffers an acute episode during pregnancy, start therapeutic doses of heparin to maintain PTT 1.5 2.5 times normal or low molecular weight heparin 1 mg/kg twice a day
   7. If using molecular weight heparin, anti-factor Xa levels should be checked every trimester to maintain through levels of 0.5–1.1 U/ml.

thrombocytopenia and osteopenia. The risks of bleeding and osteopenic fracture increase with increasing doses of heparin, thus providing rationale for using prophylactic doses in patients who have no history of thrombosis. Osteopenic fracture occurs in 1% to 2% of women treated with anticoagulant doses of unfractionated heparin during pregnancy. Therefore, calcium and vitamin D supplementation and weight-bearing exercises are encouraged. Heparin-induced thrombocytopenia occurs in up to 5% of patients treated. Platelet counts should initially be followed for three weeks, because the complications resulting from heparin therapy are detectable within 21 days of starting treatment.

Low molecular weight heparin has been used safely during pregnancy (Dulitzk et al 1996; Hunt et al 1997) and appears promising in the treatment of APS. The recommended dose of enoxaparin is 1 mg/kg administered subcutaneously in two equal doses, 12 hours apart, to accomplish full anticoagulation. However, due to increased plasma volume and renal blood flow in the pregnant patient, the pharmacokinetics of enoxaparin are altered by pregnancy. Thus, intermittent monitoring of anti-factor Xa levels should be performed to ensure adequate dosing. The target anti-factor Xa level for full anticoagulation using low molecular weight heparin is 0.5 to 1.1 U/ml. Low molecular weight heparin appears to carry less risk for osteopenia and thrombocytopenia than unfractionated heparin. However, it is more expensive and has a longer half time, making it less convenient. If possible, heparin should not be used in combination with high-dose prednisone because of an increased risk of ostepenic fractures and lack of improvement in fetal outcome with combination therapy (Branch et al 1992).

Immunoglobulin therapy: Immunoglobulin therapy has usually been reserved for women with overt disease, heparin-induced thrombocytopenia, or both. It is used when other first-line therapies have failed, especially in the setting of pre-eclampsia and fetal growth restriction (Cowchock 1996; Heilmann et al 2003). Immunoglobulin is administered in doses of 0.4 g/kg intravenously daily for 5 days. This is repeated monthly, or is given as a single dose of 1 g/kg each month. Immunoglobulin has been evaluated in a preliminary placebo-controlled study (Branch et al 2000). This drug may cause anaphylactic reactions especially in women who have IgA deficiency due to anti-IgA antibodies.

Immunosuppressive therapy: Immunosuppressive therapy has not been well evaluated, but azathioprine and cyclosporine do not appear to improve standard therapies (Silver et al 1997). Methotrexate and cyclophosphamide are contraindicated because of their teratogenic potential (Enns 1999).

Current data suggest the most efficacious therapy to be low-dose heparin (7500 to 10,000 units administered subcutaneously, twice daily) given along with low-dose aspirin, 60–80 mg, once daily. If active lupus is also present, prednisolone may also be given.

Other aspects of management during pregnancy: Ideally, patients who have APS should undergo pre-conception counselling regarding their medical and obstetric risks. If the diagnosis is uncertain, LA and aCL should be confirmed. There is no evidence of benefit to serial testing during pregnancy or in titrating medicines to suppress antibody levels. As with other autoimmune diseases like SLE, patients who have APS should undergo intensive surveillance (weekly clinic visits and biweekly non-stress tests) for pre-eclampsia, IUGR, and uteroplacental insufficiency at the appropriate gestations. Antenatal testing may be useful in more severe cases, as early as 24–25 weeks of gestation (Druzin 1987).

Postpartum Considerations: Thromboprophylaxis (or full anticoagulation if appropriate) should be continued 6 weeks postpartum. Coumarin may be safely used while breastfeeding. After delivery, women who have APS should be counselled regarding their substantial risk for the development of non-obstetric disorders associated with aPL, because they are at increased risk of major complications such as thrombosis or development of SLE (Silver 1994). Patients who have had prior thrombosis and APS should receive lifelong anticoagulation with coumarin (Crowther et al 2003). Lifelong treatment with low-dose aspirin may decrease the risk for thrombosis in women who have not had prior thrombotic events (Erkan et al 2001).

RHEUMATOID ARTHRITIS

This is a chronic multisystem disorder of unknown cause with an immunologically mediated pathogenesis. Its prevalence is about 0.8% and women are affected three times more often than men. This is a chronic arthritis with symptoms of synovitis, fatigue, anorexia, weakness, weight loss, depression and vague musculoskeletal symptoms.

There is marked improvement in the inflammatory component of rheumatoid arthritis. Maternal immune response to paternal antigens may play a role in pregnancy induced remission of arthritis. Most women with rheumatoid arthritis improve during pregnancy, some develop new disease, and others become worse (Nelson and Ostensen 1997). Pregnancy has a protective effect in new-onset disease; conversely, there is increased likelihood of new disease onset in the first 3 months postpartum (Silman et al 1992). Barrett and co-workers (2000) reported that a flare was more common if women were breastfeeding.

There is no obvious adverse effect of rheumatoid arthritis on pregnancy outcome, including preterm labour (Kipple and Cecere 1989). It may be that large doses of aspirin or other nonsteroidal antiinflammatory drugs, typically used to treat these diseases, might adversely affect the fetus and neonate. Nonetheless, these drugs remain appropriate for treatment of symptomatic women during pregnancy. Corticosteroids are also used as indicated. Gold compounds have been used in pregnancy, but their fetal effects are largely unknown. Immunosuppressive therapy is not routinely used during pregnancy. Of these, only azathioprine should be considered for use during early pregnancy if required.

MULTIPLE SCLEROSIS

Multiple sclerosis (MS) is a multisystem disorder characterised by fibrosis of skin, blood vessels and visceral organs. Its prevalence ranges from 1 in 10,000 with a 3:1 female dominance—most patients present at 30–50 years. The association of progressive systemic sclerosis and pregnancy is uncommon. Microchimerism is believed to be involved in the pathogenesis of MS (Maloney et al 1999).

Effects on Pregnancy

Pregnancy outcome is related to the severity of the underlying disease. Maymon and Fejin (1989) reported in their review of 94 cases, exacerbations in a third of cases and 15% mortality due to hypertension, renal failure or cardiopulmonary complications. Steen (1999) reported more optimistic outcome in 214 women with MS. Major complications were renal failure. The incidence of renal crisis was the same as in non-pregnant women with MS. Risk of preterm delivery, fetal growth restriction were increased. Women with diffuse scleroderma or with hypertension, renal, cardiac or pulmonary involvement fare poorly. Pregnancy termination may be considered in the presence of worsening renal or cardiac disease.

Women with multiple sclerosis who are considering pregnancy need to be aware that certain drugs used to treat multiple sclerosis should be avoided during pregnancy and while breastfeeding. These drugs can cause birth defects and can be passed to the fetus via blood and to an infant via breast milk. Among them are prednisone, corticotropin, azathioprine, cyclophosphamide, diazepam, phenytoin, carbamazepine and baclofen.

However, most women find that multiple sclerosis relapses or attacks are 2–3 times more common than usual in the first six months after childbirth. There is no evidence that pregnancy and childbirth affect the overall course of the disease one way or the other. Also, while multiple sclerosis is not in itself a reason to avoid pregnancy and poses no significant risks to the fetus, physical limitations can make child care more difficult. Child care assistance is strongly recommended. Multiple sclerosis does not influence childbirth or breastfeeding ability; however, if the woman is taking immunotherapy, pregnancy and breastfeeding are not recommended.

No special management is needed during labour and delivery. For cesarean delivery, epidural anesthesia is preferred as chances of aspiration are higher due to esophageal dysfunction.

Women who use steroids for acute MS exacerbations may continue to use them during pregnancy. The use of prednisone in a woman who is breastfeeding should be carefully monitored.

In general, pregnancy does not appear to affect the long-term clinical course of MS. Women who have MS and wish to have a child can usually do so successfully—the neurologist and the obstetrician should provide continuous advice and management.

References

Adams KM and JL Nelson. 2004. Microchimerism: An investigative frontier in autoimmunity and transplantation. *JAMA* 291:1127–1131.

Aggarwal N, H Sawhney, K Vasishta, S Chopra and P Banbery. 1999. Pregnancy in patients with systemic lupus erythematosus. *Aust N Z J Obstet Gynecol* 39:28–30.

Alarcon Segovia D, ME Perez-Vazquez, AR Villa, C Drenkard and J Cabiedes. 1992. Preliminary criteria for the antiphospholipid syndrome within systemic lupus erythematosus. *Semin Arthritis Rheum* 21:275–286.

Barrett JH, P Brennan, M Fiddler and A Silman. 2000. Breast-feeding and postpartum relapse in women with rheumatoid and inflammatory arthritis. *Arthritis and Rheumatism* 43:1010–1015.

Beeson PB. 1994. Age and sex determination of 40 autoimmune diseases. *Am J Med* 96:457–462.

Bierman FZ, L Baxi, I Jaffe and J Driscoll. 1988. Fetal hydrops and congenital complete heart block: response to maternal steroid therapy. *J Pediatr* 112:646–648.

Bobrie J, F Liote, P Houillier, JP Grunfeld and P Jungers. 1987. Pregnancy in lupus nephritis and related disorders. *Am J Kidney Dis* 9:339–343.

Branch DW, R Andres, KB Digre, NS Rote and JR Scott. 1989. The association of antiphospholipid antibodies with severe pre-eclampsia. *Obstet Gynecol* 73:541–545.

Branch DW, AM Peaceman, M Druzin, RK Silver, Y El-Sayed, RM Silver et al. 2000. A multicenter, placebo-controlled pilot study of intravenous immune globulin treatment of antiphospholipid syndrome during pregnancy. *Am J Obstet Gynecol* 182:122–127.

Branch DW, JR Scott, NK Kochenour and E Hershgold. 1985. Obstetric complications associated with the lupus anticoagulant. *N Eng J Med* 313:1322–1326.

Branch DW, RM Silver, JL Blackwell, JC Reading and JR Scott. 1992. Outcome of treated pregnancies in women with antiphospholipid syndrome: An update of the Utah experience. *Obstet Gynecol* 80:614–620.

Brey RL, RG Hart, DG Sherman and CH Tegeler. 1990. Antiphospholipid antibodies and cerebral ischemia in young people. *Neurology* 40:1190–1196.

Buyon JP, KC Kalunian, R Ramsey-Goldman, MA Petri, MD Lockshin, G Ruiz-Irastorza et al. 1999. Assessing disease activity in SLE patients during pregnancy. *Lupus* 8:677–684.

Burkett G. 1985. Lupus nephropathy and pregnancy. *Clin Obstet Gynecol* 28:310–323.

Carmona F, J Font, R Cervera, F Munoz, V Cararachi and I Balaschi. 1999. Obstetrical outcome of pregnancy in patients with systemic lupus erythematosus. A study of 60 cases. *Eur J Obstet Gynecol Reprod Biol* 83:137–142.

Carr RE, P Henkind, N Rothfield and IM Siegel. 1968. Ocular toxicity of antimalarial drugs. Long term follow up. *Am J Ophthalmol* 66:738–744.

Caruso A, S De Carolis, S Ferrazzani, G Valesini, L Caforio and S Mancuso. 1993. Pregnancy outcome in relation to uterine artery flow velocity waveforms and clinical characteristics in women with antiphospholipid syndrome. *Obstet Gynecol* 82:970–977.

Copel JA, JP Buyon and CS Kleinman. 1995. Succesful in utero therapy of fetal heart block. *Am J Obstet Gynecol* 173:1384–1390.

Cote CJ, HJ Meuwissen and RJ Pickering. 1974. Effects on the neonate of prednisone and azathioprine administered to the mother during pregnancy. *J Pediatr* 85:324–328.

Cowchock FS, EA Reece, D Balaban, DW Branch and L Plouffe. 1992. Repeated fetal losses associated with antiphospholipid antibodies: A collaborative randomized trial comparing prednisolone with low dose heparin treatment. *Am J Obstet Gynecol* 166:1318–1323.

Cowchock S. 1996. Prevention of fetal death in the antiphospholipid antibody syndrome. *Lupus* 5(5):467–472.

Crowther MA, JS Ginsberg, J Julian, J Denburg, J Hirsh, J Douketis et al. 2003. A comparison of two intensities of warfarin for the prevention of recurrent thrombosis in patients with antiphospholipid antibody syndrome. *N Eng J Med* 349:1133–1138.

Devoe LD and RL Taylor. 1979. Systemic lupus erythematosus in pregnancy. *Am J Obstet Gynecol* 135:473–479.

Druzin ML, M Lockshin, TG Edersheim, JM Hutson, AL Krauss and E Kogut. 1987. Second trimester fetal monitoring and preterm delivery in pregnancies with systemic lupus erythematosus and/or circulating anticoagulant. *Am J Obstet Gynecol* 157:1503–1510.

Dulitzki M, R Pauzner, P Langevitz, M Pras, A Many and E Schiff. 1996. Low molecular weight heparin during pregnancy and delivery: preliminary experience with 41 pregnancies. *Obstet Gynecol* 87:380–383.

Enns GM, E Roeder, RT Chan, Z Ali Khan Catts, VA Cox and M Galobi. 1999. Apparent cyclophosphamide embryopathy: A distinct phenotype? *Am J Med Genet* 86:237–241.

Erkan D, JT Merrill, Y Yazici, L Sammaritano, JP Buyon and MD Lockshin. 2001. High thrombosis rate after fetal loss in antiphospholipid syndrome: effective prophylaxis with aspirin. *Arthritis Rheum* 44:1466–1467.

Fine LG, EV Barnett and GM Danovitch. 1981. Systemic lupus erythematosus in pregnancy. *Ann Int Med* 94:667–677.

Groves AM, LD Allan and E Rosenthal. 1996. Outcome of isolated congenital heart block diagnosed in utero. *Heart* 75:190–194.

Hahn BH. 2001. Systemic lupus erythematosus. In *Harrison's Principles of Internal Medicine,* ed E **Braunwald,** AS Fauci, DL Kasper et al, 15th ed. New York: McGraw-Hill, p1922.

Harris EN, RA Asherson, AE Gharavi, SH Morgan, G Derue and GR Hughes. 1985. Thrombocytopenia in SLE and related disorders: association with anticardiolipin antibody. *Br J Haematol* 59:227–230.

Harris EN. 1987. Syndrome of the black swan. *Br J Rheumatol* 26:324–326.

Hayslett JP and RI Lynn. 1980. Effect of pregnancy in patients with lupus nephropathy. *Kidney Int* 18:207–220.

Heilmann L, GF von Tempelhoft and K Pollow. 2003. Antiphospholipid syndrome in obstetrics. *Clin Appl Thromb Hemost* 9:143–147.

Hochberg MC. 1997. Updating the American College of Rheumatology revised criteria for the classification of systemic lupus erythematosus. *Arthritis Rheum* 40:1725.

Hughes GL. 1983. Thrombosis, abortion, cerebral disease and lupus anticoagulant. *BMJ* 287:1088–1089.

Hunt BJ, HA Doughty, G Majumdar, A Copplestone, S Kerslake, N Buchanan et al. 1997. Thromboprophylaxis with low molecular weight heparin in high risk pregnancies. *Thromb Haemost* 77:39–43.

Jacobsen S, J Peterson, S Ullman, P Junker, A Voss, JM Rassmussen et al. 1999. Mortality and causes of death of 513 Danish patients with systemic lupus erythematosus. *Scand J Rheumatol* 28:75–80.

Jimenez SA and CM Artlett. 2005. Microchimerism and systemic sclerosis. *Curr Opin Rheumatol* 17:86–90.

Julkunen H, R Kaaja, T Palosuo, C Gronhagen-Riska and K Teramo. 1993. Pregnancy in lupus nephropathy. *Acta Obstet Gynecol Scand* 72:258–263.

Jungers P, M Dougados, C Pelissier, F Kutten, F Tron, P Lesavre et al. 1982. Lupus nephropathy and pregnancy. Report of 104 cases in 36 patients. *Arch Intern Med* 142:771–776.

Khamashta MA, EN Harris, AE Gharavi, G Derue, A Gil, JJ Vazquez et al. 1988. Immune mediated mechanism for thrombosis: Antiphospholipid antibody binding to platelet membranes. *Ann Rheum Dis* 47:849–854.

Khamshta MA, G Ruiz-Irastorza and GRV Hughes. 1997. Systemic lupus erythematosis flares during pregnancy. *Rhem Dis Clin North Am* 23:15–18.

Kipple GL and FA Cecere. 1989. Rheumatoid arthritis in pregnancy. *Rheum Clin North Am* 15:213–239.

Kutteh WH. 1996. Antiphospholipid antibody associated recurrent pregnancy loss: treatment with heparin and low dose aspirin is superior to low dose aspirin alone. *Am J Obstet Gynecol* 174:1584–1589.

Lee LA. 1993. Neonatal lupus erythematosus. *J Invest Dermatol* 100:9S–13S.

Lee RM, MA Brown, DW Branch, K Ward and RM Silver. 2003. Anticardiolipin and anti-beta$_2$-glycoprotein-1 antibodies in pre-eclampsia. *Obstet Gynecol* 102:294–300.

Levine JS, W Branch and J Rauch. 2002. The antiphospholipid syndrome. *N Engl J Med* 346: 752–763.

Lima F, MA Khamashta, NM Buchanan, S Kerslake, BJ Hunt and GR Hughes. 1996. A study of sixty pregnancies in patients with the antiphospholipid syndrome. *Clin Exp Rheumatol* 14:131–136.

Lockshin MD and LR Sammaritano. 2000. Rheumatic diseases. In *Medical Disorders during Pregnancy*, ed WM Barron, MD Lindheimer, 3rd ed. St. Louis: Mosby, p355–391.

Lockshin MD. 1996. Pathogenesis of antiphospholipid antibody syndrome. *Lupus* 5:404–408.

Lockshin MD. 1989. Pregnancy does not cause systemic lupus erythematosus to worsen. *Arthritis Rheum* 32:665–670.

Lockshin MD, E Reinitz, ML Druzin, M Murrman and D Estes. 1984. Lupus pregnancy. Case control prospective study demonstrating absence of lupus exacerbation during or after pregnancy. *Am J Med* 77:893–898.

Lockshin MD. 1994. Lupus pregnancies and neonatal lupus. *Springer Semin Immunopathol* 16:247–259.

Lubbe WF, Butler WS, SJ Palmer and GC Liggins. 1983. Fetal survival after prednisone suppression of maternal lupus anticoagulant. *Lancet* 1:1361–1363.

Luster MI, HT Hayes, K Korach, AN Tucker, JH Dean, WF Greenlee et al. 1984. Estrogen immunosuppression is regulated through estrogenic responses in the thymus. *J Immunol* 133:110–116.

Lynch A, R Marlar, J Murphy, G Davila, M Santos, J Rutledge et al. 1994. Antiphospholipid antibodies in predicting adverse pregnancy outcome. A prospective study. *Ann Intern Med* 120:470–475.

Malm J, M Laurell, IM Nilsson and B Dahlback. 1992. Thromboembolic disease–critical evaluation of laboratory investigation. *Thromb Haemost* 68:7–13.

Maloney S, A Smith, DE Furst, D Myerson, K Rupert, PC Evans et al. 1999. Microchimerism of maternal origin persists into adult life. *J Clin Invest* 104: 41.

Maymon R and M Fejin. 1989. Scleroderma in pregnancy. *Obstet Gynecol Surv* 44: 530–536.

McCune AB, WL Weston and LA Lee. 1987. Maternal and fetal outcome in neonatal lupus erythematosus. *Ann Intern Med* 106:518–523.

Moddley J, V Bhoola, J Duursma, D Pudifin, S Byrne and DG Kenoyer. 1995. The association of antiphospholipid antibodies with severe early onset pre-eclampsia. *S Afr Med J* 85:105–107.

Nelson JL and M Ostensen. 1997. Pregnancy and rheumatoid arthritis. *Rheum Dis Clin North Am* 23:195–212.

Oshiro BT, RM Silver, JR Scott, H Yu and DW Branch. 1996. Antiphospholipid antibodies and fetal death. *Obstet Gynecol* 87:489–493.

Out HJ, HW Bruinse, GC Christiaens, M van Vliet, PG de Groot, HK Niuuwenhuis et al 1992. A prospective controlled multicenter study on the obstetric risks of pregnant women with antiphospholipid antibodies. *Am J Obstet Gynecol* 167:26–32.

Out HJ, HW Bruinse and RH Derksen. 1991. Anti-phospholipid antibodies and pregnancy loss. *Hum Reprod* 6:889–897.

Out HJ, CD Kooijman, HW Bruinse and RH Derksen. 1991. Histopathological findings in placentae from patients with intrauterine fetal death and anti-phospholipid antibodies. *Eur J Obstet Gynecol Reprod Biol* 41:179–186.

Packham DK, SS Lam, K Nicholls, KF Fairly and PS Kincaid-Smith. 1992. Lupus neohritis and pregnancy. *Q J Med* 83:315–324.

Parazzini F, B Acacia, D Faden, M Lovotti, G Marelli and S Cortellazo. 1991. Antiphospholipid antibodies and recurrent abortion. *Obstet Gynecol* 77:854–858.

Parke AL. 1998. Antimalarial drugs in pregnancy. *Scand J Rheumatol Suppl* 107:125–127.

Purtilo DT and JL Sulivan. Immunological bases for superior survival of females. 1979. *Am J Dis Child* 133:1251–1253.

Pattison NS, LW Chamley, EJ McKay, GC Liggins and WS Butler. 1993. Antiphospholipid antibodies in pregnancy: prevalence and clinical associations. *Br J Obstet Gynecol* 100:909–913.

Petri M, D Howard and J Repke. 1991. Frequency of lupus flare in pregnancy. The Hopkins Lupus Pregnancy Centre experience. *Arthritis Rheum* 34:1538–1545.

Petri M. 1998. Pregnancy in SLE. *Balliere's Clin Rheumatol* 12:449–476.

Rai RS, K Clifford, H Cohen and L Regan. 1995. High prospective fetal loss rate in untreated pregnancies of women with recurrent miscarriages and antiphospholipid antibodies. *Hum Reprod* 10:3301–3304.

Rosove MH, K Tabsh, N Wasserstrum, P Howard, BH Hahn and KC Kalunian. 1990. Heparin therapy for pregnant women with lupus anticoagulant or anticardiolipin antibodies. *Obstet Gynecol* 75:630–634.

Ruiz–Irastorza G, F Lima, J Alves, MA Khamshta, J Simpson, GR Hughes et al. 1996. Increased rate of lupus flare during pregnancy and the puerperium: a prospective study of 78 pregnancies. *Br J Rheumatol* 35:133–138.

Scott JR. 1977. Fetal growth retardation associated with maternal administration of immunosuppressive drugs. *Am J Obstet Gynecol* 128:668–676.

Scott JR. 2002. Risks to the children born to mothers with autoimmune diseases. *Lupus* 11:655–660.

Silman AJ, A Kay and P Brennan. 1992. Timing of pregnancy in relation to the onset of. rheumatoid arthritis. *Arthritis Rheum* 35:152–155.

Silver RM and DW Banch. 1997. Autoimmune diseases in pregnancy: systemic lupus erythematosus and antiphospholipid syndrome. *Clin Perinatol* 24:291–320.

Silver RM, ML Draper, JL Byrne, EA Ashwood, JL Lyon and DW Branch. Unexplained elevations of maternal serum alpha-protein in women with antiphospholipid antibodies: a harbinger of fetal death. *Obstet Gynecol* 1994. 83:150–155.

Silver RM, ML Draper, JR Scott, JL Lyon, J Reading and DW Branch. 1994. Clinical consequences of antiphospholipid antibodies: A historic cohort study. *Obstet Gynecol* 83:372–377.

Sletnes KE, F Wisloff, N Moe and PO Dale. 1992. Antiphospholipid antibodies in pre-eclamptic women: relation to growth retardation and neonatal outcome. *Acta Obstet Gynecol Scan* 71:112–117.

Srivatsa B, S Srivatsa, KL Johnson, O Samura, STL Lee and DW Bianchi. 2001. Microchimerism of presumed fetal origin in thyroid specimens from women: A case control study. *Lancet* 358:2034–2038.

Steen VD. 1999. Pregnancy in women with systemic sclerosis. *Obstet Gynecol* 94:15.

Urowitz MB, DD Gladman, VT Farewell, J Stewart and J McDonald. 1993. Lupus and pregnancy studies. *Arthritis Rheum* 36:1392–1397.

Walsh SW. 1985. Pre-eclampsia: an imbalance in placental prostacyclin and throboxane production. *Am J Obstet Gynecol* 152:335–340.

Warren JB and RM Silver. 2004. Autoimmune disease in pregnancy: Systemic lupus erythematosus and antiphospholipid syndrome. *Obstet Gynecol Clin N Am.* 31:345–372.

Watson RM, AT Lane, NK Barnett, WB Bias, FC Arnett and TT Provost. 1984. Neonatal lupus erythematosus: A clinical, serological and immunogenetic study with review of literature. *Medicine* (Baltimore) 63:362–378.

Wegmann TG, H Lin, L Guilbert and TR Mosmann. 1993. Bidirectional cytokine interactions in the maternal fetal relationship: Is successful pregnancy a TH2 phenomenon? *Immunol Today* 14:353–356.

Wolfe MS and JF Cordero. 1985. Safety of chloroquine in chemosuppression of malaria during pregnancy. *Br Med J (Clin Res Ed)* 290:1466–1467.

Wong KL. FY Chan and CP Lee. 1991. Outcome of pregnancy in patients with systemic lupus erythematosus. A prospective study. *Arch Intern Med* 151:269–273.

Yasuda M, K Takakuwa, A Tokunaga and K Tanaka. 1995. Prospective studies of the association between anticardiolipin antibody and outcome of pregnancy. *Obstet Gynecol* 86:555–559.

Yetman DL and WH Kutteh. 1996. Antiphospholipid antibody panels and recurrent pregnancy loss: prevalence of anticardiolipin antibodies compared with other antiphospholipid antibodies. *Fertil Steril* 66:540–546.

16

Thrombophilia in Pregnancy

Suchitra N Pandit | Sanjay B Rao | Vijay C Pawar

Thrombophilia is defined as an inherited or acquired predisposition to thrombosis. Contact between the placenta and maternal circulation is a crucial determinant for the success of any pregnancy. This is directly affected in women with thrombophilia as they have a predisposition to prothrombotic changes and thrombosis, leading to adverse outcomes in pregnancy at any gestational age. Women with thrombophilic defects have been clearly identified to have an additional increased risk of pregnancy-associated thromboembolism and other vascular lesions such as pre-eclampsia.

PREGNANCY: A HYPERCOAGULABLE STATE

Major changes in all aspects of hemostasis are seen during a normal pregnancy, including an increase in the levels of factors VIII, IX and X. A significant rise of about 50% in fibrinogen levels is often observed. In contrast, the concentration of endogenous anticoagulants including anti-thrombin III and Protein S tend to decline. This shifts the overall balance in favour of a hypercoagulable state throughout pregnancy and during puerperium (Clark et al 1998).

Classification The main subtypes of thrombophilia are inherited and acquired thrombophilia. Inherited thrombophilia is caused by Protein C deficiency, Protein S deficiency, anti-thrombin III deficiency or activated Protein C resistance. Acquired thrombophilia could be related to lupus anticoagulants or anticardiolipin antibodies.

Screening The main indications for initiating screening for thrombophilia are a history of recurrent or atypical thrombosis in the axillary, cerebral, mesenteric, portal or hepatic veins and a history of thrombosis that is not related to the use of combined oral contraceptive pills, pregnancy or surgery.

The select subgroup of women would also include those with a personal or strong family history of venous thromboembolism or a history of recurrent fetal loss. Deficiency of Protein C, Protein S or anti-thrombin III is relatively uncommon. Activated Protein C resistance (APCR) due to factor V Leiden mutation is the commonest cause of thrombophilia.

Prevalence The prevalence of thrombophilia is largely dependent on the ethnicity and country of origin. The estimated prevalence among people of European origin is 5%. This disease is much less common in other ethnic groups; it is rare in people of Asian and African descent (Rees et al 1995; Cox and

Clegg 1995). Screening should be done in the first trimester or preconceptually to allow planning of pregnancy management.

Inherited Thrombophilia

Protein C Deficiency Protein C is a vitamin K-dependent factor that circulates in plasma in an inactive state. Thrombin activates Protein C and its co-factor, Protein S. These together cleave and inactivate clotting factors Va and VIIIa (Gilham). The prevalence of heterozygous Protein C deficiency is 0.3% in the general population. It results from an autosomal dominant pattern of inheritance (Tait et al 1995). In pregnant patients with Protein C deficiency, thrombosis occurs in 25% of patients without anticoagulation and the majority of these are during puerperium.

Protein S Deficiency Protein S is a vitamin K-dependent factor. About 60% of this protein is bound to the C4 binding protein and 40% is left free. The diagnosis of Protein S deficiency is difficult to make in pregnancy because of a physiological decrease in its levels. The prevalence of Protein S deficiency remains unknown in the general population (Tait et al 1995). Two studies report that around 3% of patients with venous thromboembolism have Protein S deficiency (Koster et al 1995; Faioni et al 1997).

Anti-Thrombin III Deficiency This is a rare disorder with an autosomal dominant inheritance (Tait et al 1995). It is a more severe defect than Protein C or S deficiency. Anti-thrombin is the primary physiological regulator of fibrin formation. There are two main types of anti-thrombin deficiency. Type 1 deficiency is a quantitative reduction of qualitatively normal protein, whereas Type 2 deficiency results from the production of a qualitatively abnormal protein (Finnazi et al 1987). Most patients with this defect experience a thrombotic event before the age of 25 years (Thaler and Lechner 1981; Demers et al 1992).

Factor V Leiden and Activated Protein C Resistance Factor V Leiden deficiency is rare in the Indian population (Shetty et al 2000). Heterozygosity for the factor V Leiden mutation is the most common heritable thrombophilic defect in Europe (Rees et al 1995; Rosendaal et al 1995; Ridker et al 1997). The reported prevalence is between 2% and 15%. The significance of this condition is that it is associated with a 20-fold increased risk of thrombosis. Selective screening for factor V Leiden should be performed only in women with a strong family history of venous thromboembolism.

Prothrombin G20210A Mutation Prothrombin is a precursor of thrombin. It is encoded by a gene on the long arm of chromosome 11. This is the most recently described, heritable thrombophilic defect, with a G-to-A transition at nucleotide 20210 in the 3' untranslated region of the gene encoding prothrombin (Poort et al 1996). This leads to increased plasma prothrombin concentration and an increased risk of venous thromboembolism. The prevalence is highest in Southern Europe where it reaches up to 6.5% of the general population (Souto et al 1998).

Acquired Thrombophilic Defects

Antiphospholipid Antibody Syndrome The most important acquired thrombophilic defects are broadly grouped as antiphospholipids. These include lupus inhibitors and raised anticardiolipin antibody concentrations. The antiphospholipid syndrome can manifest in different ways—a thrombotic event, recurrent pregnancy loss before 10 weeks of gestation, a single unexplained fetal loss beyond 10 weeks of gestation, pre-eclampsia or intrauterine growth restriction before 34 weeks of gestation (Girling 2004).

Various studies have reported a ninefold increase in the risk of venous thromboembolism (Ginsberg et al 1995) with the risk of recurrence varying from 22% to 70% (Khamashta et al 1995).

Hyperhomocysteinemia Inherited hyperhomocysteinemia results from genetic defects that affect the pathway of homocysteine, which is produced by the metabolisation of the essential aminoacid methionine (D'Angelo and Selhub 1997). The acquired form of hyperhomocysteinemia can be secondary to deficiency of folate, vitamin B6 or vitamin B12 or the use of antifolate metabolism chemotherapy with methotrexate (Ubbink et al 1993). A fasting level of over15 mmol/l is significant.

Management of Pregnancy

Women who have a history of thrombophilia should provide a complete personal and family history. All risk factors should be explicitly documented. There should be objective confirmation of venous thromboembolism and a close liaison with the obstetrician and an expert in the specialised area to carefully interpret the history and investigations. These women should be given complete information pre-conceptually about the likely risks of venous thrombosis related to pregnancy.

The initial screening for thrombophilia includes activated partial thromboplastin time, prothrombin time, assays to determine anti-thrombin III levels and antiphospholipid antibodies. Prothrombin gene mutation and factor V Leiden deficiency can be detected by PCR-based testing.

Currently, there is little evidence for standardising current management of women with a history of thrombophilia. Therefore, management should be individualised. The general consensus is that these patients should receive both antepartum and postpartum thromboprophylaxis (Gilham). In women with no personal history of venous thromboembolism but with a family history of Protein S deficiency, factor V Leiden or prothrombin gene mutation, low molecular weight heparin is not required antenatally, but could be considered as a prophylaxis to be given postnatally (Walker et al 2001). Low dose aspirin has been recommended in the antenatal period (Girling 2004). Oral anticoagulation with warfarin may be introduced postpartum when the INR is within range.

Pregnancy Outcome Thrombophilia is now clearly recognised to be associated with pregnancy-related complications including recurrent miscarriages, intrauterine growth restriction, pre-eclampsia, placental abruption and intrauterine death. The main pathophysiological basis for this is placental thrombosis, which may cause infarction and alter the placental function. There is strong evidence to suggest the beneficial role of low dose aspirin and heparin in reducing rates of miscarriage.

Acute Venous Thromboembolism

Etiology The pathogenesis of acute venous thromboembolism is complex. It remains the leading cause of maternal mortality in Western nations such as the UK. Therefore, based on the report of the Confidential Enquiry into Maternal Deaths, the Royal College of Obstetricians and Gynaecologists has emphasised the importance of careful vigilance for thromboembolic events throughout pregnancy and puerperium, and the need for thromboprophylaxis in high-risk situations (Green Top Guidelines 2001).

Besides thrombophilia, the main risk factors in the etiology of venous thromboembolism are:

- Prothrombotic physiological changes in pregnancy
- A marked fall in the velocity of blood flow due to peripheral vasodilation, with its peak at 34 weeks and returning to normal within 6 weeks postnatally
- A more marked fall in blood flow velocity in women delivered by cesarean section
- A greater extent in the left femoral vein than in the right
- A predominance of left-sided deep venous thrombosis (DVT) in pregnancy (85% left versus 15% right); this is secondary to the compression of the left iliac vein by the right iliac artery and ovarian artery
- Likely trauma to pelvic veins as the fetal head traverses the pelvis
- Immobility and dehydration during labour
- Obesity, intercurrent medical conditions such as pre-eclampsia, diabetes and dehydration (Girling 2004)

Diagnosis The risk of thromboembolic disease in relation to maternal age, pregnancy and mode of delivery is shown in Table 16.1 (Girling 2004).

Clinical Features The main signs and symptoms of venous thromboembolism are leg pain, swelling, tenderness, warmth, lower abdominal pain and a raised white cell count. In a suspected pulmonary embolism, dyspnea, collapse, chest pain, hemoptysis, raised JVP and focal signs in the chest (Green Top Guidelines 2001) are usually seen.

Imaging Modalities The positive diagnosis of venous thromboembolism has implications for immediate management. The main diagnostic imaging modalities include ultrasound or x-ray with suspected DVT; a ventilation-perfusion (V-Q) scan, angiography or MRI if the chest x-ray is abnormal. The pulmonary angiogram is the gold standard for the diagnosis of pulmonary embolism. It is invasive and bears a mortality rate of 0.5% and morbidity rate of 2–4% (Gilham). Spiral CT scanning is also a useful imaging modality with minimum radiation risks to the fetus. In the acute phase, an arterial blood gas analysis should be done in the sitting or left lateral position to avoid the effects of inferior venacaval compression, which may give a false impression of hypoxia (Girling 2004). The electrocardiogram (ECG) usually lacks specificity, but the classical findings are T wave inversion and Q wave in lead III. D-dimer testing in pregnancy has limited value because of its physiological elevation. However, a low value may suggest that there is no venous thromboembolism (Green Top Guidelines 2001).

Initial Management In the initial treatment of clinically suspected DVT or pulmonary embolism, the Royal College Guidelines recommend treatment with unfractionated heparin or low molecular weight heparin until diagnosis is excluded by objective testing or treatment is strongly contraindicated. Subcutaneous unfractionated heparin is an effective alternative to intravenous unfractionated heparin for the initial management of DVT. Many systematic reviews have concluded that low molecular weight heparin is a safe alternative to unfractionated heparin as an anticoagulant in pregnancy (Ensom and Stephenson 1999; Sanson et al 1999). Due to altered pharmacokinetics, a twice daily dosage of low

TABLE 16.1: RISK OF THROMBOEMBOLIC DISEASE BY AGE, PREGNANCY AND MODE OF DELIVERY

Thromboembolic Event	*Age Under 35 Years*	*Age Over 35 Years*
Antenatal DVT	0.615	1.216
Postnatal DVT	0.304	0.72
Postnatal pulmonary embolus	0.108	0.405
DVT after Emergency LSCS	0.431	1.248
DVT after elective LSCS	0.238	0.68

molecular weight heparins such as dalteparin and enoxaparin are recommended during pregnancy (RCOG 2001). In the immediate management of venous thromboembolism, the dose of enoxaparin is 1 mg/kg twice daily, based on early pregnancy weight. It does not cross the placenta and should be continued 12 hourly until objective testing has been performed. When the diagnosis is confirmed, peak anti-Xa activity should be measured by a chromogenic substrate assay, and platelet counts should be checked. The target therapeutic range of enoxaparin is arbitrary, but in the range of 0.6–1 unit/ml (Green Top Guidelines 2001).

Special Consideration Inferior venacaval filters are reserved for patients with recurrent pulmonary embolism despite adequate anticoagulation. Surgical embolectomy is the last resort based on the decision of specialist clinicians.

Maintenance Treatment Oral anti-coagulants such as warfarin are generally avoided for maintenance treatment. This is because they readily cross the placenta and cause a characteristic embryopathy consisting of nasal hypoplasia, stippled epiphysis and abnormal facies, referred as the Conradi syndrome. Therefore, adjusted dose, subcutaneous unfractionated heparin or low molecular weight heparin are effective alternatives to oral anticoagulants in maintenance treatment.

Labour and Delivery Once in established labour, heparin should be stopped and further doses should be prescribed only by medical staff. Regional anesthesia should not be used until 12 hours after the injection, to avoid epidural hematomas. A senior anesthetist should be involved in developing local protocols and managing the case. In women delivering by cesarean section, wound drains should be considered and skin incisions should be closed by staples or interrupted sutures to allow drainage of hematomas.

Postnatal Anticoagulation Graduated compression elastic stockings should be worn for at least two years to reduce the risk of post-thrombotic syndrome. Anticoagulants should be continued postnatally for 6–12 weeks, depending on risk factors such as the underlying thrombophilia.

The Royal College has recommended thromboprophylaxis based on risk categorisation, as shown in Table 16.2 (Report of the RCOG Working Party on Prophylaxis (and Management) against Thromboembolism in Gynaecology and Obstetrics 1995).

Conclusion Inherited and acquired thrombophilias are particularly high-risk situations during pregnancy and puerperium.

Table 16.2: Risk categories and appropriate management of thrombophilia

Risk Category	*Definition*	*Management*
Low	Elective LSCS Uncomplicated pregnancy	Good hydration Early mobilisation
Moderate	Emergency LSCS Age >35 Weight >80 kg Gross varicose veins Current infection Pre-eclampsia Immobilisation prior to LSCS >4 days Major medical disease	TEDS/Heparin
High	Three or more moderate risk factors Cesarean hysterectomy Antiphospholipid syndrome H/O venous thromboembolism	TEDS + Heparin

(TEDS: Thromboembolic deterrent stockings)

There are no standard guidelines to define the exact principles of intervention. The use of a multidisciplinary approach, with the services of an expert in the specialised area, is likely to optimise the obstetric outcome and prevent life-threatening complications.

References

Clark P, J Brennand, JA Conkie et al. 1998. Activated Protein C sensitivity, Protein C, Protein S and coagulation in normal pregnancy. *Thromb Haemost* 79: 1166–70.

D'Angelo A and J.Selhub 1997. Homocysteine and thrombotic disease. *Blood* 90:1–11.

Demers C, JS Ginsberg, J Hirsh et al. 1992. Thrombosis in antithrombin III deficient persons: report of a large kindred and literature review. *Ann Intern Med* 116:754–61.

Ensom MHH and MD Stephenson. 1999. Low molecular weight heparins in pregnancy. **Pharmacotherapy** 1013–1025.

Faioni EM, C Valsecchi, A Palla et al. 1997. Free Protein S deficiency is a risk factor for venous thrombosis. *Thromb Haemost* 78:1343–1346.

Finnazi G, R Caccia and T Barbui. 1987. Different prevalence of thromboembolism in the subtypes of congenital antithrombin III deficiency: review of 404 cases. *Thromb Haemost* 58:1094.

Gilham JC. Haematological Conditions In *Obstetrics and Gynaecology*, 1st ed, 6 (5):64–79. Arnold.

Ginsberg KS, PS Wells, P Brill-Edwards et al. 1995. Antiphospholipid antibodies and venous thromboembolism. *Blood* 86:3685–91.

Girling J. 2004. Thromboembolism and thrombophilia. *Cur Obstet and Gynaecol* 14:11–22.

Khamashta MA, MJ Cuardrado, F Mujic et al. 1995. The management of thrombosis in the antiphospholipid syndrome. *N Engl J Med* 332:993–997.

Koster T, FR Rosendaal, E Briet et al. 1995. Protein C deficiency in a controlled series of unselected outpatients: An infrequent but clear risk factor for venous thrombosis. Leiden thrombophilia study. *Blood* 85:2756–2761.

Poort SR, FR Rosendaal, PH Reitsma et al. 1996. A common genetic variation in the 3' untranslated region of the prothrombin gene is associated with elevated plasma prothrombin levels and an increase in venous thrombosis. *Blood* 88:3698–703.

Rees DC, M Cox and JB Clegg. 1995. World distribution of factor V Leiden. *Lancet* 346:1133–1134.

Report of the RCOG Working Party on Prophylaxis (and Management) against Thromboembolism in Gynaecology and Obstetrics. 1995. London: RCOG.

Ridker PM, JP Miletich, CH Heenekens et al. 1997. Ethnic distribution of factor V Leiden in 4047 men and women. *JAMA* 277:1305–1307.

Rosendaal FR, T Koster, JP Vandenbroucke et al. 1995. High risk of thrombosis in patients homozygous for factor V Leiden (activated protein C resistance). *Blood* 85:1504–1508.

Royal College of Obstetricians and Gynaecologists. 2001. Thromboembolic disease in pregnancy and the puerperium: acute management. *Clinical Green Top Guideline* No: 28. London: RCOG Press.

Sanson BJ, AW Lensing, MH Prins, JS Ginsberg, ZS Barkagan, E Lavenne-Pardonge, B Brenner, M Dulitzky, JD Nielsen, Z Boda, S Turi, MR Mac Gillavry, K Hamulyák, IM Theunissen, BJ Hunt and HR Büller. 1999. Safety of low-molecular-weight heparin in pregnancy: A systematic review. *Thromb Haemost* 81(5):668–672

Shetty S, M Madkaikar, S Nair, A Pawar, S Baindur, A Pathare, K Ghosh and D Mohanty. 2000. Combined Factor V and Factor VIII deficiency in Indian Population. *Haemophilia* 6(5):504–507.

Souto JC, I Coll, D Llobe et al. 1998. The prothrombin 20210 A allele is the most prevalent genetic risk factor for venous thromboembolism in the Spanish population. *Thromb Haemost* 80:306–309.

Tait RC, ID Walker, PH Reitsma et al. 1995. Prevalence of protein C deficiency in the healthy population. *Thromb Haemost* 73:87–93.

Thaler E and K Lechner. 1981. Antithrombin III deficiency and thromboembolism. *Clin Haematol* 10:369–390.

Ubbink JB, WJ Vermaac, A van der Merwe et al. 1993. Vitamin B12, Vitamin B6 and folate nutritional status in men with hyperhomocysteinaemia. *Am J Clin Nutr* 57:47–53.

Walker ID, M Greaves and FE Preston (on behalf of the British Society of Haematologists). 2001. Guideline, investigation and management of heritable thrombophilia. *Br J Haematol* 114:512–528.

17

Hemoglobinopathies in Pregnancy

Deepika Deka | Renu Saxena | Inusha Panigrahi

Hemoglobinopathies are a heterogenous group of hemoglobin disorders, usually inherited, that affect hemoglobin structure, function or production, and thereby, oxygen delivery to tissues (Forget et al 2000; Steinberg and Benz 2000). They are of varying severity, ranging from an asymptomatic state with only a positive laboratory screening test, to a symptomatic state leading to acute hematological crisis—anemia and vaso-occlusion—and causing significant mortality and morbidity in adolescence, infancy or in utero. These most common of single-gene defects include the hemoglobin variants (due to structural abnormalities in globin; for example, sickle cell anemia—HbS, HbE and C) and the thalassemia syndromes (due to impaired globin synthesis; for example, α and β thalassemia). Variants are HbSC disease, sickle cell β thalassemia, sickle cell HbE disease, Hb Lepore, HbE β thalassemia, HbH disease and Hb Bart's disease.

More than 270 million people worldwide are heterologous carriers, and at least 300,000 affected homozygotes or compound heterozygotes are born every year (ACOG Practice Bulletin 2005). An estimated 5% of the world's population are carriers of hemoglobin disorders (Sickle Cell Disease Guideline Panel 1993). Earlier, affected individuals did not survive beyond the second decade of life or could not reproduce because of anemia or menstrual and other endocrine abnormalities associated with these conditions. With advances in medical treatment, they now enjoy an improved quality of life well into adulthood, when they may elect to start a family (Pafumi et al 2000; Rappaport et al 2004; Wanapirak et al 2004).

Pregnancy may be associated with exacerbation of disease and may place women, such as those with sickle cell anemia (HbSS), at an additional risk of obstetric complications (Rahimy et al 2000; Arora et al 2001; Odum et al 2002; Hassell et al 2005). Carrier couples could have an affected fetus; therefore, genetic screening and prenatal diagnosis (PND) by DNA mutation analysis is an important aspect of periconceptional and prenatal care (Deka 1998; Coughey 2005; Firdous 2005; Thomas et al 2005). Couples who wish to avoid prenatal diagnosis and termination of pregnancy could opt for preimplantation genetic diagnosis (PGD) (Monni et al 2004). Umbilical cord blood as an alternative stem cell source with curative potential for patients with hemoglobinopathies is under investigation, thereby indicating the usefulness of a programme for medically indicated cord blood collection and banking (Deka 1997; Reed et al 2001).

Epidemiology

Hemoglobinopathies have specific ethnic and regional predilections, being more common in areas where malaria used to be endemic, such as in the Mediterranean, Middle East, Southeast Asia, Africa and the West Indies. However, with increasing immigration and interracial marriages, the problem is now global. In India, one study estimates that there are about 42 million carriers, with 12,000 affected infants born every year (Balgir 1999). An NGO national screening programme targeting people aged 12–35 years and newborns in the Maldives established a β thalassemia prevalence rate of 18% (one in five), a 28% incidence of α thalassemia and a significantly high incidence of more than one hemoglobinopathy on individual islands (Firdous 2005). Three specific mutations accounted for 95% of thalassemia genes, ensuring a high detection rate and the cost effectiveness of the prenatal diagnosis programme. In Thailand, overall prevalence of the thalassemia trait was 25.4%; α thalassemia (SEA type) trait 6.6%, β thalassemia trait 3.7%, hemoglobin E trait 11.6%, homozygous HbE trait 0.8%, combination of α thalassemia 1 (SEA type) and β thalassemia trait 1.2%, α thalassemia and HbE trait 1.5% and β thalassemia HbE disease 0.2% (Wanapirak et al 2004).

The frequency of occurrence of various common hemoglobinopathies is as follows:

- Thalassemias are the most common genetic disorders in the world. β thalassemia has an incidence of 10–15% in the Mediterranean region, Myanmar, India, Southeast Asia and the Middle East (Angastiniotis and Modell 1998). α thalassemia has a 1–15% incidence of silent carriers in the Mediterranean, Southeast Asia, the Pacific islands and tribal populations of central and eastern India.
- Africa is the primary birthplace of sickle cell mutations; the number of newborns affected by sickle cell disease is estimated at 200,000 per year. HbS carriers in West Africa are as high as 25% of the population. Other populations with a high prevalence of sickle cell carriers are those in the Mediterranean, the Caribbean, South and Central America, Arabia and eastern India. About 0.2% of African Americans in the United States have sickle cell disease (Steinberg and Benz 2000), while 22–80% of certain tribal populations in India are affected (Balgir 1996).
- HbE is prevalent in eastern India, Southeast Asia, Thailand, Laos and Cambodia. A carrier rate of about 25–30% is seen in eastern Thailand near the Vietnamese border, which forms the 'HbE triangle' (Forget 2000), while a 7–50% carrier rate is seen in Northeast India (Balgir 1996; Piplani 2000).
- HbC has a 25% carrier rate in parts of West Africa (Angastiniotis and Modell 1998).

PATHOLOGY OF HEMOGLOBIN STRUCTURE AND FUNCTION

Hemoglobin is a tetrameric protein, composed of two polypeptide chains with a heme molecule attached to each chain. In fetal life, fetal hemoglobin (HbF) is predominant and consists of two alpha and two delta globin chains (α2/δ2). The globin genes reside on chromosomes 11 and 16. There are four α globin genes, two on each chromosome 16, and two β globin genes on chromosome 11. The globin gene is also found on chromosome 11. In the third trimester, the β and δ globin genes become active, with an increase in the amount of adult hemoglobins A (α2β2) and HbA2 (α2/δ2) produced. Infants become dependent on HbA synthesis by about 4-6 months of age, when the circulating HbF cells are slowly replaced. The normal adult hemoglobin comprises two α chains and two β chains, HbA ($\alpha_2\beta_2$, 97%) with less amount of HbA2 ($\alpha_2\delta_2$, <3.2%), and HbF ($\alpha_2\gamma_2$, <1%).

Erythrocyte hemoglobins are precisely regulated for oxygen pick-up and delivery to tissues. They are present as a viscous solution at concentrations of 33–35 g/dl normally, in the discoid-shaped RBCs, which are 7–8 μm in diameter, but have to squeeze through 3 μm calibered capillaries without being hemolysed by the mechanical and metabolic changes. The pathological hemoglobins tend to gel or crystallise, and hence bind oxygen abnormally, and readily hemolyse in stressful situations, resulting in anemia and other complications thereof.

β thalassemia is characterised by diminished production of β globin chains with compensatory accumulation and aggregation of α globin chains, increased HbA2 (α2δ2) and HbF (α2γ2), resulting in microcytic hypochromic anemia. In β° thalassemia, the most severe form, no β globin chains are present—only HbA2 and HbF are present. β+ thalassemia cases have small amounts of β globin; HbA, HbA2 and HbF are found on electrophoresis, and the symptoms are milder than in β° thalassemia. Coexistence of α thalassemia, other abnormal hemoglobins and disorders affecting HbF synthesis modify the phenotype of β thalassemia.

Over 200 mutations have been described in β thalassemia. Base substitution mutations are common in β thalassemia, whereas deletion mutations are common in α thalassemia. The five common β thalassemia mutations seen in India are IVS 1-5 (G-C), IVS 1-1 (G-T), Cd 8-9 (+G), Fr 41/42 (-TCTT) and 619 bp deletion. The frequencies of these show regional variation, but together they account for more than 90% of the mutations (Arora et al 2001).

There is significant ethnic predilection. The 619-bp deletion is common among the Sindhis, Lohanas (45–50%), Khoja and Memon Muslims from Gujarat (46.7%) and Punjabi Hindus (34.7%). IVS 1-5 (G→C) is the predominant mutation in Jains (94%), Brahmins, Patels and scheduled castes from Gujarat (58–78%) and Brahmins, Marathas and scheduled castes from Maharashtra (58–74%). The IVS 1-1 (G→T) mutation is common among Sindhis, Lohanas and Punjabi Hindus (25–32%). Codon 41/42 (-TCTT) is the dominant mutation among the Vanias from Gujarat (59.1%), though the IVS 1-5 (G→C) mutation has also been observed (22.7%).

α thalassemia is characterised by defective α globin chain synthesis. Normally, there are two α genes on each chromosome 16

Table 17.1: Occurrence of different hemoglobin disorders in the Indian population*

Condition	Frequency (%)	Groups with a Higher Predilection
β thalassemia	1–17 (avg 3.3)	Khatris, Sindhis, Bhanusalis
α thalassemia	5–13	Koya Dora and Konda Reddi tribal communities in Andhra Pradesh
HbE	1–50	Northeastern region (avg 10.9%)
HbS	0–22	Tribal populations
HbD Punjab	0.86	Punjab, Jammu and Kashmir, Uttar Pradesh

** References: Balgir RS, Piplani S, Fodde R et al.*

($\alpha\alpha/\alpha\alpha$). Trait cases ($-\alpha/-\alpha$; $--/\alpha\alpha$) may have microcytosis or mild anemia. HbH disease cases ($--/-\alpha$; $\alpha^T\alpha/\alpha^T\alpha$) may present in pregnancy with anemia with or without splenomegaly or jaundice. Usually, there is an absence of functional α globin genes ($--/--$) in Hb Bart's (γ_4), HbH (β_4) and small amounts of Hb Portland ($\zeta_2\gamma_2$) types. The α thalassemias are best diagnosed by detecting the common deletion mutations. The α thalassemia deletions $-\alpha^{3.7}$ and $-\alpha^{4.2}$ (α thalassemia 2) are present worldwide, but the α thalasemmia 1 (α^o thalassemia) deletions are present in specific geographic regions. The α^o thalassemia deletions include $--^{SEA}$, $--^{SA}$, $--^{MED}$, $--^{FIL}$, etc. HbCS with $--^{SEA}$ deletions is a major cause of HbH disease in Southeast Asia. The commonest α deletions reported from India are $-\alpha^{3.7}$, $-\alpha^{4.2}$, $--^{SA}$ and Hb Koya Dora. The gene frequency for α thalassemia is variable, being more in tribal populations from central and eastern India. For $-\alpha^{3.7}$ kb deletions, frequencies of 4% and 5% have been reported from Uttar Pradesh and Delhi, respectively, in the normal population. The $-\alpha^{4.2}$ deletions are common in eastern India but rare in North India. The $--^{SA}$ deletion is the commonest α^0 deletion found in Indian HbH disease cases. Other α^0 deletions are rare in the Indian population. Hb Koya Dora is present in up to 10% of the Koya Dora tribal community. Other point mutations reported include Hb Constant Spring and polyadenylation signal mutation. There is considerable regional variation in α mutations (Panigrahi 2004).

In sickle cell anemia, a genetic defect leads to a change in the aminoacid from glutamine to valine. This is caused by a point mutation in codon 6 of the β globin gene (GAG→GTG), resulting in sickle hemoglobin (HbS). The disorder can exist in the severe homozygous form—sickle cell disease (HbSS)—as a sickle cell trait (HbAS) or in compound heterozygous form—as sickle β thalassemia. In people of African origin, sickle HbC (HbSC) disease is also seen.

CLINICAL FEATURES IN PREGNANCY

An abnormal globin chain structure may result in unstable, abnormal oxygen binding or accelerated destruction of red cells. Pregnancy is a state of physiological anemia. The physiological hematological changes of pregnancy, increased metabolic demands and oxidative stress increases maternal anemia to a variable range of severity, leading to deficient oxygen supply to the maternal organs and fetus. Disorders of α globin synthesis may manifest in utero or at birth, while disorders of β globin synthesis usually manifest by 4–6 months of age.

Thalassemia

β Thalassemia In thalassemia major (Cooley's anemia), the lifespan of a red blood cell is shortened by hemolysis, with profound compensatory extramedullary hematopoesis and bone marrow expansion—typically, in the maxillary and frontal bones producing the 'chipmunk' facies (Benz 2001). Severe growth retardation, hepatosplenomegaly and high output cardiac failure are seen. The child is susceptible to infection, and endocrine dysfunction may occur, resulting in death in the first decade of life. Treatment with chronic blood transfusion prolongs life, but iron overload leads to hepatic and endocrine dysfunction and myocardial damage. Iron chelation and allogenic bone marrow transplantation has been used, and successful pregnancies have become a reality.

If both parents are carriers of β thalassemia, the fetus/newborn has a 1 in 4 chance of inheriting thalassemia major.

Patients with β **thalassemia intermedia** have a milder phenotype and may require blood transfusion occasionally. This is a heterogeneous group with varying clinical severity, influenced by other genetic modifiers such as α gene deletions and triplications, and factors that increase the HbF level. The patient may be homozygous or heterozygous for β thalassemia at the molecular level. They may present with amenorrhea, endocrinal problems or infertility. Some of these patients may be first identified during pregnancy.

The heterozygous cases presenting as **'thalassemia trait'** are asymptomatic. Their hemogram may show mild anemia and/or microcytosis, that is not responsive to iron. They may have gallstones or a stress-induced rise in hemolysis. In this case, they must be differentiated from iron deficiency and anemia of chronic disease.

α Thalassemias Patients with the α thalassemia trait are usually asymptomatic carriers. They resemble those with β thalassemia traits, but with hypochromia and microcytosis in addition. Patients with HbH have moderately severe 'intermedia' hemolytic anemia, commonly surviving till mid-adulthood without β thalassemia. The homozygous state of α thalassemia, Hb Bart's, is associated with almost no oxygen to fetal tissues, resulting in hydrops fetalis and death. 'Hydrops fetalis' refers to fetuses with edema due to congestive heart failure resulting from severe anemia. The peripheral smear shows large hypochromic macrocytes and numerous nucleated red cells. Affected fetuses are delivered stillborn or die shortly after delivery. Pregnancy with α thalassemia hydrops may be associated with severe pre-eclampsia (mirror syndrome), and vaginal delivery may be complicated because the baby may be large. A high incidence of postpartum hemorrhage (PPH) has been described in mothers of these infants, probably due to a massive placenta.

Sickle Cell Anemia Sickle cell disease is common in Africans and the tribal populations in central India. HbS prevalence reaches up to 80% in certain tribal groups (Table 17.1). The erythrocyte membranes are stiffened and increased viscosity is seen, resulting in cell dehydration, leakage of potassium and influx of calcium, producing the characteristic sickle shape. The sickled cells lose the pliability to traverse small capillaries; the sticky membranes (especially reticulocytes) adhere abnormally to the endothelium of small vessels, causing microvascular occlusion, tissue ischemia, acute pain (painful crisis) and gradual end organ damage or frank infarction of the spleen (splenic sequestration crisis), central nervous system (causing stroke), bones, liver, kidneys and lungs (acute chest syndrome). The abnormal red cells are hemolysed and destroyed by the spleen (Steinberg and Benz 2000; Benz 2001).

Clinical Features The clinical features of a hemolytic anemia state are hematocrit at 15–30%, significant reticulocytosis and granulocytosis especially during pain, crisis or infectious episodes. Vaso-occlusion causes acute intermittent episodes of pain, tenderness, fever and tachycardia, varying in severity and frequency. Infection, fever, abrupt changes in temperature, dehydration, hypoxia or excessive exercise can precipitate a crisis. Renal papillary necrosis may produce asymptomatic hematuria. Urological manifestations include pyelonephritis, renal papillary necrosis, hyposthenuria, renal infarction, hematuria and renal cell carcinoma.

Most women do not reach reproductive age. The most evident clinical problem is that of maternal anemia. Medical complications from sickle cell crisis remains a major disadvantage and may occur in about half the pregnant women, with pain in the lower back, chest, femoral shaft, hip joints, ribs and knees, besides a painful abdomen and headache, often making diagnosis of pregnancy complications a dilemma. Impaired oxygenation and placental sickling infarcts are thought to result in miscarriage, preterm labour, fetal death and other complications (Odum et al 2002).

Pulmonary arterial hypertension is a complication of the disease. This is associated with a maternal mortality rate of around 50% (Sun et al 2001). Pregnancy problems in 60 HbSS sickle cell disease patients in Lagos (Nigeria) were seen in 96.6% of cases, though all patients maintained a stable hematological profile, with booking, pre-delivery and postdelivery PCV of 23.2 ± SD 4.6% and 23.6 ± SD 4.5%, respectively (Odum et al 2002). Bone pain (41.4%), acute hemolysis with anemia (34.4%), malaria (22.4%), other systemic infectious (22.4%), need for blood transfusion both antenatal and postpartum (in 45% and 81.6%, respectively) and cesarean section (43.2%) were significant events (Rahimy et al 2000). Observations in West Africa indicated that *P. falciparum* malaria infection was one of the major causes of maternal morbidity, and that with improved antenatal care and patient education on nutrition, malaria prevention and early detection of bacterial infections, 58.3% (19 SS and 44 SC) of the patients did not need blood transfusion (Rahimy et al 2000). Maternal and perinatal mortality rates of 67 and 121/1000, respectively, were seen at Lagos (Odum et al 2002). This rate went as low as 1.8% (of 42 SS and 66 SC mothers) maternal deaths and 13/111 (9 SS and 4 SC) fetal deaths at Benin in West Africa (Rahimy et al 2000).

An inability to produce concentrated urine makes them unusually prone to dehydration during labour. HbHC patients are prone to sudden massive, even fatal, sickling crisis during pregnancy and particularly in the puerperium.

In patients with the sickle cell trait, no associated abnormalities are seen, but at high altitudes and low oxygen pressures, spontaneous hematuria may occur in around 1% of cases (Benz 2001). Interaction of HbS with HbD Punjab gives rise to features similar to those of sickle cell disease. Hemoglobin SC disease presents with 50% less frequency and less severe symptoms of pain crisis than homozygous HbSS. During pregnancy, women are at risk of infections—bacteriuria and pyelonephritis may occur, as well as benign hematuria, while parvovirus β_1 infection may precipitate an aplastic crisis.

There is increased risk of placental thrombosis, retained placenta and greater maternal and fetal morbidity and mortality, mainly in late pregnancy, during delivery and in the postpartal periods (Sergeant et al 2004).

Sickle cell β thalassemia patients may also experience pain crisis and other similar systemic manifestations, depending on the amount of HbA present—being milder if HbA is more than 25% of the total Hb.

Sickle cell HbE disease is a condition associated with mild hemolysis, though vaso-occlusive crisis is rare.

Other Abnormal Hemoglobins

Hemoglobin E (HbE) is the commonest Hb variant in India—second only to sickle hemoglobin (HbS)—with a prevalence of 7–50% in the northeastern regions (Balgir 1996; Piplani 2000). The abnormal hemoglobins in simple homozygous or heterozygous forms are relatively mild, but manifest with hemolytic anemia when they are present in conjunction with β thalassemia in compound heterozygous form.

Individuals with the HbE trait are asymptomatic. **Homozygous hemoglobin E** cases (HbEE) may show mild anemia, microcytosis and splenomegaly. Increased frequency of gallstones has been observed. The compound heterozygous **HbE β thalassemia** cases present with moderate to severe (transfusion dependent) phenotypes (Fucharoen and Winichagoon 2000; Panigrahi et al 2005). Some abnormal hemoglobins or hemoglobin variants in association with β thalassemia may also present with the thalassemia intermedia phenotype. **HbD Punjab** is another abnormal hemoglobin, commonly found among the North Indian population (Balgir 1996). It is more prevalent in Pakistan and northwestern India. There are reports of **Hb Lepore** from the Mediterranean region, Italy and recently from India. The frequency of this condition varies by area because of the genetic drift and coexistence of endemic malaria. Hb Lepore can coexist with β thalassemia.

Typical thalassemia indices with hypochromic microcytosis are observed in compound **HbD Punjab/β+ thalassemia** and **HbD Punjab/HbE**. HbD Punjab is also more severe when present with HbS in the compound state **(HbSD)**.

DIAGNOSIS, CARRIER SCREENING AND PRECONCEPTIONAL COUNSELLING

In populations at high risk of hemoglobinopathies, Hb electrophoresis should be done as routine prenatal screening. It is important to increase awareness of the hemoglobinopathies and **screen carriers** for many of the common hemoglobinopathies, to identify the couples in need for prenatal diagnosis (PND).

If both parents are carriers of a recessive hemoglobinopathy, the defective genes may be inherited from either side. The fetus/newborn has a 1 in 4 chance of inheriting the condition of homozygous or compound heterozygous form. Genetic counselling for carriers should focus on screening partners for any hemoglobinopathy—thalassemia, sickle disease or HbE. A definitive fetal diagnosis requires detection of causative mutations in couples at risk. This enables targeted **preconceptional and prenatal genetic counselling** for determination of the fetal genotype. Prenatal diagnosis of hemoglobinopathies in the fetus are readily available and should be discussed with the prospective parents, preconceptionally or early in pregnancy.

The severity of anemia, hypochromia and microcytosis varies depending on the amount of impaired globin alleles present (Benz 2001). Red cell indices may provide a clue to diagnosis. Low MCV with high RBC count and low RDW suggest thalassemia minor. Low MCV and low RBC count is seen in iron deficiency.

The diagnosis of many of the hemoglobinopathies is made by high performance liquid chromatography (HPLC)/Hb electrophoresis at a pH of 8.6. Whenever this is not informative/conclusive, molecular genetic methods come to the rescue. HbF levels are normally high at birth and reach adult levels within six months after birth. Normal HbA2 and HbF levels are found in small quantities in adult life—2–3.3% and 0.2–1%, respectively—(Bain 2001). Most carriers with β thalassemia have increased HbA2 levels (>3.5%), which can be detected by Hb electrophoresis, column chromatography or HPLC. Many abnormal hemoglobins can be detected in carriers by HPLC. HPLC can reliably detect HbQ India, HbD Iran, double heterozygosity for β thalassemia and HbS/HbE.

For β thalassemia, the usually recommended

strategy in carriers is to first screen for the five common β thalassemia mutations by ARMS PCR or reverse dot blot. These account for over 90% of mutations in thalassemia major in India (Arora 2001). If the patient is negative for these mutations, the less common mutations in a particular community can be screened by ARMS PCR or reverse dot blot (Fig. 17.1). If this is also negative, then a screening technique such as DGGE/SSCP can be used to screen for rare/unknown mutations to be followed by sequencing.

FIGURE 17.1: MEMBRANE STRIP SHOWING DETECTION OF MUTATIONS IN β THALASSEMIA BY REVERSE DOT BLOT TECHNIQUE. PATIENT'S RESULTS DEPICTED HERE SHOW COMPOUND HETEROZYGOSITY FOR THE IVS 1-5 (G→C) AND FRAMESHIFT 41/42 MUTATIONS

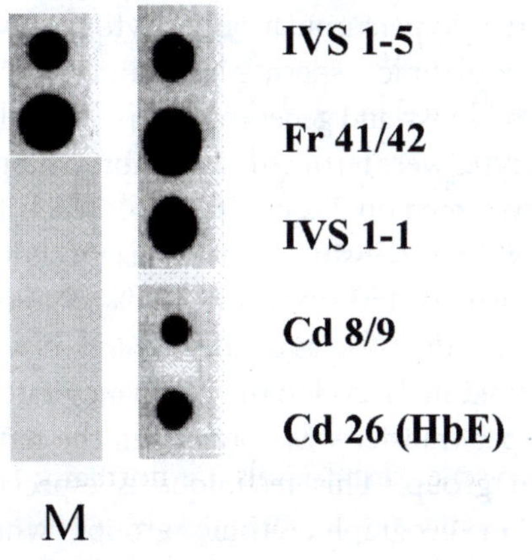

The problem arises especially in the detection of **milder α thalassemias, Hb Lepore and Hb Constant Spring.** The β thalassemia short programme (biorad) detects only Hb Bart's and HbH present in severe α thalassemia. Hb Lepore and Hb Constant Spring, which are present in low quantities in the heterozygous state, may not be reliably detected (Krishnamurti and Little 1998). The **sickle cell trait cases** can also be detected by the sickling test. Diagnosis of α thalassemia is often made in individuals with microcytic hypochromic anemia, after exclusion of β thalassemia and iron deficiency.

MATERNAL PRECONCEPTIONAL CARE

Patients with severe hemoglobinopathies contemplating pregnancy should have a thorough evaluation of their general health status and assessment of specific organ function, transfusion and chelation needs, infection screening—hepatitis B and C/HIV/cytomegalovirus (CMV)—cardiac and renal functions. Diabetes and the degree of hypersplenism should be assessed. Infertility due to hormone dysfunction such as hypogonadotrophic hypogonadism in β thalassemia major can be treated with ovulation induction and assisted reproductive techniques (Skordis 1998).

PRENATAL DIAGNOSIS

Once the mutations are identified in the couple, they can be assessed in the fetus. Prenatal diagnosis by **chorionic villus sampling** usually establishes diagnosis. PCR amplification of fetal DNA from chorionic villus samples are hybridised to allele-specific oligonucleotide probes. These probes can simultaneously detect multiple mutations accounting for 95–99% of the **α or β thalassemias** that occur in a particular ethnic population group. If mutations have not been characterised, then linkage analysis can be done using molecular markers for polymorphisms.

If mutation studies are non-informative, globin gene synthesis ratio or HPLC can be done on fetal cord blood obtained by **cordocentesis** or umbilical cord blood sampling in the second trimester, which is around 18–20 weeks (Panigrahi et al 2005). In a study from New Delhi, three out of nine affected fetuses (thalassemia major) were detected by cord blood HPLC studies. No fetal losses were reported, and the cordocentesis procedure is quite safe in experienced hands.

In non-immune hydrops fetalis without any obvious cause, testing for **α thalassemia** mutations should be done. This is accomplished by the GAP PCR technique performed on parental blood prior to pregnancy, and subsequently, in fetal chorionic villi or cord blood samples. Known point mutations can be screened by the reverse dot blot technique. Hb Bart's may be detected by HPLC on a cord blood sample. Unknown mutations require sequencing. Newer molecular techniques include real-time PCR, denaturing HPLC and microarrays (Dallapiccola 2002). These are high throughput techniques which are mostly done on a research basis. For diagnosis of complex thalassemia syndromes, heterozygosity of α thalassemia and β thalassemia or hemoglobin E has been reported to be obtained using a simultaneous multiplex PCR. This will facilitate characterisation and PND of complex syndromes in regions where α and β thalassemias and HbE are common (Siriratmanawong et al 2001).

Non-invasive PND by a simple technique to identify the presence or absence of α globin chains in fetal nucleated RBCs enriched by maternal blood at 10–26 weeks has been reported to identify 3/10 fetuses at risk (Winichagoon et al 2005). Another study reported the usefulness of non-invasive evaluation of intrahepatic umbilical venous maximum flow velocity, middle cerebral artery peak velocity, fetal liver length and spleen perimeter for diagnosis of α thalassemia, confirmed by cord blood sampling and managed by serial intrauterine fetal blood transfusions (Leung et al 2002).

Some of the reasons why PND cannot be performed include late presentation of the mother in pregnancy (>20 weeks), unavailability of partners or previous affected child for testing and unavailability of information to couples regarding available options.

PREIMPLANTATION GENETIC DIAGNOSIS (PGD)

This has been successfully used in thalassemia and sickle cell disease to achieve the birth of an unaffected fetus (Fiorentino et al 2003; Monni et al 2004; Vrettou et al 2004). After oocyte harvest and fertilisation, single-cell analysis is done at the blastomere stage or using polar body analysis. One study from Sardinia reported the experiences of 23 couples at risk of β thalassemia. All patients followed the protocol of ovarian hyperstimulation, oocyte retrieval, intracytoplasmic sperm injection (ICSI), embryo biopsy and genetic analysis. A total of 272 oocytes were fertilised, and embryo biopsy was performed on 202 embryos, of which 192 (95%) were successful. Genetic diagnosis was performed on 150 embryos (78.1%), Ninety-eight were identified as unaffected and 75 were transferred in 31 cycles; the pregnancy rate of 30.8% per transfer was obtained in the fertile women group. This technique is especially useful in geographic/ethnic groups where abortion is unacceptable due to religious or socio-cultural reasons.

CLINICAL MANAGEMENT OF HEMOGLOBINOPATHIES DURING PREGNANCY

Each hemoglobinopathy has certain specific effects on maternal/fetal outcome and complications. Hence, management should be tailored to the specific hemoglobinopathy, which is generally the same as in the non-pregnant patient.

Bone marrow transplantation for β thalassemia and sickle cell anemia, early in the course of disease, before end organ failure develops, has been shown to be curative in 80–90% of patients, with a treatment-related mortality of <10% (Benz 2001). Gene therapy and in utero stem cell transplantation for these hemoglobinopathies are still at the experimental stage.

Pregnancy is associated with exacerbation of the disease and may place women at an additional risk. Because of low family income, public health funding and local beliefs, overall treatment is still poor and, in some places, inadequate. Appropriate management by healthcare providers (hematologists, endocrinologists familiar with conditions such as sickle cell disease) and providers of high-risk obstetric care can result in successful pregnancy outcome for mother and child. The American Council of Obstetricians and Gynecologists (ACOG) and the British Committee Hematology Task Force have laid down recommendations for the screening and clinical management of hemoglobinopathies during pregnancy (ACOG Practice Bulletin 2005).

Fetal umbilical cord blood after delivery may be collected and stored/preserved for future use; CB bank programmes focussed on sibling donations for families with specific medical needs such as child with thalassemia major or sickle cell disease have been developed (Reed 2001). The aim of UCB may also be the possibility of obtaining complete marrow reconstitution in an attempt at heterologous transplantation to the mother (Pafumi et al 2000).

β Thalassemia

THALASSEMIA TRAIT: Around 30% of thalassemia trait cases in India have associated iron deficiency. A serum ferritin estimation early in pregnancy is advisable. Routine use of iron is not indicated, but iron deficiency anemia may develop during pregnancy or if bleeding occurs, requiring iron supplementation. Parenteral iron should never be given. Folic acid (5.0 mg daily) is required for defective erythropoiesis and may be given intramuscularly if required. If anemia persists, blood transfusion is indicated. Screening of the partner is done preconceptionally or early in pregnancy, and genetic counselling for prenatal diagnosis is done accordingly.

THALASSEMIA INTERMEDIA: Many patients require blood transfusions to maintain their Hb levels. Iron chelation may be given. Oxidative drugs should be avoided. Splenomegaly, if large, may be associated with dystocia at delivery. Cesarean section may be required for obstetric indications.

THALASSEMIA MAJOR: The improvement in current treatment modalities is likely to result in a steady increase in pregnancies in thalassemic women, making pregnancy a real eventuality. A precise and detailed pre-pregnancy assessment should be done for viral markers, serum ferritin, complete blood counts, liver function tests, cardiac evaluation, endocrine evaluation and RBC antigen typing. Hemoglobin should be maintained at 10 mg/dl with transfusions 2–3 times/week (Seracchioli et al 1994; Tampakoudis et al 1997). Continuation of desferrioxamine during pregnancy for iron chelation is not associated with adverse fetal outcomes and should be continued. Vitamin C should not be supplemented because it generates free radicals in iron excess states. Normally, delivery can be conducted vaginally in those without myocardial disease. Term pregnancy can be achieved, as a report of five healthy babies weighing 2.6–3.2 kg showed (Pafumi et al 2000). Those with impaired cardiac function and poor chelation have higher mortality.

α Thalassemia

THALASSEMIA TRAIT: These cases do not require any specific management, besides genetic counselling. Oral folate supplements should be given.

HBH DISEASE: These patients have features similar to β thalassemia intermedia, and cholelithiasis is common. Management is symptomatic and blood transfusions may be required.

In **Hb Bart's, hydrops fetalis,** limb abnormalities and hypospadias are reported. The obstetric complications in mothers of these fetuses include pre-eclampsia, polyhydramnios and retained placenta in 50–60% of cases. Around 33% of the affected fetuses show overt hydrops on ultrasound by 17–18 weeks of gestation (Leung et al 2002). Repeated intrauterine transfusions may salvage these fetuses.

Sickle Cell Disorders

SICKLE TRAIT: People with this trait may develop vaso-occlusive crises and anemia. Management is symptomatic.

SICKLE CELL DISEASE: Vitamins, especially folate, should be supplemented in patients with homozygous sickle cell disease. A baseline serum ferritin level should be done just before or early in pregnancy and oral iron given, if necessary. One school of thought is that regular blood transfusions at 6-week intervals are required to maintain the proportion of HbA at 60–70%, thereby reducing sickling crisis; 3—4 units of blood are given at each sitting. Though controversial for singletons, this protocol of routine prophylactic transfusion has universal consensus for twin pregnancies, which are more common in these communities. Long-term prophylactic penicillin, after splenectomy or otherwise, is recommended in pregnancy to prevent pneumococcal infection. Additionally, regular screening for urinary infection, hypertension, abnormal renal or liver function and fetal growth are mandatory.

Around 50% of sickle cell disease patients develop crisis in pregnancy. **Acute pain crisis** management involves vigorous hydration, evaluation of any precipitating cause such as infection or dehydration, and aggressive narcotic analgesia with morphine (0.1–0.15 mg/kg every 3–4 hours) or, in milder situations, with oral analgesics. Oxygen may be required to maintain adequate saturation, and acute chest syndrome may require ICU care. In severe cases, blood transfusion or exchange transfusion (ET) may be justified, though the usual crisis period of 1–7 days remains the same. Emergency ET is recommended when the patient presents late in pregnancy, is profoundly anemic or in preparation for general anesthesia. If used for analgesia, nonsteroidal antiinflammatory drugs (NSAIDS) can cause oligohydramnios and premature closure of the ductus arteriosus.

Labour should be allowed to be spontaneous unless there are other obstetric indications for cesarean section. Prostaglandins can cause increased sickling, and spinal anesthesia may precipitate a crisis. Continuous fetal heart rate monitoring during labour is important. Vigorous oral hydration should be done, hypoxia and dehydration should be avoided during anesthesia. Most maternal deaths occur in the immediate postpartum or postoperative period.

Patients with sickle cell disease are counselled to avoid oral contraceptive pills and intrauterine contraceptive devices.

Others

In the compound heterozygote states, sickle cell β thalassemia and sickle cell HbC disease, management is similar to that mentioned above. The disease is milder if the HbA2 level is above 25% and HbS is less.

PREVENTION AND CONTROL OF HEMOGLOBINOPATHIES: COST EFFECTIVENESS ANALYSIS

With increasing concern regarding rapidly expanding healthcare costs, a cost effectiveness analysis provides a methodology to assess whether marginal gains from new technology are worth the increased costs. In the area of PND, particular methodological and ethical concerns include the effect of such testing on individuals other than the patient—how screening may reassure or cause anxiety depending on the results and redundancy of screening and diagnostic methods. The existing literature has demonstrated cost effectiveness of screening and diagnosis of genetic disorders that have a higher prevalence among particular groups— diseases such as hemoglobinopathies, Down syndrome and neural tube defects (Coughey 2005). It has been realised that the heavy genetic load of hemoglobinopathies, frequent blood transfusions, high cost of treatment and management, physical trauma and the psychological and mental harassment to the patients and their families makes the preventive approach most suitable for the Indian setting (Balgir 1999).

A system wherein pregnant women were screened in general practice and a model-of-care pathway were evaluated in a primary care setting in North London. The gestational age at screening was 4.1 weeks earlier than in hospital clinics and 2.9 weeks earlier than in community midwife clinics (Thomas et al 2005). Providing pregnant SCD women patients with basic information and education about SCD—about improving the nutritional status, malaria prevention, early detection of bacterial infections and restricted use of BT—were found to be simple, cost effective approaches that could have a positive impact on SCD-associated morbidity and mortality in otherwise difficult settings (Rahimy et al 2000).

Data from the UK Thalassemia Register and the UK Register of Prenatal Diagnosis for Hemoglobin Disorders, which included fetuses known to have been diagnosed with β thalassemia major/intermedia, or HbE/β thalassemia, revealed that, of 1074 born with a disorder, 807 were alive, with bone marrow transplantation performed successfully in 117 out of 581 (20%) patients born since 1975. Despite the acceptability of PND, the proportion of affected births remained 50% higher than expected, with residents of Pakistani origin replacing Cypriots as the main risk group (Modell et al 2001).

A national surveillance register is a powerful instrument for monitoring the treatment and prevention of inherited hemoglobinopathies and for highlighting correctable shortcomings (Modell et al 2001). There is a strong case for funding for such databases, cost effective analysis of prenatal diagnosis (Coughey 2005) and antenatal screening for hemoglobinopathies in general practice and primary care settings (Thomas et al 2005) within modern health services. Health education, inclusion in school curriculum, legal requirements for screening prior to marriage, legalisation of PND and MTP, commencement of PND services, public awareness and sensitisation, effective advocacy, resource mobilisation, motivation for screening and awareness about hemoglobinopathies are measures to be advocated for the benefit of the general public.

References

ACOG Committee. ACOG Practice Bulletin. 2005. Clinical Management Guidelines for Obstetrician-Gynecologists. Number 64, July 2005 (Replaces Committee Opinion Number 238, July 2000): Hemoglobinpathies in pregnancy. *Obstet Gynecol*; 106:203–210.

Angastiniotis M and B Modell. 1998. Global epidemiology of hemoglobin disorders. *Proc Natl Acad Sci USA* 850:251–269.

Arora S, M Kabra, M Maheshwari, S Shastri, D Kaur, D Deka et al. 2001. Prenatal diagnosis of haemoglobinopathies. *Natl Med J India* 14:340–342.

Bain BJ and BJ Wild. 2001. Investigation of abnormal haemoglobin and thalassaemia. In *Practical Haematology*. 9th ed., ed SM Lewis, BJ Bain and I Bates, 231–268. London: Churchill Livingstone.

Balgir RS. 1996. Genetic epidemiology of the three abnormal hemoglobins in India. *J Assoc Physicians India* 44:25–28.

Balgir RS. 1999. Control and prevention of the genetic load of haemoglobinopathies in India. *Natl Med J India* 12:234–238.

Benz Jr. E.J. 2001. Hemoglobinopathies. In *Harrison's Principles of Internal Medicine*, 15th ed, ed E Braunwald. New York: McGraw Hill.

Coughey AB. 2005. Cost-effectiveness analysis of prenatal diagnosis: methodological issues and concerns. *Gynecol Obstet Invest* 60:11–18.

Dallapiccola B. 2002. Reliability of dHPLC in mutational screening of beta-globin (HBB) alleles. *Hum Mutat* 9:287–295.

Deka D. 1997. Umbilical cord blood at delivery: 'Waste' or 'Priceless source of stem cells'. *Obstet and Gynae Today* I:773–775.

Deka D. 1998. Chorionic Villus Sampling. *Obst & Gynae Today* III:340–342.

Fiorentino F, MC Magli, D Podini, AP Ferrarati, A Nuccitelli, N Vitale et al. 2003. The minisequencing method: an alternative strategy for preimplantation genetic diagnosis of single gene disorders. *Mol Hum Reprod* 9:399–410.

Firdous N. 2005. Prevention of thalassaemia and haemoglobinopathies in remote and isolated communities—the Maldives experience. *Ann Hum Biol* 32:131–137.

Forget BG, DR Higgs, RL Nagel et al. 2000. Disorders of hemoglobin. New York: Cambridge University Press.

Fucharoen S and P Winichagoon. 2000. Clinical and hematologic aspects of hemoglobin E beta-thalassemia. *Curr Opin Hematol* 7:106–112.

Hassell K. 2005. Pregnancy and sickle cell disease. *Hematol Oncol Clin North Am* 19:903–916.

Krishnamurti L and JA Little. 1998. Homozygous hemoglobin constant spring with normal electrophoresis—a possible cause for under-diagnosis. *Ann NY Acad Sci* 850:415–419.

Leung WC, D Oepkes, G Seaward and G Ryan. 2002. Serial sonographic findings of four fetuses with homozygous alpha-thalassemia-1 from 21 weeks onwards. *Ultrasound Obstet Gynecol* 19:56–59.

Modell B, M Khan, M Darlison, A King, M Layton, J Old, M Petrou and L Varnavides. 2001. A national register for the surveillance of inherited disorders: beta thalassaemia in the United Kingdom. *Bull World Health Organ* 79:1006–1013.

Monni G, G Cau, V Usai, G Perra, R Lai, G Ibba, V Faa, F Incani and MC Rosatelli. 2004. Preimplantation genetic diagnosis for beta-thalassaemia: the Sardinian experience. *Prenat Diagn* 24:949–954.

Odum CU, RI Anorlu, SI Dim and TO Oyekan. 2002. Pregnancy outcome in HbSS-sickle cell disease in Lagos, Nigeria. *West Afr J Med* 21:19–23.

Pafumi C, M Farina, G Pernicone, S Bandiera, A Russo, L Mangiafico and A Cianci. 2000. At term pregnancies in transfusion-dependent beta-thalassemic women. *Clin Exp Obstet Gynecol* 27:185–187.

Panigrahi I, PH Rafeeq, VP Choudhry and R Saxena. 2004. High frequency of deletional alpha-thalassemia in beta-thalassemia trait: implications for genetic counselling. *Am J Hematol* 76:297–299.

Panigrahi I, RP Ahmed, M Kannan, M Kabra, D Deka and R Saxena. 2005. Cord blood analysis for prenatal diagnosis of thalassemia major and hemophilia A. *Indian Pediatr* 42:577–581.

Panigrahi I, S Agarwal, T Gupta, P Singhal and M Pradhan. 2005. Hemoglobin E-beta thalassemia: Factors Affecting Phenotype. *Indian Pediatr* 2:357–362.

Piplani S. 2000. Hemoglobin E disorders in the north east India. *J Assoc Physicians India* 48: 1082–1084.

Rahimy MC, A Gangbo, R Adjou, C Deguenon, S Goussanou and E Alihonou. 2000. Effect of active prenatal management on pregnancy outcome in sickle cell disease in an African setting. *Blood* 96:1685–1689.

Rappaport VJ, M Velazquez and K Williams. 2004. Hemoglobinopathies in pregnancy. *Obstet Gynecol Clin North Am* 31:287–317.

Reed W, M Walters, E Trachtenberg, R Smith and BH Lubin. 2001. Sibling donor cord blood banking for children with sickle cell disease. *Pediatr Pathol Mol Med* 20:167–174.

Seracchioli R, E Porcu, C Colombi, P Ciotti, R Fabbri, V De Sanctis et al. 1994. Transfusion-dependent homozygous beta-thalassaemia major: successful twin pregnancy following in-vitro fertilization and tubal embryo transfer. *Hum Reprod* 9: 1964–1965.

Sergeant GR, LL Loy, M Crowther and M Thame. 2004. Outcome of pregnancy in homozygous sickle cell disease. *Obstet Gynecol* 103:1278–1285.

Sickle Cell Disease Guideline Panel. 1993. Sickle cell disease: screening, diagnosis, management, and counselling in newborns and infants. (Clinical Practice Guideline no. 6). Rockville (MD): Agency for Health Care Policy and Research, US Public Health Service (AHCPR Publ. No. 93-0562).

Siriratmanawong N, G Fucharoen, K Sanchaisuriya, T Ratanasiri and S Fucharoen. 2001. Simultaneous PCR detection of beta-thalassemia and alpha-thalassemia 1 (SEA type) in prenatal diagnosis of complex thalassemia syndrome. *Clin Biochem* 34:377–380.

Skordis N, S Christou, M Koliou et al. 1998. Fertility in female patients with thalassemia. *J Pediatr Endocrinol Metab* 11:935–943.

Steinberg MH and EJ Benz. 2000. Pathobiology of the human erythrocyte and its hemoglobins. In *Hematology: Basic Principles and Practice*. 3rd ed, ed J Hoffman, 356–66. New York: Churchill Livingstone.

Sun PB, W Wilburn, BD Raynor et al. 2001. Sickle cell disease in pregnancy: twenty years of experience at Grady Memorial Hospital, Atlanta, Georgia. *Am J Obstet Gynecol* 184:1127–1130.

Tampakoudis P, C Tsatalas, M Mamopoulos, T Tantanassis, JI Christakis, Z Sinakos et al. 1997. Transfusion-dependent homozygous beta-thalassaemia major: successful pregnancy in five cases. *Eur J Obstet Gynecol Reprod Biol* 74:127–131.

Thomas P, L Oni, M Alli, J St Hilaire, A Smith, C Leavey and R Banarsee. 2005. Antenatal screening for haemoglobinopathies in primary care: a whole system participatory action research project. *Br J Gen Pract* 55:424–428; Comment: 556–7, 419–420.

Vrettou G, J Traeger-Synodinos, M Tzetis, G Palmer, C Sofocleous, E Kanavakis et al. 2004. Real-time PCR for single-cell genotyping in sickle cell and thalassemia syndromes as a rapid, accurate, reliable, and widely applicable protocol for preimplantation genetic diagnosis. *Hum Mutat* 23: 513–521.

Wanapirak C, W Muninthorn, T Sanguansermsri, P Dhananjayanonda and T Tongsong. 2004. Prevalence of thalassemia in pregnant women at Maharaj Nakorn Chiang Mai Hospital. *J Med Assoc Thai* 87:1415–1418.

Winichagoon P, S Sithongdee, S Kanokpongasakdi, P Tantisirin, LF Bernini and S Fucharoen. 2005. Noninvasive prenatal diagnosis for hemoglobin Bart's hydrops fetalis. *Int J Hematol* 81:396–399.

18

Drugs in Pregnancy

Kiran Guleria

The medical needs of pregnancy are unique because of the presence of the fetus. It is important that the clinician has sufficient data to counsel patients about the risk-benefit ratio of a particular drug, for the fetus. Because few absolutes are possible in the area of human teratology, the evidence or the lack of it must be carefully weighed before a drug can be prescribed for a pregnant woman. Pregnant women need drug treatment for a wide variety of illnesses; about 35–99% of pregnant women require drugs for illnesses. About 6% take drugs in the first trimester, excluding IFA supplementation. Over the last four decades, the use of drugs prescribed during pregnancy has fallen from 80% to 35% and that of self-administered drugs from 64% to 9% (Forfar and Nelson 1973). This is primarily because of the perception of high risk by the pregnant women themselves from the information provided by pharmaceutical companies and the media about drug-induced abnormalities (Koren et al 1989, 1990). The selection of an appropriate drug from the available options requires knowledge of teratology and the altered metabolic state of pregnancy.

TERATOLOGY

Teratogenesis is defined as the dysgenesis of fetal organs as evidenced by structural or functional changes. A teratogen (Table 18.1) is an agent that acts during the embryonic or fetal period of development to produce a permanent alteration in form or function (Shepard 2001). Teratology is the study of environmental contributions to this abnormal development. In the general population, 2–3% of all newborns have major structural malformations. Of these, 10% are caused by teratogens. Teratogenesis manifests as restricted growth or death of the fetus, carcinogenesis and malformation of organ structure or function (Schardein 1993). Hadegen is the agent that interferes with normal maturation and function of organs while trophogen is an agent that alters growth. Hadegens and trophogens usually act after organogenesis and even after birth.

FOOD AND DRUG ADMINISTRATION (FDA) CLASSIFICATION

In 1979, the FDA introduced a drug classification system to discourage non-essential use of drugs in pregnancy. Drugs were classified as A, B, C, D or X according to their potential as teratogens. The definition used for risk factor assessment is categorised as follows:

Category A: Controlled studies in women fail to demonstrate a risk to the fetus in the first trimester (and there is no evidence of a

Table 18.1: Known or likely teratogens or fetal toxins

Radiation
Radioiodine
Infections
- Cytomegalovirus
- Herpes simplex virus I and II
- Parvovirus B19 (erythema infectiosum)
- Rubella virus
- Syphilis
- Toxoplasmosis
- Varicella virus
- Venezuelan equine encephalitis virus

Drugs and Environmental Chemicals
- ACE inhibitors (benazepril, captopril, enalapril, fosinopril, lisinopril, moexipril, quinapril, ramipril, trandolapril)
- Aminopterin
- Androgenic hormones
- Busulfan
- Chlorobiphenyls
- Cocaine
- Coumarin anticoagulants
- Cyclophosphamide
- Diethylstilbestrol
- Etretinate
- Fluconazole (high doses)
- Iodides
- Anesthetics
- Isotretinoin
- Indomethacin and related NSAIDs
- Lithium
- Mercury, organic
- Methimazole
- Methotrexate
- Methylene blue (after intra-amniotic injection)
- Misoprostol
- Penicillamine
- Phenobarbital
- Phenytoin
- Tetracyclines and its derivatives
- Thalidomide
- Toluene (abuse)
- Trimethadione
- Valproic acid

Maternal and Metabolic Imbalance
- Alcoholism
- Amniocentesis, early (before Day 70 post conception)
- Chorionic villus sampling (before Day 60 post conception)
- Cretinism, endemic
- Diabetes mellitus
- Folic acid deficiency
- Hyperthermia
- Phenylketonuria
- Rheumatic disease
- Sjogren's syndrome
- Virilising tumours

Possible Teratogens or Fetal Toxins
- Binge drinking
- Carbamazepine
- Cigarette smoking
- Colchicines
- Disulfiram
- Ergotamine
- Lead
- Primidone
- Quinine (suicidal doses)
- Streptomycin
- Vitamin A (high doses)
- Zinc deficiency

Unlikely Teratogens
- Agent Orange
- Aspartame
- Aspirin
- Bendectin ® (antinauseant)
- Hydroxyprogesterone
- Lysergic acid amides (LSD)
- Marijuana
- Medroxyprogesterone
- Metronidazole
- Oral contraceptives
- Progesterone
- Rubella vaccine
- Spermicides
- Video display terminals and electromagnetic waves
- Ultrasound

risk in later trimesters), and the possibility of fetal harm appears remote.

Category B: Either animal-reproduction studies have not demonstrated a fetal risk and there are no controlled studies in pregnant women, or animal-reproduction studies have shown an adverse effect (other than a decrease in infertility) that was not confirmed in controlled studies in women in the first trimester (and there is no evidence of a risk in later trimesters).

Category C: Either studies in animals have revealed adverse effects on the fetus (teratogenic, embryocidal or other) and there are no controlled studies on women, or studies on women and in animals are not available. Drugs should be given only if the potential benefit justifies the potential risk to the fetus.

Category D: There is positive evidence of human fetal risk, but the benefits from use in pregnant women may be acceptable despite the risk (for example, if the drug is needed in a life-threatening situation or for a serious disease for which safer drugs cannot be used or are ineffective).

Category X: Studies in animals or human beings have demonstrated fetal abnormalities or there is evidence of fetal risk based on human experience, or both, and the risk of the use of the drug in pregnant women clearly outweighs any possible benefit. The drug is contraindicated in women who are or may become pregnant.

Though this system is used to provide therapeutic guidance, it has led to excessive maternal anxiety and unnecessary termination of pregnancies, because many drug ratings are based only on case reports or limited animal data. Further, the drug ratings are not updated as new evidence emerges. Hence, the FDA is evaluating a labelling system based on clinical management, drug description and a summary of risk assessment, that is, an evidence-based rating system (Table 18.2).

Table 18.2: Common drugs initially teratogenic but subsequently proven safe

Drug	*Initial Evidence of Risk*	*Subsequent Evidence of Safety*
Diazepam*	Oral clefts	No increase in risk in large cohort and case control studies
Oral contraceptives	Birth defects involving the vertebrae, anus, heart, trachea,esophagus, kidney, and limbs; masculinising effects on female fetuses resulting in pseudohermaphroditism	No association between first-trimester exposure to oral contraceptives and malformations in general or external genital malformations in two meta-analyses
Spermicides	Limb defects, tumours, Down syndrome and hypospadias	No increase in risk in a meta-analysis
Salicyates	Cleft palate and congenital heart disease	No increase in risk in large cohort studies
Bendectin (doxylamine plus pyridoxine)	Cardiac and limb defects	No increase in risk in two meta-analyses

** Diazepam taken near term may cause the neonatal withdrawal syndrome or cardio respiratory instability.*

Evaluation of a Potential Teratogen

The teratogenicity of a drug for clinical use can be identified by (1) follow-up studies or (2) case control surveillance (Mitchell 2003). The following specific criteria must be met:

- The defect must be completely characterised.
- The agent must cross the placenta.
- Exposure must occur during the critical period of organogenesis.
- A biologically plausible association must exist.
- Epidemiological findings must be consistent.

Specificity: The suspected teratogen causes a defect in an animal. Specificity indicates that a substance may be teratogenic in some species but not in others. For example, thalidomide produces phocomelia in primates but not in rodents. Often, animal safety data is not necessarily applicable to humans (Table 18.3).

Fetal exposure to drugs is determined by many factors:

1. **The absorption of the agent**: Pregnancy alters absorption in many ways. For example, prolongation of gastric emptying time and increased volume of distribution is seen. Estrogen alters hepatic enzyme activity with varying effects on drug metabolism and clearance. Renal excretion is generally increased in pregnancy.
2. **Placental transfer of the drug:** Lipid-soluble and low-molecular-weight agents cross the placenta readily. The degree to which a drug is bound to the plasma proteins decides the amount available to cross the placenta, besides active placental transfer. Most drugs cross the placenta to some extent, except for large ions such as heparin and insulin.
3. **Teratogenicity and timing of the drug:** A teratogen can act by causing cell death, altering tissue growth or interfering with cellular differentiation or basic morphogenesis. Teratogen exposure in the first 2–3 weeks of conception results in an all-or-none phenomenon. The susceptibility to a teratogenic agent occurs primarily at 3–8 weeks post conception (35–70 days after the last menstrual period) and for up to 10 weeks. After this period, either growth restriction or defects of nervous or gonadal tissue are seen. During organogenesis, each system will have a different critical period of sensitivity.
4. **Dose of the drug:** At a low dose, no effects are seen while malformations occur at intermediate dosages and fetal death at higher doses. Sequential dosing may induce certain enzymes to metabolise the substance, thus causing less potential for damage as against a bolus dose, which can be extremely destructive.
5. **Route of administration**: This is also an important factor because different absorption rates are associated with different routes.
6. **Combination of drugs**: This may put a woman at a higher risk of malformation.
7. **Genetic factors:** The genetic make up can affect the individual's susceptibility to drugs. For example, fetuses with low levels of the epoxide hydrolase enzyme are more likely to manifest the fetal hydantoin syndrome.

DRUGS USED IN PREGNANCY

Antimicrobials

Penicillins The penicillin group antimicrobials are probably the safest antibiotics used during pregnancy for a wide variety of bacterial infections such as pharyngitis, otitis media, mild pneumonia, urinary tract infections and syphillis. It includes

TABLE 18.3: TERATOGENIC EFFECTS OF DRUGS IN ANIMALS AND HUMANS*		
Drug	**Effects In Animals**	**Effects In Humans**
Angiotensin-converting-enzyme inhibitors	Stillbirths and increased fetal loss in sheep and rabbits	Prolonged renal failure and hypotension in the newborn, decreased skull ossification, hypocalvaria, and renal tubular dysgenesis
Carbama-zepine	Cleft palate, dilated cerebral ventricles, and growth retardation in mice	Neural tube defects
Cocaine	Dose-dependent decrease in uterine blood flow, fetal hypoxemia, hypertension, and tachycardia in sheep; reduced fetal weight, fetal edema, and increased resorption in rats and mice	Growth retardation involving weight, length, and head circumference placental abruption and uterine rupture
Ethonol	Microcephaly, growth deficiency and limb anomalies in dogs, chickens and mice	Fetal alcohol syndrome—prenatal and postnatal growth deficiency, CNS anomalies (microcephaly, behavioral abnormalities, and mental retardation), characteristic pattern of facial features (short palpebral fissures, hypoplastic philthrum, and flattened maxilla), and major organ-system malformations; with age, facial features may become less distinctive, but short stature, microcephaly and behavioral abnormalities persist
Isotretinoin	CNS, head, limb and cardiovascular defects in rats and rabbits	Retinoid embryopathy resulting in some or all of the following abnormalities CNS defects (hydrocephalus, optic-nerve blindness, retinal defects, microphthalmia, posterior fossa defects and cortical and cerebellar defects);craniofacial defects (microtia or anotia, lowset ears, hypertelorism, depressed nasal bridge, microcephaly, micrognathia and agenesis or stenosis of external ear canals); cardiovascular defects (transposition of great vessels, tetralogy of fallot, and ventricular or atrial septal defects); thymic defects (ectopia and hypoplasia or aplasia); and miscellaneous defects (limb reduction, decreased muscle tone, spontaneous abortion and behavioral abnormalities)
Lithium	Heart defects in rats	Ebstein's anomaly and other heart defect
Methyl mercury	CNS abnormalities in rats; growth retardation, motor disturbances, microencephaly and brain lesions in rhesus monkeys	Fetal Minamata disease—diffuse neuronal disintegration with gliosis, cerebral palsy, microcephaly, strabismus, blindness, speech disorders, motor impairment, abnormal reflexes and mental retardation

Phenytoin	Cleft palate, micromelia, renal defects and hydrocephalus in rabbits, mice and rats	Fetal hydantoin syndrome—prenatal and postnatal growth deficiency, mental deficiency, short nose with broad nasal bridge, microcephaly, hypertelorism, strabismus, epicanthus, wide fontanelles, low-set or abnormally formed ears, positional deformities of limbs, hypoplasia of nails and distal phalanges, hypospadias, hernia, webbed neck, low hairline, impaired neurodevelopment and low performance scores on tests of intelligence
Thalidomide†	Limb-shortening defects in rabbits (most sensitive species)	Limb-shortening defects, loss of hearing, abducens paralysis, facial paralysis, anotia, microtia, renal malformations, congenital heart disease. Neural tube defects
Valproic acid Warfarin†	Exencephaly in hamsters and mice Maxillonasal hypoplasia and skeletal anomalies in rats	Fetal warfarin syndrome—skeletal defects (nasal hypoplasia and stippled epiphyses), limb hypoplasia (particularly in distal digits), low birth weight ($<10^{th}$ percentile), hearing loss, and ophthalmic anomalies; CNS defects with exposure after first trimester; dorsal midline dysplasia (agenesis of corpus callosum and Dandy Walker malformations) or ventral midline dysplasia (optic atrophy)

broadspectrum agents such as pipercillin and mezocillin, those combining β-lactam with B-lactamase inhibitors such as clavulanic acid, salbactam and tazobactam, and many oral and parenteral cephalosporins.

Amoxicillin and **ampicillin** have a wide margin of safety and almost no toxicity for the mother and the fetus. **Amoxicillin-clavulanate** has an expanded spectrum of activity. The extended spectrum penicillins and cephalosporins are more expensive and thus used as second-line agents in pregnancy.

Erythromycin and **azithromycin** inhibit bacterial protein synthesis and are used as first-line treatment for mycoplasma, chlamydia and community acquired pneumonia, and as an alternative for penicillin-allergic patients. Only a small amount of these macrolides cross the placenta and even then they do not cause any fetal anomaly. **Clindamycin** readily crosses the placenta but is clinically safe. It can be used as a second-line agent to treat bacterial vaginosis and anerobic infections. Up to 10% of users will develop pseudomembranous colitis. **Aztreonam**, an alternative to aminoglycoside, has no renal or ototoxicity, and **Imipenum,** which is effective against anerobes and aerobes, has no data on human safety but is not teratogenic in animals.

Nitrofurantoin is highly effective and extensively used in treating urinary infections during pregnancy. It can induce hemolytic anemia in G6PD-deficient women but has not been seen to be associated with it or congenital malformations in actual practice.

The **quinolones**—ciprofloxacin, norfloxacin, ofloxacin and enoxacin—have been used for the treatment of urinary and bowel infections in pregnancy without any teratogenic effects, although no well-controlled studies are available. Fluoroquinolones can induce reversible arthropathy in animals and is not recommended for use in pregnancy.

The commonly used **antituberculosis** drugs such as rifampicin, isoniazid and ethambutol are safe in pregnancy. **Chloramphenicol** crosses the placenta readily and, if given in large doses, can cause gray baby syndrome (cyanosis, vascular collapse and death), especially in preterm neonates. **Tetracyclines,** including doxycycline and minocycline, can cause a yellow-brown discolouration of deciduous teeth and get deposited in fetal long bones. **Aminoglycosides** (gentamycin and streptomycin) can cause nephrotoxicity and ototoxicity in the fetus, preterm neonates and adults. The trimethoprim-sulfamethoxazole combination has been associated with slightly increased risk of cardiovascular defects and hyperbilirubinemia or kernicterus in newborns, and so should not be used in the first trimester and near delivery.

Metronidazole, a nitroimidazole, is recommended by the Center for Disease Control (CDC) for the treatment of trichomoniasis and bacterial vaginosis in pregnancy. Although carcinogenic in rodents, it has not produced any birth defects in human fetuses even when used in the first trimester (Piper 1993; Burtin 1995).

Antivirals

Experience with antiviral drugs in pregnancy has grown with the emergence of HIV and AIDS. Acyclovir, valacyclovir, gancyclovir and famcyclovir are effective in the treatment of primary herpes and varicella infections. Acyclovir and valacyclovir show no increase in congenital anomalies to some extent, even when used in the first trimester for herpes, hepatitis and varicella pneumonia. There is limited information on the use of ganciclovir and famciclovir in pregnancy.

Antiretroviral Therapy The medication generally falls into three categories—nucleoside reverse transcriptase inhibitors (nRTI), non-nucleoside analog reverse transcriptase (NNRTI) and protease inhibitors (PIs). Zidovudine, zalcitabine, didanosine, stavudine, lamivudine and abacavir are the six NNRTIs that are currently approved and recommended for use in pregnancy, as there are no reports of birth defects in exposed human beings. Amprenavir, indinavir, lopinavir, ritonavir, nelfinavir and saquinavir are the PIs that can be used in pregnancy without causing congenital malformations (Table 18.4). When these two groups of drugs are combined, they lower the serum viral concentrations considerably, thereby reducing disease complications and perinatal transmission rates to 1%.

Interferons have antiviral, antineoplastic and immunomodulating actions and are used during pregnancy for the treatment of chronic myeloid leukemia, thrombocytopenia and some viral infections. These have a low potential for teratogenesis but the evidence is limited.

Antifungals

Clotrimazole, miconazole and nystatin are used to treat vaginal candidiasis during pregnancy without any congenital malformations in the fetus (Rosa et al 1987; Czeizel et al 2003). Amphotericin B is used to treat systemic histoplasmosis, cryptococcosis and candidiasis, but no congenital anomalies were noted during use in pregnancy.

Antimalarials

Chloroquine, used for the treatment of malaria and also for rheumatoid arthritis and systemic lupus erythematosus, has no adverse fetal effects. Quinine and quinidine are reserved for seriously ill patients and are not associated with increased congenital malformations (McGready et al 2002); however, mefloquine has been associated with increased risk of stillbirths (Nosten et al 1999).

Drugs for Upper Respiratory Tract Infections

The common cold is one of the most frequent, self-diagnosed and treated illness in pregnancy. Most antihistaminics such as chlorpheniramine, clemastine, dipenhydramine and doxylamine are safe in pregnancy. The newer antihistamines such as astemizole, cetrizine, loratadine and fexofenadine are used as second-line therapy, as little information is available about their use in pregnancy. The oral decongestants include pseudoephedrine, phenylepherine and phenylpropanolamine. Since there are reports of fetal gastroschisis with pseudoephedrine, it is safer to use topical decongestants in pregnancy. Cough suppressants such as codeine and dexamethorphan are not teratogenic.

Analgesics

Analgesics are the most commonly prescribed or purchased over-the-counter medicines in pregnancy. These are used for headache, malaise, soft tissue and muscular pains, joint pains and stiffness and for pain relief in labour. The drugs fall into two categories—non-steriodal antiinflammatory agents and opiods.

Non-steroidal Anti-inflammatory Drugs (NSAIDs) Aspirin is a potent prostaglandin inhibitor and fetal exposure could lead to premature closure of the ductus arteriosus. In doses of 100 mg or below per day, it has been used extensively to treat pre-eclampsia and intrauterine growth retardation without complications. Higher doses have been associated with increased risk of placental abruption or maternal and fetal bleeding.

Acetaminophen is widely used in pregnancy. It crosses the placenta but is considered safe and is used routinely in all trimesters to relieve fever and pain. Other NSAIDs include ibuprofen, naproxen and ketoprofen. Indomethacin has been employed as a tocolytic and for the treatment of hydramnios. It can, however, result in the construction of fetal ductus arterosus, decrease fetal urine output and reduce amniotic fluid volume. These effects are reversible if the drug is discontinued after 32–34 weeks.

Local analgesic applications containing methyl salicylates, menthol and ibuprofen should be used sparingly.

Narcotic Analgesics These include meperidine, morphine codeine, propoxyphene, oxycodone and hydrocodone; all of them cross the placenta but are not associated with congenital malformations. Chronic ingestion or its use, close to delivery, can cause neonatal respiratory depression and withdrawal syndrome.

The drugs commonly used for colic in pregnancy include hyoscine N-butyl bromide (Buscopan), dicyclomine hydrochloride, valethamate (Epidosin) and drotaverine. These drugs help relieve smooth muscle spasms and assist cervical dilatation in labour.

Pain Relief during Labour Pethidine is used in the early active phase of labour to relieve pain. If used within an hour of delivery, nalorphine must be administered to the mother in the second stage and to the newborn. Promethazine HCL (Phenargen) is an antihistaminic that potentiates the action of pethidine or pentazocine, the combinations provide better relief in labour.

Tramadol is available as 1–2 ml ampoules containing 50 mg/ml. This drug has a longer duration of action, effective analgesia and minimal fetal respiratory depression.

Table 18.4: Antiretroviral drugs in pregnancy

Condition	*Drug*	*Dosage*	*Comments*
HIV			
Nucleoside	Zidovudine	100 mg, 6 times a day	Rare mitochondrial toxic
reverse			effects but generally very safe
transcriptase			and should be part of standard
inhibitors	Lamivudine		regimen
	Didanosine		First-line agent with zidovudine
		150 or 300 mg bid	part of highly active anti-
	Stavudine	≥60 kg: 200 mg bid	retroviral therapy (HAART)
	Zalcitabine		therapy in pregnancy
	Nevirapine		Should not be used with
		≥60 kg: 40 mg bid	zidovudine
	Delavirdine	0.75 mg tid	Rarely indicated in pregnancy
Nonnucleoside	Indinavir	200 mg qd × 2 weeks,	Part of HAART therapy
reverse	Ritonavir	then 200 mg bid	
Transcriptase		400 mg tid	
inhibitors	Saquinavir	800 mg q8h	No human studies, not
	Nelfinavir	600 mg bid	recommended
Protease	Amprenavir or	second PI	Can be part of HAART therapy
inhibitors(PI)	lopinavir	600–1200 mg tid	Use in low dosago
		750 mg tid	Can be part of HAART therapy
		-----	Can be part of HAART therapy
			No studies in humans

Anesthetic Agents

The agents currently used as general and local anesthetics are non-teratogenic. Though they cross the placenta and have systemic absorption, the exposure in pregnancy is brief and non-toxic and so does not result in adverse fetal outcome. The '—caine' local anesthetics may result in fetal bradycardia and, rarely, hyperthermia. However, to be on the safer side, all elective operative interventions in pregnancy are scheduled in the second trimester.

Anticoagulants

Thromboembolism is a leading cause of morbidity and mortality in pregnancy and postpartum; being very common in the West. Anticoagulation is required for thromboembolism, valvular heart disease, inherited thrombophilia and acquired thrombophilias such as antiphospholipid antibody syndrome. The commonly used anticoagulants are coumarin, unfractionated heparin and low-molecular-weight heparin (LMWH).

Thromboembolism occurs in 1 in 1000 pregnancies. Heparin is used with a target activated partial thromboplastin time (aPTT) of 1.5–2.5 times the control, and switched to subcutaneous heparin after 3–5 days. For inherited and acquired thrombophilias, unfractionated heparin or LMWH is used. Both types of heparin do not cross the placenta and are not teratogenic, but patients can develop heparin-induced thrombocytopenia or osteopenia on prolonged use.

The oral anticoagulant warfarin sodium is a known terotogenic and can easily cross the placenta; so it should not be used in pregnancy. Warfarin can cause embroyopathy (nasal hypoplasia, bilateral optic atrophy, blindness, mental retardation), spontaneous abortions and stillbirths.

A number of thrombolytic agents such as urokinase, streptokinase, alteplase and tissue plasminogen activators have been safely used in pregnancy.

ANTIEMETICS

Morning sickness or nausea and vomiting occur in as many 90% of pregnancies. Unless the complaint is excessive, it is better to avoid medication and try simple measures such as diet alterations and small, frequent meals.

Antiemetics are prescribed if the patient does not respond to conservative measures or shows clinical and biochemical signs of dehydration. She may even require hospitalisation, IV fluids and electrolyte and glucose correction. Among the commonly used drugs are doxylamine and pyridoxine, piperazines (meclizine and cyclizine) and phenothiazines (chlorpromazine, prochlorperazine, pro-methazine and metoclopramide). None of these drugs is associated with adverse fetal effects. Ondensetron is an expensive drug and has not been used very often in pregnancy. It is reserved for the treatment of hyperemesis refactory to other medications.

Reflux or heartburn is another common complaint in up to 80% of women in pregnancy. This condition can be treated by elevating the head while sleeping, eating small frequent meals and taking antacids as the first line of therapy. Histamine (H_2 blockers) antagonists including cimetidine, famotidine and ranitidine are compatible with pregnancy but should be given at least one hour after or before antacids. Proton pump inhibitors (omeprazole, rabeprazole, lansoprazole) are relatively new agents and should be used with caution in pregnancy.

ANTIEPILEPTICS

Epilepsy is the most common neurological disorder during pregnancy, affecting about 0.15% of women. All antiepileptic drugs (AEDs) cross the placenta and are potential teratogens. The physiological changes of pregnancy alter the metabolism and bioavailability of these drugs and hence there is a need for revision of drug dosage during pregnancy. About 1 in 250 fetuses is exposed to AEDs, which are now thought to be the cause of congenital malformations in offsprings of women with epilepsy and not the epilepsy itself, as has been conjectured in the past. The incidence of epilepsy is 8–9% in the treated subjects.

Phenytoin (dilantin) is associated with 'fetal hydantoin syndrome', which includes microcephaly, mental retardation, IUGR, craniofacial and limb defects and performance delays. Carbamazepine (tegretol) causes similar defects and, in addition, increases the risk of spina bifida to about 0.5–1.0%. Valproic acid is associated with facial, central nervous system (lumbosacral spina bifida 1–2%), cardiac, limb and genitourinary anomalies. Phenobarbitones have similar fetal defects. AEDs are also known to suppress the neonatal synthesis of vitamin K-dependent clotting factors, thus predisposing newborns to bleeding.

Information about the safety of newer antiepileptics such as felbamate, gabapentin, oxcarbazepine, tiagabin and vigabatrin is limited (Briggs et al 2002). Some of these drugs may prove to be safe as they do not have any antifolate effects. However, lamotrigine and topiramate belong to different drug classes and are associated with teratogenic risks, though lower than in traditional drugs (Briggs et al 2002; Sabers et al 2004), and should be avoided in pregnancy. All young epileptic women contemplating pregnancy should take 5 mg folic acid daily and continue this dose throughout pregnancy and lactation. It is preferable to use monodrug, minimum effective dose therapy, to reduce the incidence of malformations. The pregnancy should be carefully monitored with serum alpha fetoprotein (AFP) and ultrasonic screening to check for fetal defects. If necessary, medical termination may need to be advised. Vitamin K should be prescribed and serum levels of drugs monitored, if facilities are available. With a multidisciplinary approach, satisfactory obstetric outcome is possible in 90% of cases.

Antihypertensives

Hypertension complicating pregnancy is an important cause of maternal and perinatal mortality and morbidity. A large number of drugs have been used in pregnancy.

Methyl dopa is the most widely used agent during pregnancy and is entirely safe. Hydralazine also does not have any adverse fetal effects. Sodium nitroprusside and clonidine have been used to treat acute severe hypertension in pregnant women without adverse fetal effects.

Among the beta-adrenergic antagonists, propranolol and labetalol have been used in pregnancy. There appear to be conflicting reports about the association of beta-blockers with fetal growth restriction and neonatal hypoglycemia (Crooks et al 1998; Reprotox 2003).

Antihypertensives such as ACE inhibitors are contraindicated in pregnancy. Among calcium channel blockers, nifedipine in an oral dose of 5–10 mg produces rapid control of blood pressure; however, sublingual administration is not recommended as it causes sudden hypotension and may result in myocardial infarction. Verapamil has been associated with fetal cardiac depression and possible fetal defects when used in the first trimester.

Diuretics are prescribed during pregnancy to treat chronic hypertension and pulmonary edema. Thiazide diuretics can cause neonatal thrombocytopenia, bleeding and electrolyte disturbances when given near time of delivery. Acetazolamide, spironolactone, ethacrynic acid and furesamide are not commonly used in pregnancy and have no adverse fetal effects.

Antiparasitic Agents

Metronidazole is recommended for the treatment of trichomoniasis and bacterial vaginosis in pregnancy. Choloroquine, quinine and mefloquine are used as first line antimalarials for treatment and chemoprophylaxis. Pyrimethamine, along with sulpadiazine for treatment of toxoplasmosis, does not increase the frequency of malformations in newborns, and spiramycin has no embryo–fetal adverse effects.

Mebendazole, used for treating helminthes and neurocysticercosis, is teratogenic in animals at very high doses. However, evidence suggests that there is no increased risk in humans. Thiobendazole is a second-line therapy for which human studies are lacking. Pyrantal pamoate, used for treatment of ascariasis, is safe in pregnancy.

Asthma Medication

Asthma is the commonest chronic respiratory condition in pregnancy, complicating about 5% of them. Most medications for the treatment of asthma can be used safely in pregnancy.

Short-acting β-sympathomimetic agents are the first line of treatment for acute asthma exacerbations. Albuterol, terbutaline and metaproterenol inhalers are commonly used and are safe for the fetus. Long-acting β-sympathomimetics such as salmeterol are also available and safe.

Inhaled glucocorticoids are also used as first-line therapy. They act by reducing inflammation. These include beclomethasone, fluticasone and others. Inhaled steroids are not teratogenic whereas systemic glucocorticoids, used for acute exacerbations, may increase the risk of cleft lip or palate. In the presence of the above mentioned agents, the role of theophylline has reduced markedly as it has a narrow therapeutic window. Theophylline is otherwise non-teratogenic and can be used safely in pregnancy.

Cromolyn sodium is used for long-term therapy in patients with atopy and has shown no teratogenic effects. The leukotriene receptor anatagonists and lipoxygenase inhibitors are new agents, but human testing data is sparse and so it should be avoided in pregnancy.

In labour with acute asthma, propped-up position, oxygen, correction of dehydration and acidosis, bronchodilator, aerosols and nebulisers should provide relief. Besides this, epidural analgesia is the method of choice for pain relief and anesthesia for cesarean section. Use of $PGF_2\alpha$ and methylergometrine should be avoided.

Cardiac Medications

Cardiac glycosides such as digoxin have been used to treat heart failures and rhythm disorders without any adverse effects on the fetus. Antiarrhythmic drugs are administered to the mother or the fetus to control fetal tachycardia (Harrigan 1981; Weiner 1988). Quinidine, several beta-blockers and other antiarrhythmic drugs such as local anesthetics and calcium channel blockers all cross the placenta and have been used to treat fetal arrhythmia without adverse effects.

Hormones

Early exposure of the fetus to androgens may result in congenital adrenal hyperplasia, masculinised female external genitalia and abnormal male genital growth. Of the testosterone derivatives used as contraceptives, medroxyprogesterone acetate/DMPA or norethindrone may result in female fetus masculinisation in less than 1% of exposures. Inadvertent use of danazol in early pregnancy is reported to cause virilisation of female fetuses in 40–57%, and the extent is dose-related. Most estrogens, used as contraceptives currently, do not affect the fetus. There is little information regarding GnRH exposure in early pregnancy in women treated for infertility, but oral contraceptives have not been associated with any abnormality.

Diethylstilbestrol (DES) produced structural and functional abnormalities in up to half of exposed female fetuses resulting in cervical ectropion, vaginal adenosis, a twofold increase in vaginal and cervical intraepithelial neoplasia, hypoplastic, T-shaped uterine cavity, cervical collars, hoods, septa and withered fallopian tubes and poor reproductive outcomes (Kaufman 2000).

Exposed male fetuses have increased risk of epididymal cysts, microphallus, cryptorchidism and testicular hyperplasia (Klip 2002).

Antineoplastic Agents

Cancer complicates 1 in 1000–1500 pregnancies. The most common malignancies are cancers of the cervix and breast, lymphoma, melanoma, leukemia and cancers of the ovary and colon. Since chemotherapeutic drugs act on rapidly dividing cells and are potentially harmful to the fetus, especially in the period of teratogenesis and later on during the development of the brain in the second and third trimesters, a delivery plan must be determined because both maternal and neonatal blood counts are depressed. Most classes of chemotherapeutic drugs such as alkylating agents and antimetabolites are teratogenic. The Taxols including paclitaxel use in pregnancy, is scarce. Cisplatin has been used in the second and third trimesters and may result in growth restriction. Hence, the treatment of pregnant woman with cancer must be individualised in consultation with the oncologist and perinatologist.

IMMUNOSUPPRESSANTS

Azathioprine is used primarily after organ transplantation and is not teratogenic. There is a risk of growth restriction, immune suppression and pancytopenia in exposed neonates. New immunosuppressants such as cycloserine appear to be safe for the fetus but tacrolimus may cause fetal problems such as preterm delivery, growth restriction, hyperkalemia and nephrotoxicity.

PSYCHOTROPIC DRUGS

Depression (15%) and schizophrenia (8–10%) are common in the reproductive years; so there are concerns about teratogenesis, neonatal withdrawal and long-term behavioural problems. Hence, a balance must be struck between the risks and benefits to the mother and the fetus.

Tricyclic agents have a long history of use in pregnancy and there is no evidence of clear adverse effects on the fetus or neonate (Rowe 1973). The most commonly used antidepressants are serotorin re-uptake inhibitors (SSRIs), which include fluoxetine and newer agents such as fluvoxamine, paroxetine and sertraline. Fluoxetine is safe for the fetus and the neonate, however, the experience with newer agents is insuffcent to judge their safety; but since this group of antidepressants has fewer side effects, it is a good choice for antenatal women.

MAO inhibitors are best avoided in pregnancy because of severe adverse reactions and hypertensive crisis. **Mood stabilisers,** especially lithium, valproic acid and carbamazepine, have been identified as teratogens in the past. Initial reports linked the Epstein anomaly with maternal lithium exposure but now it is not considered as a major teratogen. Since lithium can have toxic fetal effects such as diabetes inspidus, hypothyroidism and hypoglycemia, it is better avoided till 8 weeks of gestation and even then, monitoring of serum levels is a must. **Benzodiazepines** (diazepam, lorazepam and midazolam) have not been linked with fetal defects in humans, but can cause cleft palate in rodents.

Birth defects in humans are thought to be caused by the additive effects of alcohol and other substance abuse. These drugs can cause neonatal depression, somnolence and withdrawal symptoms. Alprazolam has a similar effect during pregnancy. **Antipsychotic** agents such as phenothiazines are associated with minimal teratogenic potential. Haloperidol is classified as having unknown but potientially worrying effects during lactation.

VITAMINS AND MINERALS

Prenatal multivitamins are commonly prescribed by many healthcare providers. Women who eat a balanced diet meet most of the daily recommended allowances except for folate and iron. Additional requirements are necessary in women with eating disorders, poor vegetarians, substance abusers or those with multiple pregnancy, anemia, etc. The only clear teratogen is vitamin A, which when used at a dose of more than 10,000 units/day, can cause cranial and neural crest anomalies. It would be prudent not to exceed 5,000 IU/day in supplements. Isotretinoin, an isomer of vitamin A used for dermatological disorders, is a potent teratogen. First trimester exposure is associated with fetal loss and a 26-fold increase in malformations in survivors. The malformations typically involve the cranium, face, heart, CNS and thymus. Hence, a mistake-proof method of contraception is required prior to beginning therapy. Etretinate is used orally to treat psoriatics and has a long half life; hence, it should not be used by women planning pregnancy, and after concluding treatment, the women should wait for at least two years before conceiving.

Recreational Drugs

Recreational drug use in pregnancy is a major problem in the West, with 7.5–13% of the population involved in the use of these substances. Cocaine and alcohol are potent teratogenic substances, but risks of other abused substances are confounded by other factors such as poor maternal health, malnutrition, infections and polydrug substances. Further, the presence of contaminants, diluents and impurities in these illegal drugs has serious independent side effects on the mother and the fetus.

Nicotine in tobacco decreases uteroplacental flow and increases risk of preterm birth, IGUR and sudden infant death syndrome. Maternal alcohol use can cause fetal alcohol syndrome.

Marijuana (hashish) though not associated with anomalies in humans, can cause low birth weight. Cocaine use causes increased risk of placental abruption, preterm premature rupture of membranes (PPROM) and low birth weight. The risk of congenital anomalies and long-term neurobehavioural effects is not clear. Amphetamines, methamphetamines and methylamphetamine (speed, ice, crank, crystalmeth), used to dilute illicit drugs, have not been associated with defects in humans but can cause symmetrical fetal growth restriction. Similarly, problems such as IUGR, severe perinatal complications, mild developmental delays, behavioural problems, withdrawal symptoms and occasional seizures are observed in 40–80% of newborns. The same fate awaits mothers who are addicted to heroin.

Lysergic acid amides (LSD) have been linked with increased frequency of chromosomal breakage in somatic cells of the mother as well as the exposed newborn. Phencyclidine (PCP) or angel dust can cause neonatal withdrawal symptoms, behavioural problems and developmental abnormalities. 'Ts and blues' (a mixture of pentazocine and tripelennamine) has not been associated with increased incidence of congenital anomalies.

Radiation

The two major concerns in women who require diagnostic imaging during pregnancy are exposure to ionising radiation and the effects of contrast agents. From the data derived from the atomic bombing of Hiroshima and Nagasaki, it has been extrapolated that a threshold dose of 5 rads is required to affect the developing fetus. This dose may be lethal in the preimplantation period; malformations occur between 9–60 days. Mental retardation occurs at around 61–104 days post conception, with a still higher threshold of 12 rads. Computed tomography increases the risk of leukemia 1.5–2-fold for every exposure of 1–2 rads in the mid- and third trimesters (Table 18.5).

In nuclear medicine cases, fetal dose will be less than 1 rad, except for sodium iodide,

TABLE 18.5: RADIATION EXPOSURE TO THE FETUS IN DIAGNOSTIC STUDIES (1 RAD = 1000 MILLIRADS)

Chest x-ray	2–8 millirads
Dental x-rays	<1 millirad
Mammography	7–10 millirads
Abdominal x-ray	200–700 millirads
Lumbar spine x-ray	300–600 millirads
Hip x-ray	200–500 millirads
Upper GI series	100–550 millirads
Barium enema	800–1300 millirads
Intravenous pyelogram	600–1000 millirads
Cholecystography	100 millirads
CT head	50 millirads
CT chest	1,000 millirads
CT abdomen	3000–4000 millirads
CT pelvimetry	250 millirads
Cardiac catheterisation	<500 millirads

Ga67 and iodinated red blood cells. Iodine[131] can cause fetal thyroid damage and goitre. Technetium[99] can cross the placenta but the amount of radiation is small. Magnetic resonance imaging (MRI) involves exposure to magnetic fields rather than ionising radiation. Only a few studies evaluating the effect of MRI on the fetus have shown absence of deleterious effects, though it should be reserved for clearly warranted indications.

ALTERNATIVE THERAPY

Alternative therapies include acupuncture, acupressure, massage, aromatherapy and herbal preparations. The risks and safety of herbal remedies are difficult to estimate; so they should be avoided in pregnant women. Patients should be asked about the use of complimentary medicines and, if required, efforts should be made to find out the constituents and safety of each component.

COUNSELLING ABOUT TERATOGENIC RISKS

A number of lay publications misinform women by assigning risks to drugs not known to be teratogenic in humans. Many physicians are also unfamiliar with the current literature on safety of drugs in pregnancy and may encourage termination of a pregnancy just to be on the safe side. Hence, physicians counselling women in pregnancy should make sure that they clearly understand the nature and magnitude of a risk with a drug. In addition, the same information about the nature and magnitude of a teratogenic risk may prompt different decisions by different women. During counselling, it is important to ensure that women understand the concept of baseline teratogenic risk and additional fetal or perinatal risk associated with the medical condition.

The counsellor should also communicate the same information to the woman's physician to avoid conflicting advice. For up-to-date, evidence-based information on safety and risks of drugs in pregnancy, the Internet may be used to gather teratogenic information.

Prescribing in Pregnancy: General Principles

1. Since fetal safety is a major concern,

effective drugs that have been in use for long periods should be preferred over newer alternatives.
2. Drugs doses at the lower end of the therapeutic range should be prescribed to minimise the fetal risks.
3. Pregnant women should be discouraged from taking over-the-counter drugs.
4. Many factors including the stage of pregnancy can influence the risk to the fetus; so drugs should be taken only when the benefit outweighs the risks and the drug is prescribed by a properly qualified physician.

References

Briggs GG, RK Freeman and SJ Yaffe. 2002. *Drugs in pregnancy and lactation*, 6th ed. Baltimore: William and Wilkins.

Briggs GG, RK Freeman and SJ Yaffe. 2005. *Drugs in pregnancy and lactation – a reference guide to fetal and neonatal risk*, 7th ed. Philadelphia: Lippincott Williams and Wilkins.

Burtin P, A Taddio, O Ariburnu et al. 1995. Safety of metronidazole in pregnancy: A meta-analysis. *Am J Obstet Gynecol* 172:525.

Crooks BN, SA Deshpande, C Hall et al. 1998. Adverse neonatal effects of maternal labetalol treatment. *Arch Dis Child Fetal Neonatal Ed* 79:150.

Czeizel AE, Z Kazy and E Puho. 2003. A population based case control teratological study of oral nystatin treatment during pregnancy. *Scand J Infect Dis* 35:830.

Forfar JO and MM Nelson. 1973. Epidemiology of drugs taken by pregnant women. *Clin Pharmacol Ther* 14:632.

Harrigan JT, JJ Kangos, KR Sikka et al. 1981. Successful treatment of fetal congestive failure secondary to tachycardia. *N Engl J Med* 304:1527.

Kaufman RH, E Adam, EE Hatch et al. 2000. Continued follow-up of pregnancy outcomes in diethylstilbestrol-exposed offspring. *Obstet Gynecol* 96:483.

Klip H, J Verloop, JD van Gool et al. 2002. Hypospadias in sons of women exposed to diethylstilbestrol in utero: A cohort study. *Lancet* 359:1102.

Koren G and A Pastuszak. 1990. Prevention of unnecessary pregnancy termination by counselling women on drug, chemical and radiation exposure during first trimester. *Teratology* 41:657–661.

Koren G, M Bologa, D Long, Y Feldman and NH Shear. 1989. Perception of teratogenic risk by pregnant women exposed to drugs and chemicals during the first trimester. *Am J Obstet Gynecol* 160:1190–1194.

McGready R, KL Thwai, T Cho et al. 2002. The effects of quinine and chloroquine antimalarial treatments in first trimester of pregnancy. *Trans r Soc Trop Med Hyg* 96:180.

Mitchell AA. 2003. Systemic identification of drugs that cause birth defects: A new opportunity. *N Eng J Med* 349:26.

Nosten ME, M Vincenti, J Simpson et al. 1999. The effects of mefloquine treatment in pregnancy. *Clin Infect Dis* 28:808.

Piper JM, EF Mitchell and WA Ray. 1993. Prenatal use of metronidazole and birth defects: No association. *Obstet Gynecol* 82:348.

Reproductive Toxicology Center. 2003. Reprotox: Tretinoin.

Rosa FW, C Hernandez and WA Carlc. 1987. Griseofulvin teratology, including two thoracopagus conjoined twins. *Lancet* 1:171.

Rowe I. 1973. Prescriptions of psychotropic drugs by general practitioners: Antidepressants. *Med J Aust* 1:642.

Sabers A, M Dam, B A-Rogvi-Hansen et al. 2004. Epilepsy and pregnancy: Lamotrigine as main drug used. *Acta Neurol Scan* 109:9.

Schardein JL. 1993. *Chemically induced birth defects.* 2nd ed. New York: Marcel Dekker.

Shepard TH. 2001. *Catalog of Teratogenic Agents*, 10th ed. Baltimore, Johns Hopkins University Press.

Weiner CP and MIB Thompson. 1988. Direct treatment of fetal supraventricular tachycardia after failed transplacental therapy. *Am J Obstet Gynecol* 152:362.

Selected teratogen information websites and books are listed below:

http://www.motherisk.org
http://www.apregistry.com
http://www.otispregnancy.org
http://www.tiu.edu/obgyn/info/cp.cfm
http://www.massgeneral.org/aed
http://www.perinatology.com/exposures/druglist.html.
http://www.vh.org/Patients/IHB/ObGyn/MedicinesPregnancy.html.
http://nccam.nih.gov/
http://www.herbalgram.org/

Weiner CP and C Buhimschi. 2004. *Drugs for pregnant and lactating women.* Philadelphia: Churchill Livingstone.

19

Multiple Pregnancy

Akhila Vasudeva

Introduction

The occurrence of multiple births has increased due to older age at childbearing and fertility enhancing therapies (Endres and Wilkins 2005). Multiple gestations occur at the rate of 3% of all pregnancies (ACOG Practice Bulletin 2004).

Genesis of Twinning

Dizygotic twins (two-thirds of all twins) result from the fertilisation of two separate ova by two sperms. The zygotes are genetically dissimilar. Monozygotic twins (one-third of all twins) result from the fertilisation of a single ovum by a sperm. The ovum then divides to form two genetically similar zygotes. In monozygotic twins, the timing of division determines the mode of development of the placenta and the fetuses:

- Division in the first 72 hours after fertilisation results in dichorionic, diamniotic twin gestation (about one-third of monozygotic twins).
- Division between the fourth and eighth day will produce monochorionic, diamniotic twin gestation (two-thirds of monozygotic twins) as shown in Figs 19.1(a) and (b).
- Division after the eighth day results in a monoamniotic, monochorionic twin pregnancy (<4% of monozygotic twins).

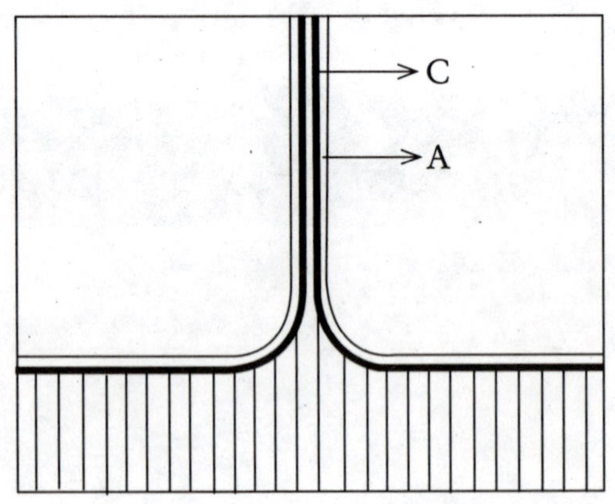

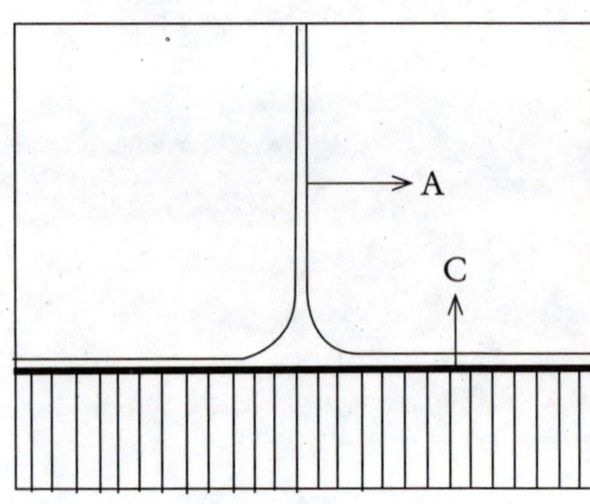

Figures 19.1(a) and (b): Line diagram showing chorionicity in twin gestation.
1(a): Dichorionic diamniotic twin gestation showing twin peak sign.
1(b): Monochorionic diamniotic twin gestation showing lambda or T sign
A - Amnion; C - Chorion

- Finally, division after the twelfth day (after the embryonic disc is completed) results in conjoint twin gestation of varying degrees of fusion of twins (one in 400 monozygotic twins).

Factors Associated with Multiple Gestation

The frequency of monozygotic twins is a relatively constant, 3–5 per 1000 births (MacGillivray 1986). This is not affected by race, heredity, maternal age or parity, all of which affect the incidence of dizygotic twinning.

Maternal family history is strongly associated with dizygotic twinning. In Asia, twinning is less common than in the West, where it is seen in 1 in 155 births (MacGillivray, 1986). The frequency of dizygotic twinning increases with greater parity and maternal age, peaking at the age of 37. A BMI of 30 or more is associated with a higher incidence of twinning (Basso 2004).

Infertility treatment increases both dizygotic as well as monozygotic twin gestations (Wenstom et al 1993). The incidence of multiple pregnancy with clomiphene ranges 1.83–17% and with hMG–hCG treatment, 18–53% (Schenker et al 1981). Risk of multiple pregnancy increases from 1.4% with a single embryo transfer to 24.1% with the transfer of four embryos (Jodie and Caroline 2005). All the maternal physiological changes are exaggerated in multiple pregnancy.

Diagnosis of Multiple Pregnancy

Specific risk factors must be elicited and evaluated during history-taking. Exaggerated fundal height, multiple fetal parts, palpation of two fetal heads and auscultation of two separate fetal heart sounds are characteristic.

Ultrasound in Multiple Pregnancy

First trimester sonography identifies two characteristic, separate sacs. Ideally, two fetal heads or two abdomens should be seen in the same scanning plane. Ultrasound is used to detect chorionicity/amnioticity, diagnose fetal abnormalities including growth derangements (growth restriction, discordant growth), enable cervical assessment and provide fetal surveillance throughout gestation.

Opposite genders of fetuses suggests dizygosity. Fetuses are monozygotic if they are monoamniotic or monochorionic. However, if they are dichorionic and diamniotic, they could be either monozygotic or dizygotic.

Fetuses are dichorionic if separate chorionic sacs are clearly identified by vaginal sonography by the fifth week of pregnancy (Ana and Ashley 2005). Two separate placentas with a thick (≥2 mm) and multilayered (≥3 layers) intertwine membrane suggests a dichorionic pregnancy. If a triangular tissue of placenta is found between two layers of membrane, when two placentas are placed side by side, it is called the twin peak/Lambda sign. This suggests dichorionicity (Fig. 19.2). This is best elicited between 10 and 14 weeks of gestation and might disappear after 20 weeks of gestation (Sepulveda et al 1996).

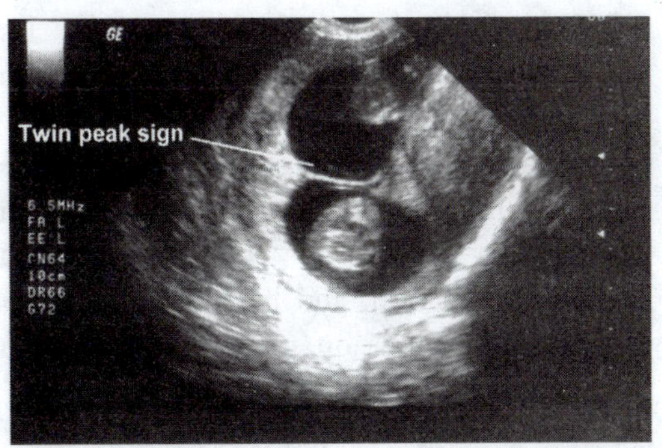

Figure 19.2: Dichorionic diamniotic twin gestation showing the 'twin peak' sign

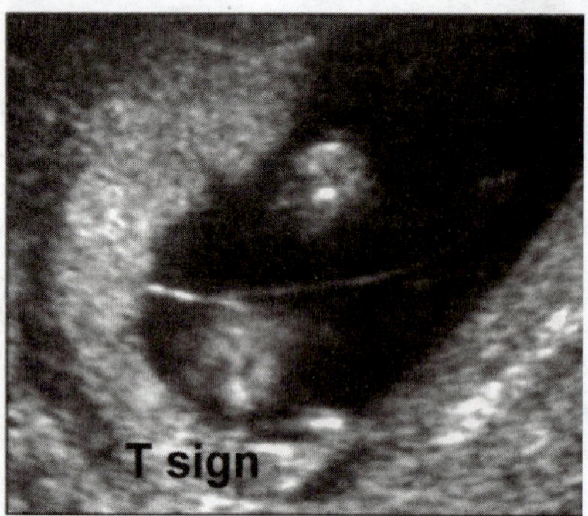

FIGURE 19.3: MONOCHORIONIC DIAMNIOTIC TWIN GESTATION SHOWING 'T' OR 'LAMBDA' SIGN

In monochorionic pregnancy, the dividing membrane is thin (<2 mm) and consists of only two layers. There would be a T sign near the placental attachment to the membrane with no chorionic tissue between the layers of membrane (Fig. 19.3). The abovementioned signs taken together can be used to predict zygosity and chorionicity with more than 91% sensitivity and specificity (Scardo et al 1995).

When a twin pregnancy is diagnosed in the second trimester, opposite genders or separate placental masses indicate dichorionicity. Fetuses with the same gender or a single placental mass indicate further evaluation. Evaluation of the intertwine membrane and the membrane take-off site provides less accuracy (90%) in determining chorionicity in the second trimester (Ana and Ashley 2005).

Assessment of chorionicity helps in distinguishing between twin-to-twin transfusion syndrome (TTTS) and fetal growth restriction, and has implications for selective termination/multifetal reduction (Jodie and Caroline 2005).

Nuchal Translucency Screening

The combination of nuchal translucency measurement and maternal age yield similar sensitivity and false-positive rates in a dichorionic pregnancy as those for singleton pregnancies (Sebire et al 1996). The false-positive rate is higher for monochorionic twins, with discordancce for nuchal translucency measures as a possible indicator of early onset TTTS (Nicolaides et al 1999). Twins also have a higher incidence of congenital abnormalities (Jodie and Caroline 2005).

PREGNANCY OUTCOMES OF TWIN GESTATIONS

'Vanishing Twin' In about 20–70% of twins diagnosed in the first trimester, one twin is 'lost' by the second trimester (Landy et al 1986). The fetal loss rate is greater among monochorionic twin gestations (12.2%) than dichorionic twin gestations (1.8%) (Sebire 1997). Prognosis for the remaining fetus is good (Fig. 19.4). However, it can lead to raised maternal serum and amniotic fluid alphafetoprotein, and elevated amniotic fluid acetylcholinesterase levels, which should be cautiously interpreted in these pregnancies (Winsor et al 1987).

Anomalies Major malformations complicate 2.12% of twin pregnancies compared to 1.05% among singleton pregnancies. Minor malformations complicate 4.13% of twin

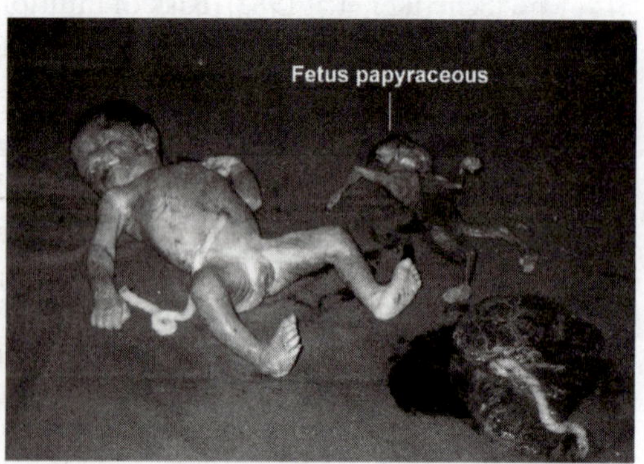

FIGURE 19.4: MONOCHORIONIC TWIN GESTATION SHOWING SINGLE PLACENTA AND ONE FETUS AS FETUS PAPYRACEOUS

pregnancies when compared to 2.45% among singleton pregnancies (Allen and Timothy 2005). The risk of malformations is 3.1% among monozygotic twins. This risk is only 1.9% among dizygotic twins (Allen and Timothy 2005).

Birth Weight Birth weights are lower among multiple gestations than in singletons because of intrauterine growth restriction and preterm delivery. Suboptimal implantation/placentation early in pregnancy may be seen. Also, there is also uterine crowding later in pregnancy. These two factors play a significant role in restricting fetal growth (Allen 2005). The growth of twins is similar to that of singletons up to 28–30 weeks, after which they lag behind, and this lag persistently increases till term (Arbuckle et al 1993). However, most clinicians believe that singleton growth curves can be used for twins to evaluate growth abnormalities (Errol et al 2005).

Duration of Gestation The more the number of fetuses, the earlier the delivery. About 50% of all twins are delivered by 36 weeks (Luke 1994). The mean gestational age at delivery is 33.5 weeks for triplets and 31 weeks for quadruplets (Berkowitz et al 1996).

Preterm Delivery The incidence of preterm delivery varies between 30% and 50% among twins and can be as high as 80% among higher order multiple gestations (Jodie and Caroline 2005). Preterm delivery occurs due to spontaneous preterm labour (54%) or preterm premature rupture of membranes (PPROM) (22%), or could be indicated for maternal/fetal conditions (23%) (Gardner et al 1995).

'Term' Twin Pregnancy Twins are considered 'post term' after 38 weeks because intrauterine growth restriction and perinatal death rates increase substantially after this period. The lowest incidence of perinatal death (10.5 per 1000 infants) is seen at 38 weeks in twin pregnancies. This corresponds to a similar incidence in singleton pregnancies at 43 weeks (Minakami and Satol 1996).

Increased maternal morbidity with multiple births includes hyperemesis, early onset/severe hypertension, gestational diabetes, anemia, antepartum and postpartum bleeding, preterm labour, abnormal placentation, polyhydramnios and difficulties in labour.

Antepartum Management of Twin Gestation The specific objectives of antepartum management of twin gestation are to safeguard maternal health from the unusual burden, prevent extreme prematurity and appropriately manage fetal growth restriction.

Nutrition and Weight Gain Women who carry twins must consume 150 kcal/day more than women with a singleton pregnancy, 30 mg of iron and 300 μg of folic acid per day after the twelfth week of gestation (Allen and Timothy 2005). One study suggests vitamin C supplementation to maintain the integrity of amniotic membranes, thereby reducing the incidence of PPROM (Casaneuva et al 2005). The US Institute of Medicine (IOM) recommends that women carrying more than one fetus be given a daily supplement that contains 15 mg zinc, 2 mg copper, 250 mg calcium, 2 mg vitamin B6, 300 μg folic acid, 50 mg vitamin C, 5 μg vitamin D and 30 mg iron after 12 weeks of gestation (Brown and Carlson 2000).

The following recommendations are made for micronutrient supplementation for women carrying multiple fetuses (Barbara 2005):

- One multivitamin daily with 100% of non-pregnant RDA for the first trimester, including 400 μg of folic acid. Double the dose for the second and third trimesters.

- 3 g of calcium per day
- 1.2 g of magnesium per day
- 45 mg of zinc per day
- Consider supplementation with an additional 1 g of vitamin C and 400 IU of vitamin E for prevention of pre-eclampsia.

The National Academy of Sciences suggests that women carrying twins should aim at a weekly weight gain of about 0.75 kg during the second and third trimesters, which is equivalent to a total gain of 16–20.5 kg (Luke et al 1993; Fagen 2003). A low rate of gain before 24 weeks (<0.39 kg/week), regardless of the rate of gain after 24 weeks, is significantly associated with poor intrauterine growth and higher morbidity (Luke 1993).

Genetic Testing

The risk of fetal aneuploidy among monozygotic twins is the same as that expected for the maternal age with singleton gestation. However, among dizygotic twins, the abovementioned risk is twice that expected for the maternal age (Wapner 1995). The recent American College of Obstetrics and Gynecologists (ACOG) Practice Bulletin suggests that a woman carrying twins at the age of 33 years has the same risk as a singleton pregnancy in a 35-year-old woman. The reliability of serum biochemical screening against aneuploidy/neural tube defects is not clearly known in twin gestation as these markers are elevated. Biochemical screening is associated with Down syndrome detection rates of at least 15% less than in singleton pregnancies. Nuchal translucency measurements provide better detection rates of 75–85%, with a false-positive rate of 5% (Melissa et al 2005).

Prenatal diagnostic procedures in twin gestations should be performed under ultrasound guidance (Wapner 1993). Detailed sonography prior to the procedure is done, so that fetal and placental positions are well mapped. After aspirating the necessary amniotic fluid, 1 ml of indigo carmine dye is injected into the sac so that each sac is tested only once. Indigo carmine has not been associated with fetal risks (Cragan et al 1993). When one sac completely overlies the other, a single-needle technique should be considered (Meredith et al 2005). The issue of higher pregnancy loss rate following multifetal amniocentesis is not clear (Meredith et al 2005). Multifetal chorionic villus sampling is a technically challenging procedure. However, it is probably advantageous when selective termination or multifetal pregnancy reduction is required (Meredith et al 2005).

Medical Disorders

Hypertensive disorders in twin gestations are more common, earlier in onset and more severe than in singleton gestations. Moreover, the risk of pre-eclampsia among nulliparous twin gestations is 14 times more than the risk among parous singleton gestations (Coonrod et al 1995). Multiple pregnancy is a risk factor for the development of acute fatty liver of pregnancy (Cynthia et al 2005). Conflicting data and lack of clear-cut evidence means that there is nothing to suggest increased incidence of gestational diabetes among women carrying twin fetuses (Cynthia et al 2005).

Anemia One study reported that there was a fourfold increase in the risk of anemia in twin pregnancies when compared to singletons pregnancies (Blickstein et al 1995). Women carrying twin fetuses require 1.8 times more iron than those carrying one fetus (Maria et al 2005).

Antepartum Hemorrhage Women with twins are at increased risk of developing antepartum hemorrhage, both due to placenta previa and abruption (Ananth et al 2001, 2003).

Antepartum Surveillance

Ultrasound Surveillance Serial ultrasounds at an interval of 2–4 weeks are recommended to identify fetal growth restriction and growth discordancy (D'Alton and Mercer 1990). Amniotic fluid is assessed by measuring either the deepest vertical pocket in a sac or the overall amniotic fluid index (AFI). Normative AFI measurements have been established based on 282 sets of uncomplicated twin pregnancies (Porter et al 1996).

Oligohydramnios may indicate underlying uteroplacental insufficiency or twin-to-twin transfusion syndrome and requires further evaluation. Similarly, polyhydramnios may indicate twin-to-twin transfusion syndrome or fetal anomaly and requires evaluation.

Tests of Fetal Well-being Assessment of amniotic fluid and biophysical profile are difficult and may be inaccurate in twin gestations. Therefore, non-stress test and Doppler velocimetry are more reliable tests of fetal well-being (Devoe and Ware 1995). The use of serial umbilical artery Doppler velocimetry has been shown to be beneficial in improving perinatal outcome among high-risk twin pregnancies (Jodie and Caroline 2005).

Duplex Doppler ultrasound, used to measure umbilical venous flow and systolic/diastolic ratios, can predict concordant and discordant growth in twin pairs (Gerson et al 1987).

Prevention of Preterm Delivery A potential preventive strategy is to reduce the background uterine activity and prevent the occurrence of known causes of stress, especially infectious diseases (John 2005). Three types of interventions can be used to reduce the baseline uterine activity—bed rest, progesterone and prophylactic tocolytic therapy.

Routine hospitalisation and bed rest This has not been found to be useful in prolonging twin and triplet pregnancies, though bed rest is definitely helpful as a good adjunctive care along with other measures. Current studies do not show any significant difference in mean gestational age at delivery or perinatal outcomes among those hospitalised and not hospitalised, though there was some difference in neonatal birth weight (Crowther et al 1990; Adams 1998).

Cervical length measurements A closed cervical length of ≤25 mm at 24 weeks has been shown to be a predictor of spontaneous preterm labour. Similarly, a cervical length of 3.5 cm or more throughout the second trimester is highly unlikely to result in preterm labour before 34 weeks. However, no intervention has been found to be of proven benefit to affect the outcome so far. Therefore, the clinical usefulness of routine cervical length measurement has been questioned (Souka et al 1999; ACOG Practice Bulletin 2001).

Fetal fibronectin A positive fetal fibronectin in cervical secretions at 28–30 weeks is shown to be a predictor of birth prior to 32 weeks. However, it is unclear if this knowledge helps to bring down preterm births (Wennerholm et al 1997). The value of this test lies primarily in its negative predictive value. About 99% of patients with a negative FFN test do not deliver within seven days (Errol et al 2005).

Home uterine activity monitoring Home uterine activity monitoring (HUAM) was not shown to be effective in predicting preterm labour (US Preventive Services Task Force 1993) and is currently not recommended in twin pregnancies.

Prophylactic tocolytic therapy Cuurent literature has not shown any benefit of prophylactic betamimetic therapy in reducing the occurrence of preterm labour in twin gestations (Allen and Timothy 2005). Treatment with oral tocolytics did not affect the crescendo of uterine activity occurring before preterm labour (Ashworth et al 1990). It should also be remembered that tocolytic therapy is associated with more complications in twin gestations.

Current evidence is insufficient for the usage of 17-hydroxy progesterone for preterm labour prophylaxis in twin gestations, though this has been successfully used for those with a history of recurrent preterm delivery (Errol et al 2005). However, given the absence of proven alternatives, progesterone use may be appropriate in high-risk cases such as those with prior spontaneous preterm delivery.

Cervical circlage Statistically significant reduction in preterm birth has not been shown when mid-trimester cervical encirclage was performed for shortened cervix in twin gestations (Newmann et al 2002). Similarly, prophylactic circlage has not shown statistically significant reduction of preterm delivery among triplet pregnancies (Allen 2005).

Corticosteroid therapy Corticosteroids are recommended for enhancement of lung maturity in multiple gestations in preterm labour and impending delivery (< 34 weeks) (NIH Publication 1994). Data supports the use of corticosteroids between 28 and 34 weeks in triplet pregnancies to reduce the incidence of hyaline membrane disease of the newborn (Pons et al 1998).

Fetal lung maturation Mostly, pulmonary maturation is synchronous among twin pairs as measured by the L/S ratio. However, data regarding the acceleration of lung maturity among multiple fetuses is conflicting (Allen and Timothy2005).

Tocolytic therapy Acute tocolysis is difficult and more risky in twin gestations. A higher drug dosage is required and multiple drugs may be needed for successful tocolysis followed by a long period of maintainance (John 2005).

Preterm Premature Rupture of Membranes (PPROM) Twin gestations complicated by PPROM remote from term are managed expectantly as in the case of singleton gestations (Allen and Timothy 2005). When PPROM among twin and singleton gestations were managed expectantly, no significant differences were seen with respect to latency to delivery, maternal infectious morbidity or perinatal morbidity (Mercer et al 1993). PPROM near term is managed in a similar manner to that of singleton gestations, which is most often delivery.

However, management of PPROM at a pre-viable gestational age is not clear. Options range from expectant management to termination of the entire pregnancy. Expectant management results in an extremely high pregnancy loss rate and exposes the mother to the risks of infection and complications of prolonged bed rest. In addition, high neonatal mortality and morbidity due to infection and prematurity is seen. Hence, an individualised approach is recommended (George and Sreedhar 2005).

Vaginal Birth after Cesarean Section A study done on 210 twin gestations, all with one prior lower segment cesarean section scar on the uterus, shows that maternal and neonatal outcomes among those who underwent elective cesarean and those who undertook a trial of labour were similar (Miller et al 1996).

Complications Unique to Multifetal Gestations

Monoamniotic Twins Monoamniotic twins constitute 1% of monozygotic twin gestations.

Pseudomonoamniotic twinning can occur, either spontaneously or following invasive procedures. The following are the ultrasound criteria for the diagnosis of monoamniotic twins (George and Sreedhar 2005):

- Single placenta and same sex fetuses
- No dividing membrane visualised
- Adequate amniotic fluid surrounding each fetus
- Both fetuses move freely within the uterine cavity

Monoamniotic twin gestations are associated with higher mortality (50%), mainly because of the often unpredictable cord entanglement, the reported incidence is 22–57% (Roque et al 2003). Recent literature suggests that many fetal deaths occur before 32 weeks and therefore, prophylactic preterm delivery, which is practiced by many, may not be indicated (Tessen and Zlatnik 1991). A safe time for delivery should probably be decided by the NICU facility.

Cord entanglement is diagnosed when a mass of cord is seen between the two fetal bodies (Sebire et al 2000). Regular NST and Doppler ultrasound have been used to diagnose cord entanglement. More intense fetal monitoring has been employed following diagnosis of cord entanglement, so that cord occlusion can be diagnosed and prompt delivery can be performed. However, sudden death may not be prevented, and there is no evidence that such monitoring improves the outcome (Jodie and Caroline 2005). The optimal route of delivery in monoamniotic twins remains unclear, though cesarean section has been recommended in general (Allen and Timothy 2005).

Conjoint Twins The incidence of conjoint twins is 1in 57,000 deliveries or 1 in 200 monozygotic twins (Hanson 1975). They are grouped according to the shared body part:

- Caudal (ischiopagus)
- Cephalic (craniopagus)
- Anterior (thoracopagus)—most common
- Posterior (pygopagus)

Early sonography shows a single amniotic sac with a bifid fetal pole that moves as one; the fetuses remain in the same position, relative to each other, despite changes in position (Alisa et al 2005).

A mid-trimester ultrasound scan should diagnose the problem and accurately describe the shared organs so that counselling and optimal obstetric care can be given. Prognosis depends on the separability of vital organs between the twins, and the presence of additional malformations. Polyhydramnios, secondary to circulatory imbalances, is a common complication (affecting up to 50% of cases). This may necessitate amnioreduction (George and Sreedhar 2005).

Termination can be offered if the problem is diagnosed early in pregnancy and the twins are inseparable. Otherwise, fetal echocardiography should be performed and pediatric surgeons should be consulted about optimal management. Fetuses are delivered by elective cesarean section once lung maturity is attained (van den Brand et al 1994).

Twin Reversed Arterial Perfusion (Trap): Acardiac Twin Gestation This occurs in approximately 1 in 100 monozygotic twins or 1 in 35, 000 births (Jodie and Caroline 2005). It results from vascular communications between the twins in monochorionic twin gestation. When arterial pressures in one twin exceed that of the other, there is a reversal of blood flow in the perfused twin. The pump twin suffers from cardiac overload resulting in congestive cardiac failure and growth restriction. The 'used blood' from the donor twin is shunted to the iliac vessels of the recipient thereby perfusing the lower part of the body more than the upper part. This leads to incomplete morphogenesis of the upper part of the body, resulting in malformations such as an acardiac twin.

The main perinatal problems associated with acardiac twinning are pump twin congestive cardiac failure, hydramnios, hydrops and preterm delivery (Allen and Timothy 2005), in addition to the possibility of long-term neurological sequelae. Overall, the perinatal mortality for the pump twin was found to be 55% in a series of 49 such cases (Moore et al 1990). The mortality of the recipient was 100%.

Second trimester ultrasound scans may show the acardiac fetus as a tissue mass with heterogenous echotexture, or as a fetus that has undergone in utero demise. Doppler ultrasound of umbilical vessels may help in their diagnosis (Alisa et al 2005).

Fetal surveillance is recommended, with intervention advocated with the development of fetal hydrops or polyhydramnios (Jodie and Caroline 2005). Reports of serial amniocentesis and use of indomethacin have been made. The mainstay of treatment would be to disrupt vascular communications. This has been performed by percutaneous umbilical cord ligation using endoscopic and sonographic guidance at around 20 weeks. The mode and timing of birth would depend on fetal compromise and presentation, with the possibility of the grossly enlarged acardiac twin obstructing labour (Jodie and Caroline 2005).

Twin-to-twin Tranfusion Syndrome (TTTS) TTTS complicates about 5–25% of monochorioic diamniotic twin gestations and is associated with significant perinatal mortality and morbidity. Unbalanced vascular communications are seen in the placenta, leading to unidirectional flow from the donor to the recipient twin. As a result, the donor twin becomes anemic, oligohydramniotic and growth restricted while the recipient twin develops polycythemia, polyhydramnios and hydrops. A study by Bajoria et al (1995) suggests that twins with TTTS are likely to have deep, rather than superficial, anastomoses.

Fetal Central Nervous System Injury Twin pregnancies complicated by acute TTTS are at increased risk of central nervous system (CNS) injury resulting in microcephaly, porencephaly, cerebral palsy and multicystic encephalomalacia (Allen and Timothy 2005). Death of one of the monochorionic twins, later in gestation, causes a relaxed circulation in the dead twin, which leads to acute TTTS. The survivor suffers from massive blood loss/hypotension, which may lead to degeneration of brain tissue and its consequences (Hecher et al 1994). Thus, cerebral damage in the survivor may be the result of acute TTTS rather than DIC (Fusi et al 1991). Cerebral ischemic complications can set in immediately after the death of the first twin, and at least two weeks should pass before the CNS lesions can be visualised by sonography/MRI. Therefore, prompt delivery of the surviving twin may not prevent CNS morbidity (Langer et al 1997).

Diagnosis of TTTS TTTS is diagnosed antenatally using the following criteria:

- Monochorionic twin gestation with placental vascular anastomoses
- Same sex fetuses with inter-twin weight difference of more than 20%
- Polyhydramnios of the larger twin and oligohydramnios of the smaller twin
- Hemoglobin difference of more than 5 g/dl (cordoscentesis)

The accuracy of such diagnostic criteria is nearly 44% (Bruner and Rosemond 1993). The pulsatility index (PI) of the renal artery was significantly lower and urine output significantly higher in the polyhydramniotic twin than in the oligohydramniotic twin

(Mari et al 1993). This polyhydramnios-oligohydramnios sequence is responsible for pulmonary hypoplasia, growth restriction and contractures for the stuck twin, and hydrops and preterm premature rupture of membranes for the recipient. A discrepancy in umbilical cord diameter and abnormal umbilical artery (in the donor)/or abnormal venous Doppler waveforms (in the recipient) may be seen in TTTS. In the case of 'stuck twin', the dividing membrane is shrink-wrapped around the stuck fetus, which does not move freely in the amniotic cavity. This condition may be difficult to differentiate from monoamniotic twins. TTTS is not the only cause for stuck twin, and genitourinary abnormalities should be ruled out in these fetuses (Alisa et al 2005).

It is worthwhile considering fetal blood sampling to determine discordant hemoglobins among the twin pairs before planning invasive procedures (Allen and Timothy 2005).

Perinatal Survival in TTTS Overall, perinatal survival is around 21–65%, which depends on gestational age at diagnosis and at delivery, and the severity and progression of the disease. The watershed for survival appears to be delivery at 28 weeks (Guncombe et al 2003).

Volume overload can cause hypertension and myocardial hypertrophy, and about 10% of recipients have chronic cardiac problems. Once abnormal Doppler waveforms are seen, the risk of death or neurological impairment is high (Richard and Mark 2006).

Quintero staging system (Quintero et al 1999) describes the five stages of TTTS as follows:

Stage 1: Polyhydramnios oligohydramnios sequence alone

Stage 2: Urine in donor's bladder not visible

Stage 3: Critically abnormal Doppler waveforms in either twin

Stage 4: Ascitis or frank hydrops in either twin

Stage 5: Demise of either twin

Stage 3 is the largest group and it comprises a very broadspectrum of severity. The Cincinnati modification of the Quintero staging system (Ursula and Timothy 2005) uses fetal echocardiographic assessment of the recipient twin to stage these patients so that fetal TTTS-induced cardiomyopathy is taken into account, to determine the response to therapy.

Treatment of Pregnancies Complicated by TTTS

Serial amnioreduction is one of the treatment modalities which aims at decompressing the polyhydramnios sac of the recipient twin, thereby reducing the incidence of preterm labour. Also, the cycle of increasing interfetal blood transfer is disrupted, and this may result in reversal of unidirectional flow associated with TTTS. It may also help in increasing uterine artery blood flow.

Various studies have shown improved perinatal survival with serial amnioreduction (Mahony et al 1990; Garry et al 1996). However, there is an increased incidence of various pregnancy complications associated with serial amnioreduction, such as placental abruption, intraamniotic infection, preterm premature rupture of membranes, preterm labour/delivery and fetal injury. This procedure is indicated in the presence of clinically tense polyhydramnios, amniotic fluid index of more than 40 cm or significant maternal discomfort.

Another treatment modality is fetoscopic neodymium—YAG laser occlusion of superficial placental vascular communications. This is intended to disrupt interfetal transfer and also enable functional elimination of the involved cotyledon (De Lia et al 1990; Lundvall et al 1999). A few complications such as limb necrosis, congenital skin loss and placental vessel laceration have been reported following laser coagulation.

Recent trials comparing laser coagulation

with amnioreduction have reported better pregnancy outcome and less fetal neurological morbidity in the laser group than in the amnioreduction group (Quintero et al 2003). However, amnioreduction is readily available, cheaper and less invasive; laser is available only in select institutions and requires specialised training.

Encouraging results have been reported following fetoscopic microseptostomy, which is the intentional puncture of the intervening membrane between the two twin fetuses in an attempt to equalise the pressure between the two sacs (Johnson et al 2001).

Various techniques including fetoscopic diathermy have been attempted to achieve permanent arrest of blood flow through the cord of the target fetus so that a severely damaged fetus can be selected and subjected to selective fetocide (Challis et al 1999). This procedure can be offered up to 26 weeks when a fetus is deemed to be preterminal, or whenever it is classified to be in stage 3 or 4 of TTTS (Richard and Mark 2006).

Stage-based treatment approaches are described by several authors, with amnioreduction and septotomy used for early disease, and laser treatment or cord occlusion reserved for more severe disease (Richard and Mark 2006).

Ursula et al propose a sequential treatment approach. Presentation after 24 weeks is managed by amnioreduction/ microseptostomy. Those who present earlier are initially managed similarly; however, laser therapy is required once the disease progresses. Fetoscopic cord occlusion is reserved for advanced irreversible TTTS cardiomyopathy in the recipient twin.

Discordant Growth Unequal intrauterine growth of twin fetuses is usually apparent in late second or third trimester. This is seen in 5–15% of twins and 30% of tripets. Significant risk factors incude monochorionicity, pre-eclampsia and antepartum bleeding (Errol et al 2005). Perinatal morbidity is directly proportional to the degree of growth discordancy and morbidities are caused by fetal growth restriction, respiratory distress and hyperbilirubinemia. If discordancy is apparent in the first trimester, there is an increased risk of congenital malformations in the fetuses (Weissman et al 1994; Demissie et al 2002).

Etiology In monochorionic twins, discordancy is usually caused by TTTS. In dichorionic twins, different genetic growth potentials of dizigotic twins or suboptimal placentation of one twin due to in utero crowding could be the cause.

Diagnosis Diagnosis is by serial ultrasound scans wherein weight discordancy is calculated by dividing the difference in the weights of the twin fetuses by the weight of the largest twin. Literature so far suggests that a weight discordancy of 20–25% is clinically significant and associated with adverse perinatal outcome (Hollier et al 1999).

Management Management involves regular monitoring to detect the progression of discordancy and performance of fetal well-being tests. Once significant fetal stress is detected, a decision about delivery may have to be taken (Allen and Timothy 2005).

Demise of One Twin The demise of one twin remote from term is more frequent in monochorionic than in dichorionic twin gestations because of placental vascular communications. Studies have revealed overall incidence of single fetal demise as 6.2%, the specific incidences were 8.4% in monochorionic twins and 4.1% in dichorionic twin gestations (Saito et al 1999). The incidence of perinatal complications in the surviving twin, such as perinatal death and cerebral damage, was significantly more common among monochorionic twins than in dichorionic twins (30% and 10%, respectively). The proposed etiology in monochorionic twins is rapid blood loss from the survivor to the relaxed circulation of the dead twin, rather than DIC, as thought earlier (Allen and Timothy 2005). Specific problems seen in the survivors are microcephaly, hydrocephaly, porencephaly, cerebral atrophy, cerebral palsy, renal necrosis and intestinal atresia. The characteristic cystic periventricular leukomalacia, which is thought to be responsible for cerebral damage is reported in 40–50% of such pregnancies (Pharoah and Adi 2000). Risk of preterm labour also increases following single fetal demise, regardless of chorionicity. Overall, 50–80% of surviving co-twins are delivered before term (George and Lynn 2004). In addition, there is a risk of maternal DIC following single fetal demise, which is reported to be of low incidence and transient by some authors, but as high as 25% by others (Landy and Weingold 1989). Parental psychological impact should also not be forgotten.

Single fetal demise is not an indication for immediate termination of pregnancy, regardless of chorionicity. Few studies support expectant management with close fetomaternal monitoring as they did not show increased morbidity with such management (Santema 1995). Also, immediate delivery has not been shown to prevent acute TTTS and neurological morbidity in few other studies (Langer 1997). Corticosteroids are given and fetal well-being is monitored. Serial ultrasounds and MRI, performed 2–3 weeks after the demise, may be used to detect multicystic encephalomalacia antenatally (George 2005). Detailed parental counselling is essential and the possibility of undetectable neurological damage should be explained. Periodic surveillance for maternal DIC is recommended. Elective delivery should be considered at 37 weeks of gestation with cesarean section reserved for obstetrical indications.

In monochorionic twins with impending death of one fetus, preterm delivery may be indicated to prevent neurological damage to the survivor, or to salvage both fetuses if possible (George and Sreedhar 2005). The outcome of the surviving twin is usually unaffected in dichorionic twin pregnancies.

Multifetal Pregnancy Reduction (MFPR)

MFPR involves nonselective reduction of one or more fetuses in higher order multiple gestations, to reduce the risk of adverse maternal and perinatal outcomes. This procedure is utilised frequently, as IVF has become commonplace.

MFPR is done transvaginally or transabdominally using ultrasound assistance; potassium chloride is commonly used to achieve asystole (Berkowitz et al 1996). Prior knowledge of chorionicity is essential. The transabdominal procedure is done 10–13 weeks after the period when spontaneous loss of embryo may occur. Chorionic villus sampling can be performed before the procedure so that chromosomally normal fetuses are chosen to be left behind (Meredith et al 2005).

MFPR is clearly associated with better pregnancy outcome in quadruplets and higher order multiple gestations (Allen 2005). Better pregnancy outcome is seen with triplets undergoing MFPR than those managed expectantly (Lipitz et al 1996), and benefits of the procedure exceed the risks involved.

Unintended pregnancy loss rate of 5.4% and preterm delivery are two complications associated with MFPR (Stone et al 2002). However, MFPR improves the outcome of multifetal pregnancies above and beyond a reduction in the total pregnancy loss rates (Meredith et al 2005).

Higher incidence of fetal growth restriction and growth discordance has been reported following MFPR; therefore, specific surveillance is required for these complications (Depp et al 1996). Maternal serum alphafetoprotein (MSAFP) cannot be used as a screening tool in these pregnancies, as their levels are usually elevated following the procedure (Berkowitz et al 1996).

Selective Termination Selective termination of one of the fetuses is performed when a chromosomal, structural or genetic abnormality is identified in the fetus using ultrasound or an invasive prenatal diagnostic test, with the intention of optimising the outcome of the normal fetus (Meredith et al 2005).

The risks associated with continuing a pregnancy with an anomalous fetus in a twin gestation include higher risk of preterm delivery and fetal demise with subsequent complications. Selective termination in this setting appears to be a reasonable management option (Malone and D'Alton 1997).

Alexandra et al (Berkowitz et al 1996) list the following indications (other than anomalous fetus) for selective termination in monochorionic, diamniotic twin gestations:

- TRAP sequence
- Early severe TTTS/IUGR

Determination of chorionicity and precise identification of the affected fetus are vital preprocedural considerations. The procedure is almost the same as in MFPR. In monochorionic twin pregnancies, various techniques have been used to interrupt umbilical cord blood supply, including fetoscopic cord ligation, laser ablation and diathermy, and radiofrequency ablation (Berkowitz et al 1996). Selective termination in experienced hands is a safe procedure at any gestational age (Meredith et al 2005).

Multiple Pregnancy: Labour And Delivery

This is a well-recognised high-risk area with the following potential complications:

- Fetal malpresentations
- PROM/cord prolapse
- Abruption
- Preterm labour
- Incordinate uterine action
- Uterine atony
- Postpartum hemorrhage
- Asphyxia of second twin

Timing of delivery Delivery by week 38–39 seems to be optimal for an uncomplicated twin gestation (Allen and Timothy 2005).

Prerequisites

- One-to-one care
- Skilled obstetrician, capable of intrauterine manipulations
- Well-equipped delivery room/OT readily available/ultrasound machine
- Skilled pediatricians/anesthetist
- Good intravenous access/blood products

Labour induction/augmentation Multifetal gestation as such is not a contraindication for labour induction (ACOG Practice Bulletin 1999). Labour augmentation with dilute oxytocin infusion can also be done safely (Fausett et al 1997).

Fetal monitoring Continuous electronic monitoring of the heart rate of both fetuses must be done, separately and simultaneously, throughout labour (Allen and Timothy 2005).

Analgesia during labour Epidural analgesia is beneficial because it can be extended for intrauterine manipulations/operative delivery. Preloading with intravenous fluids and lateral positioning are very important.

Mode of Delivery Ultrasonography should be done at onset of labour to evaluate fetal positions and weights, which determine the mode of delivery. Combinations of fetal presentations in the order of decreasing frequency are cephalic–cephalic, which is the most common, followed by cephalic–breech, cephalic–transverse and breech–breech.

Vertex-Vertex: Vaginal delivery is appropriate in this situation. The presentation of the second twin is determined by examination/ultrasound, oxytocin infusion/timely AROM can be done. Cesarean section is performed for indications such as non-reassuring fetal status of twin B or cord prolapse (ACOG Practice Bulletin 2004).

Vertex-Nonvertex: Literature supports vaginal delivery if the first twin is cephalic, irrespective of the lie and presentation of the second, provided the second twin weighs < 2 kg (Simpson and Alcon 1997). However, some evidence suggests that this policy may be associated with slightly increased mortality and morbidity in the second twin due to perinatal asphyxia (Andrew and Gordon 2004), and this must be included in patient counselling/decision.

Data is currently insufficient to advocate either routine abdominal or routine vaginal delivery of the second twin whose birth weight is < 1500 g, although cesarean section is performed more frequently in such situations (Davison et al 1992; ACOG Practice Bulletin 2004; Allen and Timothy 2005). However, if twin B weighs more than 1500 g, current evidence suggests that vaginal delivery is a safe option (ACOG Technical Bulletin 1998; Winn et al 2001). The available options are assisted vaginal breech delivery and external/intrauterine manipulations followed by breech extraction or vertex delivery.

Twin A Nonvertex: The recommended mode of delivery is cesarean section (ACOG Practice Bulletin 2004). Especially when twin A is breech and twin B is cephalic, interlocking, though rare, may result in perinatal death in 25% of cases (Andrew and Gordon 2004).

Time Interval between Delivery of Twins Strict time interval restriction may not be necessary between the delivery of two twins, as long as maternal and fetal well-being are ensured, uterine monitoring is done and progressive descent occurs (Allen and Timothy 2005). However, progression of labour should be monitored/judicial augmentation be done to optimise the interval. This is because lengthy intervals are known to be problematic to the second twin (Leung et al 2002).

Active management of the third stage of labour is recommended after the birth of the second twin (Prendivillie 2004).

Delayed Delivery of the Second Twin (Asynchronous Birth) This is a rare situation wherein one of the twin fetuses is delivered preterm (previable), uterine contractility ceases and the next fetus is delivered days to weeks later. The efficacy of aggressive management, often practiced in this situation, including cerclage, antibiotics, tocolysis, steroids, etc., is unclear.

Candidates must be carefully selected, considering all contraindications, counselled and monitored for sepsis (Alisa et al 2005).

Triplets, Higher Order Multiple Gestations (HOM) The maternal risks of HOM gestations can be listed as follows (Patricia and Fergal 2004):

- Preterm labour
- Prolonged hospitalisation increasing risks of thromboembolism, osteopenia and psychological distress
- Severe pre-eclampsia/gestational diabetes
- Cesarean section
- Obstetric hemorrhage
- Anemia and other nutritional deficiencies
- Hyperemesis
- Acute fatty liver of pregnancy

- Intrahepatic cholestasis

Preterm labour and growth restriction are much more common in HOM gestation. The more the number of fetuses, the earlier the delivery.

Micronutrient supplementation at higher dosages is essential. Adequate weight gain is very important. Aggressive manipulation of background uterine activity with bed rest, psychological reassurance, maintenance tocolysis, cervical assessment and timely encirclage will reduce the incidence of preterm labour. Management is directed at delaying delivery until 34 or 35 weeks, if at all possible (John 2005).

In general, triplets and higher order multiple gestations, when viable, are delivered by cesarean section, as several complications may arise during their delivery (Allen and Timothy 2005).

References

Adams SM, JS Sholl, EI Haney et al. 1998. Perinatal outcome associated with outpatient management of triplet pregnancy. *Am J Obstet Gynecol* 178: 843–847.

Alisa B, Modena and B Vincenzo. 2005. Antepartum management of multifetal pregnancies. *Clin Perinatol* 32(2): 443–454.

Allen A and RBJ Timothy. 2005. Management of multiple pregnancy: prenatal care- part-II. *Obstet Gynecol Survey* 60(8):538–548.

Allen A and RBJ Timothy. 2005. Management of multiple pregnancy: labor and delivery. *Obstet Gynecol Surv* 60(8):550–554.

Allen A and RBJ Timothy. 2005. Management of multiple pregnancy: prenatal care—part 1. *Obstet Gynecol Survey* 60(8):527–536.

American College of Obstetricians and Gynecologists. 1998. Special problems of multiple gestation. *ACOG Technical Bulletin No. 253*. Washington, DC: ACOG.

American College of Obstetricians and Gynecologists. 1999. Induction of labor. *ACOG Practice Bulletin No. 10*. Washington, DC: ACOG.

American College of Obstetricians and Gynecologists. 2001. Assesment of risk factors for preterm birth. *ACOG Practice Bulletin No 31*.Washinton, DC: ACOG.

American College of Obstetricians and Gynecologists. 2004. Multiple Gestation: Complicated Twin, Triplet, and High Order Multifetal Pregnancy. *ACOG Practice Bulletin No. 56*. Washington, DC: ACOG.

American College of Obstetricians and Gynecologists. 2004. Multiple gestation: Complicated twin, triplet and high order multiple pregnancy. *ACOG Practice Bulletin No. 56*. Washington, DC: ACOG.

Ana M and SR Ashley. 2005. Ultrasound in multiple gestations: Twins and other multifetal pregnancies. *Clin Perinatol* 32(2):329–354.

Ananth C, J Smulian, A Vintzileos et al. 2001. Placental abruption among singleton and twin births in the United States: risk factor profiles. *American Journal of Epidemiology* 153(8):771–778.

Ananth C, K Demissie, J Smulian et al. 2003. Placenta previa in singleton and twin births in the United States, 1989–1998: a comparison of risk factor profiles and associated conditions. *Am J Obstet Gynecol* 188:275–281.

Andrew B and S Gordon. 2004. Mode of delivery of twins. *The Obstetrician and Gynecologist* 6:222–226.

Arbuckle TE, R Wilkins and GJ Sherman. 1993. Birth weight percentiles by gestational age in Canada. *Obstet Gynecol* 81:39–46.

Ashworth MF, SF Spooner, DAA Verkuyl et al. 1990. Failure to prevent preterm labor and delivery in twin pregnancy using prophylactic oral salbutamol. *Br J Obstet Gynecol* 97: 878–882.

Bajoria R, J Wigglesworth and NM Fisk. 1995. Angioarchitexture of monochorionic placentas in reaction to the twin-twin transfusion syndrome. *Am J Obstet Gynecol* 172: 856–863.

Barbara L. 2005.Nutrition in multiple gestations. *Clin Perinatol* 32(2):403–430.

Basso O, EA Nohr, A Christensen et al. 2004. Risk of twinning as a function of maternal height and body mass index. *JAMA* 291:1564–1566.

Berkowitz RL, L Lynch, J Stone et al. 1996. The current status of multifetal pregnancy reduction. *Am J Obstet Gynecol* 174: 1265–1272.

Blickstein I, R Goldschmit and S Lurie. 1995. Hemoglobin levels during twin versus singleton pregnancies: parity makes the diference. *J Reprod Med* 40: 47–50.

Brown JE and M Carlson. 2000. Nutrition and multifetal pregnancy. *J Am Diet Assoc* 100: 343–348.

Bruner JP and RL Rosemond. 1993. Twin–twin transfusion syndrome: a subset to the twin oligohydramnios–polyhydramnios sequence. *Am J Obstet Gynecol* 169: 925–930.

Casaneuva E, C Ripoll, M Tolentino et al.2005. Vitamine C supplementation to prevent preterm rupture of chorioamniotic membranes: a randomized trial. *Am J Clin Nutr* 81: 859–863.

Challis D, E Gratacos and JA Deprest. 1999. Cord occlusion techniques for selective termination in monochorionic twins. *J Perinatol Med* 27: 327–338.

Consensus development conference on the effect of corticosteroids for fetal maturation on Perinatal Outcomes, Feb–March 1994. 1994. *Report on Public Health Service and NIH.* Pub. No 95-3784:1–8.

Coonrod DV, DE Hickok, K Zhu et al. 1995. Risk factors for pre-eclampsia in twin pregnancies: a population based cohort study. *Obstet Gynecol* 85: 645–650.

Cragan JD, ML Martin, MJ Khoury et al. 1993. Dye use during amnioscentesis and birth defects (letter). *Lancet* 341: 1352.

Crowther CA, DAA Verkuyl, JP Neilson et al. 1990. The effects of hospitalization for rest on fetal growth, neonatal morbidity and length of gestation in twin pregnancy. *Br J Obstet Gynecol* 97: 872–877.

Cynthia G, S Joanne and AD Keith. 2005. Maternal complications of multifetal pregnancy. *Clin Perinatol* 32(2): 431–442.

D'Alton ME and BM Mercer. 1990. Antepartum management of twin gestation: ultrasound. *Clin Obstet Gynecol* 33: 42–51.

Davison L, TR Easterling, JC Jackson et al. 1992. Breech extraction of low birth weight second twins: Can cesarean section be justified. *Am J Obstet Gynecol* 166:497–502.

De Lia JE, DP Cruikshank and WR Keye. 1990. Fetoscopic neodymium: YAG laser occlusion of placental vessels in severe twin-twin transfusion syndrome. *Obstet Gynecol* 75:1046–1063.

Demissie K, CV Ananth, J Martin et al. 2002. Fetal and neonatal mortality among twin gestations in the United States: the role of intrapair birthweight discordance. *Obstet Gynecol* 100:474–480.

Depp R, GA Macones, MF Rosenn et al. 1996. Multifetal pregnancy reduction: evaluation of fetal growth in remaining twins. *Am J Obstet Gynecol* 174: 1233–1240.

Devoe LD and DJ Ware. 1995. Antenatal assessment of twin gestation. *Semin Perinatol* 19: 413–423.

Endres L and I Wilkins. 2005. Epidemiology and biology of multiple gestations. *Clin Perinatol* 32:301–314.

Errol R, E Valentine and SP Joong. 2005. Maternal physiology and complications of multiple pregnancy. *Semin Perinatol* 29(5):338–345.

Fagen C. 2003. Nutrition during pregnancy and lactation. In *Krause's Food, Nutrition and Diet Therapy*, 167–195. Philadelphia: WB Saunders.

Fausett MB, WH Barth Jr, BA Yoder et al. 1997. Oxytocin labor stimulation of twin gestations: effective and efficient. *Obstet Gynecol* 90: 202–204.

Fusi L, P Mcparland, N Fisk et al. 1991. Acute twin-twin transfusion: a possible mechanism for brain damaged survivors after intrauterine death of a monochorionic twin. *Obstet Gynecol* 78: 517–521.

Gardner MO, RL Goldenberg, SP Cliver et al. 1995. The origin and outcome of preterm twin pregnancies. *Obstet Gynecol* 85: 553–560.

Garry D, A Lysikiewicz, J Mays et al. 1996. Intra amniotic pressure reduction in twin-twin transfusion syndrome. *Am J Obstet Gynecol* 174: 311.

George G and LS Lynn. 2004. Diagnosis and management of obstetric complications unique to multiple gestations. *Clin Obstet Gynecol* 47(1):163–180.

George M and G Sreedhar. 2005. Diagnosis and Management of Obstetrical Complications Unique to Multiple Gestations. *Semin Perinatol* 29 (5):282–293.

Gerson AG, DM Wallace, NK Bridgens et al. 1987. Duplex Doppler ultrasound in the evaluation of growth in twin pregnancies. *Obstet Gynecol* 70: 419–423.

Guncombe GJ, JE Dickinson and SF Evans. 2003. Perinatal characteristics and outcomes of pregnancies compicated by twin–twin transfusion syndrome. *Obstet Gynecol* 101: 1190–1196.

Hanson J. 1975. Incidence of conjoining twinning. *Lancet* ii: 1257.

Hecher K, E Jauniaux, S Campbell et al. 1994. Artery-artery anastomoses in monochorionic twins. *Am J Obstet Gynecol* 171: 570–572.

Hollier LM, DD McIntire and KJ Leveno. 1999. Outcome of twin pregnancies according to intrapair birthweight differences. *Obstet Gynecol* 94: 1006–1010.

Jodie MD and AC Caroline. 2005. Evidence based care of a women with multiple pregnancy. Best Practice and Research *Clin Obstet Gynecol* 19 (1):131–153.

John PE. 2005. Management of high order multiple gestation. *Clin Perinatol* 32(2):387–402.

John PE. 2005. Preterm labor in twins and high-order multiples. *Obstet Gynecol Clin N Am* 32:429–439.

Johnson JR, KQ Rossi and RW O'Shaughnessy. 2001. Amnioreduction versus septostomy in twin-twin transfusion syndrome. *Am J Obstet Gynecol* 185: 1044–1047.

Landy HJ and AB Weingold. 1989. Management of a multiple gestation complicated by an antepartum fetal demise. *Obstet Gynecol Surv* 44(3):171–176.

Landy HJ, S Weiner, SL Corson et al. 1986. The 'vanishing twin': ultrasound assessment of fetal disappearance in the first trimester. *Am J Obstet Gynecol* 155: 14–19.

Langer B, E Boudier, B Gasser et al. 1997. Antenatal diagnosis of brain damage in the survivor after the second trimester death of a monochorionic and monoamniotic co-twin. *Fetal Diagn Ther* 12: 286–289.

Leung T, W Tam, T Leung et al. 2002. Effects of twin-to-twin delivery interval on umbilical cord blood gas in the second twin. *Brit J Obstet Gynecol* 109(2): 1424–1425.

Lipitz S, J Uval, R Achiron et al. 1996. Outcome of twin pregnancies reduced from triplets compared with nonreduced twin gestations. *Obstet Gynecol* 87: 511–514.

Luke B, J Minogue, FR Witter et al. 1993. The ideal twin pregnancy: patterns of weight gain, discordancy and length of gestation. *Am J Obstet Gynecol* 169: 588–597.

Luke B. 1994. The changing pattern of multiple births in the United States: maternal and infant characteristics, 1973 and 1990. *Obstet Gynecol* 84: 101–108.

Lundvall L, L Skibsted and N Graem. 1999. Limb necrosis associated with twin–twin transfusion syndrome treated with YAG laser coagulation. *Acta Obstet Gynecol* 78:349–352.

MacGillivray I. 1986. Epidemiology of twin pregnancy. *Semin Perinatol* 10:4–8.

Mahony BS, CN Petty, DA Nyberg et al. 1990. The 'stuck twin' phenomenon: ultrasonographic indings, pregnancy outcome, and management with serial amniocentesis. *Am J Obstet Gynecol* 163: 1513–1522.

Malone FD and ME D'Alton. 1997. Management of multiple gestations complicated by a single anomalous fetus. *Curr Opin Obstet Gynecol* 9: 213–216.

Mari G, B Kirshon and A Abuhamad. 1993. Fetal renal artery flow velocity waveforms in normal pregnancies and pregnancies complicated by polyhydramnios and oligohydramnios. *Obstet Gynecol* 81:560–566.

Maria E, F Laiza and C Esther. 2005. Twin pregnancies: Eating for three? Maternal nutrition update. *Nutrition Reviews* 63 (9):295–302.

Melissa C, C Bush and DM Fergal. 2005. Down syndrome screening in twins. *Clin Perinatol* 32(2): 373–386.

Mercer BM, LG Crocker and WF Pierce. 1993. Clinical characteristics and outcome of twin gestation complicated by preterm rupture of membranes. *Am J Obstet Gynecol* 168: 1467–1473.

Meredith R, AE Keith and S Joanne. 2005. Invasive procedures in multifetal pregnancies. *Clin Perinatol* 32(2): 355–372.

Miller DA, P Mullin, D Hou et al. 1996. Vaginal birth after cesarean section in twin gestation. *Am J Obstet Gynacol* 175: 194–198.

Minakami H and I Satol. 1996. Reestimating date of delivery in multifetal pregnancies. *JAMA* 275: 1432–1434.

Moore TR, S Gale and K Benirschke. 1990. Perinatal outcome of 49 pregnancies compicated by acardiac twinning. *Am J Obstet Gynecol* 163: 907–912.

Newmann RB, RS Krombach, MC Myers et al. 2002. Effect of cerclage on obstetrical outcome in twin gestations with a shortened cervical length. *Am J Obstet Gynecol* 186: 634–640.

Nicolaides K, N Sebire and R Snijders. 1999. *The 11–14 Weeks Scan: The Diagnosis of Fetal Abnormalities*. New York: The Parthenon Publishing Group.

Patricia CD and DM Fergal. 2004. Maternal complications associated with multiple pregnancy. *Clin Obstet Gynecol* 47(1): 227–236.

Pharoah PO and Y Adi. 2000. Consequences of in utero death in a twin pregnancy. *Lancet* 355(9215):1597–602.

Pons JC, C Chariemain, E Dubreiul et al. 1998. Management and outcome of triplet pregnancy. *Eur J Obstet Gynecol Reprod Biol* 76: 131–132.

Porter TF, GA Dildy, JR Blanchard et al. 1996. Normal values for amniotic fluid index during uncomplicated twin pregnancy. *Obstet Gynecol* 87: 699–702.

Quintero RA, JE Dickinson, WJ Morales et al. 2003. Stage based treatment of twin–twin transfusion syndrome. *Am J Obstet Gynecol* 188: 1333–1340.

Quintero RA, WJ Morules, MII Allen et al. 1999. Staging of twin-to-twin transfusion syndrome. *J Perinatol* 19: 550–555.

Richard PS and LD Mark. 2006. Review, twin–twin transfusion syndrome. *The Obstetrician and Gynecologist* 8: 1–6.

Roque H, GJ Gillen, E Funai et al. 2003. Perinatal outcomes in monoamniotic gestations. *J Matern Fetal Neonatal Med* 13 (6): 414–421.

Saito K, Y Ohtsu, K Amano et al. 1999. Perinatal outcome and management of single fetal death in twin pregnancy: a case series and review. *J Perinatol Med* 27: 473–477.

Santema GJ, AM Swaak and HCS Wallenberg. 1995. Expectant management of twin pregnancy with single fetal death. *Br J Obstet Gynecol* 102:26–30.

Scardo JA, JM Ellings and RB Newman. 1995. Prospective determination of chorionicity, amnionicity, and zygosityin twin gestation. *Am J Obstet Gynecol* 173: 1376–1380.

Schenker JG, S Yarkoni and M Granat. 1981. Multiple pregnancies following induction of ovulation. *Fertil Steril* 35: 105–123.

Sebire N, R Snijders, H Abraha et al. 1996. Screening trisomy 21 in twin pregnancies by maternal age and fetal nuchal translucency thickness at 10- 14 weeks of gestation. *Br J Obstet Gynaecol* 103: 999–1003.

Sebire NJ, A Souka, H Skentou et al. 2000. First trimester diagnosis of monoamniotic twin pregnancies. *Ultrasound Obstet Gynecol* 16(3):223–5.

Sebire NJ, RJM Snijders, K Hughes et al.1997. The hidden mortality of monochorionic twin pregnancies. *Br J Obstet Gynaecol* 104: 1203–1207.

Sepulveda W, N Sebire, K Hughes et al. 1996. The Lambda sign at 10–14 weeks of pregnancy as a predictor of chorionicity in twin pregnancies. *Ultrasound in Obstetrics and Gynecology* 7: 421–423.

Simpson LJ and MC Alcon. 1997. Multiple Pregnancy. In *Management of labor and delivery*, ed RK Creasy, 395–413. London: Blackwell Science.

Souka AP, V Heath, S Lint et al. 1999. Cevical length at 23 weeks in twins in predicting spontaneous preterm delivery. *Obstet Gynecol* 94: 450–454.

Stone J, K Eddleman, L Lynch et al. 2002. A single centre experience with 1000 consecutive cases of multifetal pregnancy reduction. *Am J Obstet Gynecol* 187: 1163–1167.

Tessen JA and J Zlatnik. 1991. Monoamniotic twins. A retrospective controlled study. *Obstet Gynecol* 77: 832–835.

Ursula FH and MC Timothy. 2005. Twin-twin transfusion syndrome: Where do we go from here? *Semin Perinatol* 29: 296–304.

US Preventive Services Task Force. 1993. Home uterine activity monitoring for preterm labor. *JAMA* 270: 371–376.

van den Brand SFJJ, JG Nijhuis and WJ van Dongen. 1994. Prenatal ultrasound diagnosis of conjoined twins. *Obstet Gynecol Surv* 49: 656–662.

Wapner RJ, A Johnson, G Davis et al. 1993. Comparison between second trimester amnioscentesis and first trimester chorionic villous sampling. *Obstet Gynecol* 82: 49–57.

Wapner RJ. 1995. Genetic diagnosis in multiple pregnancies. *Semin Perinatol* 19: 351–362.

Weissman A, R Achiron, S Lipitz et al. 1994. The first trimester growth discordant twin: an ominous prenatal finding. *Obstet Gynecol* 84: 110–115.

Wennerholm U, B Hom, BI Mattsby et al. 1997. Fetal fibronectin, endotoxin, bacterial vaginosis and cervical length as predictors of preterm birth and neonatal morbidity in twin pregnancies. *Br J Obstet Gynecol* 104 (2):1398–1404.

Wenstom KD, CH Syrop, DG Hammitt et al. 1993. Increased risk of monochorionic twinning associated with assisted reproduction. *Fertil Steril* 60:510–514.

Winn HN, J Cimino, J Powers et al. 2001. Intrapartum management of nonvertex second-born twins: a critical analysis. *Am J Obstet Gynecol* 185: 1204–1208.

Winsor EJT, BST Brown, ER Luther et al. 1987. Deceased co-twin as a cause of false positive amniotic fluid AFP and AChE. *Prenat Diagn* 7:485–489.

20

Prolonged Pregnancy

Shripad Hebbar

Introduction

Post-term, postdates, prolonged and postmature are the terms accepted by the World Health Organization (1994) to describe a pregnancy that continues beyond 42 weeks, or 294 days, from the first day of the last menstrual period. Imprecision in terminology, along with varying definitions of the upper limit of normal pregnancy, makes the search for information in published literature difficult. Hence, the term 'prolonged pregnancy', which is an apt description of this condition, is used in this chapter.

The estimated date of confinement, or due date, for normal pregnancies is calculated as 38 weeks after conception, or 40 weeks after the first day of the last normal menstrual period (assuming a 'normal' 28-day menstrual cycle). Prolonged pregnancy has traditionally been defined as a pregnancy that extends two weeks or more beyond the estimated day of confinement. Approximately 18% of pregnancies in the United States extend beyond 41 weeks, while 7% extend beyond 42 weeks. The perinatal mortality rate doubles by 42 weeks of gestation (4–7 against 2–3 per 1000 deliveries), rises fourfold by 43 weeks, and five to sevenfold by 44 weeks.

Prolonged pregnancy has gained prominence in the last decade as a probable high-risk condition after widespread use of antenatal testing. The policy of routine induction of labour at 41 weeks has contributed to a decline in the incidence of prolonged pregnancy from 4.6% to 2.8% in New South Wales.

Etiology

The incidence of prolonged pregnancy is often overestimated because of an error in determining the patient's due date. The use of the last menstrual period (LMP) to determine the gestational age is fraught with inaccuracy. The biological variations in the follicular and luteal phases of the menstrual cycle add to the problem (Table 20.1).

Labour is a poorly defined, biological process that involves fetal, placental and maternal signals. Recent research suggests that human parturition is determined by the placental release of the corticotrophin-releasing hormone (CRH) and that women who have low levels of this hormone are more likely to deliver beyond their due date.

A defect in the fetal hypothalamic–pituitary–adrenal axis contributes to loss of normal mechanisms that initiate labour at term. Abnormalities of the central nervous system, such as anencephaly have been associated with prolonged pregnancy, for the same reason. The role of fetal adrenal glands in the initiation of labour was highlighted by Naeye, who documented marked adrenal hypoplasia in 10 out of 19 post-term fetuses with lethal congenital malformations.

Low estrogen level at term has also been implicated in the etiology of prolonged pregnancy. Sulfatase and aromatase are the key enzymes of estrogen biosynthesis in the human placenta. Placental sulfatase deficiency (X-linked recessive disorder) leads to prolongation of pregnancy and difficulties in both cervical ripening and labour induction.

Other suggested risk factors are primiparity, sedentary lifestyle and previous history of prolonged pregnancy. The role of primary prostaglandins (such as PGE2 and PGF2) as uterine stimulants is well established. Recently, it has been suggested that the use of NSAIDs during pregnancy may lead to prolonged pregnancy by their action on prostaglandin synthesis.

Risks of Prolonged Gestation

Prolonged pregnancies are associated with numerous adverse outcomes (Table 20.2).

Fetal risks are generally related to uteroplacental insufficiency, intrauterine hypoxia and oligoamnios. Prolonged pregnancies are associated with a higher rate of intrapartum fetal heart rate abnormalities, meconium staining of the amniotic fluid, low umbilical artery pH and low 5-minute Apgar scores.

Oligoamnios (AFI <5 cm) has been reported in 10–15% of prolonged pregnancies. It has been hypothesised that fetal hypoxemia may result in redistribution of blood flow with decreased renal perfusion and diminished fetal urine production. A vicious cycle could develop with oligoamnios causing cord compression, resulting in further hypoxemia, oligoamnios and fetal heart rate abnormalities. Severe intrauterine hypoxia

Table 20.1: Causes of Prolonged Gestation

1. Errors in estimation of expected date of delivery
2. Maternal factors
   a. Biological variability in follicular phase of menstruation
   b. Primiparity
   c. Previous history of prolonged pregnancy
   d. ? Sedentary lifestyle, use of NSAIDs
3. Fetal factors—Congenital malformations (for example, anencephaly, adrenal hypoplasia)
4. Placental factors—Sulphatase deficiency

Table 20.2: Risks Associated with Prolonged Pregnancy

Neonatal risks	*Maternal risks*
• Asphyxia • Aspiration • Bone fracture • Perinatal death • Peripheral nerve paralysis • Pneumonia	• Emergency cesarean delivery • Cephalopelvic disproportion • Cervical rupture • Dystocia • Dysfunctional labour • Postpartum hemorrhage • Puerperal infection

Olesen AW, Westergaard JG, Olsen J. 1978–1993. Perinatal and maternal complications related to postterm delivery: a national register-based study. Am J Obstet Gynecol 2003; 189:224.

results in relaxation of rectal sphincters and hence, meconium staining of liquor leading to meconium aspiration syndrome.

Not surprisingly, fetal macrosomia is also more common in post-term infants, leading to a greater risk of dysfunctional labour, cephalopelvic disproportion, cesarean delivery and shoulder dystocia. Finally, post-term fetuses are more likely to die within the first year of life. Although peripartum complications (such as meconium aspiration syndrome) account for the deaths of some of these infants, the vast majority are unexplained.

In first describing fetal dysmaturity (postmaturity) syndrome in 1954, Clifford included subcutaneous wasting, cutaneous peeling, dry cracked skin, absence of vernix (stage I postmaturity), meconium staining and birth asphyxia (stage II postmaturity), and respiratory distress, convulsions and neonatal death (stage III postmaturity) in a post-term infant. He attributed these changes to placental senescence and dysfunction. Of late, researchers have been using this term to describe infants with intrauterine growth restriction resulting from chronic uteroplacental insufficiency.

This syndrome complicates roughly one in five prolonged pregnancies. It is linked with increased risk of umbilical cord compression from oligoamnios, no reassuring antepartum or intrapartum fetal testing, meconium aspiration and short-term neonatal complications such as hypoglycemia, seizures and respiratory insufficiency.

A prolonged pregnancy does not affect the fetus alone. Usually overlooked, maternal risks of prolonged pregnancy (Table 20.2) include labour dystocia, cesarean delivery and third or fourth degree perineal laceration. All of these complications appear to be related to fetal macrosomia.

Diagnosis

Diagnosis of prolonged gestation should be made on the basis of the best available estimation of the duration of gestation at the time of delivery. It is now apparent that the clinical estimation of gestational age is inferior to sonographic measurements obtained in early pregnancy. Numerous studies have shown that the incidence of prolonged pregnancy drastically falls by as much as one-fifth if ultrasound dating is used. The error in gestational dating by LMP is mainly due to poor recall by the patient. It is, however, important to recognise that even when the LMP is recalled with certainty, it is not a good predictor of ovulation, and that physiological variations in the duration of the follicular phase may result in an error that favours an overestimation of the true gestational age. Table 20.3 lists the methods used to confirm term pregnancy when LMP is not reliable.

Fetal Surveillance Beyond Term

Women who opt for conservative management beyond 41 weeks are generally advised to participate in some form of fetal assessment while awaiting spontaneous onset of labour. These tests include fetal movement counting, NST, ultrasound assessment of amniotic fluid, biophysical profile and Doppler studies. However, it should be remembered that, to date, no programme of fetal testing has been shown to completely eliminate the risk of stillbirth. On the other hand, false-positive tests may lead to unnecessary interventions that are potentially hazardous to the gravid woman.

Fetal movement counting should be done on a daily basis and any reduced movements should lead to further intensive monitoring. Two randomised trials, involving more than 68,000 women, have proved that routine formal fetal movement counting alone does not reduce the incidence of intrauterine death in late pregnancy.

Antenatal cardiotocography (CTG) has been widely used for more than 20 years to monitor high-risk pregnancies on a biweekly basis. Recent systematic reviews involving four large, randomised, controlled trials have suggested that antenatal CTG does not have a significant effect on perinatal outcome. It must be remembered that a reactive NST provides only short-term reassurance about fetal well-being, probably 24 hours at most.

It has been well documented that an AFI of less than 5 cm is indicative of oligoamnios and should be considered an indicator for termination of pregnancy. A recent meta-analysis involving 18 series and 10,551 patients has suggested that AFI <5 cm is associated with an increased risk of cesarean delivery for fetal distress and low Apgar score. However, it should be remembered that up to 50% of patients, who are diagnosed with oligoamnios by ultrasound, have a normal volume of amniotic fluid upon artificial rupture of membranes.

A biophysical profile usually includes ultrasound monitoring of fetal movements, tone and breathing, amniotic fluid volume and an assessment of fetal heart rate by electronic monitoring. The primary disadvantages of biophysical profile scoring are the time required to perform the test and the need for an experienced sonographer. This can be alleviated to some extent by adopting a modified biophysical profile wherein only NST and AFI values are used. A recent systematic review concluded that there was not enough evidence from randomised trials to suggest that biophysical profiles could be used as a test of fetal well-being in high-risk pregnancies. Though observational studies have indicated that low biophysical scores identify babies at high risk of adverse outcomes, this should not be interpreted as sufficient proof to prevent these outcomes.

Recently, Doppler ultrasound has been applied to investigate fetal circulation, in an attempt to identify perturbations that may be associated with adverse outcomes. Pulsatility index (PI) for the fetal middle cerebral artery (MCA), renal artery, umbilical artery, inferior vena cava (IVC) and ductus venosus have been studied. A recent study concluded that oligoamnios in prolonged pregnancies was associated with arterial redistribution of fetal blood flow, typifying the brain sparing effect, with decreased resistance in the MCA and increased resistance in the fetal IVC.

Timing of Induction

In the early 1970s, obstetric units in some countries routinely offered induction at term. Four randomised trials compared the policy of routine induction at 40 weeks with expectant management and found no major benefits.

Many trials in the past have compared

Table 20.3: Confirmation of Term Gestation

- Fetal heart tones have been documented for 20 weeks by nonelectronic fetoscope or 30 weeks by Doppler.
- It has been 36 weeks since a positive serum or urine hCG pregnancy test was performed by a reliable method.
- An ultrasound measurement of the crown-rump length, obtained at 6–12 weeks of gestation, supports a gestational age of at least 39 weeks.
- An ultrasound scan obtained at 13–20 weeks of gestation, confirms a gestational age of at least 39 weeks as determined by clinical history and physical examination.

the outcome of induction of labour at 41 weeks versus expectant management, the largest being the Canadian Multicenter Post-term Pregnancy Trial (CMPPT) Group in 1992. The expectant management group had a significantly higher rate of cesarean deliveries resulting from fetal distress, but there was no difference between the groups in the rate of cesarean deliveries resulting from dystocia. Again, no differences were found in neonatal morbidity outcomes. Subsequently, the Society of Obstetricians and Gynecologists of Canada (SOGC) issued guidelines in 1997, encouraging the routine induction of labour at 41 weeks of gestation. A systematic Cochrane Review of 19 RCTs found that induction of labour was associated with benefits such as reduced risk of perinatal death, decreased incidence of meconium stained liquor and no increased cesarean rates.

Interestingly, an updated ACOG evidence-based guideline released in 1997 does not describe an upper gestational age limit for expectant management. It does, however, recommend that fetal health assessments should begin by 42 weeks of gestation.

Management

Despite many years of research, the optimal management of prolonged pregnancy is still controversial. However, these pregnancies have traditionally been considered to be at increased risk of adverse perinatal outcome, and it should not be forgotten that, unlike preterm labour and birth, the risks associated with prolonged pregnancy can be almost entirely prevented by timely delivery.

Figure 20.1: Management of prolonged pregnancy

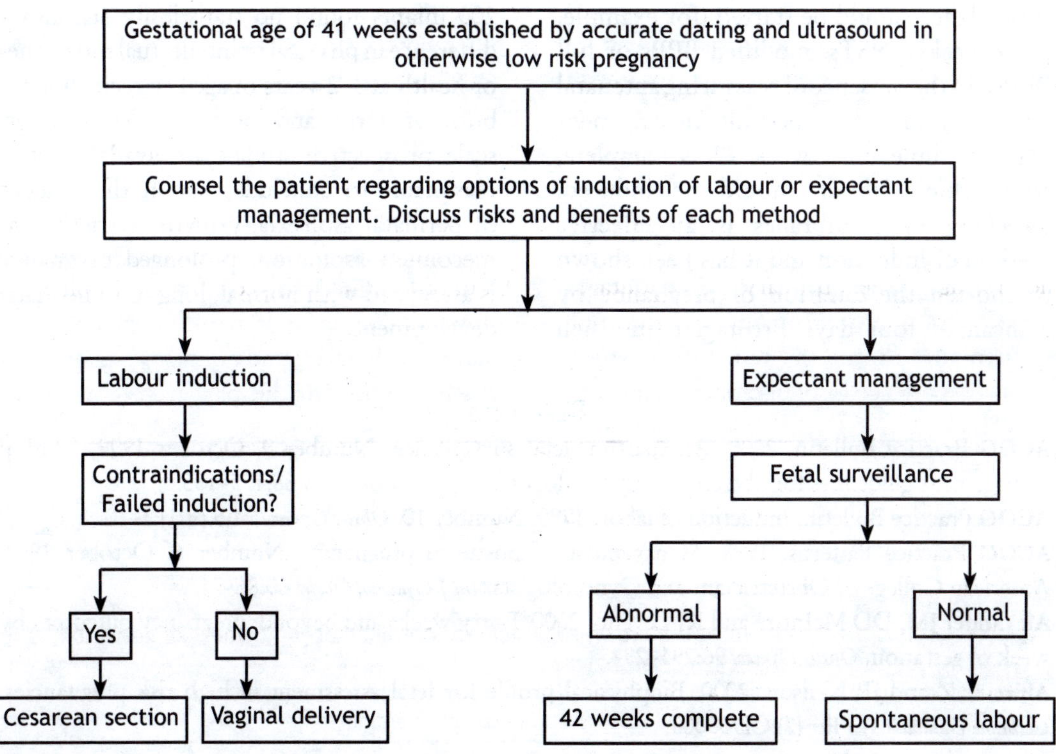

Initially, it is critical to establish an appropriate estimation of gestational age. At a minimum, the criteria to ensure fetal maturity must be met before labour induction can be considered (Table 20.2).

Pregnancies complicated by gestational diabetes, hypertension or other high-risk conditions should be managed according to the specific guidelines. An algorithm for the management of low-risk, prolonged pregnancies is given in Figure 20.1.

The risks and benefits of labour induction versus expectant management should be discussed with the patient at 41 weeks of gestation. With appropriate obstetric and neonatal care, the absolute mortality rate is low in both options. If the patient desires labour induction and there are no contraindications, the procedure can be scheduled immediately. If she desires continued expectant management, antenatal surveillance should be started (for example, twice-weekly NSTs, modified BPPs or full BPPs). In the presence of reassuring antenatal fetal surveillance, expectant management may continue until week 42 is complete, after which labour should be induced. Sweeping of membranes is an effective method of induction and it has been shown to shorten the duration of pregnancy by a mean of four days. Prostaglandins such as dinoprostone (PGE_2) and misoprostol (PGE_1 analogue) have been extensively used and are more effective and safe in prolonged pregnancy for induction of labour.

Influence of Prolonged Pregnancy on Infant Development

Although prolonged pregnancy has been associated with a twofold to sevenfold increase in perinatal morbidity and mortality, few investigators have addressed the question of long-term outcome for post-term infants. The existing information, spanning several decades, is confounded by several factors, such as different treatment eras, different population demographics, limited predictive value of testing preschool children, absence of term controls, retrospective nature of many surveys and unreliable criteria used to define prolonged pregnancy.

One prospective study of more than 200 infants found no statistically significant difference in physical or intellectual milestones or health at 1–2 years of age between children born at term and post-term. Until large-scale prospective studies are available, it is reasonable to conclude that in the absence of perinatal asphyxia, growth restriction or meconium aspiration, prolonged pregnancy is associated with normal, long-term neonatal development.

Refeences

ACOG Practice Bulletin. 2000. Antepartum fetal surveillance. Number 9, October 1999. Clinical management guidelines for obstetrician-gynecologists. *Int J Gynaecol Obstet* 68:175–185.

ACOG Practice Bulletin. Induction of labor. 1999. Number 10. *Obstet Gynecol* 94(5 pt 1):1–10.

ACOG Practice Patterns. 1998. Management of postterm pregnancy. Number 6, October 1997. American College of Obstetricians and Gynecologists. *Int J Gynaecol Obstet* 60:86–91.

Alexander JM, DD McIntire and KJ Leveno. 2000. Forty weeks and beyond: pregnancy outcomes by week of gestation. *Obstet Gynecol* 96:291–294.

Alfirevic Z and JP Neilson. 2000. Biophysical profile for fetal assessment in high risk pregnancies. *Cochrane Database Syst Rev* (2):CD00003.

Boulvain M and O Irion. 2000. Stripping/sweeping the membranes for inducing labour or preventing post-term pregnancy. *Cochrane Database Syst Rev* (2):CD000451.

Breart G, J Gourjard, F Maillard, C Chavigny et al. 1982. Comparison of two obstetrical policies with regard to artificial induction at term. A randomised trial. *J Obstet Biol Reprod (Paris)* 11:107.

Campbell MK, T Ostbye and LM Irgens. 1997. Post-term birth: risk factors and outcomes in a 10-year cohort of Norwegian births. *Obstet Gynecol* 89(4):543–548.

Chauhan SP, M Sanderson, NW Hendrix, EF Magann and LD Devoe. 1999. Perinatal outcome and amniotic fluid index in the antepartum and intrapartum periods: A meta-analysis. *Am J Obstet Gynecol* 181(6):1473–1478.

Clifford SH. 1954. Postmaturity, with placental dysfunction; clinical syndrome and pathologic findings. *J Pediatr* 44:1–13.

Cotzias CS, S Paterson-Brown and NM Fisk. 1999. Prospective risk of unexplained stillbirth in singleton pregnancies at term: population based analysis. *BMJ* 319:287–288.

Crowley P, C O'Herlihy and P Boylan. 1984. The value of ultrasound measurement of amniotic fluid volume in the management of prolonged pregnancies. *Br J Obstet Gynaecol* 91(5):444–448.

Crowley P. 2004. Interventions for preventing or improving the outcome of delivery at or beyond term. *Cochrane Database Syst Rev* (3):CD000170.

Divon MY, AD Marks and CE Henderson. 1995. Longitudinal measurement of amniotic fluid index in postterm pregnancies and its association with fetal outcome. *Am J Obstet Gynecol* 172(1 Pt 1): 142–146.

Eden RD, LS Seifert, A Winegar and WN Spellacy. 1987. Postdate pregnancies: a review of 46 perinatal deaths. *Am J Perinatol* 4(4):284–287.

Eden RD, LS Seifert, A Winegar and WN Spellacy. 1988. Maternal risk status and postdate pregnancy outcome. *J Reprod Med* 33(1):53–57.

Egarter CH, E Kofler, R Fitz and P Husselein. 1989. Is induction of labour indicated in prolonged pregnancy? Results of a prospective randomised trial. *Gynecol Obstet Invest* 27:6.

Gardosi J and RT Geirsson. 1998. Routine ultrasound is the method of choice for dating pregnancy. *Br J Obstet Gynaecol* 105(9):933–936.

Gardosi J, T Vanner and A Francis. 1997. Gestational age and induction of labour for prolonged pregnancy. *Br J Obstet Gynaecol* 104(7):792–797.

Grant A, D Melbourne, L Valentine and S Alexander. 1989. Routine formal fetal movement counting and risk of antepartum late death in normally formed singletons. *Lancet* 12;2(8659):345–349.

Hannah ME, WJ Hannah, J Hellmann, S Hewson, R Milner and A Willan. 1992. Induction of labor as compared with serial antenatal monitoring in post-term pregnancy. A randomized controlled trial. The Canadian Multicenter Post-term Pregnancy Trial Group. *N Engl J Med* 11; 326(24):1587–1592.

Hilder L, K Costeloe and B Thilaganathan. 1998. Prolonged pregnancy: evaluating gestation-specific risks of fetal and infant mortality. *Br J Obstet Gynaecol* 105:169–173.

Hollis B. 2002. Prolonged pregnancy. *Curr Opin Obstet Gynecol* 14:203–207.

Lee HY. 1997. A randomised double-blind study of vaginal misoprostol vs dinoprostone for cervical ripening and labour induction in prolonged pregnancy. *Singapore Med J* 38(7):292–294.

Liggins GC. 2000. The role of the hypothalamic-pituitary-adrenal axis in preparing the fetus for birth. *Am J Obstet Gynecol* 182(2):475–477.

Mannino F. 1988. Neonatal complications of postterm gestation. *J Reprod Med* 33:271–276.

Naeye RL. 1978. Causes of perinatal mortality excess in prolonged gestations. *Am J Epidemiol* 108(5):429–433.

Neldam S. 1986. Fetal movements as an indicator of fetal well-being. *Dan Med Bull* 33(5):213–221.

Nguyen TH, T Larsen, G Engholm and H Moller. 1999. Evaluation of ultrasound-estimated date of delivery in 17,450 spontaneous singleton births: do we need to modify Naegele's rule? *Ultrasound Obstet Gynecol* 14(1):23–28.

Olesen AW, JG Westergaard and J Olesen. 2003. Perinatal and maternal complications related to postterm delivery: a National register-based study, 1978–1993. *Am J Obstet Gynecol* 189:222–227.

Pattison N and L McGowan. 2000. Cardiotocography for antepartum fetal assessment. *Cochrane Database Syst Rev* (2):CD001068.

Rabe T, R Hosch and B Runnebaum. 1983. Sulfatase deficiency in the human placenta: clinical findings. *Biol Res Pregnancy Perinatol* 4(3):95–102.

Roberts CL and D Taylor Henderson-Smart. 1999. Trends in births at and beyond term: evidence of a change? *Br J Obstet Gynaecol* 106: 937–942

Rosen MG and JC Dickinson. 1992. Management of post-term pregnancy. *N Engl J Med* 326:1628–1629.

Sande HA, J Tuveng and T Fonstelien. 1983. A prospective randomized study of induction of labor. *Int J Gynaecol Obstet* 21(4):333–336.

Selma B, R Kokkali and T Oscan. 2000. Fetal arterial and venous Doppler parameters in the interpretation of oligohydramnios in postterm pregnancies. *Ultrasound Obstet Gynecol* 15(5):403–406.

Shame J. 1988. Influence of prolonged pregnancy on infant development. *J Reprod Med* 33(3): 277–284.

Shime J, CL Librach, DJ Gare et al. 1986. The influence of prolonged pregnancy on infant development at one and two years of age: a prospective controlled study. *Am J Obstet Gynecol* 154: 341–345.

Smith GC. 2001. Life-table analysis of the risk of perinatal death at term and post term in singleton pregnancies. *Am J Obstet Gynecol* 184:489–496.

Smith R. 1999. The timing of birth. *Sci Am* 280(3):68–75

Society of Obstetricians and Gynecologists of Canada. 1997. SOGC clinical practice guidelines. Post-term pregnancy.

Spellacy WN, S Miller, A Winegar et al. 1985. Macrosomia maternal characteristics and infant complications. *Obstet Gynecol* 66:158–161.

Treger M, M Hallak, T Silberstein et al. 2002. Post-term pregnancy: should induction of labor be considered before 42 weeks? *J Matern Fetal Neonatal Med* 11:50–53.

Tylleskar J, O Finnstrom, I Leijon, S Hedenskog and G Ryden. 1979. Spontaneous labor and elective induction–a prospective randomized study. I. Effects on mother and fetus. *Acta Obstet Gynecol Scand* 58(6):513–518.

Vorherr H. 1975. Placental insufficiency in relation to postterm pregnancy and fetal postmaturity. Evaluation of fetoplacental function; management of the postterm gravida. *Am J Obstet Gynecol* 123:67–103.

21

Pre-eclampsia and Eclampsia

Vani Ramkumar

Introduction

Hypertensive disorders of pregnancy constitute the most common medical disorder encountered by obstetricians. The incidence is 7–10%, of which pre-eclampsia/eclampsia constitutes 70% and chronic hypertension 30%. The incidence of eclampsia is one in 100 to 1 in 2000 pregnancies. It remains one of the leading causes of maternal death worldwide, accounting for 15–20% of maternal deaths, in developing as well as developed nations (August 1999).

Pre-eclampsia/eclampsia is a multiorgan disorder unique to human pregnancy. It is a common, dangerous and poorly understood condition. Pritchard stated that the presence of chorionic villi in certain women incites vasospasm, hypertension and serious organ dysfunction, especially of the placenta, kidneys, liver and sometimes the brain (Ramin 1999). In eclampsia, cerebral involvement and convulsions are seen. The clinical course is progressive and characterised by continuous deterioration that is arrested only by delivery. This disease must be detected in the early stages and managed appropriately for improved maternal and fetal outcome.

Classification

The Report of the National High Blood Pressure Education Program Working Group on High Blood Pressure in Pregnancy (2000) has classified these hypertensive disorders as follows:

- Gestational hypertension
- Pre-eclampsia
- Eclampsia
- Pre-eclampsia superimposed on chronic hypertension
- Chronic hypertension

The Working Group (2000) has recommended that the term 'gestational hypertension' replace 'pregnancy-induced hypertension' to describe cases in which elevated blood pressure (BP), without proteinuria, develops in women after 20 weeks of gestation and the BP levels return to normal postpartum. As many as one quarter of women with gestational hypertension develop proteinuria, that is, pre-eclampsia (Saudan et al 1998).

Definition

The classic features of pre-eclampsia are hypertension with proteinuria or edema, or both. The condition occurs after 20 weeks, most often in nulliparas, and the diagnosis is more easily made when women have well-documented normotension in early pregnancy. A BP reading of >140/90 mm Hg (two readings, 6 hours apart) with a proteinuria of 300 mg/L in 24-hour urine or 1 g/L in two random specimens, 6 hours apart, with edema or weight gain is diagnostic of pre-eclampsia. In addition, when convulsions or coma occurs, it is known as eclampsia.

The criteria of increase in BP levels above the baseline of >30 mm Hg systolic, >15 mm Hg diastolic or >20 mm Hg mean arterial pressure are no longer used (Moldenhauer and Simbai 2003). According to the Working Group (2000), women who demonstrate an elevation of more than 30 mm Hg systolic or 15 mm Hg diastolic above the baseline 'warrant close observation'. It is important to note that choosing the appropriate size cuff will help to render more accurate readings. Based on recent evidence, Korotkoff V should be used as a measure of diastolic BP. Although validated electronic devices can be used, a mercury sphygmomanometer is preferred because it is the most accurate device.

Many women have mid-pregnancy blood pressure levels as low as 90/60 mm Hg. Failure to appreciate that seemingly 'normal' levels of BP can be abnormal is one reason why the diagnosis of pre-eclampsia may be missed in the early stages.

Proteinuria is one of the classic laboratory features of pre-eclampsia; and although it frequently appears late in the course of the disease, its presence greatly bolsters the diagnosis. The degree of proteinuria may fluctuate widely over any 24-hour period, even in severe cases. Therefore, a single random sample may fail to demonstrate proteinuria. Poor perinatal outcome is usually seen in patients who have hypertension plus proteinuria (Hauth et al 2000).

Edema frequently accompanies normal gestation. Sudden and rapid weight gain often precedes overt manifestations of the disease. On the other hand, severe disease can occur even in the absence of edema (the 'dry' pre-eclamptic). Lower extremity edema is the most typical form. Pathological edema is seen in nondependent regions such as the face, hands, abdominal wall or lungs.

Coma is extremely rare, but when it occurs in the setting of pre-eclampsia/eclampsia, it is a harbinger of a poor prognosis.

Etiopathology

The etiology is still largely unknown. Hence, treatment remains a challenge and is mainly empirical. For many years, the hypertensive disorders of gestation were labelled toxemia of pregnancy. This term was used because it was felt that all the varieties of this disorder had a circulating toxin as a common etiological agent. This has now been proved to be untrue. Recent evidence suggests that there may be several underlying causes or predispositions leading to the signs of hypertension, proteinuria and edema—findings that allow us to make the diagnosis of the 'syndrome' of pre-eclampsia.

The immunological theory states that the primary problem lies in the placental bed. It could be because of a lack of blocking antibodies or an antigenic overload, as in hyperplacentosis. Poor spiral artery remodelling is frequently cited as the initiating feature in pre-eclampsia (Zhou 1997). Normal placentation involves invasion of the spiral artery walls by endovascular trophoblasts which migrate in a retrograde fashion, involving first the decidual segment in the second month of gestation and then the myometrial segments in the fifth month, causing considerable disruption at all layers of the vessel wall. Loss of the endothelial and muscular layers makes these vessels unresponsive to vasomotor stimuli. The arteries, therefore, remain thick-walled and muscular; the diameters in the myometrial segments being half of those measured during normal pregnancy. It has been suggested that the primary event for the development of pre-eclampsia is a failure of the second wave of trophoblast invasion at 16–20 weeks of gestation that is responsible for the destruction of the muscularis layer of the spiral arterioles. To be more precise, the primary invasion of trophoblasts is partially impaired, and the second wave fails to occur, or is limited. This failure is, most likely, a result of an immunologically induced error in the cell surface receptors of the trophoblast. The placental dysfunction leads to widespread vasospasm and endothelial injury. Obstruction of the spiral arteriolar lumen by atherosis (foam cells in the damaged vessel wall) may impair placental blood flow. These changes are not specific to pre-eclampsia and also occur in intrauterine growth restriction (IUGR) without pre-eclampsia.

Compared with other circulating cells in the body, trophoblast cells do not express the classic HLA antigens; rather, they express a non-classical antigen, HLA-G, which may have an important role in protecting the placenta from the deleterious effects of a local maternal immune response. Placental tissue from pre-eclamptic pregnancies express less, or different, HLA-G and researchers postulate that this may result in a breakdown in maternal tolerance to the immunologically foreign placenta.

The observation that pre-eclampsia occurs primarily in nulliparous women, whose subsequent gestations tend to be uncomplicated thereafter, unless there is a change in paternity, has been cited as evidence of alterations in immune response as a factor in pathogenesis. Epidemiological reports also indicate that the prevalence of pre-eclampsia decreased in women who received heterologous blood transfusions, practiced oral sex or had a long period of cohabitation that preceded an established pregnancy, suggesting that prior exposure to paternal antigens might be protective.

Endothelial dysfunction evidence for endothelial dysfunction has been demonstrated in pre-eclampsia and this is thought to be a consequence of placental ischemia and/or immune maladaptation (Dekker and Sibai 1998). An exaggerated inflammatory response, T helper-1 (Th-1) cytokines and subsequent oxidative stress have been proposed as the final common pathway in the causation of inappropriate endothelial cell activation/damage (Roberts and Hubel 1999). In a setting of reduced placental perfusion, low density lipoproteins (LDLs) are easily oxidisable and are protected from circulating antioxidants by preferentially accessing the subendothelial space. Once oxidised, the LDLs alter membrane proteins and phospholipids, thereby modifying endothelial cell wall integrity and function. Oxidised LDLs may also impair nitric oxide-mediated vasorelaxation (Witztum 1994). Transfer of this oxidative stress to maternal systemic circulation from decidual vessels can be explained by activation of neutrophils and monocytes in the intervillous spaces, which then generate free radicals on contact with the endothelium (Roberts and Cooper 2001). The large trials of antioxidants, currently underway, may provide further insight into the pathogenetic relevance of free radical species.

Thromboxane The ratio between **thromboxane** (released from platelets) and prostacyclin (released from the vessel wall) is altered in favour of the former.

Vascular sensitivity There is an increase in **vascular sensitivity**, as is evident from the angiotensin II sensitivity test. The underlying mechanism responsible for the increased vascular reactivity is presumed to result from alterations in the normal interactions of vasodilatory (prostacyclin, nitric oxide) and vasoconstrictive (thromboxane A_2, endothelin) substances. The vasospasm and subsequent hemoconcentration are associated with contraction of the intravascular space. Because of capillary leak and decreased colloid oncotic pressure, attempts to expand the intravascular space in these women with vigorous fluid therapy may result in elevation of the pulmonary capillary wedge pressure and even pulmonary edema.

LOWER INTRAVASCULAR VOLUMES Patients with pre-eclampsia have **lower intravascular volumes** and less tolerance for the blood loss associated with delivery. The reduced plasma volume contraindicates the use of diuretics. This is also the reason for the presence of IUGR.

SLOW DISSEMINATED INTRAVASCULAR COAGULATION A **slow disseminated intravascular coagulation** occurs. According to Sibai (2002), abnormalities of aberrant platelet and vessel wall interactions are thought to be caused by microangiopathy. Damage to the endothelial cells of the vessel wall triggers an increase in platelet aggregation. This in turn gives way to changes in the production of various coagulation factors, which ultimately results in increased thrombin and fibrin formation.

RENAL LESION The typical **renal lesion** is glomeruloendotheliosis, which is the swelling of the glomerular capillary endothelial and mesangial cells. Renal perfusion in pre-eclampsia is less than in normal pregnancy. Uric acid secretion predominantly decreases because of the enhanced tubular reabsorption and decreased renal clearance, resulting in a higher than normal plasma level in pre-eclampsia. Plasma uric acid levels generally correlate with the severity of disease, and high levels have been associated with poor fetal outcome. In one study, the mean uric acid level of normal pregnant women was 3.8 mg/dl, whereas it was 6.7 mg/dl in pre-eclampsia, with levels reaching 9 mg/dl in severe cases.

CHANGES IN EYE, LIVER AND BRAIN Changes also occur in the fundus of the **eye, liver and brain**. Findings at fundoscopy include vasospasm, hemorrhages, exudates, papilledema and retinal detachment. If immediate delivery is achieved, retinal detachment is reversible. Hepatic damage can range from mildly elevated liver enzyme levels to subcapsular liver hematomas and hepatic rupture. Eclamptic convulsions are perhaps the most disturbing central nervous system (CNS) manifestation of severe pre-eclampsia. The exact etiology of eclampsia is unknown, but it is thought to be attributed to coagulopathy, fibrin deposition and vasospasm. Radiological studies may show evidence of cerebral edema and hemorrhagic lesions, particularly in the posterior hemispheres, which may explain the visual disturbances seen in pre-eclampsia. Other CNS abnormalities include headaches and visual disturbances such as scotomata, blurred vision and, rarely, temporary blindness.

TRANSMISSION The transmission from mother to daughter is through **HLA DR4.** Daughters are 4–5 times more likely to develop the syndrome than daughters-in-law. How the genotype results in the characteristic placental lesion is not known but is thought to involve an immunological defect resulting in failure to establish tolerance to the fetal allograft.

There are three levels of pathology of pre-eclampsia (Chamberlain 1995). The primary pathology is of the placental bed. The secondary pathology comprises the subclinical signs, while the tertiary pathology comprises crises caused by the progression of secondary pathology, leading to decompensation of one system or another; for example, eclampsia, retinal detachment and the HELLP (hemolysis, elevated liver enzymes, low platelets) syndrome.

Risk Factors for Pre-eclampsia (Dekker et al 1995)

Patient-related factors

- Nulliparity
- Extremes of age
- Family history of pre-eclampsia
- Past history of pre-eclampsia
- Specific underlying maternal disorders
  - Essential hypertension
  - Underlying renal disease
- Obesity
- Insulin resistance/Diabetes
- Thrombophilias
- Autoimmune disorders (for example, systemic lupus erythematosus)

Partner-related factors

- Primipaternity
- Limited sperm exposure
  - o Donor insemination
  - o Oocyte donation
- Partner who fathered a pre-eclamptic pregnancy in another woman

Pregnancy-associated factors

- Multiple pregnancy
- Hydrops fetalis
- Chromosomal anomalies (trisomy 13, triploidy)
- Hydatidiform mole

Women with thrombophilias, both inherited and acquired, may be more likely to develop pre-eclampsia. This tendency has been seen in women with antiphospholipid antibody (APLA) syndrome, factor V Leiden deficiency, activated protein C resistance and hyperhomocysteinemia. Hyperhomocysteinemia is a risk factor for pre-eclampsia, presumably because of the toxic effect of homocysteine on the endothelium. It may therefore be of value to check the status of folic acid and vitamins B6 and B12 in women with adverse pregnancy outcome, as a deficiency of these vitamins can lead to acquired hyperhomocysteinemia. The association of the APLA syndrome with early severe pre-eclampsia has been established. Thrombophilias may contribute to uteroplacental thrombosis that is frequently seen in pre-eclampsia (Said and Dekker 2003).

Higher levels of triglycerides and lipoproteins have been found in women with severe pre-eclampsia, with or without the HELLP syndrome, when compared to healthy pregnant women. They postulated that triglyceride-rich particles might play an important role in thrombin generation and platelet aggregation.

Pre-eclampsia is characterised by the unpredictable nature of its clinical course. Women with mildly elevated BP and even minimal proteinuria can rapidly progress to eclampsia.

- The HELLP syndrome occurred in 20% of women with severe pre-eclampsia (Sibai 1990). As with severe pre-eclampsia, the HELLP syndrome is associated with an increased risk of adverse outcomes, including placental abruption, renal failure, subcapsular hepatic hematoma, recurrent pre-eclampsia, preterm delivery, and even fetal or maternal death.
- Approximately 20% of eclamptic patients and 15% of patients with the HELLP syndrome are normotensive (Anumba and Robson 1999).
- 'Atypical eclampsia' is the term given to the absence of high BP or if the convulsion occurs after the seventh postpartum day.

- It is important to emphasise that pre-eclampsia is a multisystem disorder, but the organ system that is likely to be predominantly affected cannot be predicted. Thus, hypertension is only one sign, albeit the most common one, of pre-eclampsia.

The one thing that is universally accepted is that a placenta is required for the development and maintenance of pre-eclampsia; and delivery is the ultimate cure (Walker 1998).

Predictive Tests

Though the following tests are recommended, they are of limited use:

- *Roll over test*: A hypertensive response (elevation of diastolic BP by at least 20 mm Hg) induced by having women at 28–32 weeks of gestation assume the supine position after lying laterally recumbent predicts gestational hypertension (Gant et al 1974).
- *Angiotensin sensitivity test*: A woman destined to get pre-eclampsia will respond to less than 8 ng/kg/min of an angiotensin infusion due to an alteration in vessel wall refractoriness (Gant et al 1974). This test is done between 26 and 30 weeks.
- *Platelet volume*: Thrombocytopenia and platelet dysfunction are integral features of pre-eclampsia. Increased destruction causes platelet volumes to increase because of relatively younger, and therefore larger, platelets (megakaryocytes) entering the circulation. Ahmed and associates (1993) found high platelet volumes to be a marker of impending pre-eclampsia but with a substantive overlap with normotensive women. In a study by Hutt (1994), a mean platelet volume ≥11 Fl at 28 weeks of gestation was found to be associated with subsequent pre-eclampsia. He stated that platelet consumption is a late finding in pre-eclampsia, but increased platelet turnover may be an early marker of pre-eclampsia.
- *Serum fibronectin*: Endothelial cell activation is the likely cause of elevated serum cellular fibronectin levels in some women with pre-eclampsia (Halligan et al 1994). In one study, though levels rose within 12 weeks in those destined to get pre-eclampsia, the positive predictive value was only 29%; however, the negative predictive value was 98% (Chavarria et al 2003).
- *Uterine artery Doppler velocimetry*: Uterine artery impedance between 18 and 26 weeks has been used as an early screening test for women at risk of pre-eclampsia. The presence of a high systolic–diastolic ratio and persistence of diastolic notch may predict pre-eclampsia or IUGR (Irion et al 1998).
- *Antithrombin III levels*: Antithrombin, which binds to and inactivates thrombin, is reduced, in keeping with thrombin generation, and correlates with maternal and perinatal outcome.
- *Urinary kallikrein excretion*: Inactive urinary kallikrein–creatinine ratio of ≤170 between 16 and 20 weeks of pregnancy predicts future development of pre-eclampsia. The sensitivity of this test is 70% and specificity is 86% (Miller 1996). Protein C inhibitor is decreased by kallikrein, which is elevated due to activation of the intrinsic coagulation pathway.
- *Urinary calcium excretion*: Pre-eclampsia is characterised by marked reduction in the fractional excretion of calcium, leading to striking hypocalciuria. The hypocalciuria may be due to increased distal tubular calcium reabsorption, or alternatively,

enhanced proximal tubular reabsorption, as seen with sodium, may be found. A urinary calcium level of <12 mg/dl is associated with a sensitivity of 91%.

- *Ambulatory BP monitoring*: Alterations in circadian BP variability are present as early as the first trimester in women who later develop pre-eclampsia.

Diagnosis

Once the diagnosis is made, admission is mandatory. The following investigations are done—complete hemogram, platelet count, peripheral smear, urine routine and culture, 24-hour urine protein, renal and liver function tests, glucose tolerance test and fundoscopy. The tests of fetal well-being include ultrasound (to assess gestational age and estimated fetal weight, and to detect IUGR, vesicular mole, multiple pregnancy, hydramnios and macrosomia). After 32 weeks of gestation, the serial use of the 'kick' count, non-stress test, biophysical profile and Doppler is mandatory.

Hemoconcentration supports diagnosis of pre-eclampsia and is an indicator of the severity of the condition. Hemoglobin values may be decreased, however, if hemolysis accompanies the disease. Signs of microangiopathic hemolytic anemia (for example, schistocytes) on blood smear favour diagnosis of pre-eclampsia and may be present when BP is only mildly elevated. Decreased levels of platelet count suggest severe pre-eclampsia. Most cases of pre-eclampsia are associated with only mild elevations in serum creatinine. Rising levels, especially when associated with oliguria, suggest severe pre-eclampsia. Increased levels of serum uric acid aid in the differential diagnosis of pre-eclampsia and may reflect the severity of the disease. Elevated levels of lactic acid dehydrogenase (present in erythrocytes in high concentration) are associated with hemolysis and hepatic involvement, and suggest severe pre-eclampsia.

Pre-eclampsia is considered severe if one or more of the following criteria are present:

- Blood pressure of 160 mm Hg systolic or higher or 110 mm Hg diastolic or higher on two occasions at least 6 hours apart while the patient is at rest
- Proteinuria of 5 g or higher in a 24-hour urine specimen or 3+ or greater on two random samples collected at least 4 hours apart
- Oliguria of less than 500 ml in 24 hours
- Cerebral or visual disturbances
- Pulmonary edema or cyanosis
- Epigastric or upper-right quadrant pain
- Impaired liver function
- Thrombocytopenia: platelet count $\leq 100{,}000/mm^3$
- Fetal growth restriction

It is vital that severe pre-eclamptic patients be evaluated and treated at a tertiary institution.

Management

Management is concerned with the maximisation of the duration of pregnancy without unnecessarily jeopardising maternal or fetal well-being (Greg 2004).

- Admission and rest: In a study that evaluated the physiological changes among women who had pre-eclampsia, a regimen of complete hospitalised bed rest was compared with one of liberal ambulation (Greg 2004). Renal function did not improve, whereas placental function showed some suggestion of improvement. Bed rest allowed earlier detection of impending morbidity, and thus, earlier intervention (Mathews et al 1982).
- BP monitoring

- Urine albumin and urine output daily
- Fetal monitoring
- Watch for signs of imminent eclampsia
- Role of antihypertensives: If the BP levels persistently stay at 150/100 mm Hg, alphamethyldopa, a central-acting alpha adrenergic false neurotransmitter (agonist) is started at a dose of 250 mg, thrice a day. This can be increased to up to 500 mg, four times a day. This is considered as the drug of choice because of extensive experience and well-documented maternal and fetal safety. About 15% of patients display side effects such as tiredness, loss of energy, dizziness, depression, flushes, headache, vomiting and palpitations. Methyldopa is best avoided in the postnatal period, as depression is a side effect. Nifedipine, 5 mg thrice daily orally, can also be given. This acts by blocking calcium influx into smooth muscle cells, thus interfering with excitation–contraction coupling. Side effects are transient and include facial flushing, headache and warm, sweaty extremities. Oral labetalol (200–1200 mg in 2–3 divided doses) is a beta-blocker and may cause reduced cardiac output to the uterus while long-term use may cause IUGR. Angiotensin converting enzyme inhibitors are contraindicated in pregnancy as they can cause neonatal anuric renal failure, neonatal death and fetal loss in animals.
- Reasons to deliver. Approximately 50% of women with mild pre-eclampsia, remote from term, will develop severe pre-eclampsia. Patients with mild pre-eclampsia are at risk of developing eclampsia suddenly, without warning, and with minimal BP elevations. Another risk is abruptio placenta. However, both these risks are less than 1%.

In mild pre-eclampsia, the use of antihypertensive agents appears to reduce the occurrence of severe hypertension, but offers no immediate benefit to the fetus. Strict bed rest, pharmacological intervention for BP control and use of magnesium sulphate as prophylaxis for seizures remain unproven management options in mild pre-eclampsia (Livingston et al 2003). Pregnancy is terminated at 38 weeks by inducing labour or by elective cesarean section if cephalopelvic disproportion is seen, or earlier if it becomes severe.

Should the disease progress from mild to severe, or if there is any indication of fetal compromise, including non-reassuring fetal heart rate, oligohydramnios or growth restriction, the patient should be evaluated for delivery. Serial laboratory evaluation of platelet counts and liver enzyme values should be performed every 3–7 days to monitor for worsening disease. Patients should be instructed to monitor daily fetal movements and undergo twice-weekly non-stress test and amniotic fluid index; weekly biophysical profile, Doppler and ultrasound for fetal growth should be done every 3–4 weeks.

Once the diagnosis of severe pre-eclampsia is established, the only cure is termination of pregnancy. The benefits of delivery must be weighed against the potential risks of continuing the pregnancy.

The indicators for termination of pregnancy are as follows:

- BP persistently 160/110 mm Hg
- Proteinuria >5 g in 24 hours
- Headache, visual changes
- Epigastric pain
- Compromised renal function
- HELLP syndrome

- Oliguria <500 ml in 24 hours
- Pulmonary edema, abruptio placenta, eclampsia
- IUGR with abnormal Doppler
- Evidence of fetal distress including repetitive late decelerations, biophysical profile <4 on two occasions four hours apart, severe oligohydramnios, IUGR <5th percentile for gestational age
- Fetal death, spontaneous labour, rupture of membranes
- Gestational age ≥34 weeks

Management of Severe Pre-eclampsia It is very important to know the precise age of the fetus.

Before 24 weeks of gestation, termination of pregnancy is recommended. The preferred mode is induction of labour, provided the high BP levels are reasonably controlled and the patient does not have a 'toxic' clinical appearance.

The management of severe pre-eclampsia in the mid-trimester (25–32 weeks) is indeed a challenge. (Fathima and Moodley 2000) Steroids (dexamethasone 12 mg intramuscularly, two injections, 12 hours apart) can be given to hasten lung maturity and delivery delayed for 24 hours, if possible. This period requires extensive fetal and maternal surveillance. Aggressive management with delivery may result in high neonatal mortality, while conservative management may be associated with an increase in maternal complications. In a study by Odendaal (1990), expectant management, when compared to aggressive management, resulted in a statistically significant prolongation of gestational age by a mean value of 7.1 days, reduction in neonatal ventilation (11% versus 33%), reduction in total neonatal complications (33% versus 75%) and no increase in maternal mortality.

Expectant management of severe pre-eclampsia before 32–34 weeks of gestation, defined solely by proteinuria (≥5 g/24 hours), is justified in an effort to prolong gestation. Patients ≥33 weeks should be delivered. It is important to obtain diastolic BP levels of 95–105 mm Hg and to subsequently induce labour (provided there are no contraindications to induction such as contracted pelvis or severe IUGR), but the threshold for resorting to a cesarean section should be low. During cesarean delivery, it is not uncommon to find moderately large accumulation of ascitic fluid in the peritoneal cavity of women with pre-eclampsia.

The objectives in management are as follows

- Prevention of complications such as pulmonary edema, renal failure, cardiovascular accidents and abruptio placentae.
- Prevention of convulsions, as this is associated with an increased risk (10 times) of maternal mortality as well as of perinatal mortality.
- Delivery of a healthy neonate with minimal maternal morbidity.

Patients with pre-eclampsia tolerate blood loss poorly because of volume contraction, and type-specific blood should be readily available for transfusion, if needed. If the patient is delivering vaginally, she should be assisted in the second stage of labour to avoid a rise in maternal BP with each uterine contraction. Appropriate steps should be taken to minimise postpartum hemorrhage in patients who develop uterine atony while receiving continuous magnesium sulphate infusion. Methylergonovine (methergine) is contraindicated in these patients.

Antihypertensives in Severe Pre-eclampsia: Three short-acting antihypertensive agents (intravenous hydralazine or labetalol, and short-acting sublingual or oral nifedipine) are commonly used to control acute, very high BP in women who may require cesarean section and who receive magnesium sulphate (Working Group 2000). Hydrallazine can be given at a dose of 5–10 mg intravenous (IV) every 20 minutes up to a maximum dose of 30 mg. Labetalol is given at 10–20 mg IV, then 40–80 mg every 10 minutes up to a maximum dose of 300 mg, a continuous infusion of 1–2 mg/min may also be used. Sublingual nifedipine is now not used because of fear of intractable hypotension. Nifedepine is given 10 mg orally and can be repeated in 30 minutes, followed by 10–20 mg every four hours, with a maximum dose of 240 mg/24 hours. Intravenous sodium nitroprusside can be used in refractory hypertension, fetal cyanide poisoning is a risk with prolonged treatment.

Care should be taken not to reduce the BP too rapidly, because a marked decrease in mean arterial pressure may lead to reduced renal and placental perfusion. All three antihypertensive agents have their proponents and detractors. Hydrallazine may cause headache, nausea and vomiting and maternal hypotension (Magee 1999). Uncertainty exists about how safe short-acting calcium channel blockers are for the mother (Cutler 1998). Nifedipine, when used in conjunction with magnesium sulphate, may result in marked hypotension because of the compounded effects of the magnesium ion on calcium channel functions. When used for treating hypertension in patients with coronary artery disease or diabetes, these agents have been associated with increased cardiovascular morbidity and mortality. The withdrawal of short-acting nifedipine from some markets has been lamented by many experts in the field of pregnancy hypertension. Labetalol has been used extensively in pregnancy and has a favourable side effect profile. However, specific concerns have been raised about the risk of fetal bradycardia with parenteral labetalol (Stevens and Guillet 1995).

Most patients will show improvement within the first 24 hours postpartum. If hypertension persists after delivery, the patient may need to continue taking antihypertensive medication after being discharged. Patients should be seen every week or so as outpatients, until they become normotensive. If hypertension persists beyond 6 weeks postpartum, a diagnosis of chronic hypertension should be entertained.

The HELLP Syndrome Weinstein coined the acronym HELLP in 1982 to aid clinicians in recognising this group of patients with remarkable hepatic involvement by severe pre-eclampsia (Weinstein 1982). Indeed, the features of the HELLP syndrome are very similar and sometimes difficult to distinguish from those of other microangiopathic syndromes that may develop in late pregnancy, such as hemolytic uremic syndrome and thrombotic thrombocytopenic purpura. The latter disorders are characterised by vascular endothelial cell damage, elicited by unknown antigens or toxic substances. Differentiation of these disorders from the HELLP syndrome is important because the latter is treated by urgent delivery, whereas hemolytic uremic syndrome or thrombotic thrombocytopenic purpura may require plasma infusion or plasmapheresis.

Sibai has noted that most patients with the HELLP syndrome present preterm with hypertension and proteinuria and report epigastric and upper-right quadrant pain (1990). Around 30% of HELLP cases develop postpartum.

The following criteria are used to establish the diagnosis of the HELLP syndrome (Sibai 2002):

Hemolysis
- Abnormal peripheral blood smear
- Increased bilirubin ≥1.2 mg/dl
- Increased lactate dehydrogenase (LDH) >600 IU/l

Elevated liver enzymes
- Increased SGOT ≥72 IU/l
- Increased LDH >600 IU/l

Thrombocytopenia
- Platelet count <100,000/mm^3

The incidence of the HELLP syndrome is also higher in pre-eclamptic patients who have been managed conservatively. Liver rupture is rare, with a high mortality rate and requires large amounts of blood and platelet transfusions, laparotomy drainage and packing. Most obstetricians consider the development of the HELLP syndrome as an indication for urgent delivery, because the laboratory abnormalities can reach life-threatening levels with profound thrombocytopenia and extremely elevated levels of hepatic enzymes.

The first priority is to assess and stabilise the maternal condition, particularly coagulation abnormalities. The patient should receive magnesium sulphate for seizure prophylaxis and antihypertensives for acute control of BP. During the observation period, maternal and fetal condition is assessed. Finally, a decision has to be made if immediate delivery is indicated.

High-dose corticosteroid therapy (10 mg IV dexamethasone every 6 hours for two doses, followed by 6 mg IV dexamethasone every six hours for two additional doses) has been shown to improve maternal laboratory findings. It appears to alter the final steps in endothelial cell disruption (Ascarelli 1998).

Platelet transfusions are indicated, either before or after delivery, in all patients with the HELLP syndrome in the presence of significant bleeding from puncture sites, wounds, intraperitoneal, extensive ecchymosis, and so on. Further, transfusion is indicated in all antepartum patients whose platelet count is less than 20,000/mm^3. Correction of profound thrombocytopenia is particularly important before cesarean section. The HELLP syndrome can be classified based on platelet count as Class 1 (<50,000), Class 2 (50,000–100,000) and Class 3 (100,000–150,000). These classes have been used to predict the rapidity of postpartum recovery.

Thrombophilia and Pre-eclampsia The combination of aspirin and heparin or low-molecular-weight heparin is effective in recurrent fetal loss in the APLA syndrome and could be considered for women with inherited thrombophilias and a history of severe pre-eclampsia, IUGR, abruptio placentae, or fetal loss, although no controlled studies on the subject are currently available.

Seizure Prophylaxis Magnesium sulphate can be used in the management of severe pre-eclampsia to prevent the first fit. There are no appropriate clinical tests to assess which women are at risk of convulsions, and to date, there is little evidence that the benefits outweigh the risks (Chein et al 1996). Coetzee (1998) concluded in his study that eclampsia occurs 11 times less often, in women with severe pre-eclampsia treated in a special care tertiary unit, when magnesium sulphate is administered.

Anesthesia and Analgesia Continuous epidural analgesia is undoubtedly of benefit for vaginal and operative delivery in pre-eclampsia. Regional anesthesia confers the dual benefits of effective analgesia and stabilisation of BP. By preventing an increase in catecholamine release, further elevations in BP values during uterine contractions are avoided. It abolishes excessive maternal bearing down during the second stage of labour and thus allows controlled delivery. Further, there is some evidence to suggest that it may improve uteroplacental perfusion (Pritchard et al 1984). The patient should be fully conscious with an adequate cardiac preload, and coagulopathy should be excluded prior to insertion of an epidural catheter. If general anesthesia is indicated, the following risks should be borne in mind:

i) possible presence of laryngeal edema, which makes intubation difficult and hazardous;
ii) the pressor response to intubation, which may precipitate an arrhythmia or pulmonary edema;
iii) risk of aspiration;
iv) decrease in uteroplacental blood flow which may be hazardous if the fetus is growth retarded; and
v) neuromuscular blockade (drug interactions may take place if the patient has received magnesium sulphate).

Invasive hemodynamic monitoring may prove beneficial in pre-eclamptic women with severe cardiac disease, severe renal disease, refractory hypertension, oliguria or pulmonary edema.

Eclampsia Eclampsia literally means 'flashing lights'. It is defined as the presence of new onset grand mal seizures in a woman with pre-eclampsia.

Regardless of the time of onset, the convulsive movements usually begin around the mouth in the form of facial twitchings. After a few seconds, the entire body becomes rigid in a generalised muscular contraction. This phase may persist for 15–20 seconds. Suddenly the jaws begin to open and close violently, and soon thereafter, the eyelids as well. The other facial muscles and body muscles alternately contract and relax in rapid succession. So forceful are the muscular movements that the woman may throw herself out of her bed, and if not protected, her tongue might be bitten by the violent action of the jaws. This phase, in which the muscles alternately contract and relax, may last about a minute. Gradually, the muscular movements become less intense and less frequent, and finally the woman lies motionless. Throughout the seizure, the diaphragm is fixed and breathing does not occur. For a few seconds, the woman appears to be dying from respiratory arrest, but she then takes a long, deep, stertorous breath, and breathing is resumed. Unless treated, the first convulsion is usually the forerunner of others, which may vary in number from one or two in mild cases to even continuous convulsions (status epilepticus) in untreated severe cases. After a seizure, coma ensues (Cunningham et al 2005).

The seizures and mental status changes of eclampsia are related to hypertensive encephalopathy. With neuroimaging after an eclamptic seizure, cerebral edema is the most common finding; but intracranial hemorrhage and petechiae are the major findings after maternal death due to pre-eclampsia.

Other causes of seizures, in addition to eclampsia, include a bleeding arteriovenous malformation, ruptured aneurysm or idiopathic seizure disorder. These diagnoses may be more likely in cases in which new onset seizures occur after 48–72 hours postpartum (ACOG Practice Bulletin 2002). Eclampsia can occur antepartum (50%), intrapartum

(25%) or postpartum (25%). In 1994, the incidence of postpartum eclampsia was 10%, and in a 2002 study, it was reported to be 25%. Many antepartum and intrapartum cases are now prevented. Although uncommon, temporary blindness (lasting a few hours to a week) also may accompany severe pre-eclampsia and eclampsia (Cunningham et al 1995). Other nervous system manifestations include headache, blurred vision, scotomata and hyperreflexia.

General management: Lighting should be kept low and noise to a minimum. The bed should have padded railings. No attempt should be made to shorten or abolish the initial convulsion, and maternal injury should be prevented during the convulsion. Adequate oxygenation is to be maintained and the risk of aspiration minimised. Suction is to be employed and the lungs auscultated after the convulsion to ensure they are clear. Prophylactic antibiotics should be given and maternal acidemia corrected. One-to-one nursing is mandatory.

Antihypertensive management: Nifedipine is useful for acute control of BP. Drugs that can be given intravenously include hydrallazine, labetalol, sodium nitroprusside and diazoxide.

Anticonvulsant management: See below.

Obstetric management: This depends on the presence of fetal heart sounds and the gestational age. Vaginal delivery is the preferred route after an eclamptic seizure. Profound hypoxia and the development of lactic acidemia following convulsions adversely affect the fetus. Fetal bradycardia (profound fetal bradycardia lasting 3–5 minutes has been documented) frequently occurs during an eclamptic seizure; usually, this can be managed by maternal treatment and cesarean delivery is not necessary (Ramin 1999). Persistence beyond 10 minutes should prompt an evaluation for uterine hyperstimulation or placental abruption. Once the patient is stabilised, the method of delivery should depend in part on factors such as the fetal status, gestational age, fetal presentation and the findings of the cervical examination.

A cesarean section is recommended in the following situations:

i) all deeply unconscious patients (unless delivery is imminent)
ii) all uncooperative patients due to restlessness
iii) if vaginal delivery is unlikely to occur within 6–8 hours from onset of the first eclamptic seizure
iv) presence of an obstetric indication for cesarean section or
v) fetal distress (Fathima 2000).

A general anesthetic is recommended for cesarean sections unless the patient is fully conscious and co-operative, has had a single seizure, the BP is well controlled and blood biochemistry is satisfactory. The anesthetist should be informed of all the drugs that have been used.

If the patient is delivering vaginally, she should be assisted in the second stage of labour. Further, ergometrine is contraindicated in the third stage. In the postpartum period, the first 24–48 hours are especially important as the BP may fluctuate and the patient is still at risk of developing complications. Major fluid shifts occur during this period. Antihypertensives are usually required for 24–48 hours and need to be gradually decreased. Magnesium sulphate is administered for 24 hours after delivery. Neonatal assessment is important, especially in preterm deliveries, abruptio placenta or maternal coagulopathy.

Anticonvulsant Management: The regimen

varies with the country.

UK: Diazepam 20 mg IV load followed by a dilute infusion 80 mg/L, titrated to sedation was being used in UK until 1992. The use of large doses of diazepam (>30 mg) during labour is associated with loss of beat-to-beat fetal heart rate variability and significant neonatal morbidity including respiratory depression, apnea, hypotonia, cold stress and poor suckling.

USA: Magnesium sulphate is the drug of choice for the treatment and prophylaxis of eclampsia in the USA.

Others: Phenytoin 500–1000 mg IV, followed by 500 mg IV or oral as indicated four and 12 hours later, may be used. Diazepam 10 mg IV was used for immediate control of seizures.

The use of magnesium sulphate has consistently aroused controversy despite many years of experience with its use. The Eclampsia Trial Collaborative Group (1995) evaluated the efficacy and safety of magnesium sulphate, diazepam and phenytoin. Of the 1680 randomised women, 453 were assigned to magnesium sulphate versus 452 to diazepam and 388 women to magnesium sulphate versus 387 to phenytoin. The magnesium sulphate group had a 52% lower risk of recurrent seizures compared to diazepam and a 67% lower risk than phenytoin. The Collaborative Eclampsia Trial has now provided irrefutable evidence of the superiority of magnesium sulphate over diazepam and phenytoin for the prevention of recurrent seizures in women with eclampsia.

The magnesium sulphate schedule for severe pre-eclampsia and eclampsia is as follows:

- 4 g IV as 20% solution (not to exceed 1 g/min).
- If convulsions persist after 15 minutes, give up to 2 g more IV as a 20% solution at the above mentioned rate
- 10 g 50% intramuscular (IM), one half in each buttock
- 5 g 50% IM every 4 hours in alternate buttocks
- Monitor patellar reflex, respiration and urine output.
- Discontinue 24 hours after delivery or after last fit.
- About 10% of patients will have recurrent seizures.

This regimen was carried out by Pritchard and colleagues. The injection should be given deep in the upper outer quadrant of the buttock, with a 3-inch, 20 gauge needle; the addition of 1 ml of 2% lidocaine minimises discomfort. One advantage of the IM route has been the uniform attainment of therapeutic serum levels. The IV regimen as described by Zuspan is a 4-g loading dose followed by a maintenance infusion of 1 g/h for 24 hours.

Magnesium sulphate toxicity:

Plasma magnesium

10 mEq/l : Patellar reflex disappears
>10 mEq/l : Respiratory depression
>12 mEq/l : Respiratory arrest

Ideal serum levels of magnesium have the range of 4–5 mEq/L. The dose can also be titrated clinically by keeping the deep tendon reflexes minimally reactive. Treatment of toxicity is with calcium gluconate (10 ml of 10% solution) 1 g IV, while simultaneously withholding magnesium sulphate. This medication should be administered slowly to avoid hypotension or bradycardia. In addition, in case of cardiorespiratory arrest, the patient should be intubated immediately and managed with assisted ventilation until resumption of spontaneous respiration. A serum magnesium level should be obtained.

There are no absolute contraindications

to magnesium therapy other than perhaps myasthenia gravis and heart muscle damage, particularly if associated with conduction defects (Idama 1998).

Magnesium sulphate is the best as unlike epilepsy, eclampsia most likely does not arise from an eclamptic locus in the brain. It is probably a result of vasospasm and subsequent cerebral edema (Ramin 1999). Magnesium sulphate is a potent vasodilator, especially in the cerebral vasculature; as is evident in a Doppler examination of the middle cerebral artery.

With magnesium use, laryngeal reflexes are usually intact, which protects against aspiration pneumonia. Injection abscess can occur with the intramuscular route. Magnesium is almost solely excreted by the kidneys and after 4 hours, about 50% of the infused dose is excreted in the urine. Extreme caution should be exercised in patients with serum creatinine levels above 1.3 mg/dl. A good rule of thumb is to give half the stated dose and to monitor the serum magnesium levels. Phenytoin can be used as an alternative.

Use of magnesium sulphate along with calcium channel blockers can cause hypotension and neuromuscular blockade. In two case reports, profound muscle weakness and respiratory arrest were associated with concomitant use of nifedipine and magnesium sulphate (Snyder and Cardwell 1989; Ben Ami 1994). However, no such blockade was reported in the Magpie trial (2002) in which 29% of women allocated to receive magnesium sulphate also received nifedipine (MAGPIE stands for Magnesium Sulphate for Prevention of Eclampsia). Therefore, any risk of neuromuscular blockade is likely to be low, and the effect is reversible with calcium gluconate.

The use of magnesium sulphate is associated with a high rate (15–67% in various trials) of minor side effects such as feeling warm, flushed skin, nausea or vomiting, muscle weakness, dizziness and irritation at the site of injections. Life-threatening magnesium toxicity is extremely rare with correct dosing and proper monitoring of the patient during magnesium sulphate therapy (Sibai 2005). The IV regimen avoids painful IM injections. However, it necessitates close maternal surveillance with availability of appropriate resuscitation facilities.

Seizure activity that fails to abate or that resumes after appropriate loading and maintenance doses of magnesium sulphate is a rare event. Intravascular sodium amobarbital in small doses of up to 250 mg can be used.

Complications Intrauterine growth restriction, abruptio placenta, renal failure, HELLP syndrome, retinal detachment, cerebral hemorrhage, cardiac failure, pulmonary edema, bronchopneumonia and postpartum psychosis are complications of pre-eclampsia/eclampsia.

Hemoconcentration, or lack of normal pregnancy-induced hypervolemia, is an almost predictable feature of severe pre-eclampsia/eclampsia. An appreciable fall in BP very soon after delivery most often means excessive blood loss, and not sudden dissolution of vasospasm. When oliguria follows delivery, the hematocrit should be evaluated frequently to help detect excessive blood loss and guide appropriate blood transfusion.

Postnatal Assessment At the sixth week of postnatal assessment, the presence of hypertension or proteinuria necessitates referral to a physician for further investigations. Pregnancy should be advised only if the BP and renal function tests return to normal. It is important to counsel the patient on booking early in future pregnancies. The advantages include possible administration of low dose aspirin and detection of pre-eclampsia as early as possible. Long-term prognosis and counselling for future pregnancies (including contraception) must be discussed.

Recurrence Careful follow-up studies performed over 30 years ago in Scotland reported a risk of recurrent pre-eclampsia in 3.4% of second pregnancies in women who had pre-eclampsia with their first pregnancies. The risk of recurrent hypertension without proteinuria was even higher, approaching 25%. More recent investigations suggest that if pre-eclampsia occurred early in the first pregnancy (in the second trimester), the risk of recurrence may be as high as 60%. Interestingly, if there is a change in paternity, the risk of pre-eclampsia in multiparas is almost as high as it is for the first pregnancy (August 1999).

Patients with pre-eclampsia are more prone to vascular disease and chronic hypertension later in life. Both early onset disease and recurrent disease are associated with an increased prevalence of chronic hypertension or renal problems.

Prevention

- Diet containing fish oil has been tried as it has unsaturated fatty acids.
- Oral calcium carbonate of 2 g per day has also been tried in women with low calcium intake but may not be necessary if calcium intake is adequate.
- The role of low dose aspirin (50–150 mg/day) in women at high risk of pre-eclampsia, particularly those with previous severe pre-eclampsia before 28 weeks, and those with marked abnormalities in uterine Doppler studies at both 18–20 weeks and 24 weeks gestation, remains controversial (Golding 1998).
- Antioxidant supplementation with vitamin C (1000 mg per day) and vitamin E (400 mg per day) has shown promise in one study, but will require further confirmation by larger studies. It lowers the incidence of pre-eclampsia in high-risk populations.

Imitators of Severe Pre-eclampsia/eclampsia There are many imitators of severe pre-eclampsia, HELLP and eclampsia (Sibai 2004):

- Acute fatty liver of pregnancy
- Thrombotic thrombocytopenic purpura
- Hemolytic uremic syndrome
- Exacerbation of lupus erythematosus
- Immune thrombocytopenic purpura
- Thrombophilias
- Cholecystitis/Pancreatitis
- Systemic viral sepsis (disseminated herpes)
- Systemic inflammatory response syndrome (sepsis)
- Hemorrhagic or hypotensive shock
- Stroke in pregnancy/postpartum

Conclusion

While prevention of pre-eclampsia/eclampsia must await an understanding of its etiology, improvement in antenatal care, together with active management of the disease when it develops, will improve both fetal and maternal prognosis.

There may be a role for outpatient management of a select subset of mild pre-eclamptic patients in certain select populations (Helewa et al 1993). The patient should be compliant, report warning symptoms, have a nurse check her BP and come to day care twice a week.

Ensuring the well-being of the mother does not always ensure the most favourable fetal outcome, therefore clinical management is challenging, and decisions regarding the timing of delivery have profound lifelong effects on both the mother and the child. When severe pre-eclampsia, with or without the HELLP syndrome, is found in a woman carrying a preterm fetus (usually less than 32 weeks gestation), careful delay of delivery can be attempted. This should be done only in tertiary care centres by specialists. Eclampsia warrants prompt delivery regardless of gestational age.

The principles of treatment have changed little over the past three decades, despite better understanding of its pathophysiology. Outcomes are improving, however, primarily because of early recognition, close maternal and fetal surveillance, seizure prophylaxis, judicious use of antihypertensive therapy and timely delivery.

The promising early results of prophylactic agents such as aspirin and calcium supplements have not been confirmed in large randomised controlled trials. Therapeutic strategies aimed at rescuing the endothelial dysfunction of pre-eclampsia with agents, such as vascular endothelial growth factor and placental growth factor and prostacyclins, should be tested in patients with severe disease to determine if pregnancy may be safely continued (Dvorak 2002).

References

ACOG Practice Bulletin. 2002. Diagnosis and Management of Preeclampsia and Eclampsia. Number 33. *Int J Obstet Gynecol* 77:67–75.

Ahmed Y, B van Iddekinge, C Paul et al. 1993. Retrospective analysis of platelet members and volumes in normal pregnancy and in preeclampsia. *Br J Obstet Gynaecol* 100:216.

Anumba DOC and SC Robson. 1999. Management of preeclampsia and the HELLP syndrome. *Curr Opin Obstet Gynecol* 11:149–156.

Ascarelli MH, V Johnson, WL May et al. 1998. Individually determined postpartum magnesium sulphate therapy with clinical parameters to safely and cost-effectively shorten treatment for preeclampsia. *Am J Obstet Gynecol* 179:952–956.

August P. 1999. Hypertensive disorders in pregnancy. In *Medical complications during pregnancy,* 5th ed, ed **GN Burrow,** TP Duffy, 53–77. Philadelphia: WB Saunders Company.

Ben Ami M, Y Giladi and E Shalev. 1994. The combination of magnesium sulphate and nifedipine: a cause of neuromuscular blockade. *Br J Obstet Gynaecol* 101:262–263.

Chamberlain G. 1995. *Turnbull's Obstetrics.* 2nd ed. London: Churchill Livingstone.

Chavarria ME, L Lara-Gonzalez, A Gonzalez-Gleason et al. 2003. Maternal plasma cellular fibronectin concentration in normal and preeclamptic pregnancies: A longitudinal study for early prediction of preeclampsia. *Am J Obstet Gynecol* 189:1212.

Chein PFW, KS Khan and N Arnott. 1996. Magnesium sulphate in the treatment of eclampsia and preeclampsia: an overview of the evidence from randomised trials. *Br J Obstet Gynaecol* 103: 1085–1091.

Coetzee EJ, J Dommisse and J Anthony. 1998. A randomised controlled trial of intravenous magnesium sulphate versus placebo in the management of women with severe pre-eclampsia. *Br J Obstet Gynaecol* 105: 300–303.

Cunningham FG, CO Fernandez and C Hernandez. 1995. Blindness associated with preeclampsia and eclampsia. *Am J Obstet Gynecol* 172: 1291–1298.

Cunningham FG, KJ Leveno, SL Bloom, JC Hauth, LC Gilstrap III, KD Wenstrom, eds. 2005. *Williams Obstetrics.* 22nd ed, 762–808. New York: McGraw Hill.

Cutler JA. 1998. Calcium-channel blockers for hypertension – uncertainty continues. *N Eng J Med* 338:679–681.

Dekker GA and BM Sibai. 1998. Etiology and pathogenesis of pre-eclampsia: current concepts. *Am J Obstet Gynecol* 179:1359–1375.

Dekker GA JI de Vries, PM Doelitzsch, et al. 1995. Underlying disorders associated with severe early-onset pre-eclampsia *Am J Obstet Gynecol* 173:1042–1048.

Dvorak HF. 2002. Vascular permeability factor/vascular endothelial growth factor: a critical cytokine in tumor angiogenesis and a potential target for diagnosis and therapy. *J Clin Oncol* 20:4368–4380.

Eclampsia Trial Collaborative Group. 1995. Which anticonvulsant for women with eclampsia? Evidence from the Collaborative Eclampsia Trial. *Lancet* 345:1455–1463.

Fathima P and J Moodley. 2000. Treatment of severe preeclampsia/eclampsia syndrome. In *Progress in Obstetrics and Gynecology 14,* ed Studd J, 102–119. London: Churchill Livingstone.

Gant NF, S Chand, RJ Worley et al. 1974. A clinical test useful for predicting the development of acute hypertension in pregnancy. *Am J Obstet Gynecol* 120:1.

Golding JA. 1998. A randomized trial of low dose aspirin for primipara in pregnancy. The Jamaica Low-Dose Aspirin Study Group. *Br J Obstet Gynaecol* 105: 293.

Greg AR. 2004. Hypertension in pregnancy. *Obstet Gynecol Clin N Am* 31:223–241.

Halligan A, J Bonnar, B Sheppard et al. 1994. Haemostatic, fibrinolytic, and endothelial variables in normal pregnancies and preeclampsia. *Br J Obstet Gynaecol* 101:488.

Hauth JC, MG Ewell, RJ Levine et al. 2000. Pregnancy outcomes in healthy nulliparas who developed hypertension. Calcium for Preeclampsia Prevention Study Group. *Obstet Gynecol* 95:24.

Helewa M, M Heaman, MA Robinson and L Thompson. 1993. Community-based home care programme for the management of pre-eclampsia. *Can Med Assoc J* 149:829–834.

Hutt R, SO Ogunniyi, MHF Sullivan et al. 1994. Increased platelet volume and aggregation precede the onset of pre-eclampsia. *Obstet Gynecol* 83:146.

Idama TO and SW Lindow. 1998. Magnesium sulphate: a review of clinical pharmacology applied to obstetrics. *Br J Obstet Gyneco;* 105:260–268.

Irion O, J Masse, JC Forest and JM Moutquin. 1998. Prediction of pre-eclampsia, low birth weight for gestation and prematurity by uterine artery blood flow velocity waveform analysis in low risk nulliparous women. *Br J Obstet Gynaecol* 105:422–429.

Livingston JC, LW Livingston, R Ramsey, BC Mabee and BM Sibai. 2003. Magnesium sulfate in women with mild preeclampsia: a randomized controlled trial. *Obstet Gynecol* 101(2):217–220.

Magee LA, MP Ornstein and P von Dadelszen. 1999. Fortnightly review: management of hypertension in pregnancy. *BMJ* 318:1332–1336.

Mathews DD, V Agarwal and TP Shuttleworth. 1982. A randomized controlled trial of complete bed rest versus ambulation in the management of proteinuric hypertension during pregnancy. *Br J Obstet Gynaecol* 89(2):128–131.

Miller J et al. 1996. Urinary kallikrein creatinine ratio in the prediction of preeclampsia. *Br Obstet Gynaecol* 103:421–26.

Moldenhauer JS and BM Sibai. 2003. Hypertensive disorders of pregnancy. In *Danforth's Obstetrics and*

Gynecology, 9th ed, ed JR Scott, RS Gibbs, BY Karlan, AF Haney, 257–271. Philadelphia: Lippincott Williams and Wilkins.

Odendaal HJ, RC Pattinson, R Bam et al. 1990. Aggressive or expectant management for patients with severe preeclampsia between 28 and 34 weeks gestation: a randomized controlled trial. *Obstet Gynecol* 76:1070–1075.

Pritchard JA, FG Cunningham and SA Pritchard. 1984. The Parklands Memorial Hospital protocol for treatment of eclampsia: evaluation of 245 cases. *Am J Obstet Gynecol* 148:951–963.

Ramin KD. 1999. The prevention and management of eclampsia. *Obstetrics and Gynecology Clinics of North America* Vol 26, No 3: 489–501.

Roberts JM and CA Hubel. 1999. Is oxidative stress the link in a two-stage model of pre-eclampsia? *Lancet* 354:788–789.

Roberts JM and DW Cooper. 2001. Pathogenesis and genetics of preeclampsia. *Lancet* 357:53–56.

Said J and G Dekker. 2003. Preeclampsia and thrombophilia. *Best Practice and Research Clinical Obstetrics and Gynecology* 17:3:441–458.

Saudan P, MA Brown, ML Buddle and M Jones. 1998. Does gestational hypertension become pre-eclampsia? *Br J Obstet Gynaecol* 105:1177–1184.

Sibai BM. 1990. The HELLP syndrome (hemolysis, elevated liver enzymes, and low platelets): much ado about nothing? *Am J Obstet Gynecol* 162:311–316.

Sibai BM. 2002. Hypertension. In Obstetrics *Normal and Problem Pregnancies*. 4th ed, ed SG Gabbe, JR Niebyl, JL Simpson, 945–1004. New York: Churchill Livingstone.

Sibai BM. 2004. Imitators of severe pre-eclampsia/eclampsia. *Clin Perinatol* 31: 835–852.

Sibai BM. 2005. New developments in preeclampsia. *Clinical Obstetrics and Gynecology* 48:2:482–485.

Snyder SW and MS Cardwell. 1989. Neuromuscular blockade with magnesium sulfate and nifedipine. *Am J Obstet Gynecol* 161:35–36.

Stevens TP and R Guillet. 1995. Use of glucagon to treat neonatal low-output congestive heart failure after maternal labetalol therapy. *J Pediatr* 127:151–153.

The Magpie Trial. 2002. Do women with preeclampsia, and their babies, benefit from magnesium sulphate? The Magpie trial: a randomized placebo-controlled trial. *Lancet* 359:1811–1890.

Walker JJ. 1998. Current thoughts on the pathophysiology of preeclampsia/eclampsia. In *Progress in Obstetrics and Gynecology 13*, ed Studd J, 177–85. Edinburgh: Churchill Livingstone.

Weinstein L. 1982. Syndrome of hemolysis, elevated liver enzymes, and low platelet count: a severe consequence of hypertension in pregnancy. *Am J Obstet Gynecol* 142:159–167.

Witztum JL. 1994. The oxidation hypothesis of atherosclerosis. *Lancet* 344:793–795.

Working Group on High Blood Pressure in Pregnancy. 2000. Report of the National High Blood Pressure Education Program Working Group on High Blood Pressure in Pregnancy. *Am J Obstet Gynecol* 183:S1–S22.

Zhou Y, CH Damsky and SJ Fisher. 1997. Pre-eclampsia is associated with failure of human cytotrophoblasts to mimic a vascular adhesion phenotype. One cause of defective endovascular invasion in this syndrome? *Journal of Clinical Investigation* 99:2152–2164.

22

Antepartum Hemorrhage

Prashanth K Adiga | Pratap Kumar N

Introduction

Antepartum hemorrhage (APH) complicates approximately 3% of pregnancies. It has important consequences for the obstetric patient and her fetus. The current definition of APH is, any bleeding from the genital tract that occurs during pregnancy, from the time of potential viability to the delivery of the fetus. APH can cause sudden, unexpected and significant bleeding, which can potentially be dangerous to both the mother and the fetus.

Classification of Antepartum Hemorrhage

APH can be classified into (i) placenta previa, (ii) abruptio placentae, and (iii) bleeding due to other causes, each of which constitutes one-third of the cases of APH.

Assessment of Bleeding

History It is important to document the initial assessment of the severity of the bleeding and the patient's condition at a centre with maternal, neonatal and surgical services. History taking should include identifying the risk factors for placental abruption or placenta previa and determining the amount of bleeding, the presence or absence of abdominal pain, uterine contractions and any history of abdominal or vaginal trauma. Placental location should be assessed if the patient has previously undergone an ultrasound examination.

The physical examination should include an assessment of the hemodynamic status of the mother. Evidence of hypovolemic shock may include pallor and restlessness with cold, clammy extremities. The maternal pulse rate and blood pressure should be measured and the presence of fetal heart sounds needs to be established. If there are any signs of hemodynamic instability, priority must be given to immediate maternal resuscitation with intravenous fluids. If the fetal heart cannot be auscultated or if the fetus is in distress, it is likely that the patient has suffered a severe abruptio placentae. During abdominal examination, the clinician must look for uterine tenderness, fundal height more than the period of gestation and irritable or hard woody consistency of the uterus, all of which are signs of abruptio placentae. A cardiocotography (CTG) should be obtained to assess the well-being of the fetus. The management of acute obstetric hemorrhage is shown below (Walker et al 1994).

Abruptio placentae Abruptio placentae is the premature separation of a normally implanted placenta before the delivery of the fetus. It is a serious condition that contributes significantly to maternal and perinatal morbidity and mortality. It is a major cause of third trimester bleeding (Saftlas at al 1991) and complicates 0.5–3.0% of pregnancies (Spinillo at al 1994).

Classification/Grading Placental abruption can be broadly classified into three grades that correlate with clinical and laboratory findings. The grading of abruptio placentae is shown in Table 22.1 (Sher 1978).

Grade I placental abruption is found in approximately 40% of cases, grade 2 in 45% and grade 3 in 15% of cases (Hurd 1983). In severe cases of abruption, the diagnosis is obvious. Milder forms are more difficult to diagnose with certainty.

Risk Factors The risk factors for abruptio placentae are given below:

- Age >35 years
- Pre-eclampsia
- Pre-pregnancy hypertension
- Smoking
- Rupture of membranes >24 hours
- Cocaine abuse

Maternal age: Advanced maternal age is associated with a risk of abruption. The unadjusted risk of abruptio placentae for women over the age of 35 years was 2.2 times the risk for women aged 19–34 years (Williams et al 1991). Kramer et al found the incidence of abruption varying significantly according to the maternal age, with higher rates among both teenage mothers and mothers aged 35 years or more (Kramer et al 1997).

Management of Acute Obstetric Hemorrhage

- Secure venous access and insert central venous pressure monitor
- Summon additional help
- Collect blood samples for cross-matching and coagulation screen
- Contact hematologist and blood bank
- Maintain blood volume with unmatched blood if necessary (same ABO and Rh D group as patient)
- Seek and deal with the source of bleeding
- Perform blood product replacement treatment if necessary

Pre-eclampsia: Pre-eclampsia and eclampsia are major risk factors for placental abruption. Ananth et al found a relative risk of 3.8 for placental abruption in patients with severe pre-eclampsia (Ananth et al 1997).

Pre-pregnancy hypertension: Pre-pregnancy hypertension is a risk factor for placental abruption. A relative risk of 2.8 for placental abruption in patients with chronic hypertension with superimposed pre-eclampsia (Ananth et al 1997).

Smoking: Maternal tobacco use, both during and before pregnancy, is linked strongly to abruption. Raymond and Mills found that with every 10 cigarettes smoked each day, there is a 20% increased risk of abruption (Raymond and Mills 1993). In a meta-analysis, Ananth et al estimated a 90% overall increased risk of abruption due to

Table 22.1: Grading of abruptio placentae

Grade I: Mild	*Grade II: Intermediate*	*Grade III: Severe*
Diagnosis of this class of abruptio placentae is made retrospectively upon post-partum detection of a small retroplacental clot.	Diagnosis is based on the classical features of abruptio placentae with uterine hypertonicity, but the fetus is still alive.	The fetus is dead. This grade is further subdivided into: **Grade IIIa,** where overt coagulopathy is absent and **Grade IIIb,** where overt coagulopathy is present.

Source: Sher G, 1978

tobacco use, and suggested that rates could fall by 15–25% with cessation of smoking in pregnancy (Ananth et al 1997).

Premature rupture of membranes (PROM): This has been associated with abruption. A study by Ananth et al found that women presenting with PROM must be placed under close monitoring to reduce the risk of placental abruption (Ananth et al 1996).

Cocaine abuse: Maternal cocaine use is associated with a significantly higher risk of placental abruption than in the general population. Hulse et al found a strong association (OR 3.92, 95% CI, 2.77–5.46) between maternal cocaine use and the incidence of abruption (1997). Animal models suggest a dose-dependent rate of placental abruption in relation to the amount of cocaine given (Hulse et al 1997).

Clinical Diagnosis The classical signs and symptoms of abruptio placentae are as follows:

- Vaginal bleeding may or may not be present.
- Abdominal pain is poorly localised and increases in severity.
- Uterine tenderness may be present.
- Uterine contractions may be seen.
- **Clinical features of shock** (tachycardia with weak and thready pulse, hypotension, cold and clammy skin) may be seen depending on the degree of placental separation and uterine spasm.
- If the abruption is severe, the uterus contracts tonically so that fetal parts cannot be felt. The uterus becomes tense and tender.
- The fetus may be **dead** with no detectable fetal heart beat.
- Features of **DIC** in severe cases, which manifest as bleeding from the injection sites and gums, hematuria and ecchymosis, may be seen.

Not all of these symptoms and signs are always present, and the absence of the same does not exclude the diagnosis of abruptio placentae.

In a prospective study by Hurd et al, vaginal bleeding was present in only about 78% of cases, uterine tenderness or pain in 66% and high-frequency contractions or uterine hypertonus in 34% of patients who were later confirmed to have an abruption. Idiopathic preterm labour was the initial diagnosis in 22% of patients, until other signs such as bleeding or fetal distress developed (Hurd et al 1983).

In severe cases of placental abruption, the diagnosis is generally obvious. Milder forms are more difficult to diagnose with certainty. **An abruption is often a diagnosis of exclusion in mild cases.**

An ultrasound will help to exclude placenta previa and to detect retroplacental clots. Ultrasound evidence of hemorrhage is found only in 50% of patients. Ultrasound can identify three predominant locations for abruptions (Nyberg et al 1987)—subchorionic, retroplacental and preplacental. The size and location of the placental abruption has prognostic significance. A large retroplacental hemorrhage is associated with a greater than 50% fetal mortality, whereas a large subchorionic hemorrhage is associated with a 10% fetal mortality (Nyberg et al 1987).

Management The investigations that need to be done are listed below:

- Hemoglobin with PCV
- Blood grouping, typing and cross-matching
- Urgent coagulation screen
- Full blood and platelet count

- Renal function tests
- Liver function tests

A woman diagnosed with abruptio placentae has a potentially dangerous condition. With placental abruption, blood loss is always **underestimated** and replacements should take this into account. As bleeding may largely be retroplacental, several litres of blood may be concealed behind the placenta. Therefore, the amount of blood released from the vagina before delivery is no indicator of the extent of placental detachment or of subsequent blood loss. It is important that urine output is measured hourly, as abruptio placentae is one of the common causes of acute renal failure. So an in-dwelling catheter should be placed.

The basic principle in the management of placental abruption is **prevention or correction of hypovolemia with expeditious vaginal delivery whenever possible.**

The three As in the management of abruptio placentae are as follows:

- Adequate blood transfusion to replace the blood lost.
- Accelerate the process of labour by amniotomy and augmentation with oxytocin.
- Anticipate complications such as coagulation failure, renal failure and postpartum hemorrhage.

Prevention/Correction of Hypovolemia and Coagulation Defects Bleeding and coagulation defects cannot be controlled until after delivery. Replacement of blood volume should be done to maintain renal perfusion. **Blood is the best fluid to replace blood loss.** Although the depleted coagulation factors should be replaced, the consumption of factors will occur until the uterus is emptied (Walker et al 1994).

Fresh frozen plasma (1 litre) is often sufficient to correct the coagulation defect, but severe depletion of fibrinogen (<0.8 g/l) requires the infusion of 10–15 units of cryoprecipitate. Thrombocytopenia (platelet count less than 50 x 10^9/l) will require correction by transfusion of platelet concentrates. Further coagulation investigations and platelet counts are required to monitor the response (Walker et al 1994).

Decision to Deliver the Fetus This will depend on the maternal and fetal conditions, gestational age and cervical status. If the fetus is immature, the patient is hemodynamically stable, and the abruption is mild; an expectant management with close observation can be undertaken (Baron and Hill 1998). Several studies have reported the use of magnesium sulphate tocolysis in managing preterm gestation with an abruptio placentae.

Vaginal delivery is preferred if the mother is relatively stable and the fetus can tolerate the delay and stress of labour. In parous women, amniotomy may be enough to stimulate labour and enable prompt delivery, but others may need oxytocin infusion.

If there are signs of fetal distress or if vaginal delivery is not imminent or seems likely to be difficult, cesarean section may be necessary. In this case, replacement of blood volume and coagulation factor is essential.

The principles of the management of severe abruptio placentae with coagulopathy are as follows:

- **Expeditious vaginal delivery**
- **Replacement of the blood lost**
- **Monitoring and correcting of electrolyte and acid base disturbances**
- **Management of DIC and fibrinolysis**
- **Management of PPH**

In a nutshell, the clinical features and management of abruptio placentae are as given below.

Surveillance in subsequent pregnancies A woman with a history of abruption in a prior pregnancy is at risk of developing abruption in the next pregnancy. In a study by Rasmussen et al, 104 placental abruption events recurred among 2748 deliveries subsequent to the initial placental abruption, or 38/1000 (95% CI=31.2–45.9) (Rasmussen et al 2001). Patients at risk of recurrent abruption would benefit from monitoring of placental function or fetal growth or by using other antenatal tests reflecting fetal health. In patients at risk of a recurrence of placental abruption, monitoring up to three months before the gestational age of the initial abruption is necessary (Rasmussen et al 2001).

Placenta Previa

Placenta previa is one of the important causes of antepartum hemorrhage, along with abruptio placentae. Maternal and fetal morbidity and mortality from placenta previa are considerable. Placenta previa develops when the placenta is inserted wholly or in part into the lower segment of the uterus. The incidence of placenta previa varies from 0.28% to 1.96% (Ananth and Smulian 1997).

Classification The classification of placenta previa has evolved from the historical grades I–IV to the major and minor types. Major placenta previa is a condition where the placenta encroaches, either wholly or partly, on the internal os. If the placenta is merely low lying, but does not involve the os, it is called minor placenta previa. Placenta previa may be divided into four main types, which are further divided into the major and minor, varieties. **Types 1 and 2 anterior** are minor while **Type 2 posterior and Types 3 and 4** are major (Table 22.2).

Risk Factors The risk factors for placenta previa are as follows:

- Maternal age
- Previous cesarean section
- History of placenta previa in a previous pregnancy
- History of previous abortions

Maternal age: The occurrence of placenta previa increases with maternal age and was found to be lowest in women aged 20–29 years, and highest in women older than 35 years (Rasmussen et al 2000).

Previous cesarean delivery: There is a strong association between having a previous cesarean delivery and the subsequent development of placenta previa. Relative risks were 4.5% for one cesarean delivery, 7.4% for two prior cesarean sections, 6.5% for three and 44.9% for four or more prior cesarean sections, respectively (Ananth and Smulian 1997).

Placenta previa in a previous pregnancy: This is an independent risk factor. Women

Table 22.2: Types of placenta previa

Type	Degree of Placenta Previa
1	Placenta is in the lower uterine segment but the lower edge does not reach the internal os
2	Lower edge of the placenta reaches the internal os but does not cover it
3	Placenta covers the os asymmetrically
4	Placenta covers the os symmetrically

with previous history of placenta previa have a tenfold risk of developing the condition in the next pregnancy. This could be due to defective decidual vascularisation, and it is reasonable that women with a history of placenta previa have increased risk of having a recurrent placenta previa (Rasmussen et al 2000).

History of previous abortions: Pregnant women with a history of abortions are at a higher risk of developing placenta previa. Zhang and Savitz reported that the risk of placenta previa was 1.6% for women with one abortion, 2.3% for two abortions and 3.7% for three or more abortions (1993).

Clinical Features

Symptoms

- Abdominal pain
- Severe shock with symptoms beyond vaginal blood loss
- Vaginal bleeding, usually old blood

Signs

- Shock
- Spasm of the uterus, described as woody
- Tender uterus
- Fetal parts hard to feel
- Often no fetal heart is heard

Emergency Treatment

Treat the shock

- Give oxygen
- Insert intravenous lines
- Arrange cross-match of 6 units of blood
- Give morphine (if the fetus is dead)

Deliver the fetus

- By cesarean section (if the fetus is alive and gestation is mature)
- By rupturing the membranes (if the cervix is ripe or the fetus is dead)

Treat disseminated intravascular coagulopathy

- Urgent hematological consultation
- Check platelet count
- Give cryoprecipitate (fresh frozen plasma)
- Transfuse with fresh blood if available

CLINICAL FEATURES

- Classical presentation of placenta previa is **painless vaginal bleeding.** Its onset is often without warning. The bleeding is thought to be associated with the development of the lower uterine segment, and the myometrium of the lower uterine segment is unable to contract adequately to stop the bleeding.
- **The degree of shock will vary directly with the amount of blood lost by the patient.** Pallor, tachycardia and hypotension may be present, depending on the degree of blood loss.
- The uterus is relaxed and the fetal parts are easily palpable. The fetal heart sounds are easily heard. Fetal death in placenta previa is uncommon.
- Some patients have uterine contractions in addition to the bleeding.
- Few women present with a **persistent transverse lie** or **breech presentation** in late pregnancy, and this is attributed to the position of the placenta in the lower segment which prevents stabilisation of the head.

Note: The possibility of placenta previa should always be considered in such cases and an ultrasound scan requested (Chamberlain 1991).

DIAGNOSIS Placenta previa should be suspected in any patient who presents with vaginal bleeding beyond 24 weeks of gestation (Baron and Hill 1998). **No vaginal examination**

should be performed on any woman who bleeds in late pregnancy, until placenta previa has been excluded by ultrasonography (Chamberlain 1991).

Ultrasound: Transvaginal ultrasound (TVS) is safe in the presence of placenta previa and is more accurate than a transabdominal ultrasound in locating the placenta. Leerentveld et al demonstrated high levels of accuracy of TVS in 100 women suspected of placenta previa with a sensitivity of 87.5%, specificity of 98.8%, positive predictive value of 93.3% and negative predictive value of 97.6% (Leerentveld et al 1990).

MANAGEMENT Once placenta previa is diagnosed, the aim of treatment is to maintain the pregnancy until the fetus is mature enough to be delivered. **Cesarean section is the recommended mode of delivery for major placenta previa,** whereas for minor placenta previa, an attempt at vaginal delivery is deemed appropriate (Leerentveld 1990). Bhide et al reported the probability of vaginal delivery at a given placental edge-internal os distance (Bhide and Thilaganathan 2004). This study found that the likelihood of successful vaginal delivery increased with increasing placental edge-internal os distance. The rate of cesarean section was 90% when the placental edge-internal os distance was between 0.1 cm and 2 cm, and about 37% when the placental edge was more than 2 cm from the internal os.

The treatment of choice for a preterm patient (24–36 weeks) **who is not actively bleeding is expectant management** (Baron and Hill 1998). However, if the hemorrhage is severe, cesarean section should be performed, despite fetal immaturity.

Adherent Placenta Adherent placenta is an abnormally firm attachment of the placental villi to the uterine wall with the absence of the normal intervening decidua basalis and fibrinoid layer of Nitabuch. Three variants of this condition are recognised. In **placenta accreta,** the placenta is directly attached to the myometrium, whereas in **placenta increta,** the placenta may extend into the myometrium. In **placenta percreta,** the placenta may extend throughout the entire myometrium. Placenta accreta occurs in approximately 1 in 2500 deliveries (Miller et al 1997).

The risk factors for placenta accreta include placenta previa with or without previous uterine surgery, prior myomectomy, prior cesarean delivery, Asherman syndrome, submucus leiomyomata and maternal age greater than 35 years (Clark et al 1985). Women who have had two or more cesarean deliveries with anterior or central placenta previa have a nearly 40% risk of developing placenta accreta (Clark et al 1985).

The ultrasound features of placenta accreta are as follows:

- The thinning or absence (<1 mm) of the normal hypoechoic myometrial zone in the anterior lower segment is suggestive of abnormally adherent placenta.
- The presence of lacunar vascular spaces within the placental parenchyma resulting in a **swiss cheese appearance**. This has a sensitivity of 93% in the gestational age timeframe of Weeks 15–40 (Comstock 2005).
- The border between the bladder and myometrium is normally **highly echogenic** and smooth. In placenta accreta, interruptions or bulging can occur. This is a specific sign, but not a sensitive one, as bulging or interruptions are not present in every patient with placenta accreta. Secondly, patients who have had cesarean section often develop increased vascularity in the space between the myometrium and the bladder because the flap is retracted

before the incision is made into the uterus. In addition, this area is exposed to blood products. Therefore, it would be important to differentiate between bulging due to enlarged or increased number of vessels and actual growth through the myometrium (Comstock, 2005).

- The usual dark line between the myometrium and the placenta is thought to represent the decidua basalis. Since the decidua is absent in placenta accreta, it has been suggested that the absence of this line indicates placenta accreta. This line is absent in normal patients with anterior placenta and hence has a low sensitivity and positive predictive value of 7% and 6%, respectively (Comstock 2005).
- The extension of placental tissue (with the same echogenicity as placental parenchyma) beyond the uterine serosa.

The **colour Doppler** criteria suggestive of placenta previa accreta are as follows (Chou et al 2000):

- A diffuse lacunar flow pattern exhibiting diffusely dilated vascular channels scattered throughout the entire placenta and the surrounding myometrial or cervical tissues
- A focal lacunar flow pattern showing irregular, sonolucent vascular lakes with turbulent lacunar flow, distributed regionally or focally within the intraparenchymal placental area
- Interphase hypervascularity with abnormal blood vessels linking the placenta to the bladder with high diastolic arterial blood flow
- Markedly dilated peripheral subplacental vascular channel with pulsatile venous-type flow over the uterine cervix
- Absence of subplacental vascular signals in the areas lacking the peripheral subplacental hypoechoic zone

Management A high degree of suspicion and preparation is essential to avoid intraoperative catastrophes. Backups for the vascular surgeon and urologist are essential. A vertical incision should be used. The intraoperative signs of placenta accreta/percreta are as follows:

- Distorted/Deformed lower uterine segment
- Placental tissue invading the uterine serosa
- Massive hypervascularisation of the lower uterine segment in a patient with placenta previa
- Invasion of other structures by the placenta and obvious abnormal blood vessels extending from the pelvic side walls to the lower segment (Hudon and Belfort 1998)

Profuse hemorrhage can occur when attempting to separate the placenta; therefore, no attempts should be made to remove the placenta in cases of obvious increta or percreta. Before any attempt is made to dislodge the placenta, **prophylactic ligation or balloon occlusion/embolisation** of the uterine or hypogastric arteries should be performed to reduce blood loss. The uterus should be hemostatically closed, oxytocic agents should be administered and **a hysterectomy** should be performed. The following surgical principles should be used when performing a cesarean section–hysterectomy for placenta percreta (Hudon and Belfort 1998):

- Pedicles should be double-clamped to avoid back bleeding.
- Pedicles should be doubly ligated and adequate length should be left to avoid retraction.
- Blunt dissection should be avoided in the region of the bladder, as significant bleeding can result from hypervascularity and abnormal blood supply of the lower uterine segment and overlying bladder.

- An intentional cystostomy can be extremely helpful in cases where the bladder is especially adherent.
- There is no place for supracervical hysterectomy in cases of placenta_previa with placenta accreta, because the cervical region is often the area of predominant bleeding. Meticulous hemostasis of the vaginal cuff (running locked stitch) is very important.
- The adnexa should be conserved, if possible.

Conservative Management of Placenta Accreta This should be considered for women desiring a future pregnancy and whose vaginal bleeding is not excessive (Buckshee and Dadhwal 1997). The successful use of **methotrexate** in the conservative management of placenta accreta was first described by Arulkumaran et al in 1986. Systemic methotrexate 50 mg as an intravenous infusion (total dose 250 mg) was administered on alternate days and the placental mass was expelled on Day 11 postnatally (Arulkumaran et al 1986). Gupta and Sinha have described a successful outcome using oral methotrexate (0.3 mg/kg) (1998).

Vasa Previa Vasa previa is a rare obstetric catastrophe with a reported incidence of 1 in 1275 to 1 in 8333 (Fung and Lau 1998; Oyelese et al 1999). The diagnosis is often not made during the antepartum period.

This is an uncommon condition in which the blood vessels traverse the lower uterine segment in advance of the presenting part. This condition is associated with a velamentous insertion of the cord or succenturiate placental lobe. The bleeding usually occurs at the time of rupture of membranes, and might be accompanied by fetal heart changes that can become sinusoidal in pattern. When ultrasound is done in the second or third trimester, identification of a velamentous or marginal cord insertion may help to determine the additional patients at risk. If placental cord insertion cannot be identified, colour flow Doppler may be useful.

When the source of bleeding is in doubt, and there is no evidence of fetal distress, the APT test can be done. The principle of this test is that fetal RBCs are resistant to the action of alkalis, unlike adult RBCs, which are sensitive to their action. An equal quantity of suspect and adult blood is placed separately in two test tubes in 5 ml of water so that they appear to be of the same colour. About 1 ml of 1% sodium hydroxide is added to both the test tubes. The test tube containing the adult blood will change from pink to yellow-brown in 2 minutes as the hemoglobin is denatured. Scheduled cesarean section is the preferred method of delivery when vasa previa has been identified antenatally, usually at 37–38 weeks.

Antepartum Hemorrhage of Unknown Origin Antepartum hemorrhage of unknown origin is a common antenatal complication and is diagnosed by exclusion of known causes. In a review of 307 patients with antepartum hemorrhage of unknown origin, Willocks found that the fetal loss rate was 14% (Willocks 1971). Chan et al, in a study of 718 cases with singleton pregnancies diagnosed to have antepartum hemorrhage of unknown origin, concluded that the main fetal risk associated with this condition is preterm labour and its subsequent fetal complications (Chan and William 1999). A small but significant proportion of these pregnancies might be associated with fetal congenital anomalies. A detailed anomaly scan needs to be done to rule out congenital anomalies, and these patients need to be monitored vigilantly to check for symptoms and signs of preterm labour (Chan and William 1999).

Clinical Guidelines, Recommendations and Practice Points The Royal College of Obstetricians and Gynaecologists (RCOG) have made the following recommendations (RCOG Clinical Green Top Guidelines 2001):

Grade A recommendation (requires at least one randomised controlled trial as part of the body of literature of overall good quality and consistency addressing the specific recommendation)

- Transvaginal ultrasound is safe in the presence of placenta previa and is more accurate than transabdominal ultrasound in locating the placenta (Grade A recommendation).

Grade B recommendation (requires the availability of well-controlled clinical studies but no randomised trials on the topic of recommendation)

- The mode of delivery should be based on clinical judgment in each situation, but a placenta encroaching within 2 cm of the internal os is a contraindication to attempting vaginal delivery.
- Women who have had cesarean section in a previous pregnancy and who subsequently have placenta previa should be considered at high risk of having a morbidly adherent placenta. In such cases, particular attention should be focussed on confirming or excluding this diagnosis using ultrasound imaging. When present, the inputs of senior anesthetic and obstetric specialists are vital in planning delivery.

Suggestions for Good Practice

- Prior to delivery, all women with placenta previa, and their partners, should have antenatal discussions regarding delivery and possible blood transfusion requirements and any objections or queries should be dealt with effectively.
- Blood should be available for the peripartum period—the amount required will depend on the clinical features of each individual case.
- When a woman with placenta previa is being delivered, the consultant on call for the delivery should be involved.
- Any woman going to theatre with known placenta previa should be attended to by an experienced obstetrician and anesthetist, with consultant presence readily available. An inexperienced obstetrician should not be left unsupervised when caring for these women; this is especially important in cases with higher risks of complications, namely previous uterine scars, anterior placenta previa or associated placenta accreta.
- The surgical maneuvers required in the face of massive hemorrhage associated with placenta previa cesarean sections should be performed by appropriately experienced surgeons and calling for extra help early should be encouraged and not seen as 'losing face'.

The American College of Obstetricians and Gynecologists (ACOG) committee opinion on placenta accreta (2002) is as follows:

- The patient should be counselled about the likelihood of hysterectomy and blood transfusion.
- Blood products and clotting factors should be available.
- Cell saver technology should be considered, if available.
- The appropriate location and timing for delivery should be considered to allow access to adequate surgical personnel and equipment.
- A preoperative anesthesia assessment should be considered.

Practice Points (Abruptio placentae)

(Harrington and Black 2005)

- Blood loss is frequently underestimated.
- Fetal distress and fetal death are common.
- Management is aimed at resuscitation of the mother and delivery of the fetus.
- Cesarean section is indicated for fetal distress but not for intrauterine death.
- DIC and postpartum hemorrhage are common.

Practice Points (Placenta Previa)

(Harrington and Black, 2005)

- Suspect this condition when there is painless, fresh bleeding from the vagina and a high presenting part or abnormal lie
- Remember that placental localisation at the time of the anomaly scan might be misleading.
- Resuscitate the mother and involve the senior staff (obstetric and anesthetic) early.
- Beware of the risk of postpartum hemorrhage.
- Anticipate a morbidly adherent placenta with anterior placenta previa and previous cesarean section, scan antenatally and counsel the patient appropriately.

References

ACOG Committee Opinion. 2002. Placenta accreta Number 266. *Int J Obstet Gynecol* 77:77–78.

Ananth CV, DA Savitz and MA Williams. 1996. Placental abruption association with hypertension and prolonged rupture of membranes: A methodologic review and meta-analysis. *Obstet Gynecol* 88:309–18.

Ananth CV, DA Savitz, WA Bowes et al. 1997. Influence of hypertensive disorders and cigarette smoking on placental abruption and uterine bleeding during pregnancy. *Br J Obstet Gynaecol* 104:572–578.

Ananth CV, JC Smulian, and AM Vintzileos. 1997. The association of placenta praevia with history of caesarean delivery and abortion: a metaanalysis. *Am J Obstet Gynecol* 177:1071–1078.

Arulkumaran S, CS Ng, I Ingemarsson and SS Ratnam. 1986. Medical treatment of placenta accreta with Methotrexate, *Acta Obstet Gynecol Scand* 65:285–286.

Baron F and WC Hill. 1998. Placenta praevia, Placenta abruptio. *Clin Obstet Gynecol* 41:527–532.

Bhide A and B Thilaganathan. 2004. Recent advances in the management of placenta praevia. *Curr Opin Obstet Gynecol* 16:447–451.

Buckshee K and V Dadhwal. 1997. Medical management of placenta accreta. *Int J Gynecol Obstet* 59:47–48.

Chamberlain G. 1991. ABC of antenatal care. Antepartum haemorrhage. *Br Med J* 302(6791):1526–1530.

Chan CWC and WK William. 1999. Antepartum haemorrhage of unknown origin-what is its clinical significance? *Acta Obstet Gynecol Scand* 78:186–190.

Chou MM, ESC Ho and YH Lee. 2000. Prenatal diagnosis of placenta praevia accreta by transabdominal color Doppler ultrasound. *Ultrasound Obstet Gynecol* 15:28–35.

Clark SL, PP Koonings and JP Phelan. 1985. Placenta praevia/accreta and prior cesarean section. *Obstet Gynecol* 66:89–92.

Comstock CH. 2005. Antenatal diagnosis of placenta accreta: a review. *Ultrasound Obstet Gynecol* 26:89–96.

Fung TY and TK Lau. 1998. Poor perinatal outcome associated with vasa praevia: is it preventable? A report of three cases and review of the literature. *Ultrasound Obstet Gynecol* 12: 430–433.

Gupta D and R Sinha. 1998. Management of placenta accreta with oral Methotrexate. *Int J Gynecol Obstet* 60:171–173.

Harrington D and RS Black. 2005. Massive or recurrent antepartum haemorrhage. *Curr Obstet Gynaecol* 15:267–71.

Hudon L, MA Belfort and DR Broomr. 1998. Diagnosis and management of placenta percreta: A Review. *Obstet Gynecol Surv* 53:509–517.

Hulse GK, E Milne, DR English et al. 1997. Assessing the relationship between maternal cocaine use and abruptio placentae. *Addiction* 92:1547–1551.

Hurd WW, M Miodovnik, V Hertzberg and JP Lavin. 1983. Selective management of abruptio placentaee: a prospective study. *Obstet Gynecol* 61: 467–473.

Kramer SK, RH Usher, R Pollack and M Boyd. 1997. Etiologic determinants of abruptio placentaee. *Obstet Gynecol* 89:221–226.

Leerentveld RA, ECAM Gilberts, MJC Arnold, JW Wladimiroff. 1990. Accuracy and safety of transvaginal sonographic placental localisation. *Obstet Gynecol* 76:759–762.

Miller DA, JA Chollet and TM Goodwin. 1997. Clinical risk factors for placenta praevia-placenta accreta. *Am J Obstet Gynecol* 177:210–214.

Nyberg DA, DR Cyn, LA Mack et al. 1987. Sonographic spectrum of placental abruption. *Am J Radiol* 148:161–164.

Nyberg DA, LA Mack, TJ Benedetti et al. 1987. Placental abruption and placental hemorrhages: correlation of sonographic findings with fetal outcome. *Radiology* 358:357–361.

Oyelese KO, M Turner, C Lees and S Campbell. 1999. Vasa praevia: an avoidable obstetric tragedy. *Obstet Gynecol Surv* 54: 138–145.

Rasmussen S, LM Irgens, S Albrechtsen and K Dalaker. 2001. Women with a history of placental abruption: when in a subsequent pregnancy should special surveillance for a recurrent placental abruption be initiated? *Acta Obstet Gynecol Scand* 80:708–712.

Rasmussen S, S Albrechtsen and K Dalaker. 2000. Obstetric history and the risk of placenta praevia. *Acta Obstet Gynecol Scand* 79:502–507.

Raymond E and J Mills. 1993. Placental abruption: Maternal risk factors and associated fetal conditions. *Acta Obstet Gynecol Scand* 72:633–639.

Royal College of Obstetricians and Gynaecologists (RCOG). 2001. Clinical green top guidelines. Placenta praevia: Diagnosis and management (27).

Saftlas AF, DR Olson, HK Atrash, R Rochat and D Rowley. 1991. National trends in the incidence of abruptio placentaee, 1979–1987. *Obstet Gynecol* 78:1081–1086.

Sher G. 1978. A rational basis for the management of abruptio placentaee. *J Reprod Med* 21:123.

Spinillo A, E Capuzzo, L Colonna, L Solerte, S Nicola and S Guaschino. 1994. Factors associated with abruptio placentaee in preterm deliveries. *Acta Obstet Gynecol Scand* 73:307–312.

Walker ID, JJ Walker, BT Colvin, EA Letsky et al. 1994. Investigation and management of haemorrhagic disorders in pregnancy. *J Clin Path* 47:100–108.

Williams MA, E Lieberman, R Mittendorf et al. 1991. Risk factors for abruptio placentaee. *Am J Epidemiol* 134:9:965–972.

Willocks J. 1971. Antepartum haemorrhage of uncertain origin. *Obstet Gynecol Br Common* 78:987–991.

Zhang J and DA Savitz. 1993. Maternal age and placenta praevia: a population based case control study. *Am J Obstet Gynecol* 166:641–645.

23

Low Birth Weight Babies

Hema Diwakar

Prematurity and/or growth restriction leading to low birth weight babies remains a major obstetric and neonatal challenge. The weight alone may be a poor index of neonatal health. In assessing perinatal outcome by weight, infants who weigh less than 2500 g at term are associated with a perinatal mortality rate that is 5–30 times greater than that of infants whose birth weights are at the 50th percentile. The mortality rates are 70–100 times higher in infants who weigh less than 1500 g.

Perinatal asphyxia involving multiple organ systems is one of the most significant problems in growth-restricted, low birth weight infants. Long-term follow-up studies have demonstrated that babies who suffered intrauterine growth retardation are more likely to develop hypertension, coronary artery disease and diabetes in adult life. There is growing evidence to suggest that patterns of early growth and other life course factors play an important role in the origin and development of cardiovascular disease (CVD), but current understanding of the processes that mediate these effects is limited.

Fetal growth is dependent on genetic, placental and maternal factors. The fetus is thought to have an inherent growth potential that, under normal circumstances, yields a healthy newborn of appropriate size.

The terms 'intrauterine growth restriction (IUGR)' and 'small for gestational age (SGA)' are often used interchangeably. Timely diagnosis and management of IUGR is one of the major achievements in contemporary obstetrics. If a growth-restricted fetus with low birth weight is identified and appropriate management instituted, perinatal mortality can be reduced. This underscores the need for assessment of fetal growth at each prenatal visit.

The investigations currently available allow the cause of the condition to be more precisely established, but the appropriate timing of delivery is often difficult to judge. Evidence is emerging that some forms of IUGR may be preordained early in pregnancy, such that their recognition may provide the opportunity for effective intervention. However, in most cases, diagnosis is confirmed late in the process and is likely to remain so in the foreseeable future. At the moment, therefore, the focus should be on establishing accurate diagnosis and carefully planning delivery with neonatologists to optimise the outcome.

The current therapeutic goals are to optimise the timing of delivery to minimise hypoxemia, and maximise gestational age and maternal outcome.

Definition of Fetal Growth Restriction

A fetus that has failed to achieve a specific

biometric or estimated weight threshold by a specific gestational age is said to have fetal growth restriction (FGR). The most commonly used threshold is the 10th percentile for abdominal circumference and estimated birth weight.

Classification

The classification of fetuses depends on the sex, race and genetic background and environmental factors, such as elevation above sea level. Fetuses are classified into three groups:

- Weight less than two standard deviations for gestational age.
- Weight less than the 3rd percentile for gestational age.
- Weight less than the 10th percentile for gestational age.

Approximately 70% of fetuses with a birth weight below the 10th percentile for gestational age are constitutionally small. In the remaining 30%, the cause of fetal growth restriction is pathologic.

Diagnosis

Abdominal Palpation Abdominal palpation has limited diagnostic accuracy for predicting an SGA fetus. Physical examination of the abdomen, by inspection and palpation, helps to detect only 30% of SGA fetuses. Therefore, if SGA is suspected, abdominal palpation must be supplemented with ultrasound biometric tests.

Fundal Height The symphysio-fundal height (SFH) measurement has limited diagnostic accuracy in predicting an SGA neonate. Although early studies reported sensitivity of 56–86% and specificity of 80–93% for fundal height as a predicator of SGA neonates, a large study of 2941 women found the sensitivity and specificity to be 27% and 88%, respectively. Serial measurements may improve sensitivity and specificity.

The impact on perinatal outcomes of measuring fundal height is uncertain. A systematic review found only one controlled trial with 1639 patients and showed that SFH measurement did not improve any of the perinatal outcomes measured. Low sensitivity, high false-positive rates and significant intra and interobserver variation make this test unsuitable for diagnosis. Therefore, if SGA is suspected, it is necessary to supplement fundal height measurement with ultrasound biometric tests.

The use of a customised fundal height chart improves accuracy in predicting an SGA fetus. A customised SFH chart is adjusted for physiological variables such as maternal height, weight, parity and ethnic group. Use of such charts was found to result in improvement in sensitivity (29% and 48% using non-customised and customised charts, respectively), resulting in increased antenatal detection of SGA babies with a reduction in unnecessary hospital investigations for fetal growth. Calculation of customised percentiles requires computer software. The charts can then be printed and incorporated into patient-held records at the time of booking.

Ultrasound Biometry The abdominal circumference (AC) and estimated fetal weight (EFW) can be used to diagnose SGA. These are, in fact, the most accurate diagnostic measurements to predict SGA. In high-risk women, AC at less than the 10th percentile has a sensitivity of 72.9–94.5% and specificity of 50.6–83.8%. The respective figures for EFW are 33.3–89.2% and 53.7–90.9%.

Several studies have compared various formulas for estimating birth weight. Most suffer from methodological and analytical faults. A prospective study by Chien et al compared four formulas and found the Shepard and Aoki formulas to have the best interclass correlation coefficient, with EFW showing the smallest mean difference from actual birth weight. Thus, the Shepard and Aoki formulas are recommended for estimating fetal weight. However, these formulas were validated over birth weights of 2080–4430 g and therefore, their use outside this range may be inappropriate. The Hadlock formula may be more appropriate when the fetus is expected to be very small.

Formulas for Estimation of Fetal Weight

Shepard's formula

Log 10 EFW = 1.2508 + (0.166 x BPD) + (0.046 × AC) - (0.002646 × AC × BPD)

Aoki's formula

EFW = (1.25647 × BPD3) + (3.50665 × Fetal Abdominal Area (FAA) × FL) + 6.3

Hadlock's formula

Log 10 EFW = 1.3596 - 0.00386 (AC × FL) + 0.0064 (HC) + 0.00061 (BPD × AC) + 0.0425(AC) + 0.174 (FL)

A systematic review by Chang et al found that a threshold of the 10th percentile had better sensitivity and specificity than other commonly used percentiles. One other study found the customised 8th percentile for EFW to be the optimal threshold for predicting operative delivery for fetal distress and admission to the neonatal care unit.

Customised Ultrasound Charts Serial measurements of AC and EFW are superior to single estimates of AC or EFW in the prediction of FGR and poor perinatal outcome. However, use of fetal growth alone to diagnose growth restriction (especially when the interval between the scans is less than two weeks) can lead to a high number of false-positive results.

The reference charts of fetal biometry based on cross-sectional data are commonly used for assessing growth velocity. Use of standard deviation scores, as opposed to simply viewing the growth pattern, is likely to result in a more reliable and accurate assessment of growth.

Ratio measures, such as from the head to abdominal circumference and femoral length to abdominal circumference, are poorer than AC or EFW alone in predicting SGA or neonatal ponderal index.

Placental Volume In a prospective, community-based study of maternal nutrition and fetal growth in six Indian villages, the mid-pregnancy placental volume was measured using ultrasonography and its relationship to maternal characteristics and fetal growth was studied. The relationship between placental size in mid-pregnancy and the birth parameters was found to be independent of maternal size before pregnancy or weight gain during pregnancy. Mid-pregnancy placental volume was a significant predictor of low birth weight (LBW) and stillbirths. At a given maternal weight, height or head circumference, a small mid-pregnancy placental volume was associated with smaller birth weight, neonatal length and head circumference. The results were compared with those from Southampton, where mid-pregnancy placental volume was measured using the same technique.

At 17 weeks of gestation, Indian fetal size was not very different from that in the West; head circumference was >95% and abdominal circumference and femur length were 91% of the Western standards. Placental size, however, was considerably smaller at this stage (71% of mid-pregnancy placental volume in Southampton, median, 214 ml at 17 weeks of gestation). At birth, the Indian fetuses grew to be smaller babies than those in Southampton (birth weight of 2653 versus 3440 g, 77% of Southampton), and placental weight was lower (367 versus 533 g, 69% of Southampton).

The volume of each placental segment is calculated by multiplying its average cross-sectional area by its longitudinal length. The sum of all the segmental volumes gives the total placental volume. In conclusion, the measured mid-pregnancy placental volume of pregnant women in rural India was considerably smaller than in women from Southampton, but was similar to that of American women accustomed to heavy exercise. The mid-pregnancy placental volume in Indian women was related to maternal pre-pregnancy weight and independently predicted LBW. Thus, poor placental growth in early pregnancy could at least partly explain LBW in Indian babies.

Management

Once IUGR has been detected, the management of the pregnancy should depend on a surveillance plan that maximises gestational age while minimising the risks of neonatal morbidity and mortality.

Such a goal requires the use of antenatal testing with the hope of identifying the fetus with IUGR before it becomes acidotic. It is important to develop a testing scheme, follow it up and have a high index of suspicion in this population when the test results are abnormal. The positive predictive value of an abnormal antenatal test result in fetuses with IUGR is relatively high, because the prevalence of acidemia and chronic hypoxemia is relatively high.

The protocol for antenatal testing suggested by Kramer and Weiner relies heavily on the use of umbilical artery (UA) Doppler testing, because severely abnormal Doppler findings (absent or reversed end diastolic flow) can precede an abnormal fetal rate by several weeks.

Harman and Baschat suggested a different antenatal testing strategy. This protocol integrates multiple venous and arterial Doppler measurements and the biophysical profile score. This strategy may be used in institutions where these measurements are routinely obtained by qualified technicians.

Assessment for Chromosomal Defects

When a small fetus is diagnosed, attempts have to be made to assess the risk of chromosomal defects. Up to 19% of fetuses with AC and EFW less than the 5th percentile may have chromosomal defects. The risk is higher when growth restriction is associated with structural abnormalities, normal liquor volume or normal uterine or umbilical artery Doppler. Therefore, all growth-restricted fetuses need an ultrasound anatomical survey. It may also be appropriate to offer karyotyping.

Surveillance of the Small Fetus A systematic review with meta-analysis has provided compelling evidence that the use of umbilical artery Doppler (UA Doppler) to monitor high-risk fetuses reduces perinatal morbidity and mortality. In addition, a significant reduction in the number of antenatal admissions and inductions of labour associated with Doppler use was observed. A study comparing fetal heart rate monitoring, biophysical profile and UA Doppler found that only UA Doppler had value in predicting poor perinatal outcomes in SGA fetuses. Use of Doppler does not lead to increased interventions, as the rates of positive tests are low (2.7% of all umbilical artery tests in high-risk women).There is evidence that use of Doppler ultrasound to manage SGA fetuses reduces the use of resources when compared with cardiotocography.

A variety of descriptor indices of UA Doppler, such as resistance index, systolic/diastolic ratio, pulsatility index and diastolic average ratio, are used to predict perinatal outcome. An analysis, using receiver operator curves in a study, found that resistance index had the best discriminatory ability to predict abnormal outcomes such as SGA, poor Apgar scores, abnormal cardiotocograph, umbilical cord pH and admission to a neonatal unit.

When the anomaly scan and UA Doppler are normal, a small fetus is likely to be a normal small fetus. Evidence suggests that outpatient management of such fetuses is safe. In addition, a randomised, controlled trial of two regimens of fetal surveillance for SGA fetuses with normal UA Doppler found that twice weekly monitoring compared with fortnightly monitoring, resulted in earlier deliveries and more inductions of labour with no difference in neonatal morbidity. This suggests that frequency of monitoring in SGA fetuses with normal Doppler need not generally be more than once every fortnight.

Liquor volume measure using either AFI or pocket depth can be used, as both tests have similar diagnostic accuracy.

Abnormal liquor volume has been variously defined as single, cord-free, 1 cm, 2 cm, 1 × 1 cm, 2 × 1 cm and 2 × 2 cm pockets or an AFI below the 5th percentile for the gestation or less than or equal to 5 cm. Both AFI and single pocket measurements poorly correlate with actual amniotic fluid volume. An AFI of less than 5 cm and single pocket of less than 2 cm were inadequate in the prediction of amniotic volume at less than the 5th percentile for gestation.

A systematic review with meta-analysis of 18 studies with over 10,000 patients found that an antepartum AFI of ≤5 cm was associated with an increased risk of an Apgar score of <7 at five minutes (RR = 5.2; 95% CI: 2.4–11.3). Poor correlation between AFI and neonatal acidosis was noted in the only study that examined this outcome. Other large studies have shown that a reduction in liquor volume is associated with increased perinatal mortality when compared with controls with normal liquor volume.

The biophysical profile has not been shown to improve perinatal outcome but sufficient data does not exist to rule out its value—a systematic review found only four poor-quality studies with fewer than 3000 patients. Authors of the systematic normal biophysictic review concede that to draw a meaningful conclusion about the impact of a biophysical profile on perinatal mortality, a study of more than 10,000 women would need to be made. However, there is evidence from uncontrolled observational studies that a biophysical profile in high-risk women has good negative predictive value; that is, fetal death is rare in women with a normal biophysical profile.

When primary surveillance with UA Doppler is found to be abnormal, the biophysical profile is likely to be useful, given its good negative predictive value in high-risk populations. This recommendation is further supported by evidence that, in high-risk women, the biophysical profile was rarely abnormal when Doppler findings were normal.

Use of cardiotocography (CTG) antepartum to assess fetal condition is not associated with better perinatal outcome; in fact, a systematic review of randomised trials showed that there was a trend towards increased mortality in the group receiving CTG compared to those who did not.

Computer systems for interpretation of CTG display better accuracy than clinical experts in predicting umbilical acidosis and depressed Apgar scores. However, further evaluation of this technology is required before clinical recommendations can be made regarding its widespread use.

The evidence for other antenatal interventions that have been tried in situations where continuation of pregnancy is under consideration, because of low gestational age, is summarised as follows:

- Most prenatal interventions do not show any significant effects on perinatal outcome.
- Smoking cessation programmes, particularly behavioural strategies, can be effective for a small minority of smokers in increasing birth weight, but there is no data to suggest that this intervention improves perinatal outcome.
- Although a meta-analysis of 13 trials evaluated the use of aspirin in the prevention of growth restriction and found that it reduced the incidence of FGR, only a few studies have used aspirin in the treatment of FGR. These trials are small and have shown conflicting results. Further trials are needed to assess the value of aspirin in the treatment of FGR.
- There is not enough evidence to assess the value of oxygen therapy, nutrient therapy, hospitalisation and bed rest, betamimetics, calcium channel blockers, hormonal therapy and plasma volume expansion in treating growth restriction.

Delivery

There is wide variation in practice in the timing of delivery of growth-restricted fetuses. The Growth Restriction Intervention Trial (GRIT) is an attempt to answer this issue. In August 2004, *Lancet* published data on brain development in survivors of the multicentre GRIT. The aim of this study was to identify compromised fetuses between 24 and 36 weeks of gestation and answer the question whether it was safer to deliver them immediately or to delay until there was no clinical doubt that delivery was necessary. As many as 588 such fetuses were identified in 69 hospitals in 13 European countries; of these, 296 were randomly assigned to immediate delivery and 292 to delayed delivery. The median interval between randomisation and delivery in the immediate delivery group was 0–9 days, and 4–9 days in the delay group. The authors had previously reported on the stillbirths and neonatal deaths in these pregnancies, and identified similar mortality rates before discharge between the immediate and delayed delivery groups.

The main outcomes of the current report were death and disability at or beyond two years of age. These outcome measures were recorded in 98% of immediate births and 97% of delayed births. Overall rates of death and disability were similar! 19% of immediate births and 16% of delayed births. In the subgroup of infants born at a gestation of less than 31 weeks, the outcomes appeared to improve by delaying the delivery where possible.

When end diastolic flow (PED) is present, delivery should be delayed until at least 37 weeks, provided other surveillance findings are normal. Absent or reversed end diastolic flow is associated with increased perinatal mortality and morbidity. The odds ratio for perinatal mortality in pregnancies complicated by absent end diastolic flow (AED) and reversed end diastolic flow (RED) were 4.0 and 10.6 respectively, compared with when end diastolic flow was present. The incidence of respiratory distress syndrome and necrotising enterocolitis was not increased with absent or reversed end diastolic volume, but there was an increase in cerebral hemorrhage, anemia and hypoglycemia. (Evidence level 2a).

When end diastolic flow is absent or reversed, admission, close surveillance and administration of steroids are required. If other surveillance results (biophysical profile, venous Doppler) are abnormal, delivery is indicated. If gestation is over 34 weeks, even if other results are normal, delivery may be considered.

The interval between first occurrence of AED and an abnormal CTG/biophysical profile is 1–26 days. Gestational age, presence of hypertension and venous Doppler abnormalities (notably pulsations in the umbilical vein) are key prognostic factors affecting this interval. The optimal surveillance strategy in fetuses with AED/RED is unclear. Options include daily CTG/BPP and/or venous Doppler with delivery when the CTG becomes pathological (decelerations with reduced variability), the biophysical profile becomes abnormal (less than or normal 4), there is reversal of Doppler velocities in ductus venosus during atrial contraction or umbilical vein pulsations are seen. Under these circumstances, delivery is likely to be by cesarean section.

Gestation and birth weight-specific charts can be used to determine the likelihood of survival if early delivery is required.

A study by Draper et al produced gestation and birth weight-specific survival rates from 24 weeks of gestation, taking into account factors such as fetal sex, ethnicity and singleton or twin. Use of these tables, rather than ones based on gestation or estimated birth weight alone, is likely to lead to a more accurate estimation of survival. The EPICURE study produced data on developmental disability for extremely preterm infants. Although the data was not specific to growth-restricted infants, they have provided useful information on morbidity when extremely premature delivery is considered.

Steroids should be administered if gestation is below 36 weeks. Antenatal steroids significantly reduce the incidence of respiratory distress syndrome. Delivery should take place in a unit where optimal neonatal expertise and facilities are available. A skilled resuscitator, who is trained and competent in the resuscitation of the newborn, should be present at delivery. Where possible, a neonatologist should be present at delivery, if gestation is extremely preterm or growth restriction is severe.

Intrapartum monitoring with continuous CTG is recommended. Although a systematic review of randomised trials found that intrapartum electronic monitoring did not reduce perinatal mortality, there is substantial observational data to suggest that intrapartum CTG in high-risk populations is likely to be of benefit in reducing perinatal death. Current data is insufficient to justify a policy of elective cesarean section of all SGA babies.

In all given situations, the test results need to be integrated.

In a situation where IUGR is diagnosed with brain sparing, the presence of oligohydramnios, BPS ≥6, increased IVC and DV indices and normal UV flow.

Interpretation: Proven fetal compromise, hypoxemia common, acidemia/asphyxia likely.

Recommended management: If at more than 34 weeks of gestation, deliver (route determined by obstetric factors and oxytocin challenge test results). If at less than 34 weeks of gestation, individualise treatment with admission, continuous cardiotocography, steroids, maternal oxygen, and/or amnioinfusion and then repeat testing up to three times a day, depending on status.

In a situation where test results show IUGR with accelerating compromise, BPS ≤6, abnormal IVC and DV indices, pulsatile UV flow.

Interpretation: IUGR with decompensation cardiovascular instability, hypoxemia certain, acidemia/asphyxia common, high perinatal mortality, death imminent.

Recommended management: If the fetus is considered viable by size, deliver as soon as possible at tertiary centre. Route determined by obstetric factors and OCT results. Fetus requires the highest level of neonatal ICU care.

These examples illustrate the need for careful integration of test reports and clinical findings against the backdrop of gestational age.

Management Planning at Different Gestational Ages

In essence, gestational age can be divided into five bands, each provoking a different response:

Before 26 Weeks The outcome in this group of babies is usually extremely poor. The combination of severe growth restriction and prematurity means that survival is about 30% and long-term handicap around 30–50%. It seems likely that the best incubator at this gestation is the uterus, and it seems unlikely that the baby would do better if delivered. Of course, if the mother has an additional problem such as hypertension, the baby may need to be delivered for her sake. However, in the absence of such pressure, delay is probably the correct decision. It may be worth administering steroids to the mother in any case.

26–28 Weeks This is an area of great uncertainty and possibly the one in which the results of the GRIT study will provide the most enlightenment. So long as the fetus is not clearly moribund, delivery following the use of maternal steroids would seem to be most appropriate. The results are reasonable, both in terms of mortality (85% survival) and morbidity (about 15%), and the additional risk to the mother of delivery by cesarean section seems justifiable. However, it is still unclear whether prolonged intrauterine life confers an advantage.

28–32 Weeks At this gestational age, the indications to deliver the IUGR fetus are fairly clear, although steroids should always be given for 48 hours, if possible. The closer to 32 weeks, the easier is the decision to deliver, but hasty delivery should be avoided unless the indications to do so are clear, since neonatal respiratory problems can still prove a significant problem at these gestational ages.

32–36 Weeks When severe problems of IUGR are found at this stage, delivery should be recommended. Steroids should be given, if possible, but delivery should not be delayed if the baby is clearly in difficulties.

37 Weeks and Over IUGR at this stage should be the indication for delivery as soon as is practically possible. There is no justification to wait and the route of delivery will be by cesarean section, unless the cervix is favourable.

Short-Term Outcome IUGR babies have a number of significant problems. They have difficulties in temperature control because of their small body mass to surface area, lack of glycogen stores and usually absent brown fat, which reduces their non-shivering thermogenesis. The adaptation to prolonged intrauterine hypoxia makes them prone to necrotising enterocolitis. Respiratory problems relate more to the gestational age at delivery than IUGR and, although there have always been suggestions that IUGR enhances lung maturity, the evidence is not secure.

The care of these babies can, therefore, be complex and requires sophisticated neonatal support. Such babies should, therefore, be delivered at tertiary centres, especially if prematurity is an additional factor.

Medium-Term Outcome The subsequent development of these children depends both on the extent and etiology of the IUGR and the gestational age at delivery. Outcome data with respect to survival and long-term handicap shows the significance of gestational age at the time of delivery. However, it has been suggested that being born small for dates may interfere more with intellectual development than being born early, which has an additional effect on motor function. The children who were severely IUGR at birth, typically symmetrically small, did not illustrate the catch-up growth seen when IUGR arose from a relatively short spell of uteroplacental insufficiency.

Long-Term Outcome The work of Barker and his group indicates the possibility that small for dates babies are prone to developing hypertension and non-insulin dependent diabetes as adults, and the subject has been extensively reviewed. Whether this arises from programming or as a response to intrauterine hypoxia is not clear. Certainly the babies that are 'rescued' nowadays from hostile intrauterine environments would almost certainly not have survived in the era in which those cases under study in Barker's work were born. It was the effect of LBW rather than IUGR that formed the basis of his studies, and although these babies may be part of a continuum, this remains uncertain. Nevertheless, the fact that the intrauterine environment may influence adult development is a critical and important observation that does offer some opportunity for useful intervention.

Conclusion Fetal growth restriction remains a challenging problem for all clinicians. Most cases occur in pregnancies in which no risk factors are present. Therefore, the clinicians must be alert to the possibility of a growth disturbance in all pregnancies. Complex strategy for diagnosis and assessment is necessary. The ability to diagnose the disorder and understand its pathophysiology is more important than the ability to prevent or treat its complications.

The obstetrician must have a thorough understanding of the importance of cautious management decisions in LBW babies. One must not lose sight of the goal in the management of FGR with low birth weight. Because no effective treatments are known, the aim of every obstetrician should be to deliver the most mature fetus in the best physiological condition possible while minimising the risk to the mother.

References

Alfirevic Z and JP Neilson. 1995. Doppler ultrasonography in high-risk pregnancies: systematic review with meta analysis. *Am J Obstet Gynecol* 172:1379–1387.

Alfirevic Z and JP Neilson. 1997. Biophysical profile for fetal assessment in high-risk pregnancies. *Cochrane Database Syst Rev* (4).

Aoki M. 1990. Fetal weight calculation: Osaka University method. In *Ultrasound in Obstetrics and Gynecology,* 2nd ed, Yoshihide C, ed. Kyoto: Kinpodo.

Arduini D, G Rizzo and C Romanini. 1993. The development of abnormal heart rate patterns after absent end diastolic velocity in umbical artery: analysis of risk factors. *Am J Obstet Gynecol* 168:43–50.

Bailey SM, P Sarmandal and JM Grant. 1989. A comparison of three methods of assessing inter-observer variation applied to measurement of the symphysis-fundal height. *Br J Obstet Gynaecol* 96:1266–1271.

Barker DJP. 1992. *Fetal and infant origins of adult disease*. London: BMJ Books.

Baschat AA and K Hecher. 2004. Fetal growth restriction due to placental disease. *Semin Perinatol* 28(1):67–80 [Medline].

Baschat AA and CP Weiner. 2000. Umbical artery Doppler screening for detection of the small fetus in need of antepartum surveillance. *Am J Obstet Gynaecol* 182 (1 Pt 1): 154–158 [Medline].

Baschat AA, U Gembruch, I Reiss et al. 2000. Absent umbilical artery end-diastolic velocity in growth-restricted fetuses: a risk factor for neonatal thrombocytopenia. *Obstet Gynecol* 96(2):162–166 [Medline].

Bastide A, F Manning, C Harman, I Lange and I Morrison. 1986. Ultrasound evaluation of amniotic fluid: Outcome of pregnancies with severe oligohydramnios. *Am J Obstet Gynecol* 154:895–900.

Belzian JM, J Villar, JC Nardin, J Malamud and LS De Vicurna. 1978. Diagnosis of intrauterine growth retardation by a simple clinical method: Measurement of uterine height. *Am J Obstet Gynecol* 131:643–646.

Brar H and S Rutherford. 1988. Classification of intrauterine growth restriction. *Semin Perinatol* 12(1): 2–10.

Calvert JP, EE Crean, RG Newcombe and JF Pearson. 1982. Antenatal screening by measurement of symphysis-fundus height. *BMJ* 285:846–849.

Chamberlain PF, FA Manning, I Morrison, CR Harman and IR Lange. 1984. Ultrasound evaluation of amniotic fluid volume I. The relationship of marginal and decreased amniotic fluid volumes to perinatal outcome. *Am J Obstet Gynecol* 150:245–249.

Chang TC, SC Robson, RJ Boys and JA Spencer. 1992. Prediction of the small for gestational age infant: which ultrasonic measurement is best? *Obstet Gynaecol* 45:59–62.

Chang TC, SC Robson, JA Spencer and S Gallivan. 1994. Prediction of perinatal morbidity at term in small fetuses: comparison of fetal growth and Doppler ultrasound. *Br J Obstet Gynaecol* 101:422–427.

Chauhan SP, M Sanderson, NW Hendrix, EF Magann and LD Devoe. 1999. Perinatal outcome and amniotic fluid index in the antepartum and intrapartum periods: A metaanalysis. *Am J Obstet Gynecol* 181:1473–1478.

Chien PF, P Owen and KS Khan. 2000. Validity of ultrasound estimation of fetal weight. *Obstet Gynaecol* 95:856–860.

Cnattingius S, O Axelsson and G Lindmark. 1984. Symphysis-fundus measurements and intrauterine growth retardation. *Acta Obstet Gyncol Scand* 63:335–340.

Colley NV, JM Tremble, GL Henson and TJ Cole. 1991. Head circumference/abdominal circumference ratio, ponderal index and fetal malnutrition. Should head circumference/abdominal circumference ratio be abandoned? *Br J Obstet Gynaecol* 98:524–527.

Dayal AK, FA Manning, DJ Berck, GM Mussalli, C Avila, CR Harman et al. 1999. Fetal death after normal biophysical profile score: an eighteen year experience. *Am J Obstet Gynecol* 181:1231–1236.

De Jong CL, A Francis, HP van Geijn and J Gardosi. 1999. Fetal growth rate and adverse perinatal events. *Ultrasound Obstet Gynaecol* 13:86–89.

De Jong CL, A Francis, HP van Geijn and J Gardosi. 2000. Customised fetal weight limits for antenatal detection of fetal growth restriction. *Ultrasound Obstet Gynaecol* 15:36–40.

Deter RL, FP Hadlock, RB Harrist and RJ Carpenter. 1981. Evaluation of three methods for obtaining fetal weight estimates using dynamic image ultrasound. *J Clin Ultrasound* 9:421–425.

Deter RL, RB Harrist, FP Hadlock and RJ Carpenter. 1981. The use of ultrasound in the assessment of normal fetal growth: a review. *J Clin Ultrasound* 9:481–493.

Draper ES, B Manktelow, DJ Field and D James. 1999. Prediction of survival for preterm births by weight and gestational age: retrospective population based study. *BMJ* 319:1093–1097.

Fanaroff AA, LL Wright, DK Stevenson et al. 1995. Very low birth weight outcomes of the National Institute of Child Health and Human Development Neonatal Research Network. May 1991 through December 1992. *Am J Obstet Gynecol* 173:1423–1431.

Cunningham FG, Mac Donalld PC, Grant NF, Levero KJ et al. 1997. Fetal growth restriction. In *Williams Obstetrics,* 20th ed, 839–54, Cunningham FG et al eds. Stamford, Conn: Appleton and Lange.

Gardosi J and A Francis. 1999. Controlled trial of fundal height measurement plotted on customized antenatal growth charts. *Br J Obstet Gynaecol* 106:309–317.

Grant A. 1997. Elective versus selective caesarean delivery of the small baby. *Cochrane Database Syst Rev* (2).

GROW: Gestation Related Optimal Weight. 1997. Version 2. Nottingham: PRAM.

Gudmundsson S, G Tulzer, JC Huhta and K Marsal. 1996. Venous Doppler in the fetus with absent end diastolic flow in the umbical artery. *Ultrasound Obstet Gynecol* 7:262–267.

Gulmezoglu AM and GJ Hofmeyr. 1997. Nutrient treatment for suspected impaired fetal growth. *Cochrane Database Syst Rev* (1).

Gulmezoglu AM and GJ Hofmeyr. 2000. Betamimetics for suspected impaired fetal growth. *Cochrane Database Syst Rev* CD000036.

Gulmezoglu AM and GJ Hofmeyr. 2000. Calcium channel blockers for potential impaired fetal growth. *Cochrane Database Syst Rev* CD000049.

Gulmezoglu AM and GJ Hofmeyr. 2000. Hormones for suspected impaired fetal growth. *Cochrane Database Syst Rev* CD0000109.

Gulmezoglu AM and GJ Hofmeyr. 2000. Maternal oxygen administration for suspected impaired fetal growth. *Cochrane Database Syst Rev* CD000137.

Hill LM, R Breckle, KR Wolfgram and PC O'Brien. 1986. Evaluation of three methods for estimating fetal weight. *J Clin Ultrasound* 14:171–178.

Kaaij MW, PC Struijk and FK Lotgering. 1999. Accuracy of sonographic estimates of fetal weight in very small infants. *Ultrasound Obstet Gynaecol* 13:99–102.

Kalinka J, P Sieroszewski, W Hanke, T Laudanski and J Suzin. 1999. Evaluation of the effectiveness of a low dose aspirin in the treatment of intrauterine growth retardation (IUGR). *Ginekol Pol* 70:126–134.

Karsdorp VH, JM van Vugt, HP van Geijn, PJ Kostense, D Arduini, N Montenegro et al. 1994. Clinical significance of absent or reversed end diastolic velocity waveforms in umbical artery. *Lancet* 344:1664–1668.

Leger T, C Levy-Marchal, J Bloch et al. 1997. Reduced final heights and indicators for insulin resistance iu 20 year olds born small for gestational age: regional cohort study. *BMJ* 15:341–347.

Leitich H, C Egarter, P Husslein, A Kaider and M Schemper. 1997. A meta analysis of low dose aspirin for the prevention of intrauterine growth retardation. *Br J Obstet Gynecol* 104:450–459.

Lockwood CJ and S Weiner. 1986. Assessment of fetal growth. *Clin Perinatol* 13:3–35.

Magann EF, SP Chauhan, PS Barrilleaux, NS Whitworth and JN Martin. 2000. Amniotic fluid index and single deepest pocket: weak indicators of abnormal amniotic volumes. *Obstet Gynecol* 96:737–740.

Magann EF, CM Isler, SP Chauhan and JN Martin Jr. 2000. Amniotic fluid volume estimation and the biophysical profile: a confusion of criteria. *Obstet Gynecol* 96: 640–642.

Mathai M, P Jairaj and S Muthurathnam. 1987. Screening for light-for-gestational age infants: A comparison of three simple measurements. *Br J Obstet Gynaecol* 94:217–221.

Maulik D, P Yarlagadda, JP Youngblood and P Ciston. 1991. Comparative efficacy of umbilical arterial Doppler indices for predicting adverse perinatal outcome. *Am J Obstet Gynecol* 164:1434–1439.

McCowan LM, JE Harding, AB Roberts, SE Barker, C Ford and AW Stewart. 2000. A pilot randomized controlled trial of two regimens of fetal surveillance for small for gestational age fetuses with normal results of umbical artery Doppler velocimetry. *Am J Obstet Gynecol* 182:81–86.

Murphy DJ, PL Hope, A Johnson et al. 1997. Neonatal risk factors for cerebral palsy in very preterm babies: a case control study. *Lancet* 314:404–408.

Neerhof MG. 1995. Causes of intrauterine growth restriction. *Clin Perinatol* 22: 375–385.

Neilson JP. 2000. Symphysis-fundal height measurement in pregnancy. *Cochrane Database Syst Rev* CD000944.

Ott WJ. 1988. The diagnosis of altered fetal growth. *Obstet Gynecol Clin North Am* 15:237–263.

Pattison N and L McCowan. 2000. Cardiotocography for antepartum fetal assessment. *Cochrane Database Syst Rev* CD001068.

Person B, M Stangenberg, NO Lunell, U Brodin, NG Holmberg and V Vaclavinkova. 1986. Prediction of size of infants at birth by measurement of symphysis fundus height. *Br J Obstet Gynaecol* 93:206–211.

Shepard MJ, VA Richards, RL Berkowitz, SL Warsof and JC Hobbins. 1982. An evaluation of two equations for predicting fetal weight by ultrasound. *Am J Obstet Gynaecol* 142:47–54.

Snijders RJ, C Sherrod, CM Gosden and KH Nicolaides. 1993. Fetal growth retardation: Associated malformations and chromosomal abnormalities. *Am J Obstet Gynecol* 168:547–555.

Soothill PW, RA Ajayi, S Campbell and KH Nicolaides. 1993. Prediction of morbidity in small and normally grown fetuses by fetal heart rate variability, biophysical profile score and umbilical artery Doppler studies. *Br J Obstet Gynecol* 100:742–745.

Thacker SB and DF Stroup. 2000. Continuous electronic heart rate monitoring for fetal assessment during labour. *Cochrane Database Syst Rev* CD000063.

The GRIT study group. 1996. When do obstetricians recommend delivery for a high risk preterm growth retarded fetus. *Eur Jobstet Gynecol* 67:121–126.

Tyrrell SN, RJ Lilford, HN Macdonald, EJ Nelson, J Porter and JK Gupta. 1990. Randomized comparison of routine vs highly selective use of Doppler ultrasound and biophysical scoring to investigate high risk pregnancies. *Br J Obstet Gynecol* 97:909–916.

Wood NS, N Marlow, K Costeloe, AT Gibson and AR Wilkinson. 2000. Neurologic and developmental disability after extremely preterm birth. EPICURE Study Group. *N Engl J Med* 343:378–384.

24

Preterm Labour

Jasvinder Kalra

Preterm labour and the attendant complications of preterm delivery remain a major health problem. Although preterm birth rates have risen during the past two decades the majority of this increase has been due to the aggressive management of medical and surgical disorders requiring early delivery, assisted reproductive techniques resulting in a large number of higher order multifetal gestations. The incidence of preterm birth is 10%–12% in developed countries and in the last twenty years this incidence has gradually risen from 9.5% to 12% in the United States despite extensive research efforts to reduce it (Creasy 1993). In India too the preterm birth rate is 10%–12% (Singh 1999) and is among the three most common causes of neonatal mortality; in addition, it contributes significantly to increased morbidity from respiratory distress syndrome, intraventricular hemorrhage, necrotising enterocolitis and sepsis according to the National Neonatal-Perinatal Database 2002–2003, National Neonatology Forum, India. Long-term sequelae of premature disproportionality contribute to developmental delay, visual and hearing impairment, chronic lung disease and cerebral palsy. About 40% of preterm births follow idiopathic preterm labour, 35% follow preterm predator rupture of membranes and the rest are iatrogenic because of obstetric or medical indications (Iams et al 2002).

Pathogenesis of prematurity A wide spectrum of causes and demographic factors have been implicated in preterm birth. Preterm labour, preterm ruptured membranes, pre-eclampsia, abruptio placentae, multiple gestations, placenta previa, fetal growth restriction, excessive or inadequate amniotic fluid volume, fetal anomalies, amnionitis, incompetent cervix, as well as maternal medical problems such as diabetes mellitus, asthma, drug abuse and pyelonephritis may all lead to preterm delivery. Maternal characteristics associated with preterm delivery are equally numerous—maternal race, history of previous preterm birth, low socioeconomic status, poor nutrition, low pre-pregnancy weight, absent or inadequate prenatal care, age less than 18 or over 40, strenuous work, anemia, cigarette smoking, bacteriuria, genital colonisation or infection. The multitude of clinical disorders and risk factors can be classified into two broad categories based upon the clinical presentation, maternal and fetal health and the epidemiologic profile of affected pregnant women—spontaneous and indicated preterm births. Spontaneous preterm births account for nearly 75% of all preterm births and this includes preterm labour (PTL), preterm premature rupture of membranes (PPROM) or related diagnoses such as amnionitis and incompetent cervix. Risk factors for PTL and PPROM are similar, with a few exceptions such as, women with PPROM are more likely to be indigent (Meis et al 1987), to have smoked (Hadley et al 1990) and to have experienced bleeding in the current pregnancy (Ekwo et al 1992) than women who present with PTL with intact membranes.

Indicated preterm births follow medical or obstetric disorders that place the fetus at risk (for example, acute or chronic maternal hypertension, diabetes mellitus, placenta previa or abruption and intrauterine growth retardation and these account for nearly 25% of births before 37 weeks in most reports (Meis et al 1998). The distinction between spontaneous and indicated births may not always be clear, as even in the absence of an apparent maternal disease, poor intrauterine growth with associated decidual and placental vascular lesions and fetal stress may initiate preterm labour (Hediger et al 1995; Arias et al 1993).

Epidemiology of spontaneous preterm birth Goldenberg et al (1998) in their preterm prediction study suggested that some risk factors are associated with recurrent preterm birth while others appear to be unique to the affected pregnancy. A different epidemiology has also been indicated for early preterm birth (<32 weeks) and late preterm births (>32 weeks). Early preterm birth is more likely to recur, is more strongly associated with a short cervix and the presence of fetal fibronectin in cervicovaginal secretions and is, more often, accompanied by clinical or subclinical evidence of infection and by long-term morbidity for the infant. Late preterm birth is more likely to be associated with increased uterine contraction frequency, and thus to mimic normal labour at term (Darne et al 1987).

Non-recurring Spontaneous Preterm Birth

Risk factors for non-recurring spontaneous preterm labour include:

First and second trimester bleeding Vaginal bleeding in early pregnancy is associated with increased incidence of pregnancy loss prior to 24 weeks, PTL and placental abruptions. Mercer et al (1996) reported a doubling of the risk of subsequent PTL in the presence of history of both first and second trimester vaginal bleeding.

Overdistended uterus Abnormal amniotic fluid volume and multiple gestations are known to be associated with increased risk of preterm labour due to increased uterine activity via increased formation of gap junctions, oxytocin receptors and prostaglandin and collagenase production.

However, preterm birth in multiple gestations may not always be explained by uterine distension. Tallo et al (1995) reported that women, who deliver a multifetal gestation beyond 34 weeks, are more likely to have conceived spontaneously as compared to those with assisted reproductive technology. Increased levels of maternal serum relaxin, superovulation and potential for intrauterine inoculation with vaginal microorganisms during cervical instrumentation are potential mechanisms under investigation.

Lifestyle factors Cigarette smoking, drug use and inadequate maternal weight gain during pregnancy have also been linked to PTL. Cigarette smoking results in an increased incidence of births under 34 weeks gestation, the greatest risk being to those smoking more than 20 cigarettes per day. Initially, this effect was attributed to an excess of abruptio placentae, placenta praevia and preterm PROM, but more recent epidemiological studies have shown a stronger relationship with spontaneous preterm labour (Kyrklund–Blomberg and Cnattingius 1998). Shah and Bracken (2000) have systematically reviewed the relationship between smoking and preterm birth and they too suggested a dose–response effect at mild to moderate smoking values. These recent findings suggest that smoking is a causal rather than an epidemiological factor in preterm birth.

Cocaine use increases the rate of preterm delivery (relative risk 2.4), partly as a consequence of a higher risk of abruptio placentae (Volpe 1992). Recent data (Boer et al 1993, Walkinshaw et al 1993), controlling for social factors, confirms an excess of preterm births in opiate users.

Alcohol consumption and an increased risk of preterm births remains unproven. Vigorous activity or exercise into the third trimester may increase the risk of preterm delivery (Henrikson et al 1995), although regular and moderate exercise may actually reduce this risk.

Psychological stress has been implicated in increasing the risk of preterm delivery, with a clear link between stress element of a score and preterm delivery (Copper et al 1996).

Recurring Spontaneous Preterm Birth

Early preterm birth is more likely to recur and is associated with certain factors, the interrelationship of which has partly explained some of the mechanisms of preterm delivery.

Genetic factors The recurrent, familial as well as racial nature of preterm birth suggests that genetics may play a causal role. The gene for decidual relaxin, fetal mitochondrial trifunctional protein defects or polymorphism in the interleukin-1 gene complex, β2-adrenergic receptor, or tumour necrosis factor-α (TNF-α) may be involved in preterm membrane rupture (Genc et al 2002; Landac et al 2002; Yang et al 2002; Netla et al 2003).

African-American women have double the rate of preterm delivery as that of women of other races (National Centre for Health Statistics 1999). The preterm birth rates remain higher in this group of women even when controlled for educational levels. Socio-demographic factors also do not explain the higher preterm birth rates in African-American women (Goldenberg et al 1996).

Prior preterm birth The risk of spontaneous preterm birth is increased by a history of prior preterm delivery and this recurrent risk rises as the number of prior preterm births increases (Bakketeig and Hoffman 1981). The risk of recurrent preterm delivery for women whose first delivery was preterm was three times that of those whose first neonate was born at term; further, this risk increased seven- to eightfold if the previous two deliveries were preterm (Bloom et al 2001; Bakketeig and Hoffman 1981). The likelihood of recurrent preterm birth also increases as the gestational age of prior preterm birth decreases (Mercer et al 1999). The biologic variable, cervical length and function may be a part of a constitutional factor that influences preterm birth risk in successive pregnancies (Iams et al 1998).

Infection Multiple sources such as epidemiologic, microbiologic, histologic and clinical studies have shown evidence relating infection to preterm labour and birth. Maternal and neonatal infections occur more frequently after preterm birth than term birth. Several microorganisms, including *Ureaplasma urealyticum*, Mycoplasma species, *Chlamydia trachomatis, Trichomonas*, *Escherichia coli*, group B streptococci and several anerobes have been recovered from the lower and upper genital tract and amniotic fluid of women with preterm labour and PPROM (Wahbeh et al 1984; Romero et al 1992; Martius et al 1988; Krohn et al 1991; Watts et al 1992). The strength of the association between both clinical infections and histologic amnionitis increases as the gestational age at delivery decreases, especially before 32 weeks. The same inverse relationship between gestational age and positive amniotic fluid cultures were obtained from women with preterm labour who did not have overt clinical chorioamnionitis (Watts et al 1992). Another study by Hauth et al (1998) found that both positive membrane cultures and increased amniotic fluid IL-6 levels occurred more frequently in spontaneous than indicated preterm births. Infections outside the genital tract, such as pyelonephritis and appendicitis, have also been related to preterm births. Oral bacteria and periodontitis have been found to have a strong relationship with preterm birth. Offenbacher et al (1996) found a sevenfold risk of preterm birth in women with periodontitis when compared with controls and this was further confirmed in a prospective trial by Hauth and associates (2001) who found a fourfold increase in women who delivered before 32 weeks, as also by Golpfert et al (2004) who found an association of severe periodontitis with preterm delivery.

Retrospective studies of pregnant women treated with antimicrobial drugs effective against Ureaplasma, Mycoplasma and Chlamydia had shown reduced rates of preterm delivery (McCormack et al 1987; Cohen et al 1990). However, prospective trials with the same antibiotics found no difference in the incidence of preterm delivery (Eschenbach et al 1991; Carey et al 1993). This led to consideration of association of bacterial vaginosis (BV) with preterm delivery—BV infection (an alteration of the maternal bacterial flora in which Gram-negative anerobic bacteria and Mycoplasma species replace the normally predominant lactobacilli) was found to have a strong association with preterm births (OR 2.1; 95% CI 1.5 to 3.0) as reported by Hiller et al (1995). These authors suggested that BV may result in production of cytokines with biologic effects on uterus, cervix and membranes. Subsequently, two prospective trials of antibiotic treatment of women with previous preterm delivery and presence of BV reported reduced rates of preterm delivery (Hauth et al 1995; McDonald et al 1997). However, the rate of preterm birth was not affected by treatment of these women who had asymptomatic BV in a placebo-controlled trial on 1900 women. Another study, conducted simultaneously in women with *Trichomonas vaginalis,* reported an increase in the rate of preterm birth in those randomised to receive metronidazole (Carey et al 2000). These trials indicate that the relationship between infection and prematurity is more complex than can be explained by the ascent of the organism from the lower to the upper genital tract during pregnancy, and other factors such as host defense may play a role causing preterm birth.

Cervical length The length of the uterine cervix as measured by transvaginal ultrasonography (TVS) is inversely and continuously related to the risk of preterm birth in both singleton and multiple gestations (Goldenberg et al 1996).

In women with a history of delivery before 32 weeks, Owen and associates (2001) reported a significant correlation of cervical length at 16 to 24 weeks and subsequent preterm birth before 35 weeks. In a secondary analysis of these data, Yost and colleagues (2004) found that dilatation of 2–4 mm identified during second-trimester TVS independently predicted an increase in birth prior to 35 weeks.

Prevention of preterm births Effective primary care for reduction of risk of preterm births in an entire population requires understanding of the pathophysiology of the condition and public health educational efforts to modify behaviour and eliminate risk factors. Although effective primary interventions have not been demonstrated, a programme to reduce the incidence of prematurity should include efforts to prevent smoking and sexually transmitted diseases, to avoid unplanned pregnancies through use of birth control methods, to reduce stress and improve nutrition, to avoid higher order multifetal gestations etc (Hall 2000).

The next step (secondary care) involves the identification of women at risk for surveillance and prophylactic measures such as tocolytic drugs, progesterone supplementation or antibiotics. However, none of these measures have led to any significant decline in prematurity (Goldenberg and Rouse 1998).

Identification of risk factors for preterm labour Prediction of preterm birth would ideally involve a screening test with high sensitivity and high negative predictive value. It should also enable effective intervention if the test yields a positive result. The screening tools and interventions currently available have not enabled obstetricians to decrease the incidence of preterm birth and do not satisfy the requirements of an optimal screening test. However, they may allow time for transfer of a pregnancy at risk to an appropriate tertiary referral centre, as well as the administration of glucocorticoids to enhance fetal lung maturity and antibiotic prophylaxis to reduce the risk of neonatal sepsis.

Clinical risk factors for preterm birth Efforts to create scoring systems based on clinical factors to identify pregnancies at risk have proved to be fruitless because of high prevalence of these risk factors but low sensitivity and positive predictive value (Collaborative Group on Preterm Birth Prevention 1993; Mercer et al 1996). Nevertheless, women with these major clinical risk factors should be considered to be at risk of preterm birth:

- Prior preterm delivery
- Multiple gestation
- Low pre-pregnancy weight
- Vaginal bleeding in the second or third trimester

These historical risk factors, although easily elicited, identify less than half of women who will deliver prematurely.

In a retrospective analysis of 92 women in preterm labour, anemia (32.6%), bacterial vaginosis (26%t), gestational hypertension (18.4%) and previous history of preterm labour (18.4%) were found to be the main risk factors (Roy et al 2006).

Monitoring Uterine Activity

The simplest method for assessing uterine activity relies on teaching the woman to palpate and record her own contractions. Although it is an inexpensive method, it is completely subjective and has been shown to have a poor sensitivity, with 89% of women palpating less than 50% of their contractions (Newman et al 1986). A more objective approach to uterine activity monitoring involves tocography using a pressure transducer attached to a recording device. An early case control study of women at high risk of preterm labour using daily ambulatory home uterine monitoring, showed encouraging results, with the preterm delivery rate reduced to half in the study group (Katz et al 1986).

This method obviously cannot be used in a low-risk population and is relatively expensive, time-consuming (since repeated studies for many weeks of pregnancy are required), and skill-intensive (requiring interpretation by a skilled healthcare professional). A meta-analysis, presenting data from six studies on a total of 697 pregnancies, concluded that home uterine monitoring in singleton pregnancies was associated with a 24% reduction in preterm births, 52% reduction in late presentation with cervical dilatation more than 2 cm, and a significant mean increase in birth weight of 126 g. There was, however, no difference in the admission rate to neonatal intensive care (Colton et al 1995). To overcome the bias of increased level of support by a nursing attendant in the case of women whose uterine activity was monitored at home, two studies addressed this issue in their randomised controlled trials. One of them randomised 1992 women but only 72.3% women completed this trial suggesting that there may be difficulties with compliance—this study concluded that there was no evidence that either home uterine activity monitoring or daily nursing contact improved early diagnosis of preterm labour or reduced rates of preterm birth or neonatal morbidity (Collaborative Home Uterine Monitoring Group 1995). The second randomised study by Dyson et al (1998) of 2422 women also concluded that neither daily contact nor home monitoring improved pregnancy outcome beyond that seen with weekly nurse contact. More recently, in a study of high-risk singleton pregnancies where women were monitored with home uterine monitoring and also with sonographic assessment of cervix and fetal fibronectin, the authors concluded that although the likelihood of preterm delivery is associated with increased frequency of uterine contractions, assessment is not clinically useful for predicting preterm delivery (Iams et al 2002).

Sonographic Cervical Screening

Transvaginal sonography allows an accurate assessment of cervix and has been used in a variety of situations to improve the accuracy of prediction of a woman going into preterm labour. A recent meta-analysis of antenatal transvaginal ultrasound assessment of the cervix identified 46 studies involving 31,577 pregnancies describing the effectiveness of this screening technique (Honest et al 2003). TVS is more accurate and reproducible than transabdominal sonography for assessment of cervix; however, the technique is important and a standardised technique has been described by Colombo and Iams (2000). Cervical length in a low-risk population is normally distributed, with a mean length at 23 weeks gestation of 35 to 38 mm, the 10th and 90th percentile are approximately 25 mm and 45 mm respectively. Although other cervical parameters such as cervical funneling and dilatation have also been investigated for prediction of preterm labour, these did not contribute to any additional information about the risk of preterm delivery if the cervical length was less than a screen positive of 25 mm (Hassan et al 2000; To et al 2001).

Cervical assessment in asymptomatic women at high risk of preterm labour can allow early intervention that would prevent the onset of preterm delivery. It is not currently clear what the optimum gestation for screening is, what cervical cut-off should be used to define a screen positive group or whether serial scans are more appropriate than a single scan. Cook and associates (2000) showed that cervical length less than 21 mm at less than 20 weeks gestation was associated with 95% delivery by 34 weeks gestation in women at high risk of preterm delivery. Guzman and colleagues (2001) examined 469 women at high risk of preterm delivery with singleton pregnancies serially between 15 and 24 weeks gestation and found cervical length 25 mm or less in 23.4% of women out of which 76% delivered before 34 weeks of gestation. The negative predictive value of this cut-off was 96%. Similarly, Owen et al (2001) also demonstrated that a single TVS of cervix at 16 to 19 weeks gestation with a cervical length of 25 mm or less increased the risk of preterm delivery by 35 weeks gestation, 3.3 times. In one small study of serial screening of high-risk pregnancies between 16 to 30 weeks gestation, Andrews et al (2000) found that fortnightly screening was found to be significantly helpful in prediction of preterm delivery.

Cervical assessment in asymptomatic women at low risk of preterm labour has also been assessed. Iams and associates (1996) reported a multicentre study of 2915 pregnancies and found a significant association between the risk of preterm labour and short cervix. Unfortunately, there is little evidence to suggest that screening population at low risk is useful, since an effective intervention to improve pregnancy outcome has not yet been demonstrated.

To evaluate the effects of cerclage in women with sonographically measured cervical dilatation, Owen et al (2003) summarised five retrospective cohort series and two randomised trials and found that four of the seven reports cited a beneficial effect and three showed no benefit.

Fetal fibronectin Fetal fibronectin is a glycoprotein found in amniotic fluid, placental tissue and the decidua basalis. It is normally found in cervicovaginal secretion before 16 to 18 weeks gestation, before fusion of the fetal membranes and decidua is complete. Similarly, it is found at the end of pregnancy, prior to onset of labour, but it is not normally present in cervicovaginal secretions between 22 and 37 weeks. It has been suggested that the presence of fetal fibronectin in cervicovaginal secretions in the later part of the second trimester and in the third trimester of pregnancy is due to disruption of the chorionic decidual interface and is often secondary to infection (Lockwood 1994).

Honest et al (2002) reported a large systematic review of 64 studies assessing the effectiveness of screening for preterm delivery by the detection of cervicovaginal fetal fibronectin in a total of 26,876 women. In the subset of asymptomatic women, the likelihood ratio for predicting preterm delivery before 34 weeks was 4.01 (95% CI 2.93–5.49) with a likelihood ratio for negative results of 0.78 (95% CI 0.72–0.84). Among those women who were symptomatic, the likelihood for positive results was 5.42 (95% CI 4.36–6.74) for predicting birth between 7 and 10 days of testing, with a corresponding negative likelihood ratio of 0.25 (95% CI 0.20-0.31). Another meta-analysis found that fetal fibronectin was useful in the prediction of delivery before 34 weeks with an overall sensitivity of 53% and specificity of 89% (Leitich et al 2003). In a further analysis of studies in asymptomatic women who could be divided into low risk and high risk showed that for a single test for fibronectin, sensitivity for detection of delivery prior to 34 weeks was 41% for low risk women and only 23% for high risk women with a comparable specificity of 94% for both low and high risk women. Subgroup analysis of asymptomatic and symptomatic pregnancies demonstrated that this test was more sensitive in women with symptoms of preterm labour but with a much lower specificity. The authors concluded that fetal fibronectin is a reasonably effective marker in predicting preterm delivery in the short term, particularly if there are symptoms of preterm labour.

Hincz and associates (2002) proposed a two-step test comprising of cervical length measurement, followed by fibronectin testing, if cervical length was in a range of 21 mm to 31 mm. This form of testing had an overall sensitivity of 86% with a specificity of 90% for predicting delivery within 28 days.

Screening for bacterial vaginosis in early pregnancy Despite the convincing evidence of a link between early infection with BV and preterm delivery, as mentioned earlier, screening and subsequent treatment of BV remains controversial. A recent review of the Cochrane Collaboration (McDonald et al 2003) of 10 trials of 4249 women showed that antibiotic therapy successfully treated BV but failed to reduce the risk of preterm birth before 37 weeks, with an odds ratio of 0.95 (95% CI 0.82–1.10), at 34 weeks with an odds ratio of 1.20 (95% CI 0.69–2.07), or 32 weeks with an odds ratio of 1.08 (95% CI 0.70–1.68). In those women who had a previous preterm birth, treatment of BV did not decrease the risk of subsequent preterm birth but did decrease the risk of PPROM, an odds ratio of 0.14 (95% CI 0.05–0.38). At present the role of screening for BV and then treating is not clear in low-risk population, although it has possible benefit in a high-risk population.

Periodontal disease: Periodontal infection has been found to be associated with increased risk of preterm delivery. Offenbacher and associates (1996) found a sevenfold risk of preterm birth with periodontitis, compared with controls, and this was confirmed in a prospective trial of more than 1300 women by Hauth et al (2001). The incidence of preterm birth before 35 weeks was found to be 4.9% versus 3.3% in those who had only prophylaxis in the form of single teeth cleaning and polishing compared to those who had intervention (deep root scaling and planing) and metronidazole treatment in a randomised trial of 366 women (Jeffcoat et al 2003). Two multicentre trials sponsored by the National Institute of Dental and Craniofacial Research are underway to determine whether mid-pregnancy identification and treatment of women with periodontal disease prevents preterm birth.

Other biochemical markers An association between increased maternal salivary estriol concentration and subsequent preterm birth has been described by Heine et al (1999), although it requires further evaluation. Plasma CRH, a peptide produced by syncitiotrophoblast and serum alpha-fetoprotein (Mclean et al 1999) are under investigation for prediction of a subsequent preterm labour. Preliminary data on human chorionic gonadotropin (hCG) in cervical secretions of high-risk women shows promise, with predictive values in the range of those seen with fetal fibronectin (Bernstein et al 1998).

Strategies for prevention of preterm labour A number of strategies involving the prophylactic use of certain agents have been used:

Progesterone Supplemental progesterone to prevent preterm delivery has been studied recently by daFonseca et al (2003) and Meis et al (2003) and have shown encouraging results. The most commonly used progestin has been intramuscular administration of

17α-hydroxyprogesterone caproate. In addition to this, 100 mg vaginal suppository of natural progesterone to reduce preterm delivery in high-risk women is being studied in several trials; however, so far the sample size has been insufficient to demonstrate a reduction in perinatal morbidity rate.

Tocolytics Several controlled trials of prophylactic administration of β-sympathomimetic drugs for prevention of PTL have been reported in literature. However, there is no indication that these agents decrease the incidence of preterm delivery or low birth weight in multiple or singleton pregnancies. Hence, their use in prevention/management of PTL is not recommended.

Antibiotics The role of treatment of BV has already been mentioned earlier in this chapter. In addition to this, the ORACLE trial, although not directly answering the question of the use of prophylactic antibiotics for prevention of PTL in women with intact membranes, nevertheless confirmed the generally held view that antibiotics should not be prescribed routinely for women in spontaneous labour, without evidence of clinical infection.

Corticosteroids The use of prophylactic maternal corticosteroids to enhance fetal lung maturity in women at risk for preterm delivery has currently been restricted to use in situations of threatened PTL and established PPROM if it occurs before 34 weeks of gestation. A repeat course of corticosteroids may be given at 32 weeks of gestation should delivery be imminent more than 4 weeks since the last dose of corticosteroids. Retrospective studies have suggested caution with regard to the former practice of repeated maternal corticosteroid administration in high-risk women because of possible fetal intrauterine growth retardation and neonatal neurodevelopmental impairment (Seckl et al 1997).

Diagnosis of preterm labour Traditionally, a diagnosis of preterm labour is made in the presence of persistent uterine contraction accompanied by dilatation and/or effacement of the cervix as detected by digital examination. Threatened preterm labour may be diagnosed when there are documented uterine contractions but no evidence of cervical change. Symptoms of preterm labour may be nonspecific and women treated for preterm labour may include those with symptoms of pelvic pressure, backache, and cramps similar to those in mensuration. Braxton–Hicks contractions which are irregular, non-rhythmical and painless may cause considerable confusion in the diagnosis of preterm labour. The American Academy of Pediatrics and the American College of Obstetricians and Gynecologists (1997) have proposed the following criteria to document preterm labour.

- Contractions of four in 20 minutes or eight in 60 minutes plus progressive change in the cervix.
- Cervical dilatation greater than 1 cm.
- Cervical effacement of 80% or greater.

Despite, these apparently clearly defined entities and because of the need for early management of suspected preterm labour, it is common for clinicians to make the diagnosis of preterm labour before the criteria are met. Therefore, the reported incidence of threatened preterm labour is likely to be considerably greater than the incidence of actual preterm labour. Among symptomatic women, the best predictions of preterm delivery within 24 hours to 7 days include initial cervical dilatation greater than 3 cm or effacement of 80% or more, vaginal bleeding and ruptured membranes (Macones et al 1999).

In order to increase the sensitivity of diagnosis without treating the condition unnecessarily, it is best to be 'liberal' in looking for preterm labour but 'conservative' in diagnosis and treatment. Use of fetal fibronectin in women with suspected preterm labour allows better targeting of therapy and resources. Peaceman et al (1997) showed a more than 50% likelihood of delivery within 7–14 days in women with preterm uterine activity and a positive fetal fibronectin test. More importantly, the risk of delivery within 7 days in symptomatic women without cervical change and a negative fibronectin test was found to be only 1 in 200. Vaginal ultrasound measurement of the cervix in women with preterm uterine activity has been found to be less efficient as a test than fetal fibronectin, although, predictive values of around 50% have been demonstrated with its use (Rozenberg et al 1997).

Treatment of preterm labour The ultimate goal for pregnancies complicated by preterm labour is delivery of an infant who suffers minimal possible sequelae of prematurity. Once a diagnosis of putative preterm labour is made, management includes an initial complete clinical examination and an etiological work-up, fetal fibronectin testing, ultrasound examination and possibly amniocentesis. The key clinical diagnoses to be excluded are fetal death, multiple pregnancy, uterine malformation, cervical incompetence, maternal systemic disease, infection and placental abruption. Maternal white blood counts and C-reactive protein (CRP) estimates give an index of general infection. Urine microscopy is essential to exclude urinary tract infection as a cause of preterm labour, as an appropriate antibiotic will be required and in addition to this, genital tract infection, especially group B streptococcus infections, should be tested for.

Role of amniocentesis in preterm labour Amniocentesis for diagnosis of intra-amniotic infection has been evaluated in the management of preterm labour. Romero et al (1993) found that a negative Gram stain reading was the most reliable test to exclude amniotic fluid bacteria with a specificity of 99% and a high interleukin-6 level was the most sensitive (82%). However, amniocentesis to diagnose infection has not been proven to be associated with improved pregnancy outcome in women, with or without ruptured membranes. The information given by amniocentesis may be useful clinically in determining a subset of women who are likely to deliver, are likely to be refractory to tocolysis, are at a higher risk of chorioamnionitis and are at risk of neonatal sepsis in order to provide optimal care.

Corticosteroids for Enhancement of fetal lung maturation: Liggins and Howie (1972) found that glucocorticoid therapy was effective in lowering the incidence of respiratory distress and neonatal mortality if birth was delayed for at least 24 hours after initiation of betamethasone. Steroids exert their effect via enhanced production and release of pulmonary surfactant and are also implicated in lung morphogenesis. In 1995, a National Institution of Health Consensus Development Panel recommended corticosteroids for fetal lung maturation in threatened preterm labour and there has been a nearly universal acceptance and implementation of these recommendations (Leviton et al 1999). In a subsequent meeting, the Consensus Developmental Panel concluded that data were insufficient to assess the efficacy of corticosteroids in pregnancies complicated by hypertension, diabetes, multiple gestational and fetal growth restriction, however, that it was reasonable to administer corticosteroids to these women (Bloom and Leveno 2003). They also concluded that data were insufficient to comment on benefits and risks of repeated treatments with corticosteroids. Retrospective human studies by Seckl and Miller (1997) have suggested caution with regard to the earlier practice of repeated maternal corticosteroid administration in high-risk women because of possible fetal intrauterine growth restriction and neonatal neuro-developmental impairment. More recently, adverse immediate and long-term effects have been reported with multiple course treatment with increased risk of early onset neonatal sepsis, chorioamnionitis and neonatal death (Vermillion et al 2000; Lee et al 2004). A randomised NICHD Maternal–Fetal Medicine Units Network trial of single versus weekly courses of betamethasone showed less morbidity in newborns given weekly doses who were delivered before 32 weeks (Wapner et al 2003); however, this trial was discontinued because of a negative impact on both birth weight and the incidence of fetal growth restriction with repetitive courses. A recent randomised controlled trial on single versus repeat doses of antenatal corticosteroids by Crowther et al (2006) showed reduced neonatal morbidity (respiratory distress syndrome (RDS), severe lung disease, reduced need for oxygen therapy, shorter duration of mechanical ventilation) in the multiple-dose group as a short-term outcome result. The American College of Obstetricians and Gynecologists (2001) recommends that following the initial therapy, repeated doses after one week should be given only when the threat of preterm delivery recurred and the NIH Consensus Panel (2000) recommends the use of repeated courses of corticosteroids, including rescue therapy, only as part of clinical trials. Maternal adverse effects include pulmonary edema, infection and a more difficult glucose control in diabetic women.

Betamethasone 24 mg, is administered in 24 hours in divided doses, the most popular regimen being 12 mg 12-hourly. The maximum benefit accrues if delivery occurs between 24 hours and 7 days after treatment (odds ratio 0.31). There is significant reduction in RDS, periventricular hemorrhage, necrotising enterocolitis and neonatal deaths with the use of antenatal corticosteroids.

Thyrotropin-releasing hormone which was thought to enhance surfactant synthesis when given along with betamethasone is no longer recommended, as it was found to have no benefit in decreasing the incidence of neonatal lung diseases (Ballard et al 1998). Similarly, phenobarbital and vitamin K is also no longer shown to decrease the frequency or severity of intracranial hemorrhage (Thorp et al 1995) and follow-up studies by the same authors did not show any beneficial effect on intelligence or achievement scores in children up to seven years of age (Thorp et al 2003).

Role of antimicrobials: Use of antimicrobials in the treatment of preterm labour with intact membranes has shown disappointing results, with a Cochrane meta-analysis by King and Flenady (2000) of 10 randomised trials, finding no difference in the rates of newborn RDS or of sepsis between placebo- and antimicrobial treated groups. Similar findings were observed by Goldenberg (2002) who concluded that antimicrobial treatment of women with preterm labour for the sole purpose of preventing delivery is not recommended.

Inhibition of preterm labour: Several interventions and drugs have been used to prevent or inhibit preterm labour, however, none has been found to be completely effective. Given the uncertain accuracy of diagnosis of preterm labour, as well as the relative infrequency of serious neonatal morbidity after 32 to 34 weeks, it is difficult to demonstrate with any accuracy that treatment of preterm labour with any intervention actually reduces the sequelae of prematurity in a neonate. Very few studies have compared a tocolytic drug with placebo; other studies which have compared one tocolytic to another are too restricted to allow any firm conclusions. Reviews and meta-analyses of several studies have indicated that tocolytics do not prevent preterm birth but can delay delivery in order to apply effective antenatal interventions which are known to reduce neonatal morbidity and mortality such as:

- Antepartum transfer of the mother with fetus in utero to a tertiary care hospital for a premature neonate
- Antepartum administration of corticosteroids to the mother to reduce the risk of RDS, intraventricular hemorrhage and death in the preterm neonate
- Antibiotic prophylaxis of neonatal group B streptococcal infection.

a. Bed Rest There is no evidence that bed rest, either in hospital or at home, inhibits preterm labour as reviewed by Goldenberg and colleagues (1994). On the other hand, Kovacevich et al (2000) reported an increased incidence of thromboembolic complications with bed rest of three or more days.

b. Hydration and Sedation The consequences of hypervolemia might be expected to affect uterine contractions, however, there is no published evidence that pregnancies have been prolonged through the use of hydration. Hydration has rarely been studied as a single therapy in the prevention or treatment of preterm labour. In a Cochrane Database Systematic Review (2002) which evaluated the effectiveness of intravenous hydration to avoid preterm birth and its consequences in women with preterm labour, the available data from two trials (228 women with preterm labour and intact membranes comparing intravenous hydration with bed rest alone) was found to be too little to support the use of hydration as a specific treatment for women presenting with preterm labour. There was no significant difference in the risk of preterm delivery before 34 or 32 weeks or in admission to neonatal intensive care unit. However, the reviewer suggested that women with evidence of dehydration might benefit from this intervention. On the other hand, caution concerning the use of intravenous hydration is advised because if tocolytic drugs are administered after initial intravenous hydration with large amounts of fluids, the risk for pulmonary edema increases. When sedation in the form of 8 to 12 mg of intramuscular morphine was combined with hydration and compared with bed rest in a randomised study, similar outcomes were observed in the two groups (Helfgott et al 1994)

c. Tocolytic drugs Various tocolytic agents have been used to inhibit preterm labour, the activity of an individual tocolytic agent being due to its effect on the factors like calcium and cyclic adenosine monophosphatase (cAMP) regularising the activity of enzyme myosine light chain-kinase. This enzyme is responsible for the actin-myosin interaction, which in turn, is the key process of uterine smooth muscle contraction.

The choice of tocolytics agents requires consideration of efficacy, risks and side effects for each individual patient.

- **beta-mimetic tocolytics: Of** the beta-mimetic tocolytic drugs that have been widely used over the last three decades, ritodrine and terbutaline are the two main drugs which have been used as tocolytics. Although ritodrine is the only US. Food and Drug Administration (FDA) approved drug for tocolysis, terbutaline has been more frequently used because of lower maternal side effects associated with its use. There is evidence that the beta-mimetic agents are successful in prolonging pregnancy for atleast 48 hours and perhaps longer. The recommended protocol for intravenous ritodrine therapy has been to start therapy 100 µg/min and increase by 50 µg every 10 minutes until contractions cease, side effects occur or a maximum rate of 350µg/minute is reached. The infusion is maintained at the effective level for 12 hours after contractions cease. However, due to frequent and serious maternal side effects with ritodrine, parenteral administration of this agent has been withdrawn since 1988.

Terbutaline has a longer half life than ritodrine, and as a result, has been associated with fewer side effects, although like ritodrine it can cause pulmonary edema (Angel et al 1988). Terbutaline is not FDA approved and therefore there is no manufacturer's protocol for preterm labour. Currently published protocols often employ subcutaneous administration with a usual dose of 10–25 µg every 3 to 4 hours.

Maternal side effects of beta-mimetic drugs are common and diverse. Although most side effects are mild and transient, serious maternal cardiopulmonary and metabolic complications have been reported with parenteral treatment. In a systematic review by Gyetvai et al (1999), the following adverse maternal effects were reported when compared to no treatment or placebo: palpitation (48% with beta-mimetic versus 5% with placebo), nausea (20% versus 12%), headache (23% versus 6%) and chest pain (10% versus 1%). Rare but serious and potentially life threatening adverse effects have been reported with parenteral use such as pulmonary edema. The actual incidence of this problem is difficult to estimate from literature but varies from 5% of treated women to 'a few cases' (Katz et al 1981). The cause of pulmonary edema is multifactorial and risk factors includes tocolytic therapy with beta-mimetic, multifetal gestation, concurrent glucocorticoid therapy, tocolysis for more than 24 hours and large intravenous crystalloid volume infusion. Beta-mimetics cause retention of sodium and water and can lead to volume overload and the presence of maternal sepsis also increases the risk of pulmonary edema. Symptomatic cardiac arrhythmia and myocardial ischemia have also been reported with beta-mimetic tocolytic therapy (Benedetti 1983). Beta-mimetics can produce a mild fall in diastolic blood pressure and the extensive peripheral vasodilation hinders a normal response to high volume, and therefore, should be used cautiously in cases of antepartum hemorrhage. The beta-mimetic agent may induce mild hyperglycemia in nondiabetic pregnant women and lead to gestational diabetes with prolonged use. These drugs should in general be avoided in women with diabetes or else a simultaneous intravenous insulin infusion may be required to avoid ketoacidosis. Other metabolic effects reported with use of beta-mimetics are hypokalemia, hypocalcemia, antidiuresis, altered thyroid function and elevated transaminases.

Neonatal side effects of beta-mimetics include increased risk of neonatal intraventricular hemorrhage, hypocalcemia, hypoglycemia especially if maternal infusion has been given up to two hours before delivery (Epstein et al 1979).

To summarise, although parenteral beta-mimetics can delay delivery for at least 48 hours, this delay has not proved to be beneficial. It has been suggested that this brief delay may facilitate maternal transport or affects fetal lung maturation with glucocorticoids; however, no data supports this viewpoint. Terbutaline, although not US-FDA approved, is more often used amongst beta-mimetics as a single dose subcutaneous injection of 0.25mg to facilitate maternal transfer. However, long-term oral or subcutaneous treatment has not been shown to reduce either prematurity or neonatal mortality in controlled trials. Presently, other drugs than beta-mimetics have replaced these tocolytics due to a better safety and side effect profile.

Magnesium sulphate: The precise mechanism of tocolytic activity of magnesium sulphate remains unclear. In the presence of magnesium ions in sufficient quantity, uterine muscle strips show reduced contractility. The role of magnesium sulphate is presumed to be that of a calcium antagonists either at the motor end plate reducing excitation or at the cell membrane, reducing calcium influx into the cell (Ohki et al 1997; James et al 1998). Elliott (1983) in a retrospective study found tocolysis with magnesium sulphate to be effective in 87% of cases. However, most observational studies which are small studies, are limited by the fact that many of the women diagnosed to have preterm labor did not have true preterm labor. There have been only two randomised controlled studies, of tocolysis with magnesium sulphate. Cotton et al (1984) compared magnesium sulphate, ritodrine and placebo in 54 women in preterm labour and found no difference in outcomes. Similarly, Cox and associates (1990), in a randomised study of 156 women who received either magnesium sulphate or normal saline, did not find any differences in the pregnancy outcome. There is insufficient evidence to support magnesium sulphate as an effective tocolytic and is used at most centres for its relative safety rather than for its efficacy.

Although magnesium has a low rate of serious side effects compared with other tocolytic drugs, women given this medication must be closely monitored for evidence of hypermagnesemia. Flushes, nausea, vomiting, headache, generalised muscle weakness, diplopia and shortness of breath are not rare. Life-threatening complications such as chest pain, pulmonary edema (1.1%) can occur in rare instances as reported by Elliot (1983). Magnesium sulphate should not be combined with a beta-mimetic for tocolysis, as the side effects are significantly more common when these are used together (Wilkens et al 1988).

Neonatal complications due to magnesium sulphate are generally not significant although lethargy, hypotonia and respiratory depression have been observed. Antenatal maternal magnesium treatment has been related to improved neonatal outcome in some recent studies. Nelson and Grether (1995) reported a lower rate of cerebral palsy at 3 years in a case control study where maternal magnesium treatment was given for either pre-eclampsia or preterm labour (OR, 0.14; 95% CI 0.05–0.51). In another cohort study, 519 infants with birth weight less than 1500 g were followed up. At three to five years of age, none of the 52 infants exposed to magnesium had cerebral palsy with only one having mental retardation, compared to 29 with cerebral palsy and 21 with mental retardation in infants born to 337 mothers who did not receive magnesium (Schendel et al 1996). On the other hand Murphy and colleagues (1995) observed that severe pre-eclampsia or cesarean delivery alone was protective against cerebral palsy. A recent Australian Collaborative trial of magnesium sulphate (Crowther et al 2003) reported neonatal outcomes in over 1050 women who delivered before 30 weeks, after having randomly received either intravenous magnesium sulphate or normal saline as placebo. There was a trend towards lower overall neonatal mortality and cerebral palsy at two years of age in magnesium exposed infants with non-significant differences. Significant motor dysfunction was noted in fewer survivors exposed to magnesium when compared to the control group (34 versus 6.6%)

The therapeutic dosage empirically is similar to that used for intravenous treatment of severe pre-eclampsia. A loading dose of 4–6 g is given over 20–30 minutes followed by an infusion of 2–4 g/h. Intravenous fluid should be limited to 125 ml/hr. Tocolysis is maintained for 12 hours after uterine contractions have ceased and stopped without tapering the dose. Patients treated with magnesium sulphate should be monitored with deep tendon reflexes, urinary output and magnesium levels may be checked if infusion exceeds 4 g/hr.

Indomethacin: Prostaglandins play an important role as mediators of the final pathways of uterine muscle contractions. Prostaglandins cause an increase in free intracellular calcium levels in myometrial cells and an increase in myometrial gap junction formation. Nonsteroidal anti-inflammatory drugs (NSAIDs) inhibit prostaglandin synthetase, an enzyme which converts arachidonic acid to prostaglandins. Indomethacin is one of the first NSAIDs which has been used as a tocolytic. It has been found to be superior to placebo in delaying delivery for 48 hours in randomised, placebo-controlled trials by Neibyl et al (1986) (80% versus 33%) and Zuckerman et al (1984) (95% versus 23%). In later randomised trials, no significant difference in prolongation of pregnancy was found when indomethacin was compared with ritodrine; however, the indomethacin group showed significantly fewer maternal side effects (Besinger et al 1991). In a more recent placebo-controlled randomised trial by Panter et al (1999) pregnancy was prolonged beyond 48 hours in 81% versus 56% women, but serious neonatal morbidity occurred in twice as many of the indomethacin treated infants. Maternal side effects with indomethacin are relatively infrequent as are those seen with any NSAIDs. Milder side effects include nausea, heartburn and vomiting but serious side effects such as gastrointestinal bleeding, coagulopathy and thrombocytopenia can occur. Prolonged treatment may cause renal injury. Indomethacin tocolysis is associated with potentially serious fetal and neonatal complications if the treatment protocol is not followed carefully.

Constriction of ductal arteriosus, oligohydramnios and neonatal pulmonary hypertension are the main side effects. Indomethacin inhibits prostacyclin and PGE_2 formation which is responsible for maintaining ductal vasodilation. Seven of the 14 fetuses of women treated with indomethacin between 27 and 31 weeks showed ductal constriction on Doppler studies (Moise et al 1988). The incidence of ductal arteriosus increases significantly after 32 weeks of pregnancy with less than 10% before 32 weeks to 50% after 32 weeks with more than 48 hours of exposure to indomethacin (Moise et al 1994). Although potentially serious, ductal arteriosus constriction is usually transient and reversible after discontinuation of the drug, occasionally, persistent ductus constriction with irreversible right heart failure has been reported in the neonate (Mohen et al 1992). In a review of fetal echocardiography of 61 women by Vermillion et al (1997), evidence of ductal constriction was seen in 50% of fetuses after an average of 5.1 days of indomethacin therapy, however, the ductal constriction reversed in all fetuses after medication was stopped.

Indomethacin can induce oligohydramnios, which is dose-related but reversible, however, neonatal renal insufficiency and death has been reported after prolonged administration (van der Heijden et al 1994). With long-term therapy, primary neonatal pulmonary hypertension has been reported to occur in 5% to 10% of cases (Besinger et al 1991).

In case control studies by Norton et al (1993), increased incidence of necrotising enterocolitis and intraventricular hemorrhage was observed in newborns exposed to indomethacin, however, more recent studies did not find any link between indomethacin use and intraventricular hemorrhage or necrotising enterocolitis (Muench et al 2001; Gardner et al 1996; Abbasi et al 2003).

Indomethacin is usually administered as a 50 mg loading dose orally or rectally, followed by 25 to 50 mg every six hours for 48 hours limiting its use to preterm labour before 32 weeks with women having normal amniotic fluid volume and normal renal function. If treatment is required to be given more than 48 hours, ductal flow should be evaluated with Doppler echocardiography. Indomethacin; should be discontinued if delivery is imminent. Fetal side effects have limited the use of indomethacin to brief courses of therapy in women having preterm labour before 32 weeks. A review of tocolytic efficacy and safety concluded that indomethacin was the only tocolytic for which there was convincing evidence of effectiveness with little risk when used before 32 weeks (Higby et al 1993).

Calcium channel blockers: Calcium channel blockers inhibit myometrial activity by inhibiting the entry of calcium into the cells. Nifedipine and nicardipine have been studied as tocolytics because of their selective inhibition of uterine contractions. Unlike beta-mimetics and magnesium sulphate, calcium channel blockers are rapidly absorbed after oral administration. There are no placebo controlled trials of calcium channel blockers for tocolysis; however, when nifedipine is compared with a beta-mimetic, it has been found either comparable or superior and with fewer side effects than with beta-mimetics (Kupfermine et al 1993; Papatsonis et al 1997). When combined with magnesium sulphate for tocolysis, nifedipine enhances the neuromuscular blocking effect of magnesium and thus can interfere with pulmonary and cardiac function. A Cochrane review by King et al (2003) reported fewer interruptions of treatment due to adverse effects with nifedipine compared to beta-mimetics (0% versus 7%).

Oxytocin receptor antagonist (Atosiban):

The oxytocin receptor antagonist atosiban has been compared with three different beta-mimetics (ritodrine, salbutamol and terbutaline) in a large multicentre study by Worldwide Atosiban versus Beta-agonists Study Group (2001) and atosiban was found to be associated with fewer maternal adverse effects. Evaluation of its more widespread use is awaited.

Nitric Oxide Donors These are potent smooth muscle relaxants affecting vasculature, gut and uterus. In a few small randomised trials, nitroglycerine administered orally, transdermally or intravenously has not been found to be effective or superior to other tocolytics. Maternal hypotension is a common side effect. Randomised evaluation in studies of sufficient power to test efficacy and observe rare side effects in necessary before any meaningful conclusion can be drawn with regard to safety of nitric oxide donor (Duckitt and Thornton 2003).

Recommended Management of Preterm Labour

- Confirmation of preterm labour
- For pregnancies less than 34 weeks, glucocorticoids are given for enhancement of fetal lung maturation.
- For pregnancies less than 34 weeks in women who are not in advanced labour, one can attempt inhibition of labour to delay delivery while giving corticosteroids therapy and group B streptococcal prophylaxis.
- For pregnancies at 34 weeks or more, women are monitored for progress of labour and fetal well being.

Intrapatrum Management In a preterm fetus, the risks of labour and delivery are increased. The fetal heart rate and uterine contractions should be monitored with preferably continuous electronic monitoring. Changes in fetal heart rate variability in the preterm fetus carry the same or even greater significance for risk of acidosis as in term infants. Group B streptococcus prophylaxis should be given with either penicillin G or ampicillin intravenously. An episiotomy may be needed at the time, fetal head reaches the perineum, if the vaginal outlet is not relaxed. Routine forceps delivery is not recommended as indicated by perinatal outcome data. Specialised personnel and facilities for resuscitation and care of preterm newborn should be available. The earlier hypothesis that cesarean delivery can obviate trauma from labour and vaginal delivery, thus preventing complications due to intraventricular hemorrhage, is no longer validated by recent studies. When cesarean delivery for preterm breech is chosen, an underdeveloped lower uterine segment or an inadequate incision on the uterus can lead to a traumatic delivery if adequate care is not taken.

Conclusion Factors underlying preterm labour are not fully understood and therefore prevention of preterm labour has been generally unsuccessful. Inaccurate diagnosis of preterm labour is a major impediment to appropriate care for preterm labour. Tocolytics, glucocorticoids and antibiotics are effective tertiary therapies, however, they can never be wholly effective in eliminating the morbidity and mortality due to prematurity.

References

Abbasi S, JS Gerdes, HM Sehdev et al. 2003. Neonatal outcomes after exposure to indomethacin in utero: a retrospective case cohort study. *Am J Obstet Gynecol* 189:782.

American Academy of Pediatrics and the American College of Obstetricians and Gynecologists. 1997. *Guidelines for Perinatal Care*. 4th ed. Illinois: American Academy of Pediatrics.

American College of Obstetricians and Gynecologists. 2001. Assessment of risk factors for preterm birth. *Practice Bulletin* 31.

Andrews WW, R Copper, JC Hauth et al. 2000. Mid-trimester cervical ultrasound findings predict recurrent early spontaneous delivery. *Obstet Gynecol* 95:222.

Angel JL, WF O'Brien, RA Knuppel et al.1988. Carbohydrate intolerance in patients receiving oral tocolytics. *Am J Obstet Gynecol* 159:762

Arias F, L Rodriguez, SC Rayne et al. 1993. Maternal placental vasculopathy and infection: Two distinct subgroups among patients with preterm labor and preterm ruptured membranes. *Am J Obstet Gynecol* 168:585.

Bakketeig LS and JH Hoffman. 1981. Epidemiology of preterm birth: Results from a longitudinal study of births in Norway. In *Preterm labor* ed LS Elder, CH Hendricks. London: Butterworths, p 17.

Ballard RA, PL Ballard, A Cnaan et al. 1998. Antenatal thyrotropin releasing hormone to prevent lung disease in preterm infants. *N Engl J Med* 338:493.

Benedetti T. 1983. Maternal complications of beta-sympathomimetic therapy for premature labor. *Am J Obstet Gynecol* 145:1.

Bernstein PS, R Stern, N Lin et al. 1998. Beta human chorionic gonadotropin in cervicovaginal secretions as a predictor of preterm delivery. *Am J Obstet Gynecol* 179:870.

Besinger RE, JR Niebyl, WG Keyes et al. 1991. A randomized comparative trial of indomethacin and ritodrine for the long term treatment of preterm labor. *Am J Obstet Gynecol* 164:981.

Bloom SL, NP Yost, DD Mcintire et al. 2001. Recurrence of preterm birth in singleton and twin pregnancies. *Obstet Gynecol* 98:379.

Bloom SL and KJ Leveno. 2003. Corticosteroid use in special circumstances: preterm ruptured membranes, hypertension, fetal growth restriction, multiple fetuses. *Clin Obstet Gynecol* 46:150.

Boer K, RAK Samlal, BJ Smit, ME Kreijenbroek et al. 1993. Twenty years during policy in obstetric care in Amsterdam. In *Care, concern and cure in perinatal medicine*, ed JG Kopper, TKAB Eskes, HP van Geijn, PF JH Weisenhann, Ruys, 221. Lancashire: Parthenon Press.

Carey JC, MA Klebanoff for the NICHD MFMU Network. 2000. Metronidazole treatment increased the risk of preterm birth in asymptomatic women with trichomonas (abstract 7). *Am J Obstet Gynecol* 182:S13.

Carey JC, SJ Yaffe, C Catz for the VIP Study Group. 1993. The vaginal infections and prematurity study: an overview. *Clin Obstet Gynecol* 36:809.

Cohen I, JC Veille and BM Calkins. 1990. Improved pregnancy outcome following successful treatment of chlamydial infection. *JAMA* 263:3160.

Collaborative group on Preterm Birth Prevention. 1993. Multicenter randomized, controlled trial of a preterm birth prevention program. *Am J Obstet Gynecol* 69:352.

Collaborative Home Uterine Monitoring Study (CHUMS) Group. 1995. A multicentre randomized controlled trial of home uterine monitoring:active versus sham device. *Am J Obstet Gynecol* 173:1120.

Colombo DF and JD Iams. 2000. Cervical length and preterm labor. *Clin Obstet Gynecol* 43:735.

Colton T, HL Kayne, Y Zhang et al. 1995. A meta-analysis of home uterine activity monitoring. *Am J Obstet Gynecol* 173:1499.

Cook CM and DA Ellwood. 2000. The cervix as a predictor of preterm delivery in "at risk" women. *Ultrasound Obstet Gynecol* 15:109.

Copper RL, RL Goldenberg, A Das et al. 1996. The preterm prediction study: Maternal stress is associated with spontaneous preterm birth at less than thirty-five week's gestation. National Institute of Child Health and Human Development Maternal Fetal Medicine Units Network. *Am J Obstet Gynecol* 175:1286

Cotton DB, HT Strassner, LM Hill et al. 1984. Comparison between magnesium sulfate, terbutaline and a placebo for inhibition of preterm labor: A randomized study. *J Reprod Med* 29:92.

Cox SM, ML Sherman and KJ Leveno. 1990. Randomized investigation of magnesium sulfate for prevention of preterm birth. *Am J Obstet Gynecol* 163:767.

Creasy RK. 1993. Preterm birth prevention: where are we? *Am J Obstet Gynecol* 168:1223.

Crowther CA, RR Haslam, JE Hiller et al. 2006. Australasian Collaborative Trial of Repeat Doses Of Steroids (ACTORDS) Study Group. Neonatal respiratory distress syndrome after repeat exposure to antenatal corticosteroids: a randomized controlled trial. *Lancet* 367:1913.

Crowther CA, JE Hiller, LW Doyle et al. 2003. Effect of magnesium sulfate given for neuroprotection before preterm birth: a randomized controlled trial. *JAMA* 290:2669.

daFonseca EB, RE Bittar, MHB Carvalho et al. 2003. Prophylactic administration of progesterone by vaginal suppository to reduce the incidence of spontaneous preterm birth in women at increased risk: a randomized placebo-controlled double-blind study. *Am J Obstet Gynecol* 188:419.

Darne J, HHG McGarrigle and GC Lachelin. 1987. Saliva oestriol, oestradiol, oestrone and progesterone levels in pregnancy: spontaneous labor at term is preceded by a rise in the saliva oestriol:progesterone ratio. *Br J Obstet Gynaecol* 94:227.

DIV Reproductive Health National Center for Health Statistics and CDC. 1999. Preterm singleton births – United States, 1989–96. *MMWR* 48:185.

Duckitt K and S Thornton. 2003. Nitric oxide donors for the treatment of preterm labor (Cochrane review). In *The Cochrane Library,* Issue 2. Oxford: Update Software.

Dyson DC, KH Danbe, JA Bamber et al. 1998. Monitoring women at risk for preterm labor. *N Engl J Med* 338:15.

Ekwo EE, CA Gosselink and A Moawad. 1992. Unfavorable outcome in penultimate pregnancy and premature rupture of membranes in successive pregnancy. *Obstet Gynecol* 80:166.

Elliot JP. 1983. Magnesium sulfate as a tocolytic agent. *Am J Obstet Gynecol* 147:277.

Epstein M, E Nicholls and P Strubblefield. 1979. Neonatal hypoglycemia after beta-sympathomimetic tocolytic therapy. *Pediatrics* 94:449.

Eschenbach DA, RP Nugent, AV Rao et al. 1991. A randomized placebo-controlled trial of erythromycin for the treatment of *Ureaplasma urealyticum* to prevent premature delivery. *Am J Obstet Gynecol* 164:734.

Gardner MO, J Owen, S Skelly et al. 1996. Preterm delivery after indomethacin: a risk factor for neonatal complications? *J Reprod Med* 41:903.

Genc MR, C Gerber, M Nesin et al. 2002. Polymorphism in the interleukin-1 gene complex and spontaneous preterm delivery. *Am J Obstet Gynecol* 187:157.

Goldenberg R. 2002. The management of preterm labor. *Obstet Gynecol* 100:1020.

Goldenberg RL, SP Cliver, J Bronstein et al. 1994. Bed rest in pregnancy. *Obstet Gynecol* 84:131.

Goldenberg RL, JD Iams, BM Mercer et al. 1998. The preterm prediction study: The value of new vs standard risk factors predicting early and all spontaneous preterm births. *Am J Public Health* 88:233.

Goldenberg RL, JD Iams, M Miodovnik et al. 1996. The Preterm prediction study: risk factors in twin gestations. *Am J Obstet Gynecol* 175:1047.

Goldenberg RL and DJ Rouse. 1998. Prevention of premature birth. *N Engl J Med* 339:313.

Golpfert AR, MK Jeffcoat, Andrews et al. 2004. Periodontal disease and upper genital tract inflammation in early spontaneous preterm birth. *Obstet Gynecol* 104:777.

Guzman ER, C Walters, CV Ananth et al. 2001. A comparison of sonographic cervical parameters in predicting spontaneous preterm birth in high-risk singleton pregnancies. *Ultrasound Obstet Gynecol* 18:204.

Gyetvai K, ME Hannah, ED Modnett et al. 1999. Tocolytics for preterm labour: a systematic review. *Obstet Gynecol* 94:869.

Hadley CB, DM Main, SG Gabbe et al. 1990. Risk factors for preterm premature rupture of the fetal membranes. *Am J Perinatol* 7:374.

Hall RT. 2000. Prevention of premature birth: Do pediatricians have a role? *Pediatrics* 105:1137.

Hassan SS, R Romero, SM Berry, et al. 2000. Patients with an ultrasonographic cervical length < 15 mm have nearly a 50 per cent risk of early spontaneous preterm delivery. *Am J Obstet Gynecol* 182:1458.

Hauth JC, WW Andrews, RL Goldenberg et al. 1998. Infection related risk factors predictive of spontaneous preterm labor and birth. *Prenat Neonat Med* 3:86.

Hauth JC, RL Goldenberg, WW Andrews et al. 1995. Reduced incidence of preterm delivery with metronidazole and erythromycin in women with bacterial vaginosis. *N Engl J Med* 333:1732.

Hauth JC, M Jeffcoat, SP Cliver et al. 2001. Periodontal disease and preterm birth (abstract) *Am J Obstet Gynecol* 184:S37.

Hediger ML, TO Scholl, JI Schall et al. 1995. Fetal growth and the etiology of preterm delivery. *Obstet Gynecol* 85:175.

Heine RP, JA McGregor and VK Dullien. 1999. Accuracy of salivary estriol testing compared to traditional risk factor assessment in predicting preterm birth. *Am J Obstet Gynecol* 180:S214.

Helfgott AW, DC Willis and JD Blanco. 1994. Is hydration and sedation beneficial in the treatment of threatened preterm labor? A preliminary report. *J Matern Fetal Med* 3:37.

Henrikson TB, M Hedegaard and NJ Secher. 1995. Standing and Walking at work and birth weight. *Acta Obstet Gynecol Scand* 74:509.

Higby K, EM Xenakis, CJ Paverstein. 1993. Do tocolytic agents stop preterm labor? A critical and comprehensive review of safety and efficacy. *Am J Obstet Gynecol*168:1247.

Hillier SL, RP Nugent, DA Eschenbach et al for the Vaginal Infections and Prematurity Study Group. 1995. Association between bacterial vaginosis and preterm delivery of a low birth weight infant. *N Engl J Med* 333:1737.

Hincz P, J Wilczynski, M Kozarzewski et al. 2002. Two step test: The combined use of fetal fibronectin and sonographic examination of the uterine cervix for prediction of preterm delivery in symptomatic patients. *Acta Obstet Gynecol Scand* 81:58.

Honest H, LK Bachman, JE Gupta et al. 2002. Accuracy of cervical fetal fibronectin test in predicting risk of spontaneous preterm birth: Systematic review. *Br Med J* 325:301

Honest H, LM Bachmann, A Coomarasamy et al. 2003. Accuracy of cervical transvaginal sonography in predicting preterm birth: A systematic review. *Ultrasound Obstet Gynecol* 22:305.

Iams JD, RL Goldenberg, PJ Meis et al. 1996. The length of the cervix and the risk of spontaneous preterm delivery. *N Engl J Med* 334:567.

Iams JD, RL Goldenberg, BM Mercer et al. 1998. The preterm prediction study: recurrence risk of spontaneous preterm birth. *Am J Obstet Gynecol* 178:1035.

Iams JD, Newman RB, Thom EA, et al. 2002. Frequency of uterine contractions and the risk of

spontaneous preterm delivery. *N Engl J Med* 346:250
James MFM. 1998. Magnesium in obstetric anaesthesia. *Inter J Obstet Anes* 7:115.
Jeffcoat MK, JC Hauth, NC Geurs et al. 2003. Periodontal disease and preterm birth: Results of a pilot intervention study. *J Periodontol* 74:1214.
Katz M, PJ Gill, RB Newman. 1986. Detection of preterm labor by ambulatory monitoring of uterine activity: a preliminary report. *Obstet Gynecol* 68:773.
Katz M, PA Robertson and RK Creasy. 1981 Cardiovascular complications associated with terbutaline treatment for preterm labor. *Am J Obstet Gynecol* 139:605.
King J and V Flenady. 2000. Antibiotics for preterm labor with intact membranes. *Cochrane Database Syst Rev* 2; CD000246.
King JF, VJ Flenady, DN Papatsonis et al. 2003. Calcium channel blockers for inhibiting preterm labor. Cochrane Review. In *The Cochrane Library* Issue 2. Oxford: Update Software:
Kovacevich GJ, SA Gaich, JP Lavin et al. 2000 The prevalence of thromboembolic events among women with extended bed rest prescribed as part of the treatment of preterm labor or preterm premature rupture of membranes. *Am J Obstet Gynecol* 182:1089.
Krohn MA, SL Hillier, MI Lee et al. 1991. Vaginal bacteroides are associated with an increased rate of preterm delivery among women in preterm labor. *J Infect Dis* 164:88.
Kupefermine M, JB Lessing, Y Yaron et al. 1993. Nifedipine versus ritodrine for suppression of preterm labour. *Br J Obstet Gynaecol* 100:1090.
Kyrklund–Blomberg NB and S Cnnattingius. 1998. Preterm and smoking. *Am J Obstet Gynecol* 179:1051.
Landau R, HG Xie, V Dishy et al. 2002. β2-adrenergic receptor genotype and preterm delivery. *Am J Obstet Gynecol* 187:1294.
Lee M, J Davies, D Guinn et al. 2004. Single versus weekly courses of antenatal corticosteroids in preterm premature rupture of membranes. *Obstet Gynecol* 103:274.
Leitich H and A Kaider. 2003. Fetal fibronectin – How useful is it in the prediction of preterm birth? *Br J Obstet Gynaecol* 110(Suppl 20):66.
Leviton LC, RL Goldenberg, CS Baker et al. 1999. Methods to encourage the use of antenatal corticosteroid therapy for fetal maturation: a randomized controlled trial. *JAMA* 281:46.
Liggins GC and RN Howie. 1972. A controlled trial of antepartum glucocorticoid treatment for prevention of the respiratory distress syndrome in premature infants. *Pediatrics* 50:515.
Lockwood CJ. 1994. Recent advances in elucidating the pathogenesis of preterm delivery, the detection of patients at risk and preventative therapies. *Curr Opin Obstet Gynecol* 6:7.
Macones GA, SY Segel, DM Stamilo, MA Morgan. 1999. Prediction of delivery among women with early preterm labor by means of clinical characteristics alone. *Am J Obstet Gynecol* 181:1414.
Martius J, M Krohn, SL Hillier et al. 1988. Relationships of vaginal *Lactobacillus* species, cervical *Chlamydia trachomatis* and bacterial vaginosis to preterm birth. *Obstet Gynecol* 71:89.
McCormack WM, B Rosner, Y-H Lee et al. 1987. Effect on birth weight of erythromycin treatment of pregnant women. *Obstet Gynecol* 69:202.
McDonald H, P Brocklehurst, J Parsons, R Vigneswaran. 2003. Antibiotics for treating bacterial vaginosis in pregnancy (Cochrane review). In *The Cochrane Library*. Issue 3. Oxford: Update Software.
McDonald HM, JA O'Loughlin, R Vigneswaran et al. 1997. Impact of metronidazole treatment in women with bacterial vaginosis flora (*Gardnerella vaginalis*): a randomized, placebo controlled trial. *Br J*

Obstet Gynecol 104:1391.

McLean M, A Bisits, J Davies et al. 1999. Predicting risk of preterm delivery by second trimester. Measurement of maternal plasma corticotrophin releasing hormone and alpha-fetoprotein concentrations. *Am J Obstet Gynecol* 181:207.

Meis PJ, JM Ernest, ML Moore. 1987. Causes of low birth-weight births in public and private patients. *Am J Obstet Gynecol* 156:1165.

Meis PJ, RL Goldenberg, BM Mercer et al. 1998. The preterm prediction study: Risk factors for indicated preterm birth. *Am J Obstet Gynecol* 178:562.

Meis PJ, AA Klebanoff, E Thom et al with NICHD and MFMU Network. 2003. Prevention of recurrent preterm delivery by 17 alpha-hydroxyprogesterone caproate. *N Engl J Med* 348:2379.

Mercer BM, RL Goldenberg et al. 1996. The preterm prediction study: a clinical risk assessment system. *Am J Obstet Gynecol* 174:1885.

Mercer BM, RL Goldenberg, AH Moawad et al. 1999. The preterm prediction study: effect of gestational age and cause of preterm birth on subsequent obstetric outcome. *Am J Obstet Gynecol* 181:1216.

Mohen D, JP Newnharn and LD Orsogna. 1992. Indomethacin for the treatment of polyhydramnios: a case of constriction of the ductus arteriosus. *Aust NZ Obstet Gynecol* 32:243.

Moise KJ. 1994. Effect of advancing gestational age on the frequency of fetal ductal constriction in association with maternal indomethacin use. *Am J Obstet Gynecol* 168:1350.

Moise KJ, JC Huhta, DS Sharif et al. 1988. Indomethacin in the treatment of premature labor: effects on fetal ductus arteriosus. *N Engl J Med* 319:327.

Muench V, CR Harman, AA Baschat et al. 2001. Early fetal exposure to longterm indomethacin therapy to prevent preterm delivery: neonatal outcome. *Am J Obstet Gynecol* 185:S149.

Murphy DJ, S Sellers, IZ Mackenzie et al. 1995. Case-control study of antenatal and intrapartum risk factors for cerebral palsy in very preterm singleton babies. *Lancet* 346:1449.

National Institute of Health Consensus Development Conference: Statement on Repeat Courses of Antenatal Corticosteroids 2000. Bethseda, August 17–18. Available at http//consensus.nih.gov

National Institutes of Health Consensus Development Panel. 1995. Effect of corticosteroids for fetal maturation on perinatal outcomes. *JAMA* 173:413.

Nelson KB and JK Grether. 1995. Can magnesium sulfate reduce the risk of cerebral palsy in very-low-birthweight infants? *Pediatrics* 95:263.

Netta D, A Fuks and I Godi. 2003. Polymorphism of tumor necrosis factor-alfa and preterm premature rupture of membranes. *Am J Obstet Gynecol* 189:S174.

Newman RB, RJ Gill, P Wittreich et al. 1986. Maternal perception of prelabor uterine activity. *Obstet Gynecol* 60:1172.

Niebyl JR and FR Witter. 1986. Neonatal outcome after indomethacin treatment for preterm labor. *Am J Obstet Gynecol* 155:747.

Norton ME, J Merril, BAB Cooper et al. 1993. Neonatal complications after the administration of indomethacin for preterm labor. *N Engl J Med* 329:1602.

Offenbacher S, V Katz, G Fertik et al. 1996. Periodontal infection as a possible risk factor for preterm lowbirth weight. *J Periodontol* 67:1103.

Ohki S, M Ikura and M Zhang. 1997. Identification of magnesium binding sites and the role of magnesium on target recognition by calmodulin. *Biochemistry* 36:4309.

Owen J, JD Iams and JC Hauth. 2003. Vaginal sonography and cervical incompetence. *Am J Obstet*

Gynecol 188:586.

Owen J, Yost N, Berghella V et al. 2001. Mid trimester endovaginal sonography in women at high risk for spontaneous preterm birth. *JAMA* 286:1340

Panter KR, ME Hannah, KS Amankwah et al. 1999. The effect of indomethacin tocolysis in preterm labor on perinatal outcome: a randomised placebo-controlled trial. *Br J Obstet Gynaecol* 106:467.

Papatsonis DN, HP Van Geijen, HJ Ader et al. 1997. Nifedipine and ritodrine in the management of preterm labor: a randomized multicentre trial. *Obstet Gynecol* 90:230.

Peaceman AM, WW Andrews, JM Thorp et al. 1997. Fetal fibronectin as a predictor of preterm birth in patients with symptoms: a multicenter trial. *Am J Obstet Gynecol* 177:13.

Romero R, M Sirtori, E Oyarzu et al. 1992. Infection and labor: Prevalence, microbiology and clinical significance of intraamniotic infection in women with preterm labor and intact membranes. *Am J Obstet Gynecol* 161:817.

Romero R, BH Yoon, M Mazor et al 1993 The diagnostic and prognostic value of amniotic fluid white blood cell count, glucose, interleukin-6 and Gram stain in patients with preterm labor and intact membranes. *Am J Obstet Gynecol* 169:805.

Roy KK, J Baruah, S Kumar et al. 2006. Maternal antenatal profile and immediate neonatal outcome in VLBW and ELBW babies. *Indian J Pediatr* 73:669.

Rozenberg P, F Goffinet, L Malagrida et al. 1997. Evaluatory the risk of preterm delivery: A comparison of fetal fibronectin and transvaginal ultrasonographic measurement of cervical length. *Am J Obstet Gynecol* 176:196.

Schendel DE, CJ Berg, M Yeargin-Allsop et al. 1996. Prenatal magnesium sulfate exposure and the risk for cerebral palsy or mental retardation among very low birth weight children aged 3 to 5 years. *JAMA* 276:1805.

Seckl JR and WL Miller. 1997. How safe is long term prenatal glucocorticoid treatment? *JAMA* 277:1077.

Shah NR and MB Bracken. 2000. A systematic review and meta-analysis of prospective studies on the association between maternal cigarette smoking and preterm delivery. *Am J Obstet Gynecol.* 182:465.

Singh M. 1999. Disorders of weight and gestation. In *Care of the newborn*, 5th edn, ed M Singh, 225. New Delhi: Sagar Publications.

Stan C, M Boulvain, P Hirsbrunner-Amagbaly et al. 2002. Hydration for treatment of preterm labour. *Cochrane Database Syst Rev.* CD003096.

Tallo CO, B Vohr W Oh et al. 1995. Maternal and neonatal morbidity associated with in vitro fertilization. *J Pediatr* 127:794.

Thorp J, D Ferrette-Smith, LA Gaston et al. 1995. Combined antenatal vitamin K and phenobarbitol therapy for preventing intracranial hemorrhage of newborns less than 34 weeks gestation. *Obstet Gynecol* 86:1.

Thorp JA, M O'Connor, B Beldon et al. 2003. Effects of phenobarbital and multiple dose corticosteroids on developmental outcome at age 7 years. *Obstet Gynecol* 101:363.

To MS, C Skentou, AW Liao et al. 2001. Cervical length and funneling at 23 weeks of gestation in the prediction of spontaneous preterm birth in high-risk singleton pregnancies. *Ultrasound Obstet Gynecol* 18:200.

van der Heijden BJ, C Carlus, F Nancy et al. 1994. Persistent anuria, neonatal death, and microcystic lesions after prenatal exposure to indomethacin. *Am J Obstet Gynecol* 171:617.

Vermillion ST, JA Scardo, AG Lashus et al. 1997. The effect of indomethacin tocolysis on fetal ductus arteriosus constriction with advancing gestational age. *Am J Obstet Gynecol* 177:256.

Vermillion S, D Soper and R Newman. 2000. Neonatal sepsis and death after multiple doses of antenatal betamethasone. *Am J Obstet Gynecol* 183:810.

Volpe JJ. 1992. Effect of cocaine use on the fetus. *N Engl J Med* 327:39.

Wahbeh CJ, GB Hill, RD Eden et al 1984. Intraamniotic bacterial colonization in premature labor. *Am J Obstet Gynecol* 148:739.

Walkinshaw SA, C Siney, M Kidd et al. 1993. Outcome of pregnancy in opiate dependent women within a methadone treatment programme. In *First international conference on practical obstetrics*, Paris.

Wapner RJ for the NICHHD MFMU Network. 2003. Randomized trial of single versus weekly doses of corticosteroids. *Am J Obstet Gynecol* 189:S56.

Watts DH, MA Krohn, SL Hillier et al. 1992. The association of occult amniotic fluid infection with gestational age and neonatal outcome among women in preterm labor. *Obstet Gynecol* 79:351.

Weiss G, LT Goldsmith, R Sachdev et al. 1993. Elevated first trimester serum relaxin concentrations in pregnant women following ovarian stimulation predict prematurity. *Obstet Gynecol* 82:821.

Wilkens IA, L Lynch, KE Mehaleb et al. 1988. Efficacy and side effects of magnesium sulfate and ritodrine as tocolytic agents. *Am J Obstot Gynecol* 159;685.

Worldwide Atosiban versus Beta-agonists Study group. 2001. Effectiveness and safety of the oxytocin antagonist versus beta-adrenergic agonists in the treatment of preterm labor. *Br J Obstet Gynecol* 108:133.

Yang Z, Y Zhao, MJ Benett et al. 2002. Fetal genotypes and pregnancy outcome in 35 families with mitochondrial trifunctional protein mutations. *Am J Obstet Gynecol* 187:715.

Yost NP, J Owen, V Berghella et al. 2004. Second trimester cervical sonography: Features other than cervical length to predict spontaneous preterm birth. *Am J Obstet Gynecol* 103:457.

Zuckerman H, E Shalev, G Gilag et al. 1984. Further study of the inhibition of premature labor with indomethacin. *J Perinat Med* 12:19.

25

Prelabour Rupture of Membranes

Shyamala Guruvare

Rupture of membranes at term pregnancy, with onset of labour, at or during labour, is a favourable event for the progression of labour. However, spontaneous rupture of membranes prior to onset of labour is a cause for concern. Prelabour rupture of membranes (PROM) is associated with increased risk of maternal and fetal infection, prematurity, dysfunctional labour and cesarean delivery. In addition, PROM may indicate the presence of a prevailing abnormality such as vaginal infection, malposition or cephalopelvic disproportion.

PROM may occur at or before term. When it occurs before term, it is called preterm prelabour rupture of membranes (PPROM). This constitutes 20–40% of all preterm births.

With PROM at term, 80–90% of patients deliver within 24 hours without medical intervention, while 90% of PPROM women deliver within a week (Gunn et al 1970).

Fetal Membrane

The fetal membrane is a bilayered membrane with amnion forming the inner layer and chorion the outer layer. Amnion is an avascular single-cell layer, the cells being held together by surface desmosomes and the layer strengthened by microvillar interdigitations (van Herendael et al 1978). The amnion overlies a basement membrane formed of collagen, which in turn rests on a collagen-rich extracellular matrix. The chorion is the vascular layer and is composed of trophoblastic cells arranged in 2–10 layers.

Risk Factors

Several factors have been shown to increase the risk of PROM. Infections in the form of bacterial vaginosis (Brocklehurst et al 2000), Group B streptococcal colonisation of urine (Moller et al 1984) and *Neisseria gonorrhoeae* colonisation of the cervix (Gibbs et al 1997) are proven causes of PROM. Membrane collagen degradation by bacterial collagenases and local cytokine-mediated membrane damage are the pathways for infection-induced PROM.

Cervical incompetence, over-distended uterus as in hydramnios or multiple gestations (Mercer et al 1996), connective tissue disorders, sickle cell disease, cigarette smoking, antepartum hemorrhage and prior preterm delivery (Harger et al 1990) are the other known risk factors.

Prediction

The preterm prediction study (Mercer et al 2000) found that low body mass index, pulmonary disease, contractions within two weeks, bacterial vaginosis, short cervix (≤25 mm), positive fetal fibronectin screening and a previous preterm birth caused by PROM were significantly associated with preterm birth caused by PROM in the current pregnancy. The last three factors were the strongest predictors of PROM.

Consequences of PROM

Intrauterine infection caused by ascending bacteria is one of the major threats in PPROM. Infection is a potential complication for the fetus as well as the neonate. 'Fetal inflammatory syndrome' accompanying amnionitis is found to have association with periventricular leukomalacia and consequent cerebral palsy (Yoon et al 1997).

Approximately 30% of women with PPROM have chorioamnionitis proven by microbial study. Clinical chorioamnionitis complicates 10% of the PPROM cases (Romero et al 1988).

A third of preterm deliveries (30%) are caused by PPROM. Cord prolapse, failed induction followed by cesarean delivery, variable decelerations in labour due to reduced liquor and placental abruption are the other consequences of PPROM. Prolonged severe oligohydramnios after PPROM at early gestational age (< 26 weeks) may be associated with pulmonary hypoplasia (Taylor 1984) and skeletal deformities (Nimrod et al 1984) of the fetus.

Diagnosis

A history of gushing fluids from the vagina that may persist as continuous leakage or be followed by intermittent leakage is a common presentation of PROM. Detection of clear fluid passing from the cervix or a pool of fluid in the posterior fornix confirms diagnosis on sterile speculum examination. Pressing the fundus gently during speculum examination will help demonstrate the fluid leak. In case of further doubt, a pH test showing alkalinity, a nitrazine test (orange test paper turns blue) or a ferning test may be used. Of the three, examining the smear from the posterior fornix for ferning after air-drying the slide provides a more specific diagnosis, and there is no interference from meconium or blood. A dry vulval pad that gets soaked over a few hours may also be of some help in patients in whom the leak is not consistent or significant. Oligohydramnios demonstrable by sonography may substantiate the diagnosis.

PROM at Term

PROM is a serious concern when it occurs before term. When it occurs after 37 weeks of gestation, 75–85% of women begin labour spontaneously within 24 hours. About 2–5% remain undelivered at 72 hours after PROM.

The only dilemma with term PROM is whether to wait for spontaneous onset of labour or to induce labour. If the latter option is selected, a decision will have to be made about whether to induce labour immediately or after a stipulated period of time. Considering the fact that expectant management may prolong the hospital stay and increase healthcare costs, immediate delivery is the favoured mode of management for term PROM.

Recent evidence (Hannah et al 1996) has shown that there is no significant difference in neonatal infectious morbidity or cesarean delivery rates in the groups managed by immediate and delayed (after 4 days of waiting) induction. The group with immediate oxytocin induction had the lowest incidence of chorioamnionitis, shorter interval between amniorrhexis and delivery and shorter mean duration of labour. Similarly, meta-analysis of 23 studies revealed that the lowest rate of maternal chorioamnionitis was seen in the group with immediate oxytocin induction (Mozurkewich 1997).

Digital vaginal examination can be done in term PROM to assess the cervix, which can be followed by induction of labour with intravenous oxytocin. The benefits of preinduction cervical ripening with intravaginal or intracervical prostaglandin in women with term PROM with unfavourable cervix is yet to be effectively explored. Women with anovaginal cultures that are positive for Group B streptococci (GBS) or those with unknown GBS status should receive intrapartum GBS prophylaxis.

PPROM

PPROM contributes to a third of preterm babies, which is obviously the leading cause of perinatal morbidity and mortality. Having diagnosed the rupture of membranes, accurate gestational age should be established. The patient should be thoroughly evaluated for any indication necessitating immediate termination, such as maternal chorioamnionitis. Non-assuring fetal status, placental abruption, maternal medical complications, fetal anomaly and fetal death are the other conditions that necessitate expeditious delivery.

At the gestational age of **34–37 weeks**, the risk of infection outweighs the neonatal risk of prematurity; hence, termination of pregnancy, either immediately or after a wait of 24 hours for spontaneous onset of labour, is recommended.

Pregnancies between **26 and 34 weeks** may benefit maximally from expectant management. Depending on the lowest gestational age at which a neonate can be saved in a particular neonatal unit, the lower margin can be adjusted between 24 and 28 weeks while setting the protocol for a particular centre. In this period, even a few days of prolongation will improve the neonatal outcome by making a provision for the benefit of corticosteroids. This group is best managed with corticosteroids and antibiotics, with careful surveillance for infection and fetal well-being.

Corticosteroids

The role of corticosteroids in preventing complications, especially respiratory distress syndrome and intraventricular hemorrhage, in a preterm newborn for up to 34 weeks has been proven beyond doubt. However, the role of corticosteroids in women with PPROM is controversial because of two main concerns—accelerated fetal lung maturity would take place with the rupture of the membranes and corticosteroid administration would increase the risk of neonatal infection.

A randomised, controlled trial demonstrated a significant reduction in respiratory distress syndrome (RDS) (18% versus 44%) without any apparent increase in neonatal infection when corticosteroids were given in addition to antibiotics (Lewis et al 1996). An analysis of the data from the National Institute of Child Health and Human Development (NICHD) research network showed a 30% reduction in RDS among infants with a birth weight of 501–1500 g and whose PPROM mothers had received antenatal corticosteroids (Wright et al 1995). A 49% reduction in RDS with corticosteroid administration was seen in patients with PPROM in another meta-analysis (Crowley 1992). Similarly, studies have reported significant reduction in intraventricular hemorrhage in the treated group (Morales et al 1989; Wright et al 1995). A recent meta-analysis concluded that corticosteroids administered to patients with PPROM reduced the risks of necrotising enterocolitis (NEC), intraventricular hemorrhage (IVH) and RDS without any significant increased risk of maternal or neonatal infection (Harding et al 2001).

Antibiotics

Evidence suggests that lower genital colonisation and ascending infection may play a role in PROM. Besides, infection in the form of chorioamnionitis and perinatal sepsis can complicate PROM. As already mentioned, approximately 30% of women with PPROM have chorioamnionitis proven by microbial study. Clinical chorioamnionitis complicates 10% of the cases of PPROM. There is strong evidence supporting the role of antibiotics in PPROM, which demonstrates significant pregnancy prolongation and reduction in perinatal infections (Mercer et al 1997; Kenyon et al 2001). By prolonging the pregnancy, antimicrobial therapy in PPROM reduces major complications of prematurity such as RDS, IVH, NEC and perinatal death.

The Oracle I randomised multicentre trial (Kenyon et al 2001) involving 4826 women who received antimicrobials, compared the outcome in four groups; the groups received either 250 mg erythromycin, 325 mg co-amoxclav, both erythromycin and co-amoxclav or placebo four times a day for 10 days or until delivery. The first three groups had significantly better perinatal outcome than the placebo group. However, the groups that used co-amoxclav had a significantly higher rate of NEC.

The National Institute of Child Health and Human Development–Maternal Fetal Medicine Unit Network (NICHD–MFMU) sponsored a multicentre, randomised controlled trial (Mercer et al 1997) that showed significant perinatal benefit with a combination of ampicillin 2 g and erythromycin 250 mg given intravenously every 6 hours for the first 48 hours, followed by oral treatment (amoxicillin 250 mg with erythromycin base 333 mg, every 8 hours) for five days.

The trial found a reduction in NEC with aggressive antibiotic therapy thus contradicting the results of the Oracle 1 trial. Overall, through meta-analysis it is found that there is no increased risk of NEC with antibiotics, but it is prudent to avoid amoxicillin-clavulanic acid, and also to reduce exposure to any broad spectrum antibiotics (and chorioamnionitis) by delivering women with PROM near term expediously (Mercer et al 2005).

Tocolysis

Tocolytics may be used for a short duration in PPROM while attempting to achieve the benefits of using corticosteroid and antimicrobials.

Initial Evaluation and Subsequent Monitoring

As there is a close association between vaginal colonisation and PPROM, it is worthwhile taking a vaginal swab for bacterial growth. An initial sonological evaluation offers maximum information regarding the severity of the leak (oligohydramnios), fetal condition (biophysical profile), fetal growth and estimated fetal weight. Besides, the fetal biophysical profile can be an indirect indicator of intrauterine infection.

Women on expectant management should be regularly monitored for the amount of liquor amnii and evidence of chorioamnionitis. Maternal fever, tachycardia, fetal tachycardia, uterine tenderness and foul odour of the amniotic fluid are the clinical indicators of chorioamnionitis.

Several maternal blood tests, amniotic fluid studies and fetal biophysical tests have shown clinical usefulness in diagnosing intrauterine infection. The maternal erythrocyte sedimentation rate (ESR), C-reactive protein (CRP) and leucocyte count lack sensitivity in detecting intrauterine infection. Elevated serum interleukin-6 concentration of >8 pg/ml was found to be a good predictor of histological as well as clinical chorioamnionitis (Murtha et al 1996).

The current gold standard for identifying intrauterine infection is amniotic fluid culture. However, the drawback of this test is the duration required to obtain the culture. Gram staining of the fluid is of practical value in ruling out infection. Determining the levels of interleukin-6 and interleukin-1ß can be a good diagnostic tool. Amniotic fluid leucocyte count and glucose concentration were not found to be clinically useful as they lack sensitivity. Besides these analyses, amniocentesis also offers the opportunity to study the fluid for fetal lung maturity.

Fetal non-stress test and biophysical profile studies are more feasible and practical measures of detecting intrauterine infection. A consistent association of an abnormal NST, absent fetal breathing and a low BPP score with maternal and neonatal infection has been seen. The first biophysical activities to be compromised in hypoxia or infection are fetal heart rate reactivity and fetal breathing movements (Vintzileos 1995). A normal NST has a negative predictive value of 82–93%. The predictive value is optimal when the test is conducted within 24 hours of delivery; hence NST should be performed on a daily basis. BPP may be reserved for those with non-reactive or non-reassuring NST. However, there is no consistent data to support improved neonatal outcome when delivery is based on an abnormal test (Greig 1998).

There is scope for flexibility in this group when gestational age is 32–34 weeks, wherein some fetuses may already have pulmonary maturity. If suitable facilities are available, amniotic fluid may be tested for phosphatidylglycerol, L/S ratio or surfactant albumin ratio. For this, fluid may be obtained by amniocentesis or even from the vaginal pool (Edwards et al 2000).

In **previable** PPROM, (less than 24–28 weeks) the woman should be counselled regarding poor prognosis. Mid-trimester PROM is associated with higher risk of chorioamnionitis, endometritis, placental abruption, retained placenta with postpartum hemorrhage, stillbirth, cord compression, fetal infection and fetal lung hypoplasia. The choice between expectant and expeditious management should be given to the patient herself and the case be managed accordingly. There is no specific data regarding the role of antimicrobials in prolonging pregnancy in previable PPROM.

If pregnancy could be prolonged for 2–3 weeks, the benefit of delayed corticosteroid administration may be felt. While on conservative management, fetal pulmonary growth should be followed by sonographic measurement of fetal thoracic/abdominal circumference ratio, chest circumference and pulmonary length.

Amnioinfusion

There is not enough evidence concerning the use of amnioinfusion for PROM. However, evidence supports amnioinfusion in labour for oligohydramnios to minimise cord compression (Hofmeyr 2001).

Labour and Delivery

Monitoring for evidence of infection should continue throughout labour. Cesarean delivery should be reserved for obstetric indications only, and prematurity should not be the sole indication. Intrapartum Group B streptococcal prophylaxis (ACOG 2002) is indicated for eligible cases (Table 25.1).

The antibiotic of choice is Penicillin G, 5 million units intravenously followed by 2.5 million units every 4 hours till delivery. Ampicillin 2 g loading dose followed by 1 g every 4 hours intravenously is also effective. Cefazolin, clindamycin, erythromycin or vancomycin are the other alternatives for patients with penicillin allergy. In the presence of amnionitis, the broad spectrum antimicrobial regimen should include an agent known to be active against GBS.

Chorioamnionitis

Chorioamnionitis refers to inflammation or infection of the placenta and fetal membranes (amnion and chorion). It may be histological, subclinical or clinical. PROM is one among several risk factors, the risk increasing with the duration between membrane rupture and delivery. The organisms ascend from the vagina or may sometimes be introduced during amniocentesis done as a part of management. Hence it is polymicrobial, involving *Mycoplasma hominis*, *Ureaplasma urealyticum*, bacterioides and coliforms.

Histological chorioamnionitis has little value in clinical management. Ideally, the problem should be diagnosed in the subclinical phase. As mentioned earlier, several maternal blood tests, amniotic fluid studies and fetal biophysical tests help, to some extent, in the early identification of infection.

Clinical chorioamnionitis is diagnosed in the presence of a rise in temperature to at least 37.8°C (100°F) along with two or more of the following criteria—maternal tachycardia, fetal tachycardia, uterine tenderness and foul odour of the amniotic fluid (Gibbs 1991).

Chorioamnionitis is an indication for termination of pregnancy. However, suboptimal uterine contractility, need for oxytocics to augment labour, cesarean delivery and postpartum hemorrhage should be anticipated while managing a case of chorioamnionitis in labour (Mark et al 2000).

A woman with chorioamnionitis should receive parenteral broad spectrum antimicrobials. The widely used combination is ampicillin 2 g intravenously every 6 hours plus gentamicin 1.5 mg/kg intravenously every 8 hours. Those undergoing cesarean section should, in addition, receive parenteral metronidazole or clindamycin. Parenteral antimicrobials are continued until the patient remains afebrile and asymptomatic for at least 24 hours postpartum.

Though antimicrobial treatment significantly reduces neonatal morbidity, sepsis, intraventricular hemorrhage, periventricular leukomalacia and cerebral palsy may still prevail.

Practice Points

- Infection remains as the major risk factor as well as a consequence of PROM. Clinical chorioamnionitis complicates 10% of cases of PROM.
- Preterm delivery and related perinatal complications are a major concern and a third of the preterm deliveries are caused by PROM.
- Digital vaginal examination should be deferred in women with PROM unless immediate termination is contemplated.
- Immediate induction of labour is the most favoured mode of management of PROM at term.
- Pregnancy should be terminated immediately when chorioamnionitis is diagnosed or suspected. Meanwhile, patients should receive broadspectrum antimicrobials.

TABLE 25.1: INDICATIONS FOR GBS PROPHYLAXIS

Anovaginal GBS culture positive
GBS bacteriuria in current pregnancy
Previous birth of an infant with early onset GBS disease
Unknown GBS status with PPROM
Any PROM with ≥18 hours of amniorrhexis
Maternal fever in labour ≥38°C (100.4 °F)

(Source: ACOG Committee Opinion No. 279, 2002)

- In the absence of chorioamnionitis, conservative management is offered to women with PROM. This includes monitoring for fetal well-being and for possible chorioamnionitis, corticosteroid prophylaxis and antibiotic prophylaxis.
- In labour, eligible patients should receive Group B streptococcal prophylaxis.

REFERENCES

American College of Obstetricians and Gynecologists. Prevention of early onset Group B Streptococcal Disease in Newborns. 2002. ACOG Committee Opinion No. 279. *Obstet Gynecol* 100(6):1405–1412.

Brocklehurst P, M Hannah, H McDonald et al. 2000. Interventions for treating bacterial vaginosis in pregnancy (Cochrane Review) In *Cochrane Library*, issue 1. Oxford: Update Software.

Crowley P. 1992. Corticosteroids after preterm premature rupture of membranes. *Obstet Gynecol Clin North Am* 19:317–326.

Edwards RK, P Duff and KC Ross. 2000. Amniotic fluid indices of fetal pulmonary maturity with preterm premature rupture of membranes. *Obstet Gynecol* 96:102–105.

Gibbs RS and DA Eschenbach. 1997. Use of antibiotics to prevent preterm birth. *Am J Obstet Gynecol* 177:375–380.

Gibbs RS and P Duff.1991. Progress in the pathogenesis and management of clinical intraamniotic infection. *Am J Obstet Gynecol* 164:1317–1326.

Greig PC. 1998. The diagnosis of intrauterine infection in women with preterm premature rupture of membranes (PPROM). *Clin Obstet Gynecol* 41(4): 849–863.

Gunn G, D Mishell and D Morton. 1970. Premature rupture of the fetal membranes. *Am J Obstet Gynecol* 106:469–483.

Hannah ME, A Ohlsson, D Farine et al. 1996. Induction of labour compared with expectant management for prelabour rupture of membranes at term. *N Engl J Med* 334:1005–1010.

Harding JE, J Pang, DB Knight et al. 2001. Do antenatal corticosteroids help in the setting of preterm rupture of membranes. *Am J Obstet Gynecol* 184:131–139.

Harger JH, AW Hsing, RE Tuomala et al. 1990. Risk factors for premature rupture of fetal membranes: a multicenter case-control study. *Am J Obstet Gynecol* 163:130–137.

Hofmeyr GJ. 2001. Amnioinfusion for umbilical cord compression in labour (Cochrane Review). In *The Cochrane Library*, Issue 3. Oxford: Update Software.

Kenyon S and M Boulvain. 2001. Antibiotics for preterm premature rupture of membranes (Cochrane Review). In *The Cochrane Library*, issue 3. Oxford: Update Software.

Kenyon SL, DJ Taylor, W Tarnow-Mordi et al. 2001. Broad-spectrum antibiotics for preterm, Prelabour rupture of fetal membranes: the ORACLE I randomized trial. ORACLE Collaborative Group. *Lancet* 357:979–988.

Lewis DF, K Brody, MS Edwards et al. 1996. Preterm premature ruptured membranes: A randomised trial of steroids after treatment with antibiotics. *Obstet Gynecol* 88:801–805.

Mark SP, MS Croughan-Minihane and SJ Kilpatrick. 2000. Chorioamnionitis and uterine function. *Obstet Gynecol* 95:909–912.

Mercer BM, RL Goldenberg, JD Lams et al. 1996. The preterm prediction study: Analysis of risk factors for preterm premature rupture of the membranes. *J Soc Gynecol Invest* 3:350A.

Mercer BM, M Miodovnik, GR Thurnau et al. 1997. Antibiotic therapy for reduction of infant morbidity after preterm premature rupture of membranes: a randomised controlled trial. *JAMA* 278: 989–995.

Mercer BM, RL Goldenberg, PJ Meiss et al. 2000. The preterm Prediction Study: prediction of preterm premature rupture of membranes through cervical findings and ancillary testing. *Am J Obstet Gynecol* 183:738–745.

Mercer BM, 2005. Preterm premature rupture of the membranes: current approaches to evaluation and management. *Obstet Gynecol Clin N Am* 32: 411–428.

Moller M, AC Thomsen, K Borch et al. 1984. Rupture of fetal membranes and preterm delivery associated with group B streptococci in urine of pregnant women. *Lancet* 2:69–70.

Morales WJ, JL Angel, WF O'Brien et al. 1989. Use of ampicillin and corticosteroids in premature rupture of membranes: A randomised study. *Obstet Gynecol* 73:721–726.

Mozurkewich EL and FM Wolf. 1997. Premature rupture of membranes at term: a meta-analysis of three management schemes. *Obstet Gynecol* 89:1035–1043.

Murtha AP, PC Greig, CJ Jimmerson et al. 1996. Maternal serum interleukin-6 concentrations in patients with preterm premature rupture of membranes and evidence of infection. *Am J Obstet Gynecol* 175:966–969.

Nimrod C, F Varela-Gittings, G Machin et al.1984. The effect of very prolonged membrane rupture on fetal development. *Am J Obstet Gynecol* 148:540–543.

Romero R and M Mazor. 1988. Infection and preterm labour. *Clin Obstet Gynecol* 31:553–584.

Romero R, R Quintero, E Oyarzun et al. 1988. Intraamniotic infection and the onset of labour in preterm premature rupture of membranes. *Am J Obstet Gynecol* 159:661–666.

Taylor J and T Garite. 1984. Premature rupture of membranes before fetal viability. *Obstet Gynecol* 64:615–620.

van Herendael BJ, C Oberti and I Brosens. 1978. Microanatomy of the human amniotic membranes. *Am J Obstet Gynecol* 131:872–879.

Vintzileos AM and RA Knuppel. 1995. Fetal biophysical assessment in premature rupture of the membranes. *Clin Obstet Gynecol* 38:45–58.

Wright LL, J Verter, N Younes et al. 1995. Antenatal corticosteroid administration and neonatal outcome in very low birth weight infants: the NICHD Neonatal Research Network. *Am J Obstet Gynecol* 173:269–275.

Yoon BH, JK Jun, R Romero et al. 1997. Amniotic fluid inflammatory cytokines (interleukin-6, interlukein-lb and tumour necrois factor-α), neonatal brain white matter lesions, and cerebral palsy *Am J Obstet Gynecol* 177:19–26.

26

Management of Spontaneous Labour

Rajeshwari Bhat

The mechanisms that initiate normal labour and the complex chemical and physical changes in the cervix are poorly understood. Between pregnancy and parturition, uterine function undergoes a remarkable role reversal. The quiescent myometrium becomes active and the closed cervix loses its resistance during delivery, and this process has to be repeatable for subsequent pregnancies.

Definition of Normal Birth

The World Health Organization (WHO) defines normal birth as one that is spontaneous in onset, and low risk at the start of labour and remaining so throughout labour and delivery. The infant is born spontaneously in vertex presentation between 37 and 42 completed weeks of pregnancy. After the birth, the mother and infant are in good health.

Generally, between 70% and 80% of pregnant women may be considered to be at low risk at the onset of labour. WHO recommends that during normal labour, there should be a valid reason to interfere with the natural process.

Diagnosis of Labour

Labour should be suspected or anticipated if the patient has the following symptoms:

- Intermittent abdominal pain
- Pain associated with blood-stained discharge (show)
- Watery vaginal discharge or a sudden gush of water

The onset of labour can be confirmed if cervical effacement and dilatation is seen.

Braxton Hicks contractions—painless uterine contractions—increase both in frequency and intensity towards term and can cause discomfort when the patient has a low threshold for pain. This and other causes of pain will have to be differentiated from true labour pains (Table 26.1).

First Stage of Labour

Initial assessment of the patient is done by eliciting a detailed history, performing general and obstetric examinations and by ordering the relevant investigations. High-risk pregnancies can thus be screened.

General examination of the patient includes looking for pallor, edema and jaundice. Pulse, blood pressure and temperature are also recorded. Cardiovascular and respiratory systems should be examined.

On abdominal examination, the fundal height should be measured to estimate the approximate weight of the fetus; the fetal lie

TABLE 26.1: DIFFERENCES BETWEEN TRUE AND FALSE LABOUR

	True Labour	*False Labour*
Interval between contractions	Occur at regular intervals	Occur at irregular intervals
Frequency of contractions	Increases	Remains irregular
Intensity of contractions, thus pain	Increases	Remains the same
Duration of contraction	Increases	Varies, may become less
Cervical changes	Progressive effacement and dilatation	No change
Sedation	Progress of labour is not stopped by sedation	Usually relieved by sedation

and presentation should also be noted. The level of the presenting part should be estimated in fifths. Uterine contractions are assessed by palpation with relevance to their frequency and duration over 10-minute periods. The fetal heart is auscultated after a contraction for a minimum period of one minute.

After completing the abdominal examination, a speculum is inserted carefully to visualise the fluid in the posterior fornix if the patient complains of leaking fluids from the vagina. The fluid is examined for the presence of the vernix and meconium. If the source of the fluid is unclear, it should be collected on a swab for further analysis.

Vaginal examination is then performed under aseptic precautions:

- To note the consistency, position, effacement and dilatation of the cervix
- To note the station and position of the presenting part
- To check for caput and moulding
- To assess the bony pelvis by noting the curve of the sacrum, ischial spines, side walls, subpubic arch and intertuberous diameter

Electronic Admission Test The admission test is a non-stress or contraction stress test done on patients admitted to the labour ward to identify unsuspected fetal jeopardy. In 1986, Ingemarsson and associates recommended that the test be done on all patients. However, its benefits are yet to be proved.

Investigations When the patient is admitted to the labour ward, hematocrit or hemoglobin concentration should be rechecked. Urine should be examined for proteins, ketones, sugar and leukocytes. In unbooked patients, blood grouping and typing and tests for syphilis, hepatitis B and human immunodeficiency virus should be performed.

Routine Procedures

PREPARATION OF THE VULVA AND PERINEAL REGIONS: The perineal region is washed and usually the hair on the lower part of the vulva and perineum are removed either by shaving or clipping. Pubic shaving is presumed to reduce infection and facilitate suturing, but routine use can increase the risk of infection by HIV and hepatitis virus, either to the birth attendant or to the mother.

ENEMA: Early in labour, an enema is usually given to minimise contamination by feces and, thereby, infection to the mother and child. Enemas are supposed to stimulate uterine contractions and an empty bowel is thought to allow descent of the head. However, they are uncomfortable and may cause damage to the bowel mucosa. No effects of enema on the duration of labour or neonatal or wound infection were detected.

Nutrition: Eating and drinking during labour will put women at risk of aspirating the stomach contents during anesthesia. Keeping the patient nil per oral during labour, however, does not guarantee reduced stomach contents. Routine administration of antacids during labour may not prevent Mendelson syndrome. Labour requires enormous amounts of energy. The length of labour cannot be predicted and therefore, the sources of energy need to be replenished to ensure fetal and maternal well-being. Severe restriction of oral intake can lead to dehydration and ketosis. However, if it is treated with intravenous infusion of glucose and fluids, the mean serum glucose levels will rise. This is associated with a rise in maternal insulin levels and an increase in plasma glucose levels in the baby, and it may result in a decrease in umbilical arterial blood pH. Fetal hyperinsulinemia results in neonatal hypoglycemia and raised levels of blood lactate. Offering oral fluids and light meals during labour, especially to a low-risk mother, can prevent dehydration and ketoacidosis. Routine intravenous infusions restrict the patient's freedom to move.

Urinary Bladder Function: Bladder distension must be avoided as it could lead to obstructed labour and subsequent bladder hypotonia and infection. If the bladder is readily palpated on abdominal examination, the patient should be encouraged to void. If the patient cannot void either in the bedpan or in the toilet, catheterisation is indicated.

Support in Childbirth Antenatal preparation is an essential element of quality care. According to Driscoll et al, the main purpose of antenatal preparation is to define a woman's role in labour and to teach her how to fulfill it. This comprises two components— education and training. The educational component ensures that every expectant mother has a broad understanding of the birth process. The training component aims at teaching how to achieve the satisfaction of spontaneous delivery. It is based on learning how to relax as the uterus contracts, during the second stage of labour.

Reports and randomised controlled trials on support during labour by a single person, midwife or nurse, showed that continuous empathetic and physical support during labour resulted in benefits such as shorter labour, significantly less medication and epidural analgesia, fewer Apgar scores of less than 7 and fewer operative deliveries. Support consists of praise, reassurance, measures to improve the comfort of the mother, physical contact such as rubbing the mother's back and holding her hands, explanation of what is going on during labour and delivery and a constant friendly presence.

Position and Movement During the First Stage of Labour: Several studies have shown that during the first stage of labour, the supine position affects blood flow in the uterus. The heavy uterus can compress the aorta and inferior vena cava, and reduce blood flow, which can be deleterious to the fetus. The supine position reduces the intensity of the contractions and thus interferes with the normal progression of labour. Standing up and lying down on the side are associated with greater intensity and frequency of contractions. Trials that have compared these positions to the supine have found that, on an average, patients experienced less pain and augmentation was used less frequently in the non-supine positions. Patients usually change their positions, as no position is comfortable for a long period of time. The only situation when a supine position is required is when the membranes have ruptured in the presence of a mobile head.

Pain Relief Almost all women experience pain during labour, but the responses of individual women to this pain are very different. Abnormal labour, prolonged or complicated by dystocia, induced or accelerated by oxytocics, or terminated by instrumental delivery, seems to be more painful than normal labour. Pain relief can be achieved pharmacologically. However, a non-pharmacological approach, starting during prenatal care by providing reassuring information to the pregnant woman and her partner and empathetic support before and during labour, can reduce the need for pharmacological pain relief. Touch and massage by a companion are often felt to be helpful. Other methods include attention-focussing techniques such as patterned breathing, relaxation and drawing the woman's attention away from her pain. Specific non-pharmacological methods include transcutaneous electrical nerve stimulation (TENS), use of superficial heat and cold, acupuncture and immersion in water, herbs and aroma therapy with fragrant oils. For most of these techniques, randomised trials to establish their effectiveness are not available as yet. Pharmacological pain relief in labour may use systemic agents such as pethidine, phenothiazine derivatives, benzodiazepines and others. The inhalation analgesia that is most commonly used is a combination of nitrous oxide with 50% oxygen. All agents can produce reasonable pain relief, but they have unwanted side effects.

Epidural analgesia is the most widely used form of regional analgesia in normal labour. It provides better and more lasting pain relief than systemic agents. There is a tendency for the first stage of labour to be prolonged, and oxytocin to be used more frequently when epidural analgesia is used. The number of vaginal operative deliveries was increased, especially if the analgesic effect was maintained into the second stage of labour, because of suppression of the bearing down reflex.

Obstetric analgesia has been discussed in detail in Chapter 33.

Monitoring the Maternal Condition The temperature, pulse and blood pressure should be measured every two hours. A rise in temperature may be the first sign of infection.

Monitoring Fetal Well-being in Labour

Monitoring Fetal Heart: Two methods are used to monitor the fetal heart–intermittent auscultation and continuous electronic surveillance. Intermittent auscultation can be done by using either a stethoscope or a hand-held ultrasound Doppler apparatus. The fetal heart should be auscultated after a contraction for a minimum of one minute, and at least every fifteen minutes in the first stage of labour (RCOG 2001). Intermittent auscultation is simple and the patient is free to move about at will.

Electronic fetal heart rate monitoring is used for the surveillance of high-risk pregnancies and also during labour. The monitoring is most commonly done by an external ultrasound transducer or an internal (vaginal) electrode attached to the fetal scalp, after the rupture of the membranes. The sensitivity of the method with respect to detection of fetal distress is high, but the specificity is low. The method results in a high rate of false-positive signals and therefore, a high number of unnecessary interventions, especially if used in a group of low-risk pregnant women.

Fetal Scalp Blood Sampling: It is a micro technique of sampling blood from the fetal scalp to examine the acid-base status of the blood and confirm fetal hypoxia. Its use is generally limited to high-risk cases.

Intermittent auscultation is the method of choice for monitoring the fetus during normal labour. Electronic monitoring is advantageous only in women with increased risk, such as during labour that is induced or augmented, complicated by meconium-stained amniotic fluid or any other risk factors. In the majority of labours without increased risk, electronic monitoring increases the number of interventions with no clear benefit for the fetus and with additional discomfort for the mother.

The Passage of Meconium

The passage of meconium may reflect fetal distress and is associated with intrapartum stillbirth and neonatal morbidity or death. The thick meconium that is seen after the rupture of the membranes has the worst prognosis. Undiluted meconium also reflects the reduction or absence of amniotic fluid at the time of rupturing of the membranes and should be considered a risk factor. In the presence of a normal fetal heart rate, meconium staining of amniotic fluid is not an indication for immediate delivery or fetal blood sampling, especially if it is thin staining. However, if the fetal heart rate becomes abnormal in association with thick, fresh meconium, early delivery should be considered particularly in high-risk patients.

Monitoring the Progress of Labour

Assessment of the progress of labour is made by observing the patient—her appearance, behaviour, contractions and descent of the presenting part. The most accurate method is dilatation of the cervix.

Uterine Contractions The palm of the hand is placed lightly on the uterus. The intensity of contractions is judged by the degree of firmness that the uterus achieves. At the acme of effective contractions, the finger or thumb cannot readily indent the uterus. The time at which the contractions disappear is also noted. This sequence is repeated to evaluate the frequency, duration and intensity of contractions.

Uterine contractions can also be assessed by using external and internal tocography. The instrument used for external tocography comprises a pressure sensor that detects changes in the anteroposterior diameter of the abdomen, resulting from uterine contractions. Internal tocography uses an open-ended, fluid-filled catheter connected to a previously calibrated pressure transducer. Internal tocography is useful in very obese women and in women with a previous cesarean section. In most patients, clinical assessment is satisfactory.

Descent of the Presenting Part: Descent can be assessed by abdominal palpation in terms of fetal head palpable above the pubic symphisis. A head that is felt entirely above the pubic symphysis is five-fifths (5/5) palpable, while one that is entirely below the pubic symphysis is zero-fifths (0/5) palpable (Fig. 26.1).

Vaginal examination may be used to assess the descent by relating the level of the fetal presenting part to the ischial spines of the maternal pelvis. When there is significant degree of caput or moulding, assessment by abdominal palpation is more useful than vaginal examination.

Changes in cervical effacement, dilatation

and fetal descent should be assessed by vaginal examination, which should be performed at least once every four hours during the first stage of labour and after rupture of the membranes.

Partograph: The WHO partograph has been modified to make it easier and simpler to read. The latent phase has been removed and the plotting on the partograph now begins in the active phase, when the cervix is dilated by 4 cm. The following information should be recorded on the partograph (Fig. 26.2).

Patient information: The name of the patient, parity index, hospital number, date and time of admission, time of rupture of membranes or the time elapsed since the rupture of membranes (if rupture has occurred before charting on the partograph began) should be recorded.

Fetal heart rate: This should be recorded every half hour.

Amniotic fluid: This should be recorded as I–membranes intact; R–membranes ruptured; C–membranes ruptured, clear fluid; M–meconium stained; B–blood stained fluid.

Moulding: This should be recorded as 1–sutures apposed; 2–sutures overlapped, but reducible; 3–sutures overlapped, but not reducible.

Cervical dilatation: This should be assessed at every vaginal examination and marked with a cross (X).

Alert line: A line that starts at 4 cm of cervical dilatation to the point of expected full cervical dilatation at the rate of 1 cm/hour.

Action line: A line that is parallel to and four hours to the right of the alert line.

Descent: This is assessed by abdominal palpation and recorded as a circle (0).

Hours: This refers to the time elapsed since commencement of the active phase of labour.

Time: The recorded actual time is plotted.

Contractions: These are charted every half hour; the number of contractions in a 10-minute period and their duration is recorded in seconds:

- <20 seconds
- 20–40 seconds
- > 40 seconds

Oxytocin: The amount of oxytocin per volume IV fluids in drops per minute every 30 minutes, if used, is plotted.

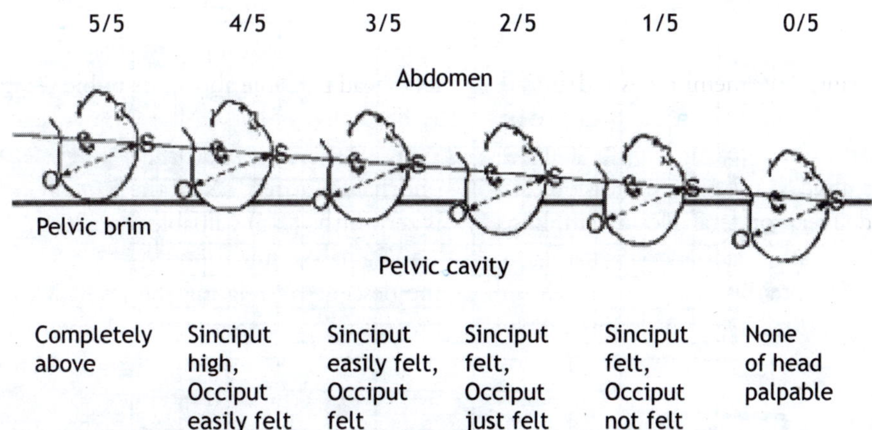

Figure 26.1: Assessment of fetal descent by abdominal palpation

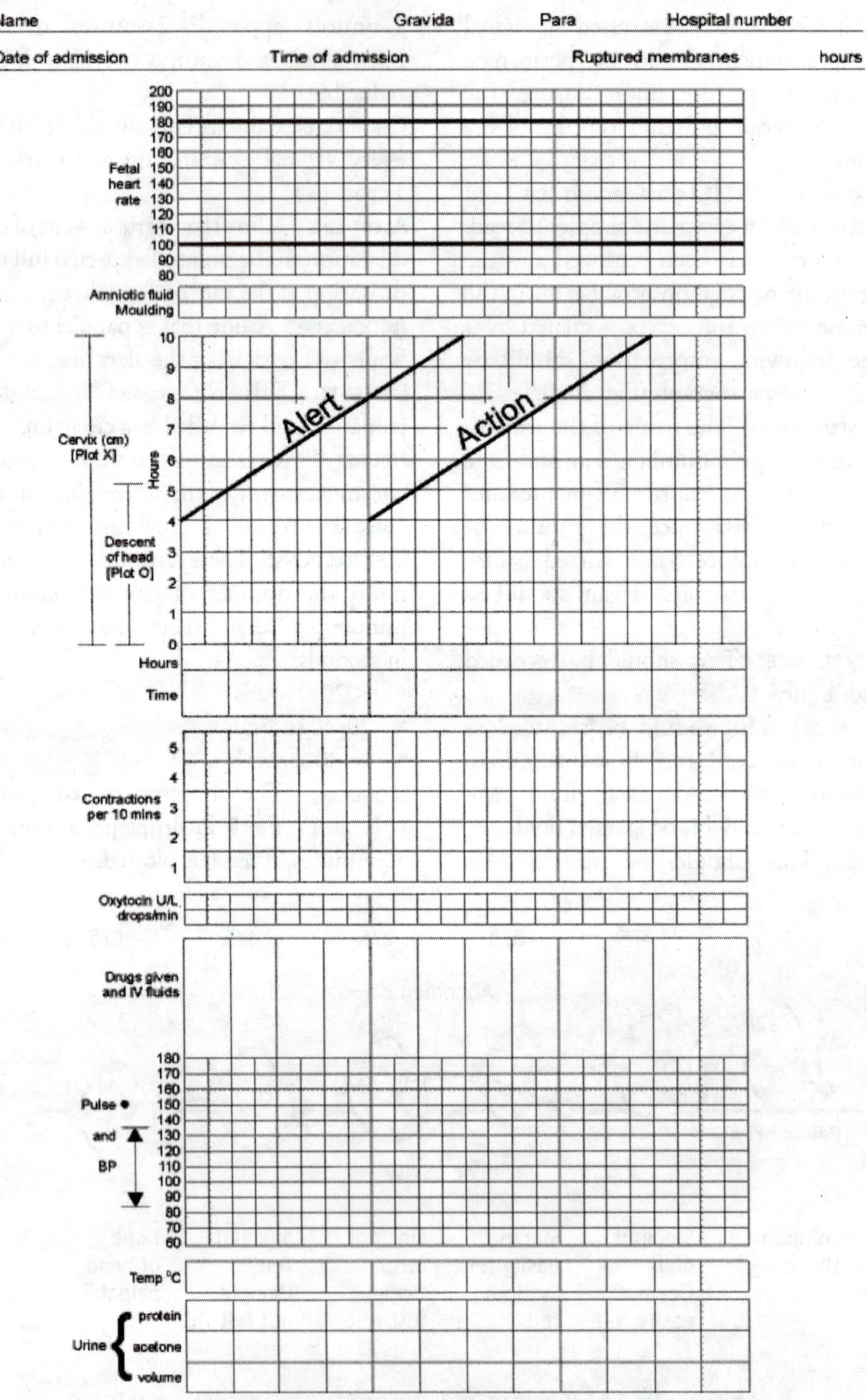

FIGURE 26.2: THE MODIFIED WHO PARTOGRAPH

Drugs: The additional drugs given should be recorded.

Pulse: This should be recorded every 30 minutes and marked with a dot (.).

Blood pressure: This should be recorded every four hours and marked with arrows.

Temperature: This must be recorded every two hours.

Urine: The protein, acetone and volume of urine should be recorded.

Findings suggestive of satisfactory progress of labour are regular contractions of progressively increasing frequency and duration, rate of cervical dilatation of at least 1 cm per hour during the active phase of labour (cervical dilatation on or to the left of the alert line) and a cervix that is applied to the presenting part.

Active Management of Labour The active management of labour was formulated by O' Driscoll et al at the National Maternity Hospital, Dublin, in 1963. The underlying philosophy is firmly based on the curtailment of the duration of exposure to stress, with avoidance of physical and emotional trauma, which is likely to follow prolonged labour. Efficient uterine action is recognised as the key factor and correct clinical diagnosis of labour is known to be of prime importance in every woman admitted to the labour ward.

Active management of labour originated as an approach to counter the widespread view that the first stage of labour was to be managed expectantly, with the interventions reserved for the second stage, often in the form of operative vaginal delivery. The new approach was meant to decrease the negative aspects of prolonged nulliparous labour and emphasised maternal expulsion of the fetus rather than delivery by traction.

Active management is not for all parturients but only for those meeting the specific inclusion criteria of nulliparity, spontaneous labour and singleton fetus at cephalic presentation at term.

The key components of this protocol are as follows:

- Special antenatal classes to prepare women for labour
- Strict criteria for diagnosing labour
- The guarantee of labour not lasting longer than 12 hours
- Artificial rupture of membranes (ARM) to be performed in all cases as soon as the diagnosis of labour is made. If there is any doubt about the diagnosis of labour, the decision to rupture the membranes should be deferred for one hour.
- Augmentation of contractions with synthetic oxytocin to be employed if dilatation does not increase at the rate of 1 cm/hour. A standard concentration of 10 units of oxytocin is to be used in all circumstances. The rate of infusion begins at 10 drops and increases by 10 drops, at intervals of 15 minutes, to a maximum of 60 drops. The total dose of oxytocin should not exceed 10 units. To guard against hypertonus, the number of contractions is not permitted to exceed 7 in 15 minutes under any circumstance.

The following conditions must be fulfilled before starting oxytocin:

- Mothers must be nulliparous
- Presentation must be vertex
- Fetus must be single
- Membranes must be ruptured
- No evidence of fetal distress must be seen
- The progress of labour is charted on a partograph
- The guarantee of the mother not being left alone, but of receiving continuous companionship from a midwifery student or medical student

- Every mother not close to an easy vaginal delivery after 12 hours to be delivered by cesarean section

The active management of labour has been the subject of controversy and debate. In the late 1980s and early 1990s, a series of trials of some of the components of active management were reported and collected by the Cochrane collaboration of Oxford. These suggested that psychological support in labour lowered the rate of cesarean section deliveries. They did not find that routine amniotomy or oxytocin, either alone or in combination, reduced the rate of cesarean delivery. Early amniotomy did not appear to provide benefits over a more conservative form of management in the context of care of nulliparous women with mild delays in the progression of labour. Six published randomised studies evaluating the effects of early amniotomy on labour outcomes were identified by Fraser et al (1992). Taken together, the results of the published trials indicate that when amniotomy is done during active labour, it is likely to result in a reduction in the duration of labour; however, it does not reduce the rates of cesarean section or operative vaginal delivery. The shortening of labour by force does not improve clinical outcome; this suggests that it is not the duration as such that gives rise to poor outcome but the pathology that underlies the delay. Among patients who had undergone amniotomy, it was found that more than 20% of contractions produced early decelerations as opposed to 3% of contractions in those who went into labour with their membranes intact.

A study by Goffinet et al in 1997 suggested that early amniotomy increases the hourly rate of severe variable fetal heart rate decelerations without evidence of an adverse effect on neonatal outcome. Amniotomy may have a detrimental effect on both the mother and the fetus, increased frequency of intrapartum infection and increased incidence of fetal distress (Mercer et al 1995). According to the WHO (1985), rupture of membranes is not required until at a fairly late stage in the delivery. Artificial rupture of membranes as a routine procedure is not scientifically justified and should be performed for specific indications only. Fraser and Sokol (1992) recommended adopting a selective approach to the artificial rupture of membranes.

Diagnosis of Poor Progress of Labour

Accurate monitoring of the progress of labour is important for the detection of prolonged labour, which is associated with adverse maternal and fetal outcome. Slow progression should be a reason for careful evaluation of the patient.

The use of a partogram for the management of labour facilitates the early detection of abnormal progress of labour and identifies the patients most likely to require intervention. A comparative study has demonstrated that clinical criteria stringently applied to the diagnosis of abnormal labour are less effective in recognising and characterising the forms of dysfunctional labour than the more objective graphicostatistical analytic approach.

There are three different patterns of abnormal progress:

- Prolonged latent phase
- Primary dysfunctional labour
- Secondary arrest of dilatation

The latent phase is usually considered to be prolonged if it lasts for more than 8 hours in nullipara and 6 hours in multipara. Primary dysfunctional labour (PDL) is diagnosed in the active phase labour when the progression of labour falls to the right of the normogram. In secondary arrest of dilatation (SACD), labour progresses satisfactorily in the early active phase, but the cervix fails to dilate or dilates slowly thereafter. More than one of these abnormal labour patterns may occur in the same patient, as their etiology is frequently common. Progress is assessed both of cervical dilatation and fetal descent.

Poor progress of labour is related to power—uterine contractions, passage (the resistance of the birth canal) and passenger (the size, position and degree of flexion of fetal head). The predominant causes are inadequate uterine contractions and, to a lesser extent, cephalopelvic disproportion or malposition or a combination of these causes. Weak contractions or minimal disproportion can be corrected by oxytocin augmentation, which causes further flexion, moulding and pelvic 'give'.

Primary dysfunctional labour (PDL) is caused by inadequate uterine activity. Secondary arrest is less common than PDL. The commonest cause of secondary arrest of dilatation is inefficient uterine activity. Disproportion usually causes SACD rather than PDL. Secondary arrest of dilatation due to inadequate uterine contractions can be corrected, resulting in vaginal delivery. However, if a diagnosis of secondary arrest is made, especially in a multiparous woman, disproportion due to the passenger or the passage should be checked. If dystocia is due to relative disproportion such as deflection or occipitoposterior position, it can be corrected by efficient uterine contractions.

Management of Poor Progress of Labour

Latent Phase of Labour: The diagnosis of the latent phase of labour is made retrospectively. A woman is said to have had false labour if the contractions cease. The diagnosis of latent phase will be confirmed when the contractions become regular and dilatation progresses beyond 4 cm. If maternal and fetal well-being is confirmed, the management of prolonged latent phase consists of explanation, reassurance, hydration, nutrition and ambulation. Unnecessary interventions such as amniotomy and augmentation with oxytocin should be avoided unless there is a clear indication for it.

Augmentation of Active Phase of Labour: The decision to augment labour should be made based on the rate of cervical dilatation recorded in the partogram, after exclusion of gross disproportion or malpresentation. Artificial rupture of membranes can be done to enhance the uterine contractions when labour progression is abnormal.

Augmentation with Oxytocin: Delay in progression of labour due to inefficient uterine contractions may be corrected by oxytocin infusion. A minor degree of disproportion caused by malposition and poor flexion of head may also be overcome by oxytocin. More forceful uterine contractions flex the atlanto-occipital joint and reduce the presenting diameter. This allows rotation of the occiput from a posterior to an anterior position. The increased force of contraction also helps moulding, reduces the presenting diameter of the head, thereby leading to an increase in the pelvic dimensions due to the descending head widening the sacroiliac and symphysis pubic joints.

During a normal pregnancy, serum oxytocin concentrations remain unchanged throughout gestation; with labour, serum plasma levels increase and then peak in the second stage. Fetch et al reported that plasma concentrations of oxytocin in normal labour are similar to those in women receiving 4–6 mU/minute by continuous intravenous infusion. From the first clinically described use of oxytocin by Theobald et al in 1948, there has been a controversy about the best and most appropriate regimen for oxytocin use. In the 1980s, Seitchik and co-workers published studies in which low dose protocols were used. They began oxytocin at 0.5–1.0 mU/minute and increased dosage by 1–2 mU/minute. They recommended an interval of 30–40 minutes for an increase in dosage. According to Satin and co-workers, labour augmentation with a high dose regimen is clearly superior to a low dose method. Many factors can account for the wide variations in responsiveness to oxytocin infusions, including differences in oxytocin receptor expression, oxytocin plasma concentration and oxytocinase concentration and activity. Clinically important predictors of required oxytocin dosage include cervical dilatation, parity and gestational age (Table 26.2).

The mechanical efficiency of uterine contractions should be defined in terms of their clinical effect, that is, the progress of cervical dilatation and descent of the head, and not in relation to the magnitude of uterine contractions. This is because normal labour progress is observed with a wide range of uterine activity in both nulliparas and

TABLE 26.2: OXYTOCIN INFUSION RATE FOR INDUCTION AND AUGMENTATION OF LABOUR (WHO)

Time since induction (hours)	*Oxytocin concentration*	*Drops per minute*	*Approximate dose (mIU/minute)*	*Volume infused*	*Total volume infused*
0.00	2.5 units in 500 ml dextrose or normal saline (5 mIU/ml)	10	3	0	0
0.50	same	20	5	15	15
1.00	same	30	8	30	45
1.50	same	40	10	45	90
2.00	same	50	13	60	150
2.50	same	60	15	75	225
3.00	5 units in 500 ml (10 mIU/ml)	30	15	90	315
3.50	same	40	20	45	360
4.00	same	50	25	60	420
4.50	same	60	30	75	495
5.00	10 units in 500 ml (20 mIU/ml)	30	30	90	585
5.50	same	40	40	45	630
6.00	same	50	50	60	690
6.50	same	60	60	75	765
7.00	same	60	60	90	855

(1 mL – 20 drops)

multiparas (Gibbs et al 1984; O' Driscoll et al 1993). Three contractions in 10 minutes is an appropriate uterine target with oxytocin titration; however, if no progress of labour is seen with this frequency of contractions, the oxytocin dose may be increased to achieve a frequency of 4–5 in 10 minutes, provided the fetal heart rate is normal. The frequency of contractions may be assessed either by external or internal tocography. A prospective controlled study did not show a better obstetric outcome when intrauterine catheters were used in augmented labour, when compared to external tocography. Wherever available, subsequent fetal surveillance should be done by electronic monitoring.

After a period of 8 hours of augmentation with adequate monitoring, the majority of nulliparous and multiparous women should deliver vaginally with little risk of intrauterine hypoxia.

Second Stage of Labour

The second stage of labour begins when the cervix is fully dilated and completely retracted past the presenting part and is no longer palpable vaginally, and ends with the delivery of the fetus.

The mean duration of the second stage is 50 minutes in nulliparous and 20 minutes in multiparas women, but it can be highly variable. Two or three expulsive forces in the second stage may be sufficient to deliver the infant in a woman of high parity with a stretched vagina and perineum. The second stage may be abnormally long in a woman with a contracted pelvis or a large fetus or with impaired expulsive efforts.

The following symptoms mark the beginning of the second stage of labour:

- The woman feels the urge to bear down, because the amniotic sac or the presenting part protrudes through the dilated cervix and presses against the rectum.
- The membranes rupture spontaneously.
- The uterine contractions and accompanying expulsive forces may last 90 seconds and recur at times after a myometrial resting phase of no more than a minute.

The second stage of labour may be divided into two phases. Phase 1 or the pelvic phase comprises full cervical dilatation to a period of passive descent of the presenting part. Phase 2 or the period of expulsion or the perineal phase begins with the arrival of the presenting part at the pelvic floor and ends with the delivery of the fetus. The uterine contractions during this phase are more frequent, intense and prolonged.

During these contractions, there is marked reduction in uteroplacental perfusion because there is less time to replenish the oxygenated blood in the intervillous space before onset of the next contraction. The descent of the fetal head into the pelvic cavity is associated with fetal head and eyeball compression, raised intracranial pressure and vagally mediated fetal heart rate decelerations and early and variable decelerations. The rate of fall of pH in the fetus is also more rapid in the second stage of labour than during than first stage. Fetuses with suboptimal antepartum energy reserve may not tolerate these added insults. Fetal hypoxia, either during pregnancy or intrapartum, remains the principal cause of both brain damage and death.

Maternal Position During the Second Stage of Labour A number of trials suggest that an upright (vertical) position or a lateral tilt during the second stage of labour shows greater advantages than a dorsal position. The upright position gives less discomfort and difficulty in bearing down, less perineal/vaginal trauma and wound infections, less frequent abnormal fetal heart rate patterns and a higher umbilical arterial pH. In one trial, a shorter duration of the second stage was observed in the upright position. An increased percentage of postpartum hemorrhage has been found in women adopting the vertical position. The lithotomy position with the legs in the stirrups was found to be less comfortable, more painful and more restrictive in movement.

Both in the first and second stage of labour, women can adopt any position they like, preferably avoiding long periods lying supine. They should be encouraged to adopt the position that they feel most comfortable in and should be supported in the positions of their choice. Birth attendants need training in performing births in other positions than the supine in order to not be an inhibiting factor in the choice of position.

Monitoring Fetal Heart Rate: For the low risk fetus, the heart rate should be auscultated every 5 minutes in the second stage of labour (RCOG 2001).

It is sometimes advised to routinely empty the bladder by catheterisation before the onset of pushing. This may cause infection of the urinary tract. Catheterisation may be difficult or traumatic if the fetal head is firmly engaged. It is advisable to encourage the woman to urinate spontaneously during the first stage of labour.

Onset of Pushing During the Second Stage: The physiological approach is to wait until the woman feels the urge to bear down herself. Trials have been done to compare early versus late pushing in normal labour in patients with epidural analgesia. As the bearing down reflex is suppressed, it is easy to delay the pushing efforts until the vertex is visible in the introitus. This procedure has been compared with pushing as soon as full dilatation is diagnosed. Delayed pushing did not show any hazardous effect on fetal or neonatal outcome. In fact, significantly more forceps deliveries occurred in the early pushing group.

Procedure of Pushing: The widely advocated practice is to encourage sustained, Valsalva bearing down efforts. The alternative is the woman's spontaneous pattern of expulsive efforts—exhalatory bearing down efforts. These two practices have been compared in several trials (Barnett and Humenick 1982; Knauth and Haloburdo 1986; Parnell et al 1993; Thomson 1993). Spontaneous pushing resulted in 3–5 relatively brief (4–6 seconds) bearing down efforts with each contraction, compared with the 10–30 seconds duration of sustained bearing down efforts, accompanied by breath holding. The latter method resulted in a shorter second stage of labour, but the mean umbilical artery pH was lower and the Apgar tended to be depressed. Thus, shorter spontaneous pushing seems to be superior.

Duration of the Second Stage One of the most controversial issues in obstetrics is that of the duration of the second stage of labour and its influence on neonatal well-being. The key question in managing the second stage of labour should be how long the patient may be allowed to labour without the fetus passing from the easily reversible respiratory acidosis into life-threatening metabolic acidosis.

Prolonged second stage of labour may lead to fetal hypoxia and a lower Apgar score at birth. It is the expulsive phase of the second stage that causes a greater and more significant fall in the fetal pH. Romer et al suggested upper limits for the duration of the expulsive forces as 45 minutes in nulliparous and 30 minutes in multiparous women.

Prolonged second stage of labour is also recognised as a risk factor for pelvic floor trauma and pressure-related nerve damage leading to medium- and long-term pelvic floor dysfunction, including symptomatic uterovaginal prolapse and urinary and fecal incontinence.

The arbitrary time limits previously imposed on the duration of the second stage of labour have been challenged because of improved intrapartum fetal monitoring techniques. Association of prolonged second stage with poor outcome is more likely to be related to injudicious use of forceps than because a defined period of time has passed.

Seizer et al have proposed a partogram for the second stage of labour. This partogram is based on a system of scoring the descent and position of the fetal head and this system can be used to study the progression of the second stage of labour and predict the mode of delivery and outcome.

Decisions about curtailing the second stage of labour should be made based on surveillance of the maternal and fetal conditions, and on the progression of labour. If there are signs of fetal distress or if the presenting part fails to descend, labour should be terminated; but if the mother's condition is satisfactory, the fetus is in a good condition and there is evidence of progress in the descent of the fetal head, there are no grounds for intervention.

Causes for Delay in the Second Stage of Labour: Many factors influence progress in the second stage—the size and shape of the pelvis, fetal weight, uterine contractions, soft tissue resistance, maternal effort and the degree of flexion and caput and moulding of the fetal head. Prolonged duration should be seen as a marker of potential obstetric problems such as inadequate expulsive forces or obstruction.

Expulsive forces may be insufficient to maintain progress in labour if epidural analgesia is used. Epidural analgesia relaxes the pelvic floor muscles and interferes with maternal bearing down efforts. It also impairs the release of oxytocin in response to the distension of the vagina and perineum. Internal rotation is therefore delayed or may fail to occur. There appears to be increased risk of uterine dysfunction with advancing maternal age and body mass index. Resistance to descent of fetal head may be caused by cephalopelvic disproportion or by soft tissue resistance. Persistent occipitoposterior position, deflexed head and macrosomic baby are associated with prolonged second stage. Pelvic masses such as ovarian tumours, myomas and pelvic kidney may cause delay in the second stage, but are rare.

Care of the Perineum: Perineal damage is one of the most frequently suffered traumas during delivery.

During delivery of the fetal head, the perineum is supported with the fingers of one hand, with the other hand applying pressure to the fetal head and controlling the speed of crowning. These measures help to, prevent or reduce damage to the perineal tissues.

There has been no formal evaluation of this strategy or the opposite, which involves not touching the perineum or head during this phase of delivery. Another technique used to reduce trauma to the perineum is massaging the perineum to stretch the tissues, during the last part of the second stage of labour. This may cause more damage to the tissues, which are already highly vascular and edematous.

Perineal Tear and Episiotomy Perineal tears occur frequently especially in primiparous women. First and second degree tears can be easily sutured under local analgesia, and usually heal without any complications. Third degree tears can have more serious consequences such as fecal incontinence or fistula and should therefore be sutured by an obstetrician.

Episiotomies are performed if there are signs of fetal distress, delay in progress of expulsive phase of second stage or threatened third degree tear. Midline episiotomies are more easily sutured and have the advantage of less scar tissue. Mediolateral episiotomies more effectively avoid the anal sphincter and the rectum. Episiotomies are given as substitutes for a ragged laceration, which is difficult to repair.

Liberal episiotomies are also used to prevent trauma to the fetal head and muscles of the pelvic floor, thus preventing urinary incontinence. However, trials do not show evidence to support this policy. Liberal use of episiotomy is associated with higher rates of perineal trauma and lower rates of women with intact perineum. There is no evidence of the protective effect of episiotomy on the fetal condition. In a follow-up study done for up to three years after birth, no influence of liberal episiotomy on urinary incontinence was found. The third degree tear rate was similar in the 'no episiotomy' and the mediolateral episiotomy groups, but higher in the midline episiotomy group. Thus, there is no reliable evidence that liberal or routine use of episiotomy has a beneficial effect. In normal delivery, there may at times be a valid indication for an episiotomy, but a restricted use of this intervention is recommended.

There is no evidence in the literature favouring a liberal policy over a restrictive policy for the use of episiotomy, both in terms of fetal (Grade C) and maternal (Grade A) indications. A number of obstetrical situations considered as at risk do not systematically indicate an episiotomy. There are, however, circumstances in which a pertinent and prudent clinical assessment will lead the obstetrician to use an episiotomy.

Timing of Cord Clamping: The umbilical cord can be clamped immediately after birth or later, and this may affect the mother and the infant. There is no evidence of a significant effect of the timing of cord clamping on the incidence of postpartum hemorrhage or on fetomaternal transfusion. If after birth the infant is placed at or below the level of the vulva, for three minutes before clamping the cord, a shift of about 80 ml of blood from placenta to the infant will be seen. The erythrocytes in this volume of blood will soon be destroyed by hemolysis, but this provides about 50 g of iron to the infant's reserve and reduces the incidence of iron deficiency anemia later in infancy.

Late clamping or not clamping at all are the physiological ways of treating the cord. The transfusion of blood from the mother to the fetus if the cord is clamped late is physiological. However, after an abnormal pregnancy or labour such as rhesus sensitisation or preterm labour, late clamping may lead to complications such as hypervolemia, polycythemia, hyperviscosity and hyperbilirubinemia.

Third Stage of Labour

The third stage of labour is the period from the delivery of the baby up to the delivery of the placenta. After delivery of the baby and cessation of umbilical cord pulsation, the placenta separates from the uterine wall through the deciduas spongiosa and is delivered through the birth canal. The placenta separates as a result of the shearing force between the placental surface and the uterine wall in the presence of uterine muscular contractions. The degree of blood loss associated with placental separation and delivery depends on how quickly the placenta separates from the uterine wall and how effectively the uterine muscle contracts around the placental blood vessels.

Management of the Third Stage of Labour: Management of the third stage of labour may be either expectant or active.

Expectant Management: Passive management of the third stage of labour involves awaiting the spontaneous contraction of the uterus and separation of placenta and membranes. Measures such as the use of nipple stimulation or postural changes may be employed. Expectant management is associated with a twofold increase in the incidence of postpartum hemorrhage and increased risk of blood transfusion when compared with active management. A poorly contracted uterus poses an increased risk of the potentially fatal complication of uterine inversion.

Active Management: It comprises the use of an oxytocic agent, which causes the uterus to contract strongly, given parenterally as the baby is born, as well as early cord clamping, and controlled cord traction. (pulling the cord to deliver the placenta as quickly as possible, combined with counter pressure upwards on the uterine body by placing a hand immediately above the symphysis pubis). Complications of oxytocics are nausea, vomiting, headache and hypertension. These complications occur more often with ergot alkaloids. Serious complications of oxytocics include cardiac arrest, intracerebral hemorrhage, myocardial infarction, postpartum eclampsia and pulmonary edema. Available evidence suggests that oxytocin is a better choice than ergot derivatives. In tropical countries, oxytocin is more stable than ergotamine or methylergometrine.

Immediate Care of the Newborn: Immediate care involves ensuring that the airway is clear, taking measures to maintain body temperature, clamping and cutting the cord and putting the baby to the breast as early as possible. Early skin-to-skin contact between the mother and infant can prevent hypothermia. Psychologically, it stimulates the mother and baby to get acquainted with each other.

Care of the Mother after Delivery of the Placenta: The placenta should be examined carefully to detect abnormalities such as infarcts, hematomas and abnormal insertion of the umbilical cord, and ensure that it is complete. If there is a suspicion that a part of the placenta is missing, preparations should be made to explore the uterine cavity. If only a part of the membranes is missing, exploration of the uterus is not necessary.

The mother should be observed carefully during the first hour postpartum. It includes the amount of blood loss, uterine fundal height and measuring pulse, blood pressure and temperature. The general well-being of the mother should also be assessed.

References

Allahabadia GN and PR Vaidya. 1992. Why deliver in a supine position? *Aus NZ J Obstet Gynaecol* 32/2:104–106

Arulkumaran S, CH Koh, I Ingemarsson and SS Ratnam. 1987. Augmentation of labour. Mode of delivery related to cervimetric progress. *Aus NZ J Obstet Gynaecol* 27:304–308

Arulkumaran S, LK Penna and K Bhasker Rao eds. 2005. The management of labour. 2nd edn. Chennai: Orient Longman Private Ltd

Cardozo LD, DMF Gibb, JWW Studd, RV Vasanth and DJ Cooper. 1982. Predictive values of cervimetric labour patterns in primigravidae. *Br J Obstet Gynaecol* 9:33–38

Chua S, A Kurup, S Arulkumaran and SS Ratnam. 1990. Augmentation of labour. Does internal tocography result in better obstetric outcome than external tocography? *Obstet Gynecol* 76: 164–167

Commentaries. 1996. Preserving the pelvic floor and perineum during childbirth—elective cesarean section? *Br J Obstet Gynaecol* 103:731–734

Crowley P, DR Elbourne, H Ashhurst, J Garcia, D Murphy and N Duignan. 1991. *Br J Obstet Gynaecol* 98:667–674

Cunningham F, J Kenneth Leveno, SI Bloom, JC Hauth, LC Gilstrap III and KD Wenstrom. 2005. Williams Obstetrics, 22nd ed. McGraw-Hill

Cunningham F, PC MacDonald, KJ Leveno, NF Gant, and LC Gilstrap III, eds. 1993. *Williams Obstetrics*, 19th ed. McGraw-Hill

Curzen P, JS Bekir, DG McLintock, and M Patel. 1984. Reliability of cardiotocography at predicting baby's condition at birth. *Br Med J* 289:1345–1347

Derham RJ and J Crowhurst. 1991. The second stage of labour: durational dilemmas. *Aust NZ J Obstet Gynecol* 31:31–36

Dudley J. 1997. Oxytocin: use and abuse, science and art. *Clin Obstet Gynecol* 40/3:516–524

Flynn AM, J Kelly, G Hollins and PF Lynch. 1978. Ambulation in labour. *Br Med J* 2:591–593

Fraser WD. 1992. Amniotomy and maternal position in labour. *Clin Obstet Gynecol* 35/3:Sep 1992

Friedman EA, KR Niswandee, R Marlene and M Ashworth. 1970. Dysfunctional labour. *Am J Obstet Gynecol* 69:219–226

Goffinet F, W Fraser, S Marcoux, G Breart, JM Moutquint and M Daris. 1997. Early amniotomy increases the frequency of fetal heart rate abnormalities. *Br J Obstet Gynecol* 104:548–553

Goodfellow CF, MG Hull, DF Swab, J Dogterom, RM Buijs. 1983. Oxytocin deficiency at delivery with epidural analgesia. *Br J Obstet Gynecol* 90:214–219

Harbert GM. 1992. Assessment of uterine contractility and activity. *Clin Obstet Gynecol* 35/3: 546–557

Hofmeyr GJ, VC Nikodem, WL Wolman, BE Chalmers and R Kramer. 1991. Companionship to modify the clinical birth environment: effects on progress and perceptions of labour and breast feeding. *Br J Obstet Gynecol* 98:756–764

Hogerzeil HV, GJA Walker, and MJ De Goeje. 1994. Oxytocin more stable in tropical climates. *Br Med J* 308:59

Johnson RA and RS Sidall. 1922. Is the usual method of preparing patients beneficial or necessary? *Am J Obstet Gynecol* 94:425–430

Kantor HI, R Rember, P Tabio and R Buchanon. 1965. Value of shving the pudendal-perineal area in daily preparation. *Obstet Gynecol* 25:509–512

Katz M, E Lunenfeld, L Meizner, N Bashan and J Gross. 1987. The effect of duration of labour on the acid-base state of the fetus. *Br J Obstet Gynecol* 94:425–430

Klaus MH, JH Kennel, SS Robertson and R Sosa. 1986. Effects of social support during parturition o maternal and infant morbidity. *Br Med J* 293:585–587

Lawrence GF, VA Brown, RJ Parsons and ID Cooke. 1982. Feto-maternal consequences of high glucose infusion during labour. *Br J Obstet Gynecol* 89:27–32

Liddell HA and PR Fisher. 1985. The birthing chair in the seond stage of labour. *Aus NZ J Obstet Gynaecol* 25:65–68

Lucas A, AA Teaynsley-Green and SR Bloom. 1980. Iatrogenic hyperinsulinism at birth. *Lancet* 1:144–145

MacDonald D, A Grant, M Sheridan-Pereira, P Boylan and I Chalmers. The Dublin randomized trial of intrapartum fetal heart monitoring. *Am J Obstet Gynecol* 152:524–539

Main DM, EK Main and DH Moore. 2000. The relationship between the maternal age and uterine dysfunction: a continuous effect throughout reproductive life. *Am J Obstet Gynecol* 182:1312–1320

Matthews CD and MR Martin. 1974. Early detection of meconium-stained liquor during laour: a contribution to fetal care. *Am J Obstet Gynecol* 120:808–811

McManus TJ and AA Calder. 1978. Upright posture and the efficiency of labour. *Lancet* 1:72–74

Meis PJ, M hall, JR Marshall and CJ Hobel. 1978. Meconium passage: a new classification for risk assessment during labour. *Am J Obstet Gynecol* 131:509–513

O'Driscoll K, D Meagher and M Robson. 2003. *Active management of labour: Dublin experience*, 4th ed. New York: Mosby

Riethmuller D, L Courtois and R maillet. 2006. Liberal versus restrictive practice of episiotomy: do there exist specific obstetrical indications for episiotomy? *J Gynecol Obstet Biol Reprod* (Paris); 35 1 Suppl): 1S32–1S39

Robinson JO, M Rosen, JM Evans, SI Revill, H David and GAD Rees. 1980. Maternal opinion about analgesia for labour. A controlled trial between epidural block and intramuscular pethidine combined with inhalation. *Anaesthesia* 35:1173–1181

Romney ML and H Gordon. 1981. Is your enema really necessary? *Br Med J* 282:1269–1271

Rutter N, A Spencer, N Mann and M Smith. 1980. Glucose during labour. *Lancet* 2:155

Satin AJ, KJ Leveno, L Sherman and DD McIntire. 1992. Factors affecting the dose response to oxytocin for labor stimulation. *Am J Obstet Gynecol* 166:1260–1261

Seitchik J, EC Alan, MA Holden and RN Maria Castillo. 1985. Amniotomy and the use of oxytocin in labour in nulliparous women. *Am J Obstet Gynecol* 153: 848–854

Sizer AR, J Evans, SM Baily and J Weiner. 2000. A second stage partogram. *Obstet Gynaecol* 96: 678–683

Sleep J and AM Grant. 1987. West Berkshire perineal management trial: three year follow up. *Br Med J* 295:749–751

Stewart P and H Spiby. 1989. A randomized study of the sitting position for delivery using a newly designed obstetric chair. *Br J Obstet Gynaecol* 96:327–333

Thornton JG. 1996. Active management of labour. *Br Med J* 313:378

Thorp JA, DH Hu, RM Albin, J McNitt, BA Meyer, GR Cohen and JD Yeast. 1993. The effect of intrapartum epidural analgesia on nulliparous labor: a randomized controlled prospective trial. *Am J Obstet Gynecol* 169: 851–858

WHO. Care in normal birth. A practical guide. Report of a Technical Working Group. Maternal and newborn health/safe motherhood division of reproductive health.

WHO, Department of Reproductive Health and Research Family and Community Health. 2003. Managing complications in pregnancy and childbirth: a guide for midwives and doctors. Geneva

27

Induction of Labour

Jayaraman Nambiar M

Induction of labour is defined as an intervention designed to artificially initiate uterine contractions and cause progressive dilatation and effacement of the cervix, resulting in the birth of the baby (RCOG 2001). The term is usually restricted to pregnancies that extend beyond the period of viability (24 weeks in the UK). Induction of labour has many therapeutic advantages when the benefits of delivery outweigh the potential risk of continuing the pregnancy. The incidence of induction of labour has been steadily increasing in obstetric practice (Martin et al 2003). The reasons for this increase is unclear. It may be partly be due to a rise in prolonged pregnancies and a trend towards elective induction of labour.

Indications for Induction of Labour

Ideally, labour should begin spontaneously at term. But sometimes, when continuation of pregnancy is dangerous either to the mother or the fetus, pregnancy has to be terminated before spontaneous onset of labour. Of all indications for induction of labour, pregnancy-induced hypertension and post-term pregnancies account for 80% of cases (Sanchez-Ramos 2005). When pregnancy is at term, induction of labour does not pose much of a problem. However, if labour is to be induced preterm, the benefits of induction should clearly outweigh the risk of prematurity.

Prolonged Pregnancy The risk of stillbirth increases steadily as pregnancy extends beyond 40 weeks. The risk of stillbirth is 3 out of every 1000 pregnancies at 42 weeks and 6 out of every 1000 pregnancies after 43 weeks (Hilder et al 1998). A similar increase in neonatal mortality is also reported. Data from one cohort (Hilder et al 1998) revealed that at 40 weeks of gestation, only 58% of women delivered when induced. This rate increased to 74% when induced at 41 weeks and to 82% when induced at 42 weeks (Hilder et al 1998). Hence, a policy of routine induction before 41 weeks would greatly increase the workload. With induction, a reduction in meconium staining of the amniotic fluid was seen when compared to that in conservative management in pregnancies extending beyond 41 weeks (Crowley 2001). Hence, a policy of routine induction at 41 weeks reduces perinatal mortality without increasing the cesarean section rates.

Pregnancy-induced Hypertension This is one of the common indications when the fetal or maternal condition warrants termination of pregnancy.

Diabetic Pregnancies Diabetic pregnancies are associated with higher perinatal mortality rates and increased risk of other complications, such as pregnancy-induced hypertension, necessitating preterm delivery. The guidelines produced by the Royal College of Obstetricians and Gynaecologists recommend induction of well-controlled diabetic pregnancies at term (RCOG 2001).

Premature Rupture of Membranes (PROM) An increased risk of maternal and neonatal infection is associated with the premature rupture of membranes. An active policy of induction of labour in PROM reduced the incidence of infectious morbidity in a study (Tan 2001).

Suspected Fetal Macrosomia It has been postulated that the induction of labour in a fetus suspected to have macrosomia will reduce the need for difficult vaginal delivery and injuries. However, the methods currently used to estimate fetal size in suspected fetal macrosomia are poorly predictive (Johnstone 1997). Only one review compared the efficacy of induction of labour at term in suspected fetal macrosomia (Irion 2001). The numbers in the trial were small but a small reduction in brachial plexus injuries and fractures in the induced group, when compared to the expectant group, were observed. However, no definitive conclusions can be drawn from this review.

Maternal Request Prior to 41 Weeks of Gestation Women may sometimes request for elective induction of labour prior to 41 weeks for an increased feeling of safety and out of a desire to shorten the duration of pregnancy (Out et al 1986). They are more likely to have had problems during their current pregnancy or complications in their past pregnancies. A potential risk of respiratory distress syndrome of prematurity is present on elective induction of labour. The American College of Obstetricians and Gynecologists does not support this practice (ACOG 1999), except when the women live a long distance away from the hospital or for psychosocial reasons. A number of studies have shown a two-to threefold increase in cesarean delivery when labour was induced electively (Maslow and Sweeny 2000; Hoffman and Sciscinone 2003; Smith et al 2003).

History of Precipitate Labour Induction of labour in women with a history of precipitate labour may help to avoid delivery outside the hospital, which is not the preferred place. One cohort study of 4976 women over a period of two years showed that 106 women had precipitate labour. No increase in the incidence of neonatal problems in the precipitate group was seen (Erkkola and Nikkanen 1978). There are no studies linking the place of birth to precipitate labour and the Royal College of Obstetricians and Gynaecologists recommends that 'No conclusions can be drawn from the available evidence in relation to the timing of induction of labour of women with a history of precipitate labour' (RCOG 2001).

Other indications for induction of labour include intrauterine growth restriction, isoimmunisation, maternal medical complications and intrauterine death of the fetus.

Contraindications for Induction of Labour

Absolute contraindications for induction of labour include a major degree of placenta previa, vasa previa, transverse fetal lie, prior classical cesarean delivery and active herpes infection. There are several other clinical situations where induction of labour is not contraindicated but caution has to be exercised. These include breech presentation, suspected cephalopelvic disproportion, maternal cardiac disease, grandmultiparity, previous lower segment cesarean section and polyhydramnios. Some of these situations will be discussed later in this chapter.

Before induction of labour, the fetal maturity should be clearly established. To avoid iatrogenic fetal prematurity, if in doubt, fetal pulmonary maturity should be documented. An ultrasound measurement of fetal crown rump length obtained at 6–12 weeks is a good indicator of fetal gestational age (ACOG 1999).

Methods of Induction of Labour

Prostaglandins PGE_2 (Dinoprostone) is the commonest prostaglandin that is used in induction of labour. Local application of PGE_2 produces direct softening of the cervix by altering the extracellular ground substance of the cervix and by forming a gap junction that is necessary for coordinated uterine contractions during labour (Uldbjerg et al 1981; Rath et al 1987). Thus, prostaglandins have the dual quality of ripening the cervix and inducing uterine contractions. Prostaglandins are available as pessary, gel and sustained release formulations. None of these formulations has any discernable advantage over the others (Kelly et al 2001).

The PGE_2 gel is commonly used in clinical practice. The recommended dose is 0.5 mg intracervically. This can be repeated every 6 hours and the maximum dose should not exceed 3 doses in 24 hours (Sanchez-Ramos 2005). There is no difference in outcome between the use of intracervical and intravaginal prostaglandins (Boulvain et al 2001). The Royal College of Obstetricians and Gynaecologists recommends intravaginal application of PGE_2 gel as a 2 mg preparation in nulliparous women with unfavourable cervix, followed by a second dose 6–8 hours later, with a maximum dose of 4 mg. In multiparous women and those with a favourable cervix, the initial dose of 1 mg is followed by a second dose six hours later, with a maximum dose of 3 mg (RCOG 2001). Intravaginal application is preferred as it causes less discomfort to the patient.

The use of PGE_2 for induction of labour is not without risk. Hyperstimulation can occur with the use of prostaglandins. Uterine hyperstimulation has been defined by the RCOG as uterine tachysystole consisting of more than 5 contractions every 10 minutes or a single contraction lasting for more than 2 minutes (RCOG 2001). Incidence of hyperstimulation with PGE_2 varies from 1% to 5% (Rayburn et al 1992; Witter et al 1992; Witter and Mercer 1996). Uterine hyperstimulation usually begins one hour after PGE_2 application but may occur up to nine hours after as well. Removal of the remaining agent may help to decrease hyperstimulation; however, irrigation is not helpful (RCOG 2001). Subcutaneous terbutaline may help to decrease hyperstimulation. Maternal side effects such as fever, vomiting and diarrhea are rare (Brindley 1988). Manufacturers of PGE_2 recommend exercising caution in patients with glaucoma, severe hepatic or renal dysfunction and asthma. However, PGE_2 by itself does not cause bronchoconstriction (ACOG 1999).

Misoprostol is a methyl ester of PGE_1. It is inexpensive and can be stored at room temperature. It has been widely used although it is not licensed for obstetric use. Misoprostol has been used orally, vaginally and sublingually for induction of labour (Hofmeyer 2003). Though various routes of misoprostol been described, it is commonly used vaginally (Hofmeyr 2001). However, there are concerns regarding the safety profile of misoprostol. Complications include uterine hyperstimulation, meconium-stained liquor, precipitate delivery, rupture of unscarred uterus and postpartum bleeding (Hofmeyr 2003). In a review, Hofmeyr states that 'personal discussion with colleagues has revealed several cases of rupture of an unscarred uterus following misoprostol usage, possibly related to higher dosages than have been used in the trials reviewed. These are usually not reported' (2001). Though vaginal misoprostol is more effective than PGE_2 (RCOG 2001), there are safety concerns regarding their use and larger trials need to be conducted before their widespread use.

Oxytocin This is a commonly used drug in the induction of labour. Traditionally, it was thought that steady rates of oxytocin should be reached within 15–20 minutes of infusion; however, recent studies have shown that it takes approximately 40 minutes for steady plasma rate concentration to be reached (Seitchik et al 1984). The effect of oxytocin on the uterus increases as pregnancy advances (Caldeyro-Barcia 1961). Oxytocin is administered as a dilute solution for induction for labour. It is used either as a low-dose or high-dose regimen. Lower dose regimens use low initial doses of oxytocin at 0.5–2 milliunits/minute and slow increments are made every 15–40 minutes. High dose regimens use a high starting dose of 3–6 milliunits/minute with intervals of increments every 15–40 minutes (ACOG 1999). High-dose regimens, though associated with more chances of vaginal delivery, appear to be linked to increased incidence of uterine hyperstimulation (Crane and Young 1998). Higher doses of oxytocin are also associated with an increase in precipitate labour (RCOG 2001). Oxytocin should not be started for six hours following administration of vaginal prostaglandins. The Royal College of Obstetricians and Gynaecologists recommends a starting dose of 1–2 milliunits/minute. This should be increased at intervals of 30 minutes (RCOG 2001).

Oxytocin should be titrated against uterine contractions aiming for a maximum of 3–4 contractions every 10 minutes. Adequate contractions usually develop with 12 milliunits/minute. The maximum licensed dose of oxytocin is 20 milliunits/minute. However, the RCOG suggests a maximum dose of 32 milliunits/minute (2001). Complications associated with oxytocin include uterine hyperstimulation, uterine rupture and water intoxication. To avoid the risk of uterine rupture, oxytocin has to be carefully used in grand multiparas and in patients with previous cesarean section. To reduce water intoxication, oxytocin should not be given in electrolyte-free solutions. Though an association between neonatal jaundice and oxytocin use has been suggested, recent trials have failed to show any clear link (Sanchez-Ramos 2005).

Mechanical Methods Mechanical methods include extra-amniotic placement of catheter transcervically or the use of hygroscopic cervical dilators. These methods, apart from leading to cervical stretching, may also release prostaglandins. Extra-amniotic placement of catheters may be used with a saline infusion and oxytocin (Culver et al 2004). It has been associated with a slower effect than with prostaglandins, but with less hyperstimulation (Boulvain et al 2001).

Though hygroscopic dilators are more cost effective, their use is associated with infection (Kazzi 1982). The Cochrane review concludes that there is insufficient data for the use of mechanical methods to induce labour (Boulvain et al 2001).

Sweeping of Membranes When performed as a routine policy at 38–40 weeks of gestation, sweeping of membranes, has been shown to reduce the incidence of post-term pregnancies and reduce the incidence of other methods of induction of labour. Sweeping of membranes is not associated with increased incidence of maternal or neonatal infectious morbidity. However, it is linked with discomfort and, sometimes, minimal bleeding. Women should be offered membrane sweeping prior to induction of labour (RCOG 2001).

Amniotomy Amniotomy may be used as a method of induction when the cervix is favourable. Used alone, amniotomy is associated with unpredictable and sometimes long intervals before delivery. However, amniotomy with oxytocin may result in shorter delivery intervals (ACOG 1999). The potential complications of amniotomy include prolapse of umbilical cord, chorioamnionitis and vasa previa.

Other Methods of Induction

There is insufficient data regarding other methods of induction such as relaxin, mifeprostone, estrogen with or without amniotomy, corticosteroids and hyalourinidase. These methods are not commonly used in clinical practice (Kavanagh 2001; Kelly 2001; Neilson 2001; Thomas 2001). When compared with placebo, breast stimulation reduces the rates of women who do not begin labour within 72 hours. Breast stimulation also reduces the incidence of postpartum bleeding. However, when used in high-risk pregnancies, it was associated with a higher perinatal mortality rate. There is no benefit from sexual intercourse for induction of labour (Kavanagh 2001).

Factors Affecting Response to Induction

The success of induction depends on the parity and state of the cervix. The state of the cervix can be evaluated by using the Bishop's score (Bishop 1964) as shown in Table 27.1.

Bishop determined that when the total score was at least 9, the likelihood for vaginal delivery was almost equal to that of spontaneous labour. There is a two-to threefold increase in cesarean section rates when the score is less than 3.

The RCOG uses a modified score developed by Calder (Calder 1974) as a scoring system to determine the success of induction. The Modified Calder system is depicted in Table 27.2. For the purpose of induction, the RCOG defined an unfavourable cervix as one with a modified Bishop's score of less than 6 (RCOG 2001).

Induction of Labour in Women with Unfavourable Cervix

An unfavourable cervix is one with a modified Bishop's score of less than 6. An unfavourable cervix has usually undergone minimal changes and is most resistant to induction. Vaginal PGE_2 is the most effective agent for induction of labour in women with unfavourable cervix (RCOG 2001; Hofmeyr 2003). Though misoprostol is more effective than PGE_2, there are serious safety concerns regarding their use in induction (Hofmeyr and Gulmezoglu 2001). As described earlier, though mechanical methods are associated with less hyperstimulation and fetal heart changes, they are not as effective as PGE_2 in inducing labour in women with unfavourable cervix. There is insufficient information regarding other methods used for the ripening of an unripe cervix.

Induction of Labour in Women with Favourable Cervix

Use of vaginal PGE_2 is associated with higher vaginal delivery rates and increased patient satisfaction than oxytocin in women with favourable cervix. The RCOG recommends PGE_2 as the initial mode of induction of labour, irrespective of cervical ripening (RCOG 2001).

Care of Women during Induction of Labour

Induction should follow only after the full informed consent of the patient. The reasons for and risks of induction should be explained to the patient. Whenever induction of labour is done, facilities for continuous electronic fetal monitoring should be made available. Fetal well-being should be established before induction of labour. When prostaglandins are used for induction, the patient should be made to lie down for 30 minutes after induction, followed by continuous fetal monitoring until fetal well-being is established, when the contractions occur. When oxytocin is used for induction, continuous electronic fetal monitoring should be ensured. If hyperstimulation occurs with prostaglandin, cessation of the drug may be helpful. When hyperstimulation occurs with oxytocin, immediate cessation of oxytocin should be undertaken. In the presence of fetal heart changes due to hyperstimulation, subcutaneous terbutaline at a dose of 0.25 mg should be given to help reduce the hyperstimulation (RCOG 2001).

Induction of Labour in Special Situations

Intrauterine Growth Restriction (IUGR)

Induction of labour in growth-retarded fetuses poses a potential problem of intrauterine asphyxia. Such fetuses are more likely to develop acidemia during labour because of uteroplacental insufficiency, lower metabolic reserves and umbilical cord compression. One study found an increase in the incidence of perinatal mortality of more than five times in IUGR pregnancies (Dobson et al 1981). Close monitoring is required for the IUGR fetus. In severe IUGR, induction of labour should not be undertaken and cesarean section is advised (Weiner 1999).

Previous Cesarean Section A potential risk of scar rupture exists in patients with previous cesarean section when labour is induced. The risk of scar rupture with

Table 27.1: Bishop's score

Cervical Feature	*0*	*1*	*2*	*3*
Dilatation cm	0	1–2	3–4	5–6
Effacement (%)	0–30	40–60	60–70	80+
Station*	–3	–2	–1/0	+1/+2
Consistency	Firm	Medium	Soft	
Position	Posterior	Mid-position	Anterior	

**Station is measured in cm relative to the ischial spines*

Table 27.2: Modified Bishop's scoring system (Calder score)

Cervical Feature	*0*	*1*	*2*	*3*
Dilatation (cm)	<1	1–2	2–4	>4
Length of cervix (cm)	>4	2–4	1–2	<1
Station*	–3	–2	–1/0	+1/+2
Consistency	Firm	Average	Soft	
Position	Posterior	Mid/Anterior		

**Station is measured in cm relative to the spines*

prostaglandins is 0.2–1.1%. The rate of vaginal delivery though remained the same as that of spontaneous labour in previous cesarean section, that is, 75% (Vause 1999). The risk of potential scar rupture will thus have to be considered before taking the patient for an elective cesarean section. The Committee on Obstetric Practice of the ACOG has concluded that the risk of uterine rupture is substantially increased following the use of vaginal prostaglandins, and their use for this purpose should be discouraged (ACOG 2002). Use of oxytocin is associated with a lesser risk of rupture than prostaglandins (SOGC 2005).

Induction of Labour in Women of High Parity This is associated with higher incidence of precipitate labour, uterine rupture and postpartum bleeding. Hence, induction of labour in higher parity has to be done carefully.

Practice Points

- Whenever the decision is made to induce labour, the benefits of induction should be clearly weighed against the risks.
- Fetal maturity should be established before induction.
- The success of induction primarily depends on the cervical score. PGE_2 should be the initial choice of induction irrespective of the cervical status of the patient.
- Though misoprostol is more effective than PGE_2 in induction of labour, there are serious safety concerns regarding their use.
- No added advantage of mechanical ripening of the cervix is seen in an unfavourable cervix.
- Caution should be exercised when inducing labour in special situations such as previous cesarean section, IUGR and grandmultiparity.

References

American College of Obstetricians and Gynecologists Committee Opinion. 2002. Induction of labour for vaginal birth after cesarean delivery. *Obstet and Gynaecol* 99:679 2001:680.

American College of Obstetricians and Gynecologists. 1999. Induction of labour. *Practice Bulletin* No.10.

Bishop EH. 1964. Pelvic scoring system for elective induction of labour. *Obstet Gynecol* 24:264–268.

Boulvain M, AJ Kelly, C Stan and O Irion. 2001. Intracervical prostaglandins for induction of labour. *Cochrane Database Syst Rev*, Issue 3.

Boulvain M, AJ Kelly, C Stan and O Irion. 2001. Mechanical methods for induction of labour. *Cochrane Database Syst Rev*, Issue 3.

Brindley BA and RJ Sokol. 1988. Induction and management of labour: basis and methods in current practice. *Obstet Gynecol Sur* 43:730–743.

Calder AA and MP Embrey. 1974. Extramniotic prostaglandin for induction of labour at term. *J Br Obstet Gynaecol Commonwealth* 81:39–46.

Caldeyro-Barcia R and JA Sereno. 1961. The response of the human uterus to oxytocin throughout pregnancy. In *Oxytocin*, ed R Caldeyro-Barcia and H Heller.

Crane JM and DC Young. 1998. Meta-analysis of low dose versus high dose oxytocin for labour induction. *J Soc Gynaecol Can* 20:1215–1223.

Crowley P. 2001. Interventions for preventing or improving the outcome of delivery at or beyond term. *Cochrane Database Syst Rev*, Issue 2.

Culver J, RA Strauss, S Brody, PC Dobson, DA Abell and NA Beischer. 1981. Mortality and morbidity of fetal growth retardation. *Aust N Z J Obstet Gynaecol* 21:69–72.

Dobson PC, DA Abell and NA Beischer. 1981. Mortality and morbidity of fetal growth retardation. *Aust N Z J Obstet Gynaecol* 21(2):69–72

Erkkola R and V Nikkanen. 1978. Precipitate labour. *Ann Chir Gynaecol* 67:150–153.

Hilder L, K Costeloe and B Thilaganathan. 1998. Prolonged pregnancy: Evaluating gestation-specific risks for fetal and infant mortality. *Br J Obstet Gynaecol* 105:169–173.

Hoffman MK and AC Sciscinone. 2003. Elective induction with cervical ripening increases the risk of cesarean delivery in multiparous women. *Obstet Gynaecol* 101:7S.

Hofmeyer JG. 2003. Induction of labour with unfavourable cervix. In *Best Practice & Research in Clinical Obstetrics & Gynaecology*, ed D Young and TF Baskett, No 17:5:777–794. Amsterdam: Elsevier.

Hofmeyr GJ and AM Gulmezoglu. 2001. Vaginal misoprostol for induction of labour. *Cochrane Database Syst Rev*, Issue 2.

Irion O and M Boulvain. 2001. Induction of labour for suspected fetal macrosomia. *Cochrane Database Syst Rev*, Issue 2.

Johnstone FD. 1997. Prediction of macrosomia in diabetic pregnancy. *Contemp Rev Obstet Gynaecol* 9:113–120.

Kavanagh J, AJ Kelly and J Thomas. 2001. Breast stimulation for induction of labour. *Cochrane Review*, Issue 4. Oxford Cochrane Library: Update Software.

Kavanagh J, AJ Kelly and J Thomas. 2001. Hyaluronidase for induction of labour. *Cochrane Database Syst Rev*, Issue 2.

Kavanagh J, AJ Kelly and J Thomas. 2001. Sexual intercourse for induction of labour. *Cochrane Database Syst Rev*, Issue 2.

Kazzi GM, SF Bottoms and MG Rosen. 1982. Efficacy and safety of Laminaria digitata for preinduction ripening of cervix. *Obstet Gynecol* 60:440–443.

Kelly AJ, J Kavanagh and J Thomas. 2001, Relaxin for induction of labour. *Cochrane Database Syst Rev* Issue 2.

Kelly AJ, J Kavanagh and J Thomas. 2001.Vaginal prostaglandin (PGE2 and PGF2a) for induction of labour at term. *Cochrane Database Syst Rev*, Issue 2.

Martin JA, BE Hamilton, PD Sutton, SJ Ventura, F Menacker and ML Munson. 2003. Births: Final data for 2002. *National Vital Statistics Reports*. Maryland: National Centre for Health Statistics, 52:10.

Maslow AS and AL Sweeney. 2000. Elective induction of labour as a risk factor for cesarean delivery among low risk women at term. *Obstet Gynecol* 95:917.

Neilson JP. 2001. Mifepristone for induction of labour. *Cochrane Database Syst Rev*, Issue 2.

Out JJ, ME Vierhout, F Verhage, HJ Duivenvoorden and HC Wallenburg. 1986. Characteristics and motives of women choosing elective induction of labour. *J Psychosom Res* 30:375–380.

Rath W, BC Adelmann-Grill, U Pieper and W Kuhn. 1987. The role of collagenases and proteases in prostaglandin induced cervical ripening. *Prostaglandins* 34:119–127.

Rayburn WF, RJ Wapner, VA Bass, E Spitberg, RD Molina, N Mandsageer and ML Yonekura. 1992. An intravginal controlled release prostaglandin E2 pessary for cervical ripening and intiation of labour at term. *Obstet Gynaecol* 79:374–379.

Royal College of Obstetricians and Gynaecologists (RCOG). 2001. Evidence-based Clinical Guideline Number: 9; London: *Royal College of Obstetricians and Gynaecologists*,

Sanchez-Ramos L. 2005. Induction of labour. In *Obstet Gynecol Clin N Am* 32:181–200.

Seitchik J, J Amico, AG Robinson and M Castillo. 1984. Oxytocin augmentation for dysfunctional labour. IV. Oxytocin pharmacokinetics. *Am J Obstet Gynecol* 150:225–228.

Smith KM, MK Hoffman and A Sciscone. 2003. Elective induction of labour in nulliparous women increases the risk of cesarean delivery. *Obstet Gynecol* 101:45S.

SOGC Clinical practice guidelines. 2005. Guidelines for vaginal birth after previous caesarean birth. *Int J Gynaecol Obstet* 89(3):319–321.

Tan BP and ME Hannah. 2001. Oxytocin for prelabour rupture of membranes at or near term. *Cochrane Database Syst Rev*, Issue 2.

Thomas J, AJ Kelly and J Kavanagh. 2001.Oestrogens with or without amniotomy for induction of labour. *Cochrane Database Syst Rev*, Issue 3.

Uldbjerg N, G Ekman, A Malmstrom, B Sporrong, U Ulmsten and L Wingerup. 1981. Biochemical and morphologicl changes of human cervix after local application of PGE_2 in pregnancy. *Lancet* 1:267–268.

Vause S and M Macintosh. 1999. Evidence based case report: Use of prostaglandins to induce labour in women with a caesarean section scar. *Br Med J* 318:1056–8.

Weiner CP and AA Baschat. 1999. Fetal growth restriction: evaluation and management. In *High risk pregnancy management option*, ed DK James, PJ Sheer, P Weiner and B Gonik. London: WB Saunders. New York: Pentagon Press.

Witter FR and BM Mercer. 1996. Improved intravaginal controlled release prostaglandin E2 insert for cervical ripening at term. The Prostaglandin E2 study group. *J Matern Fetal Med* 5:64–69.

Witter FR, LE Rocco and TR Johnson. 1992. A randomized trial of prostaglandin E2 in a controlled release vaginal pessary for cervical ripeing at term. *Am J Obstet Gyecol* 166:830–834.

28

Intrapartum Assessment of Fetal Health

Gowri Ramanathan | Sabaratnam Arulkumaran

Introduction

Labour causes stress not only for the mother but also for the fetus. During labour, uterine contractions lead to a temporary reduction of blood flow through the placental bed, resulting in decreased gas exchange and fetal oxygenation. These contractions may also cause umbilical cord compression, which could interrupt fetal oxygenation. When the uterus relaxes in between contractions, oxygenation is restored to the fetus and the fetus is able to self-resuscitate, provided there is sufficient metabolic reserve.

There are two situations that place the fetus at particular risk during labour. First, fetuses with limited reserves, that is, growth-restricted fetuses, may not be able to withstand and compensate intermittent decreases in oxygenation, which, if progressive, may lead to hypoxia. Second, even fetuses considered as being at low risk and which have normal reserves may develop hypoxia more acutely as a consequence of uterine hyperstimulation, placental abruption or cord compression. As no fetus can be categorised as being at no risk during labour, it is important to detect development of fetal hypoxia early when the process is still completely reversible, allowing timely intervention to prevent subsequent hypoxic acidemia and neurological injury.

This chapter discusses the current methods of intrapartum fetal assessment of intermittent auscultation, electronic fetal monitoring (EFM) and additional tests that complement EFM, such as stimulation tests and fetal blood sampling. The newer technological advances, fetal electrocardiogram (ECG) waveform analysis, fetal oxygen saturation monitoring, fetalscalplactatemeasurementandnear-infrared spectroscopy are also described. Significant intrapartum fetal asphyxia occurs rarely and epidemiological data suggests that only 10% cases of cerebral palsy result potentially from intrapartum causes (Nelson 1988). However, the consequences are so serious that adequate knowledge and understanding of intrapartum fetal surveillance is vital for anyone caring for women in labour.

Intermittent Auscultation

Auscultation of the fetal heart during active labour is considered as standard care universally. There remains no good evidence for fetal heart rate assessment in the latent phase of labour; however, in the event of any change in clinical condition, for example, bleeding or rupture of membranes, regular fetal heart rate assessment becomes necessary.

The National Institute of Clinical Excellence (NICE) recommends that intermittent auscultation should be offered and recommended during labour to monitor fetal well-being in healthy women with an otherwise uncomplicated pregnancy (RCOG 2001; NICE 2001). This should be performed using either a fetal stethoscope (Pinard's) or a hand-held Doppler ultrasound device for a minimum of 60 seconds after a contraction, every 15 minutes in the first stage of labour and every five minutes in the second stage of labour. The reason for auscultating after a contraction is to detect late, atypical, variable or prolonged decelerations. If during auscultation, a change in baseline fetal heart rate (FHR) is seen or if it is less than 110 bpm or greater than 160 bpm, any evidence of decelerations is observed or if any intrapartum risk factors develop (for example, meconium- or blood-stained liquor), then continuous EFM should be offered and recommended.

Despite current recommendations, maternal preference and priorities must always be considered. The aim would be to strike a balance between maximising the detection of potentially compromised babies and minimising the number of unnecessary maternal interventions. Further, as labour is a dynamic and ever-changing situation, a low-risk pregnancy antenatally or even early in labour may evolve to become a high-risk one, necessitating closer fetal assessment.

Electronic Fetal Monitoring (EFM)

Although EFM has gained widespread use in clinical practice as a means of assessing fetal well-being during labour. Over the past few decades its value has been challenged. The predictive value of EFM for adverse outcome has been shown to be low, although it has a high negative predictive value—that is to say, that while a normal EFM trace usually indicates reassuring fetal status, a non-reassuring or abnormal trace does not necessarily imply 'fetal distress' (Umstad 1993). Moreover, marked inter-observer variation in EFM interpretation has been noted (Nielsen et al 1987), with an inappropriately high operative delivery rate for non-reassuring fetal status in many units.

A meta-analysis comparing EFM during labour with intermittent auscultation, found that the use of EFM increases the odds of having a cesarean section when compared to the use of intermittent auscultation of the fetal heart (OR 1.41, 95% CI 1.23–1.61). The use of EFM, however, was associated with a reduction in neonatal seizures when compared to the use of intermittent auscultation (RR 0.51, 95% CI 0.32–0.82) (Thacker et al 2004).

The value of an admission EFM trace in a low-risk population has also been evaluated, with early research suggesting that only 0.9% of those with a reactive test had intrauterine asphyxia in labour compared to half of those with ominous traces (Ingemarsson et al 1986). A subsequent randomised controlled trial of admission EFM versus Doppler auscultation in a population of 3751 women, with no pre-identified risk factors, showed no significant difference in metabolic acidosis or any other measure of neonatal outcome (Mires et al 2001). NICE has not recommended the use of admission EFM in low-risk pregnancies (NICE 2001).

Although EFM has not been shown to improve fetal or neonatal outcome directly, a number of antenatal and intrapartum risk factors associated with the development of neonatal encephalopathy, cerebral palsy and even perinatal death have been identified. Hence, it is recommended that continuous EFM should be offered and recommended for these high-risk pregnancies (NICE 2001; RCOG 2001). Table 28.1 describes the maternal and fetal conditions that are generally used to identify high-risk situations (Steer et al 1999).

Cardiotocograph (CTG)

EFM is the recording of the FHR obtained in a continuous manner, either transabdominally, using an ultrasound transducer, or transvaginally, using a fetal scalp electrode. The FHR is recorded together with the uterine contractions, which is displayed on a cardiotocograph (CTG). To interpret the CTG, it is important to define what is normal, by considering the four features listed below.

Baseline FHR The mean level of FHR is determined over a period of 5 or 10 minutes after excluding any accelerations or decelerations. This varies with gestation, and each fetus has an individual baseline rate. The normal range for a term fetus lies between 110 bpm and 160 bpm. In the absence of infection, an uncomplicated baseline of 110–119 bpm or 161–179 bpm is probably not associated with adverse neonatal outcome if the baseline variability is normal and accelerations are present. The presence of other non-reassuring FHR features or a rise in baseline warrants further investigation.

Baseline Variability Minor fluctuations in baseline FHR are a reflection of the integrity and influence of the autonomic nervous system on the heart rate, with the ascending limb due to sympathetic activity and descending limb due to parasympathetic activity. The normal baseline variability is between 5 bpm and 25 bpm. A period of 40–90 minutes of reduced variability may be due to the fetal sleep state. Drugs acting on the central nervous system, hypoxia, brain hemorrhage, infection and chromosomal or congenital abnormality of the brain or heart may give rise to prolonged periods of reduced baseline variability.

Accelerations Accelerations are transient increases in FHR of over 15 bpm, lasting 15 seconds or more, and are usually associated with fetal movements. They may indicate the integrity of the somatic nervous system. The

Table 28.1: Maternal and fetal conditions associated with increased risk of adverse fetal outcome (Steer et al 1999)

Maternal Conditions	*Fetal Conditions*
Hypertension/pre-eclampsia	Intrauterine growth restriction
Diabetes	Post-term pregnancy
Antepartum hemorrhage	Prematurity
Maternal medical disease	Oligohydramnios/meconium-stained liquor
Previous cesarean section	Abnormal fetal Dopplers
Prolonged membrane rupture	Isoimmunisation
Induced/augmented labour	Multiple pregnancy
Epidural analgesia	Breech presentation
	Intrauterine infection

presence of more than two accelerations in a 15-minute trace is an indicator of good perinatal outcome (Krebs et al 1982). The significance of no accelerations on an otherwise normal FHR trace is, however, unclear and may be due to factors such as fetal sleep, medication, infection, brain hemorrhage and cardiac or neurological problems.

Decelerations Transient episodes of slowing of FHR below the baseline level of more than 15 bpm and lasting 15 seconds or more are termed decelerations. The duration and timing of these decelerations, in relation to contractions, forms the basis of categorisation and prognostic significance is described below.

- *Early decelerations:* Repetitive gradual slowing and recovery of FHR that corresponds with contractions is reflective of head compression and is caused by vagal stimulation. The nadir of deceleration is at the peak of the contraction. Early deceleration is only seen in the late first or second stage of labour and is not due to hypoxia.
- *Late decelerations:* Repetitive slowing of FHR, with onset from the middle to the end of the contraction with the nadir more than 20 seconds after the peak of the contraction is called a late deceleration. These are caused by reduced uteroplacental perfusion, which affects fetal oxygenation.
- *Variable decelerations:* These are intermittent periodic slowing down, rapid drop and recovery of FHR that varies in shape, size and timing in relation to contractions. These may be due to head or cord compression. 'Shouldering' (small increase in baseline FHR just before and after the deceleration) is characteristic of cord compression.
- *Atypical variable decelerations:* These are variable decelerations with any of the following additional decelerations components
  - o Loss of primary or secondary rise in baseline rate
  - o Slow return to baseline FHR after the end of the contraction
  - o Prolonged secondary rise in baseline rate
  - o Biphasic deceleration—variable followed by late decelerations
  - o Loss of variability during deceleration
  - o Continuation of baseline rate at lower level
  - o Deceleration that has a depth of >60 beats and duration of >60 seconds

  Atypical variable decelerations may result from a combination of cord compression and reduced uteroplacental perfusion.
- *Prolonged deceleration:* This is a fall in FHR to levels below the baseline that lasts 90 seconds. These decelerations are suspicious if they are <3 minutes in duration and are pathological if they last longer than 3 minutes.

In describing the FHR pattern, it is not only important to document the four features of baseline variability and presence of accelerations and decelerations, but also the interpretation of it as being either a reassuring or a non-reassuring FHR trace. Tables 28.2 and 28.3 provide a framework of CTG categorisation based on individual features of the FHR trace (NICE 2001; RCOG 2001).

The action to be taken once the trace has been categorised as suspicious or pathological depends on the stage of labour (cervical dilatation, rate of progress thus far in labour), associated risk factors and parity. Remedial actions may include continued observation, hydration, stopping oxytocin, repositioning the mother, tocolysis, fetal scalp blood sampling for pH or delivery.

Important Considerations with CTG

Fetal 'cycling' behaviour

A non-hypoxic, neurologically normal fetus will show periods of quiet sleep, seen as reduced baseline variability and perhaps occasional shallow decelerations reflecting fetal breathing. This can last 15–40 minutes and sometimes more than 90 minutes. In fact, on the contrary, the absence of 'cycling' indicates that some insult or injury may have occurred to the fetus, or that the fetus is hypoxic. Drugs, infection, cerebral hemorrhage, chromosomal or congenital abnormalities or previous brain damage should be considered in a fetus that does not exhibit 'cycling' behaviour.

Sinusoidal pattern A trace that resembles a sine wave with no other features of baseline variability, accelerations or decelerations, is seen in fetal anemia. However, it could be due to thumbsucking in a healthy fetus, in which case this pattern does not last for >90 minutes. Causes of fetal anemia such as rhesus isoimmunisation, hemoglobinopathies, fetal infection including parvovirus and feto-maternal hemorrhage should be considered.

Meconium-stained liquor The presence of meconium is an indication for continuous EFM as acidosis develops faster in the presence of meconium when the FHR is abnormal (Steer 1985). Moreover, the chances of developing an abnormal FHR pattern and acidosis are greater in the presence of thick meconium than with thin meconium-stained liquor (Arulkumaran et al 1985).

Additional Assessments of Fetal Health

About 15% of CTG recordings performed in labour are non-reassuring (RCOG 2001). Additional measures to assess fetal well-being have hence emerged, not to replace CTG but for complementary use, in an attempt to reduce unnecessary operative intervention.

Scalp Stimulation

Intrapartum FHR responses to various scalp stimulations (fetal scalp puncture, Allis clamp

Table 28.2: Classification of the individual features of the FHR trace (NICE 2001; RCOG 2001)

Feature	Baseline (bpm)	Variability (bpm)	Decelerations	Accelerations
Reassuring	110–160	≥5	None	Present
Non-reassuring	100–109 161–180	<5 for ≥40 but <90 minutes	Early deceleration Variable decelerations Single prolonged deceleration up to 3 minutes	
Abnormal	<100 >180 Sinusoidal pattern ≥10 minutes	<5 for ≥90 minutes	Atypical variable decelerations Late decelerations Single prolonged deceleration >3 minutes	The absence of accelerations with an otherwise normal CTG is of uncertain significance

Table 28.3: Classification of the CTG based on the features of the FHR trace (NICE 2001; RCOG 2001)

Category	*Definition*
Normal	A CTG whose features fall into the reassuring category.
Suspicious	A CTG whose features fall into one of the non-reassuring categories while the remainder are reassuring
Pathological	A CTG whose features fall into two or more non-reassuring categories or one or more abnormal categories.

scalp stimulation and digital scalp stimulation) and their correlation with scalp pH has been studied with promising results (Clark et al 1984). The response by an acceleration of the FHR was uniformly associated with a scalp blood pH of greater than 7.20. A meta-analysis on the performance of stimulation tests in the prediction of intrapartum fetal acidemia concluded that the likelihood ratio and 95% CIs for the prediction of fetal acidemia, given a positive test (lack of acceleration) with fetal scalp puncture, was 8.54 (CI 1.28–56.96), Allis clamp scalp stimulation was 10.4 (CI 1.47–73.61) and digital scalp stimulation was 15.68 (CI 3.22–76.24). For a negative test (presence of accelerations), the chance of acidosis with fetal scalp puncture was 0.12 (CI 0.02–0.78), with Allis clamp scalp stimulation 0.10 (CI 0.01–0.68) and with digital scalp stimulation 0.06 (CI 0.01–0.31).

Intrapartum stimulation tests are used to rule out fetal acidemia in the setting of a non-reassuring FHR pattern; however, careful continued monitoring with repeat testing during the course of labour should be performed as long as suspicious FHR patterns persist, and fetal scalp pH should be determined, whenever possible, after a positive stimulation test (lack of acceleration) (Skupski et al 2002). Further, although a reactive response is consistent with a reasonable likelihood of fetal well-being, the absence of this response does not indicate fetal compromise.

Vibroacoustic Stimulation Fetal vibroacoustic stimulation is a non-invasive, inexpensive technique that uses a device such as an artificial larynx (Smith et al 1990) or a commercially available acoustic stimulator (Umstad et al 1992), placed over the region of the fetal head on the maternal abdomen. The sound produced causes a startle reflex in the fetus with subsequent fetal heart rate acceleration (Spencer et al 1991)—an indirect evaluation of the fetal central nervous system. Safety concerns have been raised about this method of stimulation, with the risk of hearing impairment considered from a number of angles, including its plausibility given the decibel level changes in utero from the stimulus (Arulkumaran et al 1992). Long-term follow-up of infants exposed to vibroacoustic stimulation antenatally has shown no evidence of auditory impairment based on brain stem-evoked responses at two days of age (Ohel et al 1987), and lack of hearing impairment or neurological damage at 18 months, three years (Ratcliffe et al 2000) and four years of age (Arulkumaran et al 1991; Nyman et al 1992).

A systematic review of observational studies, where vibroacoustic stimulation was followed by fetal scalp pH estimation, reported likelihood ratios and 95% CIs for a positive test result (where no FHR acceleration following stimulus predicted the presence of fetal acidemia) of 5.06 (CI 2.69–9.50) and a negative test result (where FHR acceleration predicted no acidemia) of 0.32 (CI 0.19–0.55) (Skupski et al 2002). There are no randomised controlled trials that address the safety and efficacy of vibroacoustic stimulation in the assessment of fetal well-being in labour in the presence of a non-reassuring CTG trace; hence, there is insufficient evidence to base any recommendations for its routine use.

Fetal Scalp Blood Sampling (FBS)

Certain clinical situations such as placental abruption, scar rupture and cord prolapse, as well as certain CTG patterns such as a preterminal trace or prolonged unremitting fetal bradycardia, would warrant immediate delivery. However, in cases where CTG is of concern and immediate delivery is not clearly indicated, FBS should be undertaken. All pH interpretations should take into account the initial pH measurement, rate of progress of labour as well as the clinical, maternal and fetal condition.

The following actions are recommended based on the FBS result obtained (RCOG, 2001):

- pH >7.25: Reassuring. Repeat FBS if FHR abnormality persists.
- pH 7.20–7.25: Pre-acidosis. Repeat FBS within 30 minutes or consider delivery if rapid fall since last sample.
- pH <7.20: Acidosis. Immediate delivery indicated.

Analysis of FBS and pH helps to identify fetuses at risk of acidemia and has been shown to reduce the incidence of cesarean sections when used in conjunction with EFM (Thacker et al 2002). There are, however, limitations to FBS. It is invasive for both the mother and fetus, technically challenging, requires dilatation of the cervix, rupture of membranes and access to the presenting part; it is also expensive and requires a significant amount of blood. Maternal viral infections, including HIV, hepatitis and herpes simplex virus, are conditions that are associated with an increased transmission risk to the baby with the use of FBS (FIGO 1995), and is hence contraindicated. Fetal bleeding disorders such as hemophilia A are also contraindications to the use of FBS (Kadir et al 1997).

Fetal ECG Waveform Analysis

The ST analysis (STAN) or ST waveform of the fetal ECG provides continuous information about the ability of the fetal heart muscle to respond to the stress of labour (Rosén et al 2004). Like the adult ECG, fetal ECG displays P, QRS and T waves corresponding to electrical events in the heart during each heart beat. An elevation of the ST segment and T wave, quantified by the ratio between the T wave and the QRS amplitudes (T/QRS ratio), identifies the fetal heart muscle responding to hypoxia by a surge of stress hormones (catecholamines) that leads to utilisation of glycogen stored in the heart. An ST segment depression may indicate a situation where the heart is not fully capable of responding. It is important to recognise that some fetuses may not display ST changes, either because monitoring has started after ST changes have taken place or because the fetus does not display identifiable ST changes for unknown reasons. Under these circumstances, a CTG trace showing lack of variability or reactivity (preterminal pattern) will identify an adverse situation.

A Cochrane review that included three trials concluded that the use of ST waveform analysis was associated with fewer babies with severe metabolic acidosis at birth—cord pH

<7.05 and base deficit >12 mmol/l, RR 0.44, 95% CI 0.26–0.75 (Neilson 2004). This was achieved along with fewer fetal scalp samples during labour (RR 0.86, 95% CI 0.76–0.98) and fewer operative deliveries (RR 0.89, 95% CI 0.82–0.97). A recent multicentre observational study evaluated the relationships between scalp pH and CTG plus ST waveform analysis of the fetal ECG (STAN). It concluded that CTG plus ST analysis provides accurate information about intrapartum hypoxia similar to that obtained by scalp pH (Luttkus et al 2004). These findings support the use of fetal ST waveform analysis when the decision has been made for continuous EFM in labour.

Fetal Oxygen Saturation Monitoring (Fetal Pulse Oximetry)

Fetal pulse oximetry has emerged as an adjunct to a non-reassuring CTG by measuring fetal arterial oxygen saturation (SpO2). It directly measures the proportion of hemoglobin that carries oxygen, using an established, safe, non-invasive and widely-used technology found in intensive care facilities and operating theatres. A variety of fetal pulse oximetry sensors have been studied—attached to the top of the fetal head by suction (Arikan et al 2000), lying against the fetal temple or cheek (Mallinckrodt 2000; Nellcor 2004) or lying along the fetal back (OB Scientific 2002). Fetal pulse oximetry values are recorded for approximately 81% of the monitoring time (East et al 1997). Results from animal and human research suggest that when using sensors calibrated for the fetal environment, fetal oximetry values, greater than or equal to 30%, are rarely associated with fetal metabolic acidosis, even when the CTG is non-reassuring, while values less than 30% warrant consideration of interventions (Kuhnert et al 1998; Seelbach-Gobel et al 1999). Its feasibility, acceptability and usefulness have also been evaluated in busy labour ward settings (Chua et al 1999). Fetal pulse oximetry is not without its limitations. The fetal oximetry sensor may only be applied following rupture of the amniotic membranes, and at minimum 2 cm cervical dilatation.

The results of a multicentre trial, comparing conventional CTG monitoring with the addition of fetal pulse oximetry with CTG, reported no difference in the overall cesarean section rate, although the fetal pulse oximetry group had less cesarean sections performed for non-reassuring fetal status (RR 0.45, 95% CI 0.28–0.72) (Garite et al 2000). The results of recent fetal oximetry trials show no benefit in using pulse oximetry and it is doubtful whether it will be of value in clinical practice.

Fetal Scalp Lactate Measurement

The rationale of measuring fetal scalp lactate is that in hypoxia, the shift to the anerobic pathway leads to an increase in lactate production in the fetus, and the build-up of lactate appears to be related to hypoxia lasting over 10 minutes. A level of greater than 4.8 mmol/l is considered abnormal (Kruger et al 1999). Lactate measurements have been evaluated in intrapartum fetal surveillance for about 30 years; however, despite requiring less blood for analysis, fewer scalp incisions and being quicker and more likely to be successful than FBS, it was not until reliable, hand-held, microvolume devices appeared in the 1990s that it became a clinical option.

Retrospective data suggests that lactate determinations in fetal scalp blood are better than pH for predicting severe neonatal morbidity. A randomised controlled trial comparing these two measurements found lactate to be more favourable in clinical practice, in terms of less sampling failure and reduced time from the decision to do a fetal scalp blood sample to the clinician receiving the result (Westgren et al 1998). At present, a large, multicentre randomised control trial is in progress in Sweden to compare lactate and pH measurement for the clinical management of suspected fetal compromise, with the main end-points being metabolic acidemia and cord arterial blood pH at delivery of less than 7.00. Results are likely to be available in two years.

Near-infrared Spectroscopy (NIRS)

NIRS is a non-invasive optical technique aimed at directly measuring cerebral oxygenation (O'Brien et al 1993; Peebles 1997) by assessing the different absorption characteristics of oxygenated and reduced hemoglobin molecules. A device containing fibreoptic bundles in a silicone rubber moulding is placed against the side of the fetal head (Peebles et al 1992), and NIR light (750–1000 nm wavelength) is transmitted through the fetal scalp, skull and brain with the absorption calculated by measuring the reflected light (O'Brien et al 1993). Although preliminary NIRS studies have demonstrated a significant positive correlation between intrapartum mean fetal cerebral oxygen saturation and umbilical artery and vein pH at birth (Aldrich et al 1994), its use remains experimental until further technological improvements are made and tested by randomised controlled trials.

Conclusion The key to intrapartum fetal monitoring is to detect developing fetal hypoxia early in labour when the process is still completely reversible, with timely intervention preventing subsequent fetal decompensation. As no gold standard test is currently available, most units use EFM combined with a second variable to improve its specificity—most often, the pH of fetal scalp blood. With newer assessment tools becoming available and able to provide promising results, these tools will most likely gain widespread use in the near future.

References

Aldrich CJ, D D'Antona, JS Wyatt et al. 1994. Fetal cerebral oxygenation measured by near-infrared spectroscopy shortly before birth and acid-base status at birth. *Obstet & Gynecol* 84:861–866.

Arikan GM, HS Scholz, MCH Haeusler et al. 2000. Low fetal oxygen saturation at birth and acidosis. *Obstet Gynecol* 95:565–571.

Arulkumaran S, B Skurr, H Tong et al. 1991. No evidence of hearing loss due to fetal acoustic stimulation test. *Obstet Gynecol* 78:283–285.

Arulkumaran S, D Talbert, TS Hsu et al. 1992. In-utero sound levels when vibroacoustic stimulation is applied to the maternal abdomen: an assessment of the possibility of cochlea damage in the fetus. *Br J Obstet Gynaecol* 99:43–45.

Arulkumaran S, SC Yeoh, DMF Gibb et al. 1985. Obstetric outcome of meconium stained liquor in labour. *Sing Med J* 26:523–526.

Chua S, J Yam, K Razvi et al. 1999. Intrapartum fetal oxygen saturation monitoring in a busy labour ward. *Eur J Obstet Gynecol Reprod Biol* 82:185–189.

Clark SL, ML Gimovsky and FC Miller. 1984. The scalp stimulation test: a clinical alternative to fetal scalp blood sampling. *Am J Obstet Gynecol* 148:274–277.

East CE, KR Dunster, PB Colditz et al. 1997. Fetal oxygen saturation monitoring in labour: an analysis of 118 cases. *Aust N Z J Obstet Gynaecol* 37:397–401.

FIGO Study Group on the Assessment of New Technology. 1995. Intrapartum surveillance: recommendations on current practice and overview of new developments. International Federation of Gynecology and Obstetrics. *Int J Gynaecol Obstet* 49:213–221.

Garite TJ, GA Dildy, H McNamara et al. 2000. A multicenter controlled trial of fetal pulse oximetry in the intrapartum managment of nonreassuring fetal heart rate patterns. *Am J Obstet Gynecol* 183: 1049–1058.

Ingemarsson I, S Arulkumaran, E Ingemarsson et al. 1986. Admission test: a screening test for fetal distress in labor. *Obstet Gynecol* 68:800–806.

Kadir R, D Economides, J Braithwaite et al. 1997. The obstetric experience of carriers of haemophilia. *Br J Obstet Gynaecol* 104:803–810.

Krebs HB, RE Petres, LJ Dunn et al. 1982. Intrapartum fetal heart rate monitoring. VI. Prognostic significance of accelerations. *Am J Obstet Gynecol* 142; 297–305.

Kruger K, B Hallberg, M Blennow et al. 1999. Predictive value of fetal scalp blood lactate concentration and pH as markers of neurological disability. *Am J Obstet Gynecol* 5:1072–1078.

Kuhnert M, B Seelbach-Goebel, GC Di Renzo et al. 1998. Guidelines for the use of fetal pulse oximetry during labour and delivery. *Prenatal and Neonatal Medicine* 3:432–433.

Luttkus AK, H Noren, JH Stupin et al. 2004. Fetal scalp pH and ST analysis of the fetal ECG as an adjunct to CTG. A multi-center, observational study. *J Perinat Med* 32:486–494.

Mallinckrodt Inc. OxiFirst (TM) Fetal Oxygen Saturation Monitoring System. Operator's Manual. N-400 Fetal Pulse Oximeter. 2000. *Mallinckrodt Inc*, Pleasanton, CA USA.

Mires G, F Williams and P Howie. 2001. Randomised controlled trial of cardiotocography versus Doppler auscultation of fetal heart at admission in labour in low risk obstetric population. *BMJ* 322:1435–1498.

Neilson JP. 2004. Fetal electrocardiogram (ECG) for fetal monitoring during labour (Cochrane Review). *The Cochrane Library* 1. Chichester, UK: John Wiley & Sons, Ltd.

Nellcor Purital Bennett Inc (A division of TYCO Healthcare). 2004. *OxiFirst (R)* Fetal Pulse Oximetry System. http://www.nellcor.com

Nelson KB. 1988. What proportion of cerebral palsy is related to birth asphyxia? *J Pediatr* 112: 572–574.

NICE. 2001. National Institute for Clinical Excellence. The use of electronic fetal monitoring: the use and interpretation of cardiotocography in intrapartum fetal surveillance. *NICE Inherited Clinical Guideline C*, London: National Institute for Clinical Excellence.

Nielsen PV, B Stigsby, C Nickelsen et al. 1987. Intra- and inter-observer variability in the assessment of intrapartum cardiotocograms. *Acta Obstet Gynecol Scand* 66:421–424.

Nyman M, M Barr and M Westgren. 1992. A four-year follow-up of hearing and development in children exposed to in utero vibro-acoustic stimulation. *Br J Obstet Gynaecol* 99:685–688.

OB Scientific. 2002. *OBS-500* Fetal pulse oximeter. www.OBScientific.com

O'Brien PM, PR Doyle and P Rolfe. 1993. Near infrared spectroscopy in fetal monitoring. *Br J Hospital Medicine* 49:483–487.

Ohel G, E Horowitz, N Linder et al. 1987. Neonatal auditory acuity following in utero vibratory acoustic stimulation. *Am J Obstet Gynecol* 157:440–441.

Peebles DM, AD Edwards, JS Wyatt et al. 1992. Changes in human fetal cerebral hemoglobin concentration and oxygenation during labor measured by near-infrared spectroscopy. *Am J Obstet Gynecol* 166:1369–1373.

Peebles DM. 1997. Cerebral hemodynamics and oxygenation in the fetus: The role of intrapartum near-infrared spectroscopy. *Clinics in Perinatology* 24:547–565.

Ratcliffe SJ, LR Leader, GZ Heller et al. 2000. Functional regression analysis of stimulated fetal heart rate data as a predictor of infant development at 18 and 36 months. *Proceedings of the Perinatal Society of Australia and New Zealand 4th Annual Congress;* Brisbane, Australia, 318.

Rosén KG, I Amer-Wåhlin, R Luzietti et al. 2004. Fetal ECG waveform analysis. *Best Pract Res Clin Obstet Gynaecol* 3:485–514.

Royal College of Obstetricians and Gynaecologists. 2001. The use of electronic fetal monitoring: the use and interpretation of cardiotocography in intrapartum fetal surveillance. Evidence-based Clinical Guideline Number 8; *Royal College of Obstetricians and Gynaecologists*, London.

Seelbach-Gobel B, M Heupel, M Kuhnert et al. 1999. The prediction of fetal acidosis by means of intrapartum fetal pulse oximetry. *Am J Obstet Gynecol* 180:73–81.

Skupski DW, CR Rosenberg and GS Eglinton. 2002. Intrapartum fetal stimulation tests: a meta-analysis. *Obstet Gynecol* 99:129–134.

Smith CV, B Satt, JP Phelan et al. 1990. Intrauterine sound levels: intrapartum assessment with an intrauterine microphone. *Am J Perinatol* 7:312–315.

Spencer JAD, A Deans and P Nicolaidis et al. 1991. Fetal heart rate response to vibroacoustic stimulation during low and high heart rate variability episodes in late pregnancy. *Am J Obstet Gynecol* 165:86–90.

Steer PJ and P Danielian. 1999. Fetal distress in labour. In *High risk pregnancy: management options*, 2nd edn, ed DK James, PJ Steer, CP Wesner and B Gonik, 1121–1149. Edinburgh: WB Saunders.

Streer PJ. 1985. Fetal distress. In *Risks of labour*, ed. J Crawford, 11–31. Chichester : John Wiley & Sons.

Thacker SB, D Stroup and M Chang. 2002. Continuous electronic fetal heart rate monitoring for fetal assessment during labor (Cochrane review). *The Cochrane Library* 2: Update Software, Oxford.

Thacker SB, DF Stroup and M Chang. 2004. Continuous electronic heart rate monitoring for fetal assessment during labor (Cochrane Review). *The Cochrane Library* 1: Chichester, UK: John Wiley.

Umstad M, C Bailey and M Permezel. 1992. Intrapartum fetal stimulation testing. *Aust NZ J Obstet Gynaecol* 32:222–224.

Umstad MP. 1993. The predictive value of abnormal fetal heart rate patterns in early labour. *Aust NZ J Obstet Gynaecol* 33:145–149.

Westgren M, K Kruger, S Ek et al. 1998. Lactate compared with pH analysis at fetal scalp blood sampling: a prospective randomised study. *Br J Obstet Gynaecol* 105:29–33.

29

Current Management of Breech Presentation

Jyothi Shetty

Introduction

Clinicians have long recognised the excessive perinatal morbidity and mortality associated with breech-presenting fetuses. Although only 3–4% of pregnancies at term have a breech presentation, the mode of delivery has aroused much debate.

A recent randomised multicentre trial comparing planned cesarean with planned vaginal birth concluded in favour of cesarean delivery for term breech pregnancies, based on perinatal outcome (Hannah et al 2000). Even when a policy of routine elective cesarean delivery is adopted for all term infants presenting by the breech, a significant number of women will still present at a stage of labour too advanced for cesarean, while others may request a trial of vaginal delivery.

In addition, it is important to remember the technique of vaginal breech delivery, as the same principles apply to delivery of the breech through a uterine incision. It must be emphasised that a breech-presenting fetus requires similar manipulations to effect delivery, regardless of route. Poorly performed breech extraction at cesarean delivery results in injuries similar in nature to those sustained during vaginal delivery. Hence, the need to maintain and develop the skills for safe delivery of the breech-presenting fetus at cesarean delivery is high.

Incidence and Etiology

The incidence of breech presentation varies with gestational age. Nearly 25% of all fetuses will present as breech before 28 weeks (Hickok et al 1992). As term approaches, this incidence falls dramatically.

In the majority of cases of breech presentation, no specific underlying cause is generally found. Associated factors include multiparity, uterine anomalies, multiple gestation, hydrammios, placenta previa, contracted pelvis and pelvic tumours that obstruct the birth canal. Cornual implantation of the placenta is responsible in some cases for breech presentation (Fianu 1978).

Congenital malformations occur more often in breech than in vertex presentations. Collea and associates (1978) quoted a 5% risk of congenital abnormality in term breech, which is 2–3 times higher than the vertex. Lamont and colleagues (1983) in a series of preterm breeches found that 18% were congenitally abnormal. Common congenital anomalies associated with breech presentation include anencephaly, hydrocephalus and meningomyelocele. Many of these abnormalities can be detected by careful ultrasound evaluation. High rates of breech presentation are noted in certain chromosomal abnormalities including trisomies 13, 18 and 21, and myotonic dystrophy (Braun et al 1975). Thus, conditions that alter fetal muscular tone and mobility also increase the frequency of breech presentation. It is prudent to keep these facts in mind when deciding on the mode of delivery for a fetus in breech presentation.

Perinatal Morbidity and Mortality

Perinatal mortality in breech presentation is estimated to be 3–4 times that of comparable infants with vertex presentation (Rovinsky et al 1973). The excess deaths associated with breech presentation are largely due to lethal anomalies and complications of prematurity. After exclusion of these factors, the breech infant has been found to be at higher risk of asphyxia and birth trauma. The most prominent cause of fresh fetal stillbirth is asphyxia because of entrapment of the aftercoming head. Asphyxia may also be caused by prolapse of the umbilical cord, which happens in about 0.3% of frank breech, 6% of complete breech and 11% of footling breech deliveries (Myerscough 1998).

Trauma to intra-abdominal organs and/or tissues may occur with delivery if the fetus is grasped in places other than its bony pelvis. Fractures of the femur and humerus may occur during the course of delivering the legs and arms, respectively. Paralysis of the arm may follow pressure on the brachial plexus by the fingers in exerting traction, but more frequently it is caused by overstretching the neck while freeing the arms. Finally, trauma to the cervical spinal cord may occur with delivery of a breech fetus with hyperextension of the fetal head.

Management

The management of term and preterm breech-presenting fetuses will be considered separately, as small fetuses suffer from immaturity as well as trauma from the mode of delivery.

Management of Preterm Breech Presentation

Management of Preterm Breech Presentation The mortality and morbidity rates of babies delivered between 33 and 36 weeks inclusive is very low and not significantly influenced by mode of delivery, provided cesarean section is undertaken for the usual clinical indications. The main controversy about mode of delivery of the preterm breech-presenting fetus is between 26 and 32 weeks, when approximately 2% of all pregnant women with viable fetuses will deliver.

In addition to the complications of prematurity, preterm breech is at an even greater disadvantage in negotiating the pelvis than is the term breech-presenting fetus because of the disproportionately greater head circumference relative to abdominal circumference. The partially dilated cervix, which often allows for passage of the thorax, can at times entrap the head of the preterm fetus. The other potential negative factor seen in preterm breech fetuses is increased incidence of non-frank presentations with the attendant increased risk of umbilical cord prolapse.

Optimum Mode of Delivery of the Preterm Breech Most elective deliveries of the preterm breech when the woman is not in labour, are for fetal or maternal indications, when the preferred route of delivery is cesarean section. The controversy about management mainly centres on the preterm breech presentation in labour, in which the initial priorities are (i) accurate diagnosis of premature labour, (ii) confirmation of presentation and (iii) exclusion of fetal abnormalities.

It is evident that in up to 80% of cases in which the mother thinks she is in premature labour, contractions cease spontaneously and the pregnancy continues. The definitive diagnosis of labour, therefore, rests on demonstrating progressive dilatation of the cervix. Careful cervical assessment of all women in suspected premature labour is imperative to confirm or refute the diagnosis. A detailed ultrasound scan should be performed to confirm the normality of the fetus and check on the placental position at the same time.

There are no randomised studies regarding delivery of the preterm breech fetus. Penn and colleagues (1996) attempted such a study in 26 hospitals in England and discontinued the trial after 17 months because only 13 women could be recruited. Retrospective studies have yielded conflicting results. It, therefore, appears likely that the optimal mode of delivery of the preterm breech will remain uncertain for the foreseeable future.

At gestations above 32 weeks but below 37 weeks and when the fetus weighs 1500–2500 g, current evidence does not suggest any advantage in performing routine cesarean section. Under this gestation and weight but at more than 26 weeks of gestation, the optimal mode of delivery remains uncertain in the absence of any clinical feature specifically indicating cesarean section. The advantage, if any, that routine section confers on the fetus is likely to be small; otherwise it would already be obvious in the multiplicity of published data available. What is certain is that if a policy of routine cesarean section for the preterm breech fetus is followed, a number of cesarean sections will be performed unnecessarily for the fetus that is congenitally malformed, for the fetus that is over 1500 g and therefore unlikely to benefit and for some that will not actually be in established premature labour and were destined to be delivered at a later gestation. Priorities in the management of preterm breech in labour are the exclusion, as far as possible, of congenital abnormality and the participation of an experienced obstetrician during vaginal delivery (Penn et al 2006).

Management of the Term Breech

Spontaneous Version The fact that breech presentation is so uncommon at term implies that the spontaneous version usually occurs in the weeks before term and so breech presentation becomes less common as the third trimester progresses. The incidence of the spontaneous version after 32 weeks may be as high as 57% and after 36 weeks of gestation may still be as high as 25% (Westgren et al 1985). Prior to cesarean section solely for breech presentation at term, the presentation should be checked immediately before surgery by ultrasound scanning, as the chances of spontaneous version, even at this late stage, are not insignificant.

External Cephalic Version Once very popular, external cephalic version (ECV) has received renewed interest in the past two decades, coincidental with the widespread availability of ultrasound, electronic fetal monitoring and effective tocolytic agents. Recently, the American College of Obstetricians and Gynecologists (2001) recommended that efforts be made to reduce breech presentation by external cephalic version, whenever possible.

All women with an uncomplicated breech presentation after 37 weeks of gestation should now be offered ECV. The advantages of ECV at term are that most spontaneous versions would already have occurred and, in the event of a complication, rapid delivery of a mature fetus can be undertaken. This will result in fewer unnecessary attempts being made. The Cochrane Database of Systematic Reviews (Hofmyer 2000) concluded that in view of the lack of evidence of effectiveness, and reports from observational studies of unacceptably high complication rates from ECV before term, there is at present no place for ECV before term in modern obstetrics.

The Cochrane Review looked at six trials of a randomised nature and concluded that ECV at term was associated with a significant reduction in non-cephalic births (relative risk of 0.42) and a reduction in cesarean section (relative risk of 0.52). The implications of these numbers are that every 100 ECV attempts should prevent 34 breech births and 14 cesarean sections.

However, the impact of ECV on the rate of cesarean sections for this indication will depend on the success rate of ECV. This ranges from 35% to 85%, with an average of about 60% (ACOG 2000).

Factors Associated with Successful Version

Increasing parity is the most consistent factor associated with success of ECV (Zhang et al 1993). In another study, Hellstrom (1990) noted that version was more successful in a parous woman who has an unengaged fetus surrounded by a normal amount of amniotic fluid. It was also noted that the success rate was significantly lower in fetuses with extended legs and when the ammiotic fluid was reduced. Lau and associates (1997) identified three variables that predicted a failed version—an engaged presenting part, difficulty in palpating the fetal head and a uterus that is tense to palpation. In the presence of all three, there were no successes; with two, the success was less than 20%, however, if none were present, the success rate was 94%.

Technique ECV should be carried out in the labour ward where facilities for emergency cesarean section are available. An ultrasound scan should be performed to assess the liquor volume, fetal attitude and position of the fetal legs. The mother should remain awake, and cardiotocography (CTG) should be performed before and after the procedure. Rh-negative patients should receive anti-D immune globulin.

A 'forward roll' of the fetus is usually attempted first. Turning should first be attempted in the direction that increases flexion. The first step is to displace the breech from the pelvic brim. Having raised the lower pole of the fetus with the right hand, the breech is displaced to one iliac fossa, towards the side of the fetal back. The operator uses the left hand to press the fetal head towards the patient's flank. After the fetus is brought to a transverse position, the hands are changed over the fetal poles and ECV is completed.

If the forward roll fails, a backward somersault may be attempted. The fetal heart

Table 29.1: Indications and contraindications for external cephalic version

Indications
Uncomplicated breech presentation after 37 weeks of gestation
Unengaged breech

Absolute contraindications
Placenta previa
Multiple pregnancy
Congenital uterine anomalies
Significant fetal abnormality
Ruptured membranes
Conditions necessitating cesarean section

Relative contraindications
Previous cesarean section
Pre-eclampsia
Intrauterine growth restriction

rate should be observed using ultrasound regularly. A version attempt is abandoned if there is significant fetal bradycardia, discomfort for the patient or the attempt cannot be completed easily. Whether ECV is successful or not, after the procedure, a CTG is carried out again. The successful cases are managed as if they had always been cephalic, and there is no indication to offer an early induction.

Tocolysis Because of the observation that increased uterine tone decreases the chance of success of ECV, the use of tocolytics has been investigated. A variety of tocolytics have been used. The Cochrane Database reviewed six trials of routine tocolysis and showed that its use was associated with fewer failures.

In a randomised controlled trial of the use of tocolysis in ECV, Marquette and associates (1996) confirmed the efficacy of ritodrine in promoting the success of ECV in nulliparous patients but not in parous patients. They found that ritodrine increased the success rate of ECV from 25% to 43% in nulliparous women. Fernandez and co-workers (1997) also assessed the efficacy of terbutaline when compared with a placebo for ECV and found a significant decrease in non-cephalic presentations and cesarean sections because of increased chances of success with ECV. Existing evidence supports the use of uterine relaxation with a tocolytic agent, usually terbutaline 250 μg given subcutaneously, particularly in nulliparous patients.

Conduction Analgesia The use of epidural anesthesia for ECV has been controversial. Many believe that operators might apply excessive pressure to the maternal abdomen when epidural anesthesia is employed, which will make fetal compromise more likely, caused by either fetal heart rate decelerations or placental abruption.

Mancuso and collaborators (2000) conducted a randomised trial of 108 women and reported a success rate of 59% with epidural versus 33% without. Another randomised trial addressed the use of spinal anesthesia before the version attempt and found no significant difference between treatment groups (Delisle et al 2001). According to the ACOG (2000), there is not enough consistent evidence to recommend routine use of conduction analgesia.

Complications Risks of external version include transient bradycardia, abruptio placentae, cord complications, feto-maternal hemorrhage with possible sensitisation, prelabour rupture of membranes and fetal demise. Overall, it seems that complications nowadays, when compared to those reported in studies around 1970, seem to be far less frequent. One reason of this could be that anesthesia is no longer used. According to Zhang (1993), since 1980 no fetal deaths have been reported in the United States resulting directly from ECV. Scattered case reports have indicated some uncommon complications (Stine 1985; Petrikovsky 1987). Collaris and Oei (2004) concluded, based on a systematic review of 44 studies which included 7377 patients from 1990 to 2002, that ECV is a safe procedure for both the mother and the fetus.

Choice of Mode of Delivery To answer the question of the optimal route of delivery of the term breech, Hannah and associates (2000) organised the Term Breech Trial, a multinational randomised trial of planned cesarean delivery versus planned vaginal birth for term singleton frank and complete breech infants. A total of 2083 women were randomised: 1041 to planned cesarean and 1042 to planned vaginal delivery. In the planned vaginal delivery group, 57% of cases were actually delivered vaginally. Perinatal mortality/neonatal mortality and serious neonatal morbidity were significantly lower for the planned cesarean section group (1.6%) than for the planned vaginal birth group (5.0%) (relative risk 0.33). Maternal complications were similar between the groups. These relative differences between planned cesarean section and vaginal breech delivery persist even when a variety of clinical differences between groups are taken into account—parity, type of breech, estimated weight of fetus, whether the pelvis had been assessed clinically or radiologically, the degree of experience of the clinician, and a variety of other clinical parameters that are usually held to be important predictors of the success and safety of attempted vaginal delivery. The only significant interaction was between the treatment group and the countries' reported perinatal mortality/morbidity rate (PNMMR) for the combined outcome of perinatal mortality, neonatal mortality or serious neonatal morbidity rates. In countries with a low PNMMR (≤20 in 1000 births), the risk from planned cesarean section compared with planned vaginal birth was 0.4% versus 5.7%, whereas the rates in countries with a high PNMMR (>20 in 1000 births) were 2.9% versus 4.4%. This difference in the developed countries disappeared when the outcome of only perinatal or neonatal death was considered. Neonatal morbidity showed the greatest differences, with reductions in morbidity being much greater for countries with low PNMMRs than for those with high PNMMRs. It is not clear why this might be the case. Possible explanations include incomplete ascertainment of poor neonatal condition in the first week of life or death before morbidity could be recognised. However, the reduced benefit from a policy of planned cesarean section in countries with high PNMMRs might also be real, possibly because of higher levels of experience with vaginal breech delivery in those countries. Overall, this study indicated that, with a policy of planned cesarean section, for every additional 14 cesarean sections done, one baby will avoid death or serious morbidity. In countries with high PNMMR, as many as 39 additional cesarean sections would need to be done to avoid one dead or compromised baby, whereas in countries with low PNMMR, the number of additional cesarean sections required may be as low as seven.

Based on this information, the ACOG (2001) has concluded that 'patients with a persistent breech presentation at term in a singleton gestation should undergo a planned cesarean delivery'. It is important to point out that they further stated 'a planned cesarean delivery does not apply to patients presenting in advanced labour with a fetus in breech presentation in which delivery is likely to be imminent, or to patients whose second twin is in a breech presentation'. However, a number of criticisms were discussed in a series of letters to the editor of *The Lancet* and *Obstetrics and Gynecology* (Cunha-Filho and Passos 2001; Uchida and Murakami 2001; Apuzzio et al 2002). These issues include (i) the failure to consider the adverse effect of cesarean delivery on future gestations, (ii) that some of the 16 stillbirths and neonatal deaths could be excluded because their deaths were not associated with the mode of delivery and (iii) that most components included in the 'serious' neonatal morbidity do not actually portend long-term disability.

At least three contemporary single-centre studies support a trial of vaginal delivery for selected breech-presenting term fetuses. Irion and associates (1998) reported significantly fewer maternal complications, but no difference in corrected neonatal morbidity or mortality in 385 attempted vaginal breech deliveries (70% of whom were delivered vaginally), compared with that of 320 planned cesarean deliveries. Giuliani and associates (2002) reported that in their institution, vaginal breech delivery was achieved in half of 699 term breech presenting fetuses, with no short- or long-term differences in outcome for infants delivered vaginally compared with those delivered by cesarean. Alarab and associates (2004) reported no serious adverse neonatal outcomes in 146 term breech infants (one-fourth of all their breeches) who were delivered vaginally. Based on reports such as these, between 10% and 20% of singleton breeches are delivered vaginally (Cunningham et al 2005). A diligent search for any other complication, actual or anticipated, that might justify cesarean delivery has become a feature of most philosophies for managing breech delivery.

Cesarean delivery is commonly used in the following circumstances.

- Large fetus—estimated fetal weight ≥3.5 kg
- Abnormal clinical pelvimetry
- Hyperextended fetal head
- Footling breech
- Severe fetal growth restriction
- Previous perinatal death or children suffering from birth trauma
- When delivery is indicated in the absence of spontaneous labour
- Failure to progress in labour due to uterine inertia

Assessment for Vaginal Breech Delivery

The available literature stresses the importance of adhering to an appropriate protocol when assessing women for vaginal breech delivery (Table 29.2). Close consultation with the mother and partner and counselling about the implications of the choice of vaginal breech delivery versus elective cesarean section is important. It is the responsibility of the obstetrician to explain the options and the evidence to the patient and her family in the clearest possible terms. Although cesarean section is the recommended option for the vast majority of women, especially in the developed world, some women when informed of the options may still wish to attempt a vaginal delivery, and their wish should be respected.

Assisted Vaginal Breech Delivery The essence of assisted vaginal breech delivery is allowing as much spontaneous delivery by uterine action and maternal effort as possible. Operator intervention should be limited to the maneuvers described here, which are designed to correct any deviation from the normal mechanism of spontaneous delivery.

First Stage Many authors suggest that spontaneous labour increases the chances of successful vaginal delivery and if delivery is required before the onset of spontaneous labour, elective cesarean section is preferable to induction of labour.

Labour should be conducted in a labour ward with all the facilities needed to perform a cesarean section, with a full anesthetic service and senior obstetric staff available. The presence of an anesthetist is desirable in all cases of breech delivery during the second stage as, in some cases, uterine relaxation or general anesthesia may have to be induced rapidly to complete safe delivery. The intravaginal manipulations needed for breech extraction can usually be accomplished with pudendal block and local infiltration of the perineum. There is no evidence to suggest that epidural analgesia is essential for assisted breech delivery (RCOG Guidelines 2001). Total labour duration should be similar to that in cephalic presentation, although descent of the breech may be slow. The progress of labour should therefore be plotted on a partogram in the usual way. Most clinicians prefer continuous electronic monitoring of fetal heart rate and uterine contractions. When membranes are ruptured, vaginal examination should be performed to check for cord prolapse. Special attention should be directed to the fetal heart rate for the first 5–10 minutes following membrane rupture, to detect occult cord prolapse. The role of oxytocin augmentation for dysfunctional labour is debatable and less favoured. The second stage should always be confirmed by vaginal examination, because the woman frequently has a desire to bear down before the cervix is fully dilated.

Second Stage

Delivery of Breech and Legs The instrument table should be prepared in the customary manner, with the addition of Piper forceps and extra towels. The key principles of conducting vaginal breech delivery are:

- Do not be in hurry.
- Never pull from below; let the mother expel the fetus by her own effort with uterine contractions
- Always keep the fetus with the back anterior

Episiotomy is given when the breech distends the perineum. Such an episiotomy greatly facilitates the passage of the arms and the aftercoming head and allows delivery to be accomplished with less risk of asphyxia due to prolonged maneuvering. The fetus is then allowed to deliver up to the umbilicus spontaneously in flexed breech. In frank breech, manipulation is required to free the extended legs. This is done by pressing the finger into the popliteal fossa and sweeping the knee gently outwards on the fetal trunk, while at the same time flexing the knee. The anterior leg is always delivered first. Some advocate pulling down a loop of cord to avoid compression of the cord, but this should be omitted if there is resistance as it may tighten a loop around the neck or arm. The fetus is kept warm by a sterile towel wrapped around the body. The fetal back should remain anterior and any tendency to rotate backwards should be prevented.

Delivery of the Arms With uterine contractions and maternal bearing down efforts, the trunk of the fetus should be expelled and the lower border of the anterior scapula becomes visible under the pubic arch. The position of the arms should be noted. When the arms are flexed, the vertebral border of the scapula remains parallel to the vertebral column and, when extended, winging of the scapula is seen. The arms are delivered one after the other only when one axilla is visible, by simply hooking down each elbow with a finger.

One or both arms may be fully extended along the side of the head. This usually occurs due to inappropriate earlier traction placed on the fetus. Lovset's maneuvoer is an effective way of dealing with this complication. It is based on the principle that the inclination of the pelvis is such that the posterior shoulder enters the pelvic cavity in advance of the anterior shoulder. So the posterior shoulder will be below the sacral promontory when the anterior shoulder is above the symphysis pubis. The fetus is grasped around the pelvic girdle, with the thumbs overlying the lumbosacral spine and the index fingers on the iliac crests. The fetal trunk is rotated 180° keeping the back anterior and maintaining

Table 29.2: Assessment for vaginal breech delivery

Assessment of the cause of breech presentation
Exclude:
• Placenta previa
• Fibroids/pelvic tumours
• Congenital abnormality
Assessment of fetal weight and attitude
Assessment of the maternal pelvis
Clinical pelvimetry (important for medicolegal reasons)
X-ray erect lateral pelvimetry is no longer advocated
Computed tomography scanning pelvimetry and magnetic resonance imaging may be unnecessary and unreliable
Assessment of maternal condition
Exclude significant maternal disease: pre-eclampsia or diabetes

gentle downward traction. This will bring the posterior arm to emerge under the pubic arch which is then hooked out. The body is then rotated in the reverse direction keeping the back anterior to deliver the anterior shoulder under the symphysis pubis (Fig. 29.1).

Delivery of the Aftercoming Head Delivery of the head is the most crucial stage of delivery. Three methods are used to deliver the head.

Burns–Marshall method: After delivery of the arms, the fetus is suspended with partial support from the hand of the operator. The assistant applies suprapubic pressure (Kristellar's maneuver) to promote flexion of the head. Once the nape of the neck is visible—identified by the hairline—the baby is grasped by the ankles. The baby's trunk is gently lifted and swung toward the mother's abdomen. The left hand guards and slips the perineum over the fetal face. The trunk is depressed to deliver the rest of the head. This maneuver must be carefully executed and care must be taken to see that the head does not suddenly come out of the vagina. Sudden decompression of the head can lead to tentorial tears and intracranial hemorrhage.

Forceps delivery: This is the best method (Mukhopadhyay 2002). The advantage of forceps is that controlled head delivery is possible. It maintains good flexion and traction is applied directly on the head and the force is not transmitted through the neck. Long Das forceps are quite effective but Piper forceps are specially designed for this purpose. An assistant must support the fetal body during application of these forceps.

The temptation to elevate the fetal body to provide better visualisation must be resisted, because this maneuver hyperextends the neck. The fetal body should be supported parallel to the floor. The application is pelvic rather than cephalic, with the forceps being applied to the lateral aspects of the maternal pelvis. The traction of the forceps should follow the axis of the birth canal (Fig. 29.2).

Jaw flexion and shoulder traction (Mauriceau–Smellie–Veit technique): The fetus is placed on the supinated left forearm with the limbs hanging on either side. The middle and index fingers of the left hand are placed over the maxilla on each side of the nose. By this means, the head is maintained in an attitude of flexion. The ring and little fingers of the pronated right hand are placed on the right fetal shoulder, the index finger on the left shoulder and the

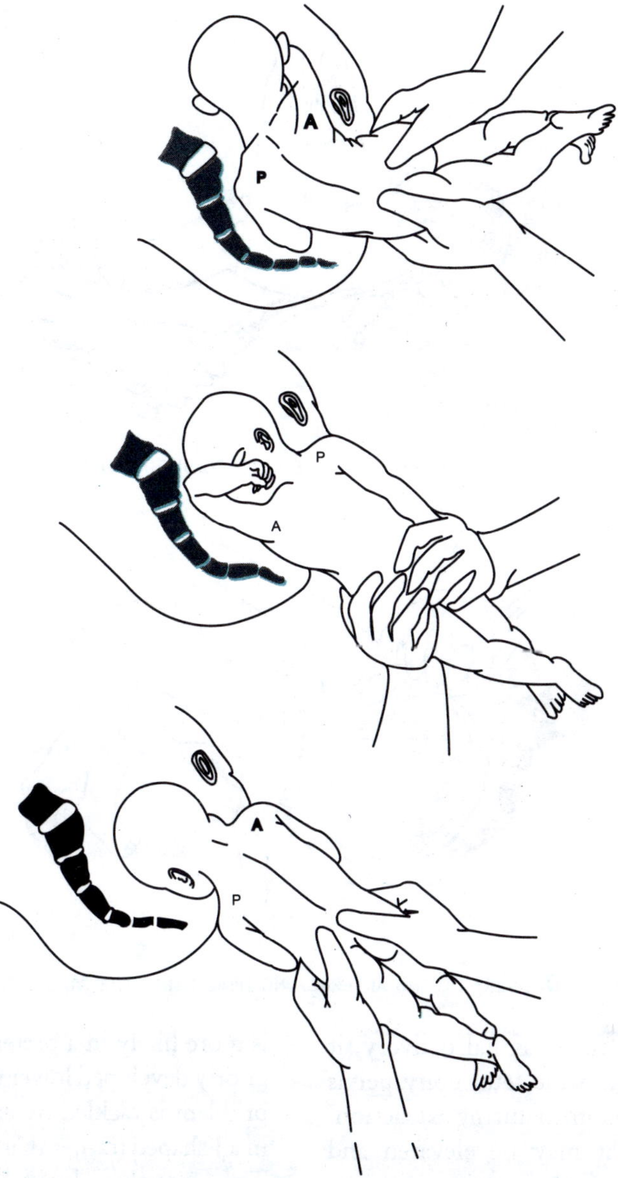

FIGURE 29.1: DELIVERING THE EXTENDED ARM BY LOVSET'S MANEUVER

middle finger on the suboccipital region (Fig. 29.3). Traction is now exerted in a downward and backward direction, until the nape of the neck is visible under the pubic arch. Gentle suprapubic pressure on the head by an assistant from above facilitates its descent into the pelvis. The body is then elevated toward the maternal abdomen, and the face, brow and eventually, the occiput emerge successively over the perineum.

Management of Cesarean Delivery

Abdominal delivery does not guarantee an atraumatic birth of the fetus in breech

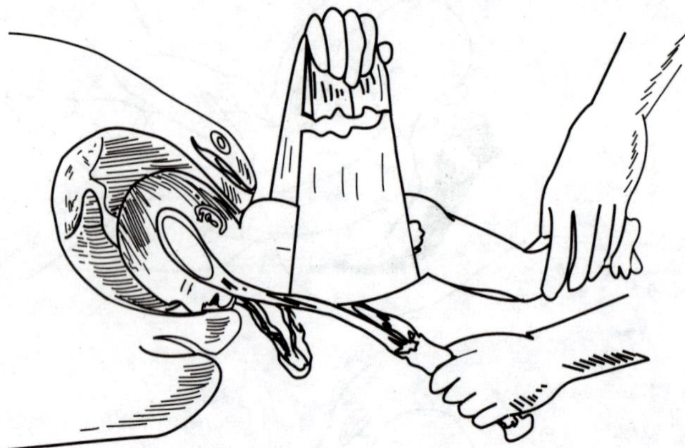

Figure 29.2: Delivery of the aftercoming head by forceps

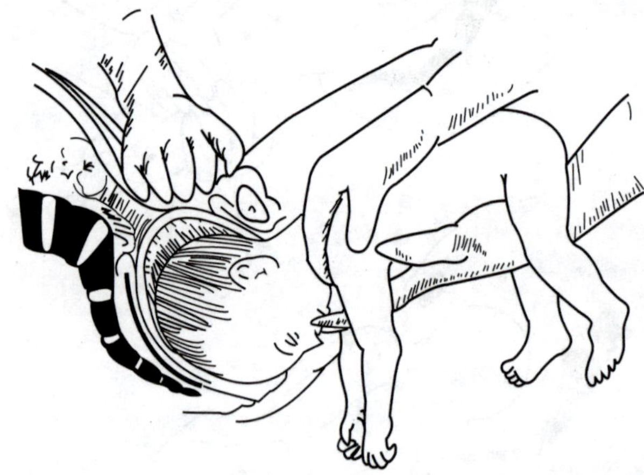

Figure 29.3: Delivery of the aftercoming head using the Mauriceau maneuver

presentation. Just as in vaginal delivery, it is important to grasp the fetal bony pelvis rather than fetal abdomen during extraction. In frank breech, it may be elevated and guided forward into the uterine incision, the right hand being used as a scoop. The complete breech is best extracted by grasping the anterior foot. The delivery is then conducted according to the rules of breech extraction.

The most serious complication is head entrapment by the uterus contracting down around the neck after delivery of the body. This is more likely in a preterm breech due to the poorly developed lower uterine segment. This problem is tackled by extending the incision in a J-shaped (rather than a T-shaped) manner. The anesthesiologist should administer general anesthesia with a halogenated agent that rapidly relaxes the uterus. This might become necessary even if the delivery is begun under regional anesthesia.

Summary

For the preterm breech in labour

- Accurate diagnosis and confirmation

of preterm labour should be done by careful vaginal examination and cervical ultrasound.

- Ultrasound should be performed to exclude congenital abnormality and placenta previa.
- There is insufficient evidence to recommend cesarean section for the preterm breech. The mode of delivery should be determined in close consultation with the woman and her family.

For term breech (37 weeks and over)

- The use of external cephalic version in the appropriately assessed woman after 37 weeks of gestation shows a clear benefit in the reduced numbers of cesarean sections and has a good safety record.
- There is now convincing evidence that women with term breech should be advised that planned elective cesarean section reduces the risk of death or serious morbidity for the fetus, with no evidence of increased morbidity in the mother.

Despite this, some women may still choose to try to deliver vaginally. Ultrasound should be performed to confirm diagnosis, check for fetal abnormalities and assess fetal attitude and estimated weight. The mother should have at least an average capacity pelvis, judged clinically. The second stage should be supervised by an experienced obstetrician.

The number of vaginal breech deliveries will fall further following the Term Breech Trial. As more and more women undergo cesarean for breech, obstetrical trainee doctors have fewer opportunities to acquire the skills of conducting a vaginal breech delivery. Hence, alternative methods of training at the earliest need to be introduced (for example, videos and training on sophisticated mannequins).

References

Alarab M, C Regan, MP O'Connell, DP Keane, C O'Herlihy and ME Foley. 2004. Singleton vaginal breech delivery at term: still a safe option. *Obstet Gynecol* 103:407–412.

American College of Obstetricians and Gynecologists. 2000. External cephalic version. Practice Bulletin No. 13. *American College of Obstetricians and Gynecologists*.

American College of Obstetricians and Gynecologists. 2001. Mode of singleton breech delivery. Committee Opinion No. 265. *American College of Obstetricians and Gynecologists*.

Apuzzio J, L Iffy and G Weiss. 2002. Mode of singleton breech delivery (letter). *Obstet Gynecol* 99: 1131.

Braun FHT, KL Jones and DW Smith. 1975. Breech presentation as an indicator of fetal abnormality. *J Pediatr* 86:419–421.

Collaris RJ and SG Oei. 2004. External cephalic version: A safe procedure? A systematic review of version related risks. *Acta Obstet Gynecol Scand* 83:511–518.

Collea JV, SC Rabin, GR Weghorst et al. 1978. The randomized management of term frank breech presentation: Vaginal delivery versus cesarean section. *Am J Obstet Gynecol* 134:186.

Cunha-Filho JS and E Passos. 2001. Term breech trial (Correspondence). *Lancet* 357:227.

Cunningham FG, KJ Leveno, SL Bloom, JC Hauth, LC Gilstrap III and KD Wenstrom, eds. 2005. *Williams Obstetrics*, 22nd ed. New York: Mc Graw Hill.

Delisle MF, A Kamani, J Douglas et al. 2001. Antepartum external cephalic version under spinal anesthesia: A randomised controlled trial. *Am J Obstet Gynecol* 185:S115.

Fernandez CO, SL Bloom, JC Smulian et al. 1997. A randomized placebo controlled trial evaluation of terbutaline for external cephalic version. *Obstet Gynecol* 90:775–779.

Fianu S and V Vaclavinkova. 1978. The site of placental attachment as a factor in the etiology of breech presentation. *Acta Obstet Gynecol Scand* 57:371–372.

Hannah ME, JW Hannah, SA Hewson, ED Hodnett, S Saigal and AR Willan. 2000. Planned cesarean section versus planned vaginal birth for breech presentation at term: a randomised multicentre trial. *Lancet* 356:1375–1383.

Hellstrom AC, B Nilsson, L Stange et al. 1990. When does external cephalic version succeed? *Acta Obstet Gynecol Scand* 69:281–285.

Hickok DE, DC Gordon, JA Milberg et al. 1992. The frequency of breech presentation by gestational age at birth: a large population based study. *Am J Obstet Gynecol* 166:851–852.

Hofmyer GJ. 2000. External cephalic version facilitation for breech presentation at term. *Cochrane Database Syst Rev*; 2:CD 000184 (Update: 2001;4:CD000184).

Irion O, PH Hirsbrunner Almagbaly and A Morabia. 1998. Planned vaginal delivery versus elective cesarean section: a study of 705 singleton term breech presentations. *Br J Obstet Gynaecol* 195: 710–717.

Lamont RF, PDM Dunlop, P Crowley et al. 1983. Spontaneous preterm labour and delivery at under 34 weeks' gestation. *Br Med J* 286:454–457.

Lau TK, KWK Lo, D Wan et al. 1997. Predictors of successful external cephalic version at term: a prospective study *Br J Obstet Gynaecol* 104:798–802.

Mancuso KM, MK Yancey, JA Murphy et al. 2000. Epidural analgesia for cephalic version: a randomised trial. *Obstet Gynecol* 95:648–651.

Marquette GP, M Boucher, D Theriault and D Rinfret. 1996. Does the use of a tocolytic agent affect the success rate of external cephalic version. *Am J Obstet Gynecol* 174:859–864.

Myerscough PR, ed. 1998. Breech presentation. In *Munro Kerr's Operative Obstetrics*, 10th ed. Delhi: AITBS Publishers.

Penn Z. 2006. Breech Presentation. In *High risk pregnancy: Management options*, 3rd ed, eds DK James, PJ Steer, CP Weiner and B Gonik, 1334–1358. New Delhi: Elsevier.

Penn ZJ, PJ Steer and A Grant. 1996. A multicentre randomised controlled trial to compare elective versus selective cesarean section for the delivery of the preterm breech infant. *Br J Obstet Gynaecol* 103:684–689.

Petrikovsky BM, HN DeSilva and FD Fumia. 1987. Erb's palsy and fetal bruising after external cephalic version: Case report. *Am J Obstet Gynecol* 157:258.

RCOG Guidelines. 2001. The management of breech presentation, April 2001. London. *Royal College of Obstetricians and Gynaecologists*,

Rovinsky JJ, JA Miller and S Koplan. 1973. Management of breech presentation at term. *Am J Obstet Gynecol* 115:497–513.

Stine LE, JP Phelan, R Wallace et al. 1985. Update on external cephalic version performed at term. *Obstet Gynecol* 65:642–646.

Uchide K and K Murakami. 2001. Term breech trial [Correspondence] *Lancet* 357:226.

Westgren M, H Edvall, E Nordstrom and E Svalenius. 1985. Spontaneous cephalic version of breech presentation in the last trimester. *Br J Obstet Gynaecol* 92:19–22.

Zhang J, WA Bowes and JA Fortney. 1993. Efficacy of external cephalic version, including safety, cost-benefit analysis and impact on the cesarean delivery rate. *Obstet Gynecol* 82:306–312.

30

Instrumental Vaginal Deliveries

Stergios K Doumouchtsis | Sabaratnam Arulkumaran

Introduction

Instrumental delivery refers to forceps-assisted or vacuum-assisted delivery. It involves the use of a vacuum extractor or obstetric forceps to allow the operator to apply traction on the fetal head and facilitate its descent along the pelvic curve. The vacuum extractor facilitates delivery by applying suction and traction to the fetal scalp with the suction cup. The forceps cradle the parietal and malar bones of the fetal skull and apply traction to these areas, as well as laterally, displacing maternal tissue.

The rate of instrumental vaginal delivery in different countries varies between 10% and 15% (Kozak and Weeks 2002; RCOG 2005). In the USA, the rate of vacuum delivery surpassed the rate of forceps delivery in 1992 (Miksovsky et al 2001; Kozak and Weeks 2002). Over the past two decades, in the United Kingdom, the use of forceps has decreased by 50% in favour of vacuum extraction or cesarean section (Patel et al 2004). In Canada, forceps delivery has decreased in the last decade from 11.2% in 1991 to 6.8% in 2001 (SOGC 2004).

The vacuum extractor (ventouse) is preferred over forceps for assisted vaginal delivery and is reported to result in a significant reduction of maternal morbidity (Chalmers and Chalmers 1989). Failure rates of less than 1% have been reported as being achievable with appropriate case selection and the correct use of a well-maintained apparatus (Bird 1982). However, recent reports have shown higher failure rates of vacuum extraction than forceps deliveries—relative risk of 1.7 (Johanson et al 2000). The higher failure rate of vacuum extraction is a concern in light of the documented risks of the use of sequential instruments for delivery (Towner et al 1999).

There are variations in obstetric practice worldwide which influence the rates and the outcomes of instrumental deliveries. These variations depend on the choice of operator, clinical indications, local policies and occasionally, maternal choice.

Indications for Instrumental Delivery

Indications for instrumental delivery in the second stage of labour may be fetal or maternal. The most common indication is poor progress in the second stage, and this is often related to malposition of the fetal head. The occipitoposterior (OP) and occipitotransverse positions (OT) occur frequently with regional anesthesia. The tone of the musculature of the pelvic floor is altered, impeding spontaneous rotation to the optimal occipitoanterior (OA) position (Hayashi 2006). Regional anesthesia has also been associated with longer second stage of labour, increased use of oxytocin, compromised maternal forces and increased incidence of instrumental vaginal deliveries. Fetal distress or presumed fetal compromise is a common indication. It may result in hypoxic brain damage or fetal death, if no intervention is undertaken.

Maternal indications are most commonly maternal distress or exhaustion, or inadequate progress of labour (SGOC 2004). Prolongation of the second stage may cause damage to the maternal pelvic floor (Baskett and Arulkumaran 2002). In these cases, it is essential to ensure that there is effective uterine activity. Medically significant conditions are less common indications. These include cardiac disease, cerebral vascular disease, pre-eclampsia, etc. Vaginal birth after previous cesarean section may be a relative indication to minimise the risk of scar rupture, if the second stage is likely to be prolonged.

Prerequisites The prerequisites to instrumental vaginal delivery include vertex presentation, full dilatation of the cervix, rupture of the membranes and full engagement of the fetal head. The relationship of the leading bony part of fetal head to the ischial spines can be misleading with vaginal examination alone because of the difficulties in assessing the contribution of the caput and moulding to the true level of descent. The abdominal assessment of the descent of the fetal head in fifths above the pelvic brim is therefore essential. The vaginal assessment of the exact position of the head is also critical and decisive for the correct application of any instrument. It is important to know the position of the vertex and whether asynclitism is present.

Other prerequisites include informed consent, appropriate analgesia, empty maternal bladder, adequate facilities and personnel, skilled and experienced operator in the use of instruments and management of possible complications, and a backup plan in case of difficulty in delivery or any adverse development.

Contraindications Instrumental vaginal delivery is contraindicated when there is incomplete cervical dilatation, non-vertex presentation, unengaged fetal head, clinical evidence of cephalopelvic disproportion, fetal coagulopathy or bone demineralisation disorder and fetal prematurity of <34 weeks. Unknown position of the fetal head is a contraindication for both vacuum and forceps delivery and the erroneous notion that the vacuum device can be used, instead of forceps in such cases, should be discouraged (McQuivey 2004).

Instrumental deliveries are classified by the station of the leading bony point of the fetal head and the degree of rotation of the sagittal suture from the midline. According to the ACOG classification, instrument-assisted deliveries are classified as **outlet** if the fetal scalp is visible without separating the labia, the sagittal suture is in an anteroposterior diameter or right or left occipitoanterior or posterior position (rotation does not exceed 45°), and the fetal head is at or on the perineum. **Low cavity** deliveries include those where the leading point of the skull is at station ≥+2 cm and not on the pelvic floor. This type is further subdivided if the rotation is ≤45° or >45°. **Mid-cavity** deliveries are those with an engaged fetal head, but the leading point of the skull is above the +2 cm station (ACOG 2000).

Vacuum Extractor

The vacuum extractor is a device comprising of a suction cup attached by tubing to a vacuum source and a handle used to apply traction to the cup. Traction is transferred to the fetal head which is pulled along the birth canal axis. Malstrom devised the stainless steel vacuum cup in the 1950s. It had rounded edges and a diameter of 60 mm, with the vacuum tubing and the traction chain attached to the centre of the upper surface of the cup (Fig. 30.1).

Bird modified the Malstrom vacuum extractor by attaching the vacuum tubing and the traction chain to the side of the cup (Fig. 30.2). This allows placement of the cup in the OP and lateral positions.

In 1973, Kobayashi introduced a single unit silastic cup with a diameter of 65 mm and a stainless steel valve that allowed the release of suction between contractions, without loss of application of the cup to the head. Although it is considered less traumatic and can shape itself to the fetal head, it is associated with a higher failure rate (Hayashi 2006). Randomised studies (Johanson et al 2000) suggest that rigid cups are more likely to result in vaginal birth than soft cups, but they are more likely to cause scalp trauma. A new device called Kiwi Omnicup (Clinical Innovations Inc, Murray, Utah, USA) is a disposable vacuum extractor with a rigid flat plastic cup and a hand pump-traction system directly applied to the vacuum cup (Fig. 30.3). This allows accurate development of negative pressure by means of an indication gauge on the traction handle.

The parturient is in the lithotomy position with adequate epidural, spinal or pudendal anesthesia. Prior to cup placement, the fetal

FIGURE 30.1: MALSTROM CUP WITH CHAIN ON THE UPPER SURFACE OF THE CUP FOR TRACTION

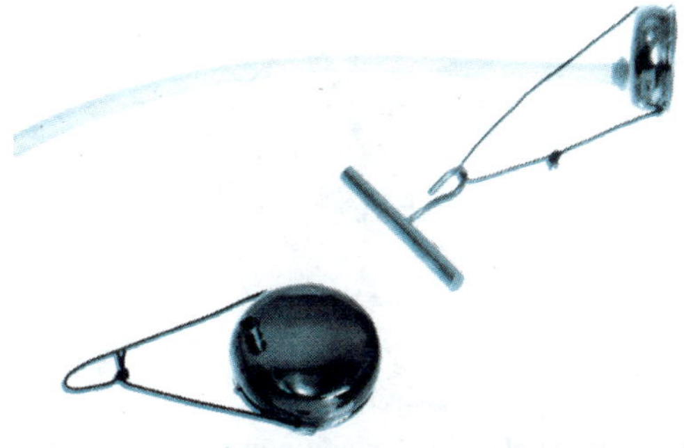

FIGURE 30.2: BIRD CUP—THE ANTERIOR CUP WITH TUBING ON THE UPPER SURFACE AND THE POSTERIOR CUP WITH TUBING ON THE SIDE OF THE CUP

presentation, amount of fetal head palpable abdominally above the symphysis pubis, and position of the fetal head and station should be confirmed. Correct placement of the cup is a major determinant of the outcome. In 1990, Vacca coined the phrase 'flexion point' to describe the site on the fetal scalp over which the centre of the vacuum cup should be placed to achieve a flexing median application. This point is located on the sagittal suture, 3 cm anteriorly to the posterior fontanelle (Fig. 30.4). Application of the vacuum cup on this point promotes synclitism and flexion of the

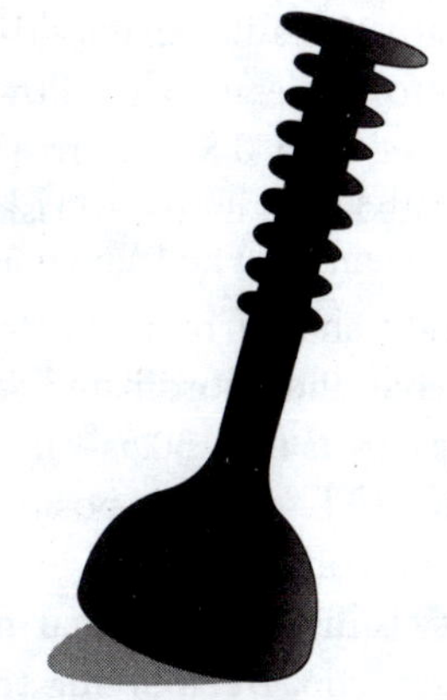

FIGURE 30.3: OMNICUP

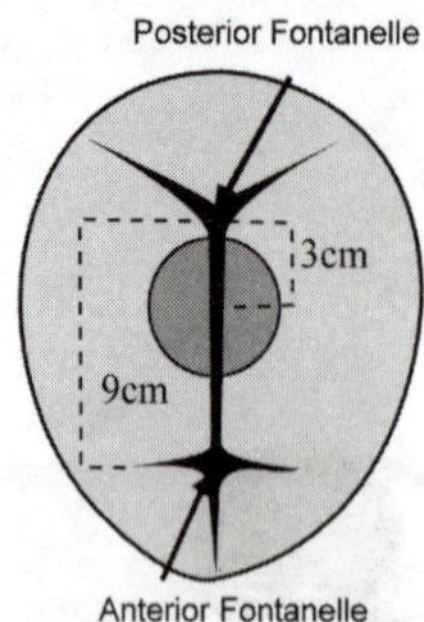

Figure 30.4: The flexion point, about 3 cm anterior to the occiput, along the sagittal suture. The cup is placed over the flexion point.

fetal head, presenting the optimal diameters of the fetal head to the maternal pelvis.

After positioning the cup, but before inducing the vacuum, the application of the cup should be checked to exclude any entrapment of maternal soft tissue between the cup and the fetal head. Apart from causing significant vaginal or cervical tears and maternal hemorrhage, entrapment of maternal tissue may cause detachment of the cup and failure of the procedure. Suction is developed by gradual increments of negative pressure and the fetal scalp is sucked into the hollow of the cup creating an artificial caput (chignon). Effective traction usually requires a negative pressure of at least 0.6 kg/cm^2 (440 mm Hg). This negative pressure enables the cup to hold firmly onto the fetal scalp, allowing traction. Pressures beyond 0.8 kg/cm^2 (588 mm Hg) are associated with increased risk of fetal head injury.

Traction should be in line with the axis of the pelvis and coordinated with maternal expulsive efforts (Fig. 30.5a–c).

In the OT or OP positions, rotation should be accomplished only by traction and not by twisting or rotational motions with the vacuum cup. By applying traction in the correct direction, flexion and asynclitism of the head can be corrected, and autorotation will occur as the head descends by virtue of the architecture of the pelvis. The use of a rotational motion is contraindicated because of the risk of scalp injury by shearing forces on the fetal head. This effect is more pronounced with the use of the metal cup than with the soft cup. Descent must begin with the initial traction effort. If the cup is dislodged, the reason for the 'pop-off' should be evaluated, and, if there are no contraindications, it must be reapplied after careful inspection of the fetal scalp for injury.

The safe parameters for the maximum number of traction attempts and the duration of a vacuum application, or the number of 'pop-offs' that can be tolerated, are not well-established. The SOGC guidelines advise that if delivery has not occurred after four contractions, the intended method of delivery should be reassessed (SOGC 2004).

Vacca suggests that three pulls for the descent phase and three pulls for the perineal phase are acceptable, provided that some progress is observed with each pull (Vacca 2002). The traction on the head is less when there is descent, compared with no descent. With efficient uterine contractions and good maternal expulsive efforts, almost all vacuum-assisted deliveries should be completed within 15 minutes. If the 20-minute limit is exceeded, the procedure should be abandoned unless delivery is imminent (McQuivey 2004). The procedure should also be abandoned if there is any evidence of fetal scalp trauma.

Forceps

Forceps are a paired instrument made of two blades that are attached to each other by the lock on the shank. The left branch is applied to the left side of the maternal

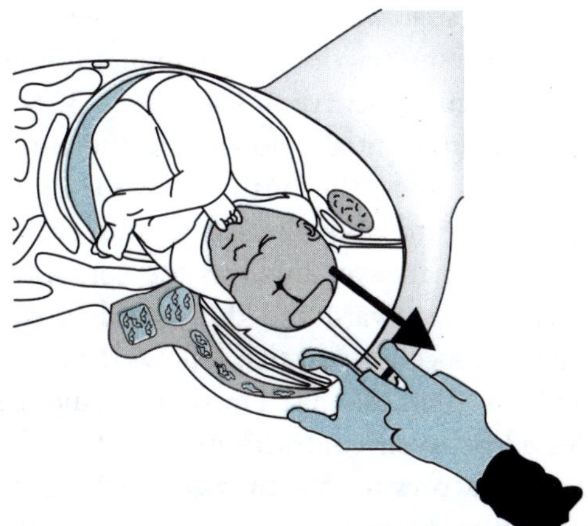

FIGURE 30. 5A: DIRECTION OF TRACTION FORCE DURING VACUUM EXTRACTION WHEN THE HEAD IS BELOW THE ISCHIAL SPINES

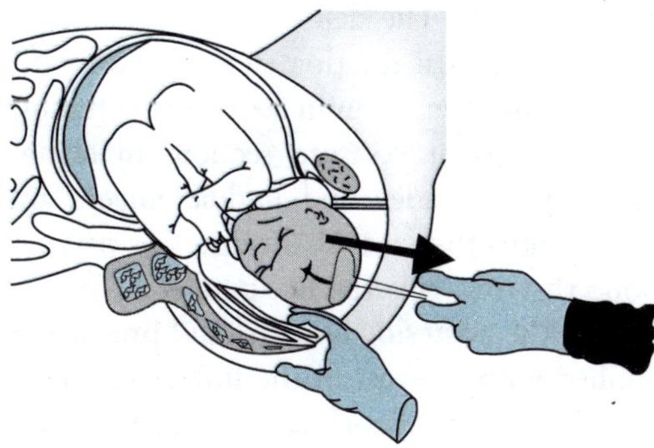

FIGURE 30.5B: DIRECTION OF TRACTION FORCE DURING VACUUM EXTRACTION IN THE LOWER PELVIC STATION

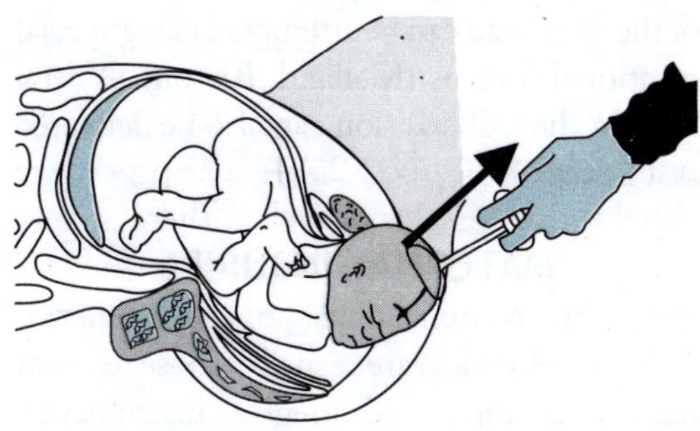

FIGURE 30.5C: DIRECTION OF TRACTION FORCE DURING VACUUM EXTRACTION ONCE THE BIPARIETAL DIAMETER HAS PASSED BEYOND THE PUBIC ARCH

pelvis using the left hand. The right branch is applied to the right side of the maternal pelvis using the right hand. There are over 700 types of forceps. They are grouped into two major categories—classical and special. Classical forceps are related to the instruments originally designed by Sir James Y Simpson (1848) and George Elliot (1858) (Hayashi 2006). This group includes the Simpson, Luikart-Simpson, Elliot, Neville-Barnes, DeLee, Anderson, Tucker-McLane, Wrigley and Naegle forceps. Classical forceps are a pair, right and left, made up of a handle, shank, lock and blade. In some types, a traction bar facilitates traction. Simpson forceps have a spread shank and a long cephalic curve. Elliot forceps have overlapping shanks and a shorter cephalic curve. In the Luikart-Simpson forceps, the blade is pseudo-fenestrated while in the Tucker-McLane forceps, it is solid.

Kielland forceps are special forceps designed for the correction of malposition and asynclitism and for rotational deliveries. The Barton forceps are used for transverse arrest in a flat pelvis, while the Piper forceps aid in the delivery of the aftercoming head in breech presentations. Other types of special forceps include the Laufe and Zeppelin, Moolgaoker and Shute.

The mechanism of action of forceps includes correction of deflexion, asynclitism or positional abnormalities of the fetal head, extraction by assisting or replacing the maternal expulsive forces, reduction of the friction between the fetal head and the birth canal and transient reduction of the resistance of the outlet by enlargement of the soft tissue of the birth canal. The main parameters that determine the outcome and associated morbidity of forceps delivery are the station of the fetal head and the degree of rotation required.

The choice of the type of forceps depends on the indication and clinical situation, preferences of the obstetrician and availability of instruments. A moulded fetal head is more accurately accommodated by the Simpson-type forceps and an unmoulded head by an Elliot-type forceps. Non-fenestrated blades are indicated in edematous soft maternal tissues to minimise risk of tearing. Face presentation with the mentoanterior position can be delivered using Kielland or Simpson forceps.

Application of the forceps to the fetal head is extremely important for a safe procedure and a successful outcome. The exact location of the sagittal suture and posterior fontanelle should be known and the final arrangement of the forceps branches should be 'ghosted' prior to insertion. The forceps should be applied gently between contractions. No force should be required, and if there is resistance, the blade should be removed and reapplied.

The blades are correctly placed when they are situated in the spaces between the fetal orbits and ears. Prior to applying traction, the obstetrician should ensure that:

- The forceps have not inadvertently penetrated the lateral vaginal walls
- The sagittal suture is perpendicular and symmetrically between the two blades
- The posterior fontanelle is palpable 2–3 cm above the plane of the shanks but not within the borders of the blade
- The handles, which should not require any pressure to close completely, are pointing straight out and not to either side (Fig. 30.6a)

No significant part of the fenestration of either blade should be palpable in front of the fetal head, that is, a space of not more than one finger between the head and the heel of the blade should be seen (Fig. 30.6b).

Once the forceps have been applied and the position of the blades checked, traction should be coordinated with maternal contractions. The axis of the traction forces should follow the pelvic curve—curve of Carus (Fig. 30.6c). The traction is initially downward and as the head descends in the birth canal, the angle moves forward and upward at the outlet. The Pajot maneuver involves the combined exertion of outward and downward forces, which produce a vector that follows the curve of Carus (Fig. 30.6d). Traction should be released between contractions to reduce the intracranial pressure and the associated vagally induced bradycardia. It is essential that the fetal heart rate is continuously monitored.

The OT position of the fetal head results in a deep transverse arrest and cephalopelvic disproportion. The delivery options include digital or manual rotation, autorotation with traction using a vacuum extractor, rotation with forceps or cesarean section. In digital rotation, the index and middle fingers are placed onto the part of the anterior parietal bone that overlaps the occipital bone in the area of the posterior fontanel and pressure is applied with the tips of the fingers to rotate the posterior fontanel upward and toward the symphysis pubis. In manual rotation, rotational pressure is applied by the hand under the posterior parietal bone and the thumb on the anterior parietal bone. Rotation of the fetal head can be attempted using special rotational forceps (Kielland, Barton). A fetal head in the OP position can also be delivered as a direct OP.

MATERNAL INJURIES

Maternal complications of instrumental vaginal deliveries are usually those of soft tissue trauma. Although instrumental delivery has been associated with a higher incidence of maternal injuries compared to spontaneous vaginal deliveries, most of the complications caused by instrumental vaginal

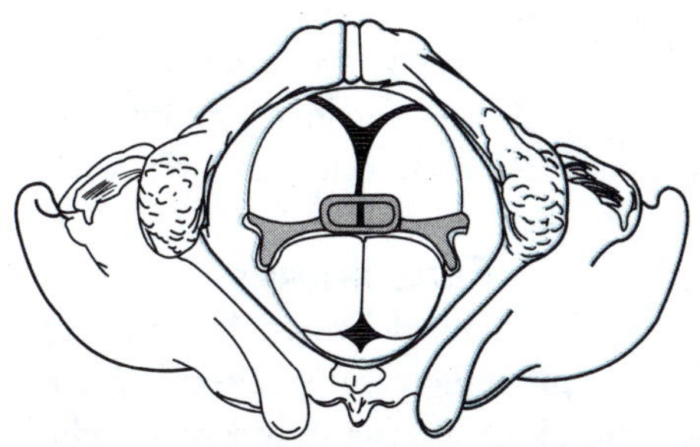

Figure 30.6a: Application of forceps on fetal head. The shank of the forceps should be in line with the sagittal suture and there should not be more than one finger space between the heel of the blades and the head.

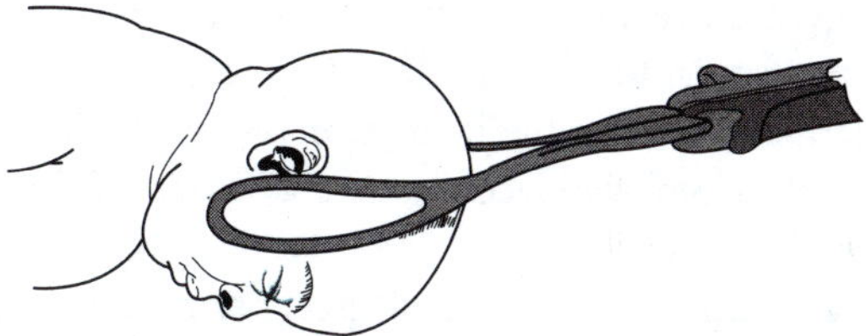

Figure 30.6b: Application of forceps on fetal head. The shank of the forceps should be 2-3 cm below the occiput, coinciding with the flexion point.

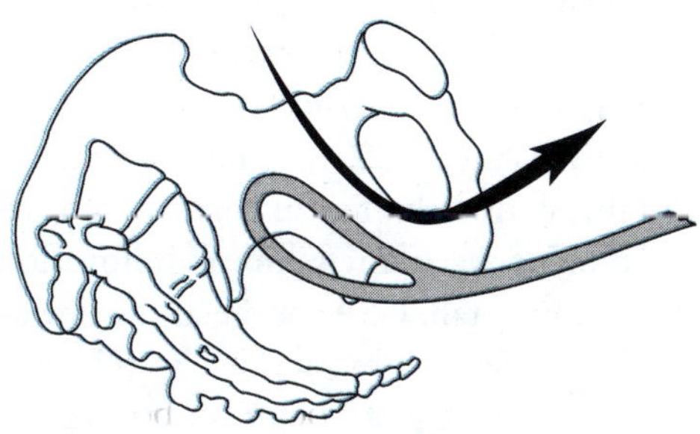

Figure 30.6c: The curve of Carus indicating the direction of traction at different levels in the pelvis

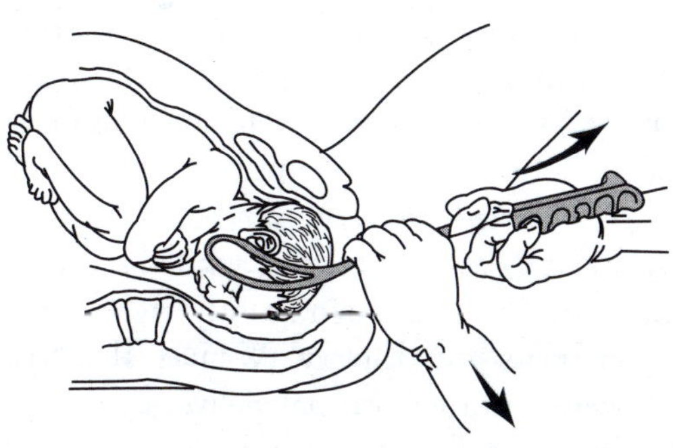

Figure 30.6d: Traction forces during forceps delivery. Pajot's maneuver and traction are used to achieve a downward and outward pull.

delivery can occur after a spontaneous vaginal delivery as well. Vaginal, cervical, labial and peri-urethral lacerations, pelvic hematomas, perineal injuries, episiotomy extension and the associated hemorrhage are the most common complications.

Maternal injury is less frequent and less extensive with the use of vacuum when compared to forceps (Johanson et al 1993; Johanson and Menon 2000; Wen et al 2001). Maternal complications of vacuum delivery include cervical lacerations, severe vaginal lacerations, periurethral lacerations (Johnson et al 2004), vaginal hematomas, and third- and fourth-degree tears (Johanson and Menon 2000). The use of forceps has been associated with a higher rate of episiotomies and third- and fourth-degree perineal and vaginal tears (Johnson et al 2004).

The most common vaginal lacerations are the posterior midline tears or the anterior peri-urethral tears. Inadvertent entrapment of the cervix or the vaginal wall with consequent lacerations can occur during an instrumental delivery. Posterior tears should be repaired if they involve more than the vaginal mucosa (Gilstrap 2002). Anterior labial and periurethral tears do not usually require repair unless they are bleeding. Injury to the bladder or to the urethra may cause urinary retention related to edema or hematoma and late fistula formation. Insertion of a Foley catheter is advisable if the tear is close to the urethra. Sidewall lacerations may extend into the ischiorectal fossae.

A third- or fourth- degree perineal tear with anal sphincter injury is a potentially severe complication of vaginal delivery which may result in anal incontinence and rectovaginal fistula formation (Hudelist et al 2005). Third-degree perineal tear and altered fecal continence occurs more frequently after forceps than vacuum deliveries (Fitzpatrick et al 2003) and in the OP positions (Damron et al 2004; Wu et al 2005). The incidence rate of third- or fourth-degree perineal tears with forceps-assisted delivery can be as high as 31% and 17%, respectively, with the use of vacuum. This rate is significantly higher than at an unassisted delivery (Wen et al 2001). However, normal vaginal delivery without evidence of sphincter injury is also associated with significant effect on anal sphincter function (Rieger et al 1997). Anal incontinence can occur regardless of the mode of delivery (Nygaard et al 1997).

Dimpfl et al (1992) suggested that vaginal delivery itself predisposes the patient for permanent stress urinary incontinence, although factors that increase trauma to the pelvic floor musculature and its innervation, including forceps and vacuum delivery, may contribute to the occurrence of urinary incontinence. Arya et al (2001) found that in primiparous women, urinary incontinence after forceps delivery is more likely to persist than with spontaneous vaginal or vacuum delivery. Liebling et al (2004) studied the symptoms of pelvic floor morbidity after difficult instrumental vaginal delivery and cesarean section during the second stage of labour and concluded that although cesarean section does not completely protect women from pelvic floor morbidity, instrumental delivery was associated with a greater prevalence of urinary symptoms and dyspareunia for up to one year after delivery.

Fetal Injuries

Nearly all infants delivered by vacuum or forceps will exhibit scalp effects. Most of these effects are transient and of no clinical significance. The more significant injuries are related to wrong placement of the instrument, excessive or poorly directed traction or cephalopelvic disproportion (McQuivey 2004).

The incidence of scalp abrasions and lacerations after vacuum extraction is 10%. The majority are superficial and of a minor degree (McQuivey 2004). The incidence of scalp abrasions is higher in infants delivered by Omnicup vacuum (Clinical Innovations Inc, Murray, Utah, USA) or metal cup devices than those delivered by silastic cup (Hayman et al 2002). Bruising of >5 cm and lacerations are more frequent in vacuum deliveries by metal cup. However, no difference between deliveries by Omnicup and the standard silastic cup was found (Attilakos et al 2005). Scalp injuries can be prevented with correct cup placement and traction, and avoidance of cup detachments or 'pop-offs' (McQuivey 2004). The use of protective covers over forceps reduces the rates of neonatal facial abrasions and skin bruises (Roshan et al 2005).

Caput succedaneum is a serosanguinous, extraperiosteal collection that extends across the midline and over the suture lines (as opposed to a cephalhematoma). It is caused by the mechanical compression of the presenting part of the fetal cranium pushing through a dilating cervix.

Vacuum extraction causes a collection of interstitial fluid and microhemorrhages (chignon) that fills the internal diameter of the vacuum cup in a 'key-in-lock' fashion. It is created by the pressure gradient between the vacuum and the mean arterial pressure of the fetus. It is less pronounced when using soft cups rather than rigid cups. The chignon is most obvious immediately following removal of the cup, but typically resolves within 12–18 hours and has no long-term sequelae (McQuivey 2004).

Cephalhematoma is a subperiosteal collection, secondary to rupture of blood vessels, between the skull and the periosteum. It does not cross a suture line and can thus be differentiated from the subgaleal hemorrhage. The mean incidence of cephalhematoma following vacuum extraction is 6% (range 1–26%) (Johanson and Menon 2000; Vacca 2002). A randomised controlled trial showed that metal cups are more likely to cause cephalhematoma than silastic cups or the Omnicup (Attilakos et al 2005). Forceps and breech deliveries are also associated with cephalhematoma (Uhing 2005). No difference in the incidence of cephalhematoma was reported in a study comparing a sequential operative vaginal delivery and cesarean section following a failed vacuum delivery (Sadan et al 2003).

Uncomplicated cephalhematomas resolve within a few weeks. Whitlow et al (2005) recommended that cephalohematomas and subgaleal hemorrhages may be prevented by observing the traction force indicators of the vacuum devices.

Subgaleal, also known as subaponeurotic hemorrhage can be a life-threatening complication that develops between the periosteum of the skull and the galea aponeurotica. The mortality of subgaleal hemorrhage approaches 25% (Amar et al 2003). The traction force applied during instrumental delivery pulls the aponeurosis from the cranium, causing subgaleal hemorrhage. Vacuum extraction (OR = 7.17; 95% CI: 5.43–10.25) and forceps delivery (OR = 2.66; 95% CI: 1.78–5.18) are risk factors associated with subgaleal hemorrhage (Gebremariam 1999). The incidence of subgaleal hemorrhage is 4 in 10,000 spontaneous vaginal deliveries and 59 in 10,000 vacuum-assisted deliveries (Uchil et al 2003). Maternal nulliparity, placement of vacuum extraction cup over the sagittal suture at a distance close to infant's anterior fontanelle and failed vacuum extraction predisposes the baby to subgaleal hemorrhage (Boo et al 2005).

A subgaleal hemorrhage presents as diffuse swelling or a fluctuant mass. It crosses suture lines and shifts dependently when the infant's head is repositioned. Loss of 20–40% of the circulating blood volume will result in hypovolemic shock (Uchil and Arulkumaran 2003).

Cranial and intracranial injuries are frequently associated with physical difficulty at delivery and the use of instruments, notably with the sequential use of different instruments (Gardella et al 2001; O'Mahony et al 2005).

Skull fractures are usually linear (affecting the parietal bones) or depressed, forming the so-called *ping-pong ball-type* fracture (Hughes et al 1999; Uhing 2005). They are caused by compression from the forceps blades or from the skull pushing against the maternal bony pelvis. A skull fracture must be suspected in any cephalhematoma or subarachnoid hemorrhage (Hughes et al 1999).

Intracranial hemorrhage in term infants can be potentially fatal or cause lifelong disability. It occurs in approximately 5-6 out of every 10,000 live births. Risk factors include forceps and vacuum delivery, precipitous delivery, prolonged second stage of labour and macrosomia (Sachs et al 1987; Pollina et al 2001).

Forceps delivery is six times more likely to be complicated by subarachnoid or subdural hemorrhage than spontaneous vaginal delivery (Jhawar et al 2003).

Epidural hemorrhage is a collection of blood in a cleavage between the calvarial bone and its inner periosteum or between the periosteal membrane and the underlying outer dura fibrous stratum. It is associated with difficult parturition and instrumental delivery in nulliparous women. Association with breech delivery has also been reported (Negishi et al 1989). Like other head injuries, epidural hemorrhage in neonates results from the mechanical forces exerted on the fetal head during birth, with or without instrumental interference (Hamlat et al 2005).

Subdural hemorrhage can be supratentorial or infratentorial and accounts for more than two-thirds of the cranial birth injuries in term neonates (Pollina et al 2001).

The incidence of subdural or cerebral hemorrhage is 2.9 in 10,000 after spontaneous delivery and 4.1 in 10,000 after cesarean section without labour. The incidence after vacuum delivery is 8.0 in 10,000, after forceps delivery, 9.8 in 10,000, after cesarean section following failed vaginal delivery and 25.7 in 10,000 and after combined vacuum and forceps delivery 21.3 in 10,000 (Towner et al 1999). These rates indicate that the injuries may be partly due to the underlying abnormality in the labour process, rather than to the mode of delivery.

Subdural hematomas have been diagnosed antenatally in utero (Hanigan et al 1985; Mateos et al 1987), and in asymptomatic newborns after uncomplicated vaginal deliveries (Holden et al 1999; Tavani et al 2003; Whitby et al 2004). The pathophysiology of a subdural hematoma involves mechanical compression and distortion of the fetal cranium during labour or *occipital osteodiastasis,* which is the separation of the squamous and lateral parts of the occipital bone, leading to rupture of the occipital sinus, direct cerebellar trauma and brainstem compression (Haase et al 2003).

Subdural hemorrhages present with apnea, unequal pupils, eye deviation, irritability, tense fontanelle, seizures and coma (Haase et al 2003; Uhing 2005). The long-term outcome depends on the size of the lesion and the presence of intraparenchymal lesions.

The incidence of subarachnoid hemorrhage after spontaneous vaginal delivery has the range of 1–1.3 in 10,000, 2.2–6 in 10,000 after vacuum extraction, 1–3.3 in 10,000 after forceps delivery and 10.7 in 10,000 after combined vacuum and forceps delivery (Towner et al 1999; Wen et al 2001).

Subarachnoid hemorrhage is most frequently caused by rupture of small veins bridging the leptomeninges (Perlman 2004). Clinical manifestations include seizures, irritability, recurrent apnea or depressed level of consciousness. Focal neurological signs may also be present.

The reported incidence of brachial plexus injury ranges between 0.13 and 3.6 for every 1000 births (Walle and Hartikainen-Sorri 1993; Gonen et al 1996; Perlow et al 1996; Graham et al 1997; Bryant et al 1998; Gilbert et al 1999; Piatt 2005). Risk factors include macrosomia, shoulder dystocia, instrumental deliveries and malpresentation (Perlow et al 1996; Ecker et al 1997; Gilbert et al 1999; Christoffersson and Rydhstroem 2002). The risk of brachial plexus injury is higher in forceps deliveries than vacuum extractions (Gilbert et al 1999; Towner et al 1999), however, other studies have shown that the risk between the two modes of delivery is similar (Wen et al 2001). Three principal types of brachial plexus injury are seen—Erb's palsy, Klumpke's palsy and injury to the entire cervical plexus. Injury to the upper plexus (Erb's palsy) involves injury to C5–C7, and accounts for approximately 90% of cases (Uhing 2005). Klumpke's palsy is rare and accounts for less than 1% of brachial plexus injury. It involves the C8 and T1 nerves. The entire plexus is involved in approximately 10% of cases, which results in a flaccid extremity with absent reflexes. Erb's palsy is associated with injury to the phrenic nerve, which is innervated with fibres from C3–C5. Klumpke's palsy is associated with ipsilateral Horner's syndrome (ptosis, miosis, anhydrosis) when there is accompanying injury to the sympathetic fibres of T1. The pathogenesis of injury often involves stretch injury when shoulder dystocia requires extreme lateral flexion and traction of the head. However, there are reports of injuries that occur when lateral flexion and traction of the head has not been applied, such as during precipitous deliveries or when there is injury to the posterior shoulder (Dunn et al 1985; Acker et al 1988; Walle and Hartikainen-Sorri 1993; Hankins and Clark 1995; Gherman et al 1999; Sandmire et al 2000; Jennett et al 2002).

Diagnosis is usually made by physical examination. Approximately 90% of brachial plexus injuries recover spontaneously (Greenwald et al 1984; Michelow et al 1994). Injuries of the fifth and sixth cervical nerve roots have good prognosis. Total plexus and lower plexus injury have poor prognosis. Initial treatment is conservative (Shenaq et al 1998). Surgical exploration may be considered in infants without recovery.

Facial nerve palsy occurs in approximately 0.06–0.7% of births (Uhing 2005). Risk factors include instrumental delivery (Towner et al 1999; Wen et al 2001) and a prolonged second stage of labour (Perlow et al 1996). The incidence of this type of injury following a spontaneous vaginal delivery is 0.3–0.4 for every 1000 births, following vacuum extraction 0.5–1.2 for every 1000 and after forceps delivery 4.5– 5.1 per 1000 (Towner et al 1999; Wen et al 2001). Forceps delivery is therefore five times more likely to cause facial nerve palsy than vacuum extraction. The pathogenesis of this injury is related to the compression of the peripheral portion of the nerve by forceps or by prolonged pressure against the maternal sacral promontory. Clinical manifestations include weakness of upper and lower facial muscles. Signs of external injury to the head and face, such as lacerations and bruising, may be present. The prognosis is good in more than 90% of the cases.

Laryngeal nerve injury causes vocal fold paralysis; 5–26% of congenital vocal fold paralysis is due to birth trauma (Cohen et al 1982; Emery et al 1984; Daya et al 2000). Forceps deliveries have been associated with an increased incidence of vocal cord paralysis (Daya et al 2000).

Upper cervical spinal cord injury is estimated to complicate approximately 1 in 80,000 deliveries (Mills et al 2001). High cervical injuries are associated most often with forceps rotation of 90° or more from the OP or OT position during vertex delivery. Menticoglou et al (1995) reported an incidence of spinal cord injury of approximately 0.7 in 1000 and suggested that these injuries are the result of 'nonphysiological torsional forces'. However, spinal cord injury has been described following cesarean section with cephalic presentation (Morgan et al 2001).

The injury is caused by longitudinal traction or rotation of the cord. Most cases of spinal cord birth injury occur without bony injury. Such an injury is termed, spinal cord injury without radiographic abnormality or

SCIWORA (Caird et al 2005). Lesions above C4 are almost always associated with apnea (Menticoglou et al 1995). In injuries between C4 and T4, the phrenic nerve and innervation to the intercostal muscles may be involved, leading to respiratory distress. In general, prognosis is poor (MacKinnon et al 1993; Menticoglou et al 1995).

In a forceps delivery, the risk of occurrence of this type of injury can be minimised by avoiding excessive torsion during rotation, rotation in the wrong direction, forceful rotation or combined rotation with traction. In a rotational delivery, the movements of traction and rotation should always be separate, unless rotation occurs spontaneously with traction. Rotation should also be avoided during a uterine contraction (Menticoglou et al 1995).

Minor ocular traumas, including retinal hemorrhages, subconjunctival hemorrhages, and lid edema are common after delivery (Holden et al 1992). Retinal hemorrhage occurs more commonly in infants delivered by vacuum than spontaneous or forceps-assisted deliveries (Berkus et al 1985; Williams et al 1993). However, hemorrhage is transient with no apparent long-term developmental or ophthalmological consequences (Johanson et al 1993).

Choice of Instrument

Studies about instrumental vaginal deliveries include prospective randomised trials that compared the outcomes after forceps deliveries and vacuum extractions (Johanson et al 1993; 1999; Johanson and Menon 2000). The comparison of these two techniques is difficult because of the differences in inclusion criteria, types of instruments or outcomes. Retrospective studies reviewed the effect of different modes of delivery on maternal and neonatal morbidity (Towner et al 1999; Johnson et al 2004). However, most retrospective studies are based on large databases which lack clinical details of importance and they may be susceptible to confounding and bias (Towner et al 1999; Wen et al 2001). A Cochrane review (Johanson and Menon 2000) suggested that vacuum is more likely to fail as the instrument of delivery than forceps.

Forceps require increased maternal analgesia and result in increased incidence of perineal trauma (Hudelist et al 2005) and episiotomy (Johnson et al 2004). Vacuum delivery is associated with less severe lacerations than forceps delivery, as well as less perineal pain at 24 hours post-delivery.

Neonatal complication rates are similar in both, forceps and vacuum-delivered groups. Cephalohematomas and retinal hemorrhages are more common in vacuum deliveries. Fetal scalp injuries, external ocular injuries and facial nerve palsies are more common with forceps deliveries. Serious complications are rare for both types of instrumental delivery but can be fatal (Towner et al 1999). Delivery by two operative interventions (cesarean section following a failed vacuum attempt or forceps attempt, or vacuum and forceps birth) is more likely to lead to a serious injury or death compared to delivery by any one of these interventions alone (Morales et al 1995; Towner et al 1999; Gardella et al 2001; Sadan et al 2003).

A five-year follow up of a randomised controlled trial did not show any significant differences between these two modes of delivery for the mother or the child (Johanson et al 1999).

The Royal College of Obstetricians and Gynaecologists recommends that the choice of instrument should be appropriate to the clinical circumstances and the operator's skills (RCOG 2005).

Sequential Instrumental Deliveries

Earlier studies that compared failed vacuum deliveries, completed either by forceps or by cesarean section, did not show important differences in maternal or neonatal outcomes (Berkus et al 1986). Two other retrospective studies did not show any difference in outcomes between successful vacuum extractions and failed vacuum extractions followed by forceps (Gray et al 1988; Ezenagu et al 1999).

Gardella et al (2001) found that the sequential use of vacuum and forceps was associated with increased incidence of intracranial hemorrhage, brachial plexus and facial nerve injury, depressed 5-minute Apgar score, assisted ventilation, seizure, fourth-degree and other lacerations, hematoma and postpartum hemorrhage. However, this was also a retrospective study based on databases and did not include information about the sequence, number of applications or duration of instrument application at the time of delivery. Fetal station was also not determined.

Comparing the risk of maternal and neonatal morbidity associated with the use of each instrument with the risk associated with the combined use of vacuum and forceps, they found a synergistic interaction effect. The neonatal outcomes are in agreement with Towner et al (1999), who demonstrated a significant increased risk of subdural or cerebral hemorrhage, subarachnoid hemorrhage and facial nerve and brachial plexus injury in sequential vacuum and forceps deliveries.

Similar findings (increased maternal and neonatal trauma after failed instrumental delivery and use of multiple instruments) were observed when excessive pulls and multiple instruments were associated with an initial attempt at vaginal delivery by an inexperienced operator (Murphy et al 2003).

More recently, Sadan et al (2003) attempted to compare the outcomes between a sequential operative vaginal delivery and a cesarean section following a failed vacuum delivery. This cross-sectional study suggested that a cesarean delivery, after a failed vacuum delivery, was associated with more postpartum anemia, meconium-stained amniotic fluid and lower pH. There was no difference in Apgar scores and the incidence of respiratory distress syndrome, cephalhematoma or jaundice. They concluded that in failed attempted vacuum delivery, the risk of injury to the neonate is increased irrespective of the chosen method of delivery and therefore, the choice of the method of delivery under the given circumstances rests on the judgement of the obstetrician.

Training

An important prerequisite for the conduction of instrumental delivery is a skilled operator. The obstetrician must be able to adequately assess the capacity of the bony pelvis, and any soft tissue obstruction; determine that the cervix is fully dilated and that the fetal vertex is engaged; and appreciate the fetal position and station. It is also important to determine flexion, asynclitism, caput and moulding. The forceps blades or the vacuum cup must be applied correctly to the fetal vertex in order to minimise the risk of injury. The amount of force used should be minimal and traction should be applied in the direction of least resistance (Gilstrap 2002).

The decrease in the number of forceps deliveries has had an impact on the residents' training opportunities. The concern for litigation has led to decreased usage and teaching in forceps delivery. This has had a major impact on training, leading to a lesser degree of technical proficiency. In turn, this may increase the incidence of complications, thereby initiating a vicious circle.

Vacuum delivery is generally perceived to be an easier technique to learn than the use of obstetric forceps; however, poor case selection and incorrect use of this technique are likely to result in increased rates of failure and complications. The RCOG recommends that only practitioners who are adequately trained, or who are under the supervision of trained practitioners, should undertake instrumental delivery (RCOG 2005).

The current educational methodology in the UK encourages the use of skills and drills scenarios with mannequins and models. Cheong et al addressed the issue of training by conducting a case-control study on the impact of formal education and training on the outcome of instrumental delivery. They concluded that there were no differences in the failure rates between the two groups. However, the introduction of an educational package resulted in a significant decrease in maternal morbidity associated with cervical, severe labial and high vaginal tears, as well as a decrease in neonatal morbidity associated with admission to special care baby unit (SCBU), severe neonatal scalp injury and facial injuries. Thus, formal education and training can be associated with improved safety for mother and baby (Cheong et al 2004).

Conclusion Obstetricians often face dilemmas in the management of labour. Careful consideration of the mode and timing of each intervention for the completion of the birth process is required. Instrumental vaginal deliveries include the risks of failure and complications. The risks of different techniques are important factors in the decision-making process. The most appropriate intervention needs to be selected after consideration of the operator's skills and experience as well as the clinical circumstances. An alternative plan that will result in a safe and expeditious birth should be made available.

References

Acker DB, KD Gregory, BP Sachs et al. 1988. Risk factors for Erb-Duchenne palsy. *Obstet Gynecol* 71 (3 Pt 1):389–392.

ACOG. 2000. Operative vaginal delivery. *Report No.: No 17*. Washington DC: American College of Obstetricians and Gynecologists.

Amar AP, HE Aryan, HS Meltzer et al. 2003. Neonatal subgaleal hematoma causing brain compression: report of two cases and review of the literature. *Neurosurgery* 52 (6):1470–1474.

Arya LA, ND Jackson, DL Myers et al. 2001. Risk of new-onset urinary incontinence after forceps and vacuum delivery in primiparous women. *Am J Obstet Gynecol* 185 (6):1318–1323.

Attilakos G, T Sibanda, C Winter et al. 2005. A randomised controlled trial of a new handheld vacuum extraction device. *Br J Obstet Gynaecol* 112 (11):1510–1515.

Baskett TF and S Arulkumaran. 2002. Intrapartum care for the MRCOG and beyond. London: RCOG Press; 63–74.

Berkus MD, RS Ramamurthy, PS O'Connor et al. 1985. Cohort study of silastic obstetric vacuum cup deliveries: I. Safety of the instrument. *Obstet Gynecol* 66 (4):503–509.

Berkus MD, RS Ramamurthy, PS O'Connor et al. 1986. Cohort study of Silastic obstetric vacuum cup deliveries: II. Unsuccessful vacuum extraction. *Obstet Gynecol* 68 (5):662–666.

Bird GC. 1982. The use of the vacuum extractor. *Clin Obstet Gynaecol* 9 (3):641–661.
Boo NY, KW Foong, ZA Mahdy et al. 2005. Risk factors associated with subaponeurotic haemorrhage in full-term infants exposed to vacuum extraction. *Br J Obstet Gynaecol* 112 (11):1516–1521.
Bryant DR, MR Leonardi, JB Landwehr et al. 1998. Limited usefulness of fetal weight in predicting neonatal brachial plexus injury. *Am J Obstet Gynecol* 179 (3 Pt 1):686–689.
Caird MS, S Reddy, TJ Ganley et al. 2005. Cervical spine fracture-dislocation birth injury: prevention, recognition, and implications for the orthopaedic surgeon. *J Pediatr Orthop* 25 (4):484–486.
Chalmers JA and I Chalmers. 1989. The obstetric vacuum extractor is the instrument of first choice for operative vaginal delivery. *Br J Obstet Gynaecol* 96 (5):505–506.
Cheong YC, H Abdullahi, H Lashen et al. 2004. Can formal education and training improve the outcome of instrumental delivery? *Eur J Obstet Gynecol Reprod Biol* 113 (2):139–144.
Christoffersson M and H Rydhstroem. 2002. Shoulder dystocia and brachial plexus injury: a population-based study. *Gynecol Obstet Invest* 53 (1):42–47.
Cohen SR, KA Geller, JW Birns et al. 1982. Laryngeal paralysis in children: a long-term retrospective study. *Ann Otol Rhinol Laryngol* 91 (4 Pt 1):417–424.
Damron DP and EL Capeless. 2004. Operative vaginal delivery: a comparison of forceps and vacuum for success rate and risk of rectal sphincter injury. *Am J Obstet Gynecol* 191 (3):907–910.
Daya H, A Hosni, I Bejar-Solar et al. 2000. Pediatric vocal fold paralysis: a long-term retrospective study. *Arch Otolaryngol Head Neck Surg* 126 (1):21–5.
Dimpfl T, U Hesse and B Schussler. 1992. Incidence and cause of postpartum urinary stress incontinence. *Eur J Obstet Gynecol Reprod Biol* 43 (1):29–33.
Dunn DW and WA Engle. 1985. Brachial plexus palsy: intrauterine onset. *Pediatr Neurol* 1 (6): 367–369.
Ecker JL, JA Greenberg, ER Norwitz et al. 1997. Birth weight as a predictor of brachial plexus injury. *Obstet Gynecol* 89 (5 Pt 1):643–647.
Emery PJ and B Fearon. 1984. Vocal cord palsy in pediatric practice: a review of 71 cases. *Int J Pediatr Otorhinolaryngol* 8 (2):147–154.
Ezenagu LC, R Kakaria and JA Bofill. 1999. Sequential use of instruments at operative vaginal delivery: is it safe? *Am J Obstet Gynecol* 180 (6 Pt 1):1446–1449.
Fitzpatrick M, M Behan, PR O'Connell et al. 2003. Randomised clinical trial to assess anal sphincter function following forceps or vacuum assisted vaginal delivery. *Br J Obstet Gynaecol* 110 (4):424–429.
Gardella C, M Taylor, T Benedetti et al. 2001. The effect of sequential use of vacuum and forceps for assisted vaginal delivery on neonatal and maternal outcomes. *Am J Obstet Gynecol* 185 (4):896–902.
Gebremariam A. 1999. Subgaleal haemorrhage: risk factors and neurological and developmental outcome in survivors. *Ann Trop Paediatr* 19 (1):45–50.
Gherman RB, JG Ouzounian and TM Goodwin. 1999. Brachial plexus palsy: an in utero injury? *Am J Obstet Gynecol* 180 (5):1303–1307.
Gilbert WM, TS Nesbitt and B Danielsen. 1999. Associated factors in 1611 cases of brachial plexus injury. *Obstet Gynecol* 93 (4):536–540.
Gilstrap LC. Gary Cunningham and JP VanDorsten. 2002. *Operative Obstetrics*. 2nd edn, ed FG Cunningham and V JP New York: McGraw-Hill.
Gonen R, D Spiegel and M Abend. 1996. Is macrosomia predictable, and are shoulder dystocia and birth trauma preventable? *Obstet Gynecol* 88 (4 Pt 1):526–529.

Graham EM, I Forouzan and MA Morgan. 1997. A retrospective analysis of Erb's palsy cases and their relation to birth weight and trauma at delivery. *J Matern Fetal Med* 6 (1):1–5.

Gray DL and DM Nelson. 1988. Cord blood acid-base status in neonates delivered by silastic vacuum cup extraction: comparison with forceps and spontaneous deliveries. *Obstet Gynecol* 71 (1):76–80.

Greenwald AG, PC Schute and JL Shiveley. 1984. Brachial plexus birth palsy: a 10-year report on the incidence and prognosis. *J Pediatr Orthop* 4 (6):689–692.

Haase R, I Kursawe, F Nagel et al. 2003. Acute subdural hematoma after caesarean section: a case report. *Pediatr Crit Care Med* 4 (2):246–248.

Hamlat A, A Heckly, M Adn et al. 2005. Pathophysiology of intracranial epidural haematoma following birth. *Med Hypotheses*.

Hanigan WC, MB Ali, TJ Cusack et al. 1985. Diagnosis of subdural hemorrhage in utero. Case report. *J Neurosurg* 63 (6):977–979.

Hankins GD and SL Clark. 1995. Brachial plexus palsy involving the posterior shoulder at spontaneous vaginal delivery. *Am J Perinatol* 12 (1):44–45.

Hayashi R. 2006. Assisted Vaginal Delivery. In *High Risk Pregnancy. Management Options*, 3rd edn, ed D James, PJ Steer, CP Weiner et al, 1514–1530. Philadelphia: Saunders Elsevier.

Hayman R, J Gilby and S Arulkumaran. 2002. Clinical evaluation of a "hand pump" vacuum delivery device. *Obstet Gynecol* 100 (6):1190–1195.

Holden KR, MO Titus and P van Tassel. 1999. Cranial magnetic resonance imaging examination of normal term neonates: a pilot study. *J Child Neurol* 14 (11):708–710.

Holden R, DG Morsman, GM Davidek et al. 1992. External ocular trauma in instrumental and normal deliveries. *Br J Obstet Gynaecol* 99 (2):132–134.

Hudelist G, J Gellen, C Singer et al. 2005. Factors predicting severe perineal trauma during childbirth: role of forceps delivery routinely combined with mediolateral episiotomy. *Am J Obstet Gynecol* 192 (3):875–881.

Hughes CA, EH Harley, G Milmoe et al. 1999. Birth trauma in the head and neck. *Arch Otolaryngol Head Neck Surg* 125 (2):193–199.

Jennett RJ, TJ Tarby and RL Krauss. 2002. Erb's palsy contrasted with Klumpke's and total palsy: different mechanisms are involved. *Am J Obstet Gynecol* 186 (6):1216–1219; discussion 9–20.

Jhawar BS, A Ranger, D Steven et al. 2003. Risk factors for intracranial hemorrhage among full-term infants: a case-control study. *Neurosurgery* 52 (3):581–590; discussion 8–90.

Johanson R and V Menon. 2000. Soft versus rigid vacuum extractor cups for assisted vaginal delivery. *Cochrane Database Syst Rev*, (2):CD000446.

Johanson RB and BK Menon. 2000. Vacuum extraction versus forceps for assisted vaginal delivery. *Cochrane Database Syst Rev* (2):CD000224.

Johanson RB, C Rice, M Doyle et al. 1993. A randomised prospective study comparing the new vacuum extractor policy with forceps delivery. *Br J Obstet Gynaecol* 100 (6):524–530.

Johanson RB, E Heycock, J Carter et al. 1999. Maternal and child health after assisted vaginal delivery: five-year follow up of a randomised controlled study comparing forceps and ventouse. *Br J Obstet Gynaecol* 106 (6):544–549.

Johnson JH, R Figueroa, D Garry et al. 2004. Immediate maternal and neonatal effects of forceps and vacuum-assisted deliveries. *Obstet Gynecol* 103 (3):513–518.

Kozak LJ and JD Weeks. 2002. U.S. trends in obstetric procedures, 1990–2000. *Birth* 29 (3): 157–161.

Liebling RE, R Swingler, RR Patel et al. 2004. Pelvic floor morbidity up to one year after difficult instrumental delivery and cesarean section in the second stage of labor: a cohort study. *Am J Obstet Gynecol* 191 (1):4–10.

MacKinnon JA, M Perlman, H Kirpalani et al. 1993. Spinal cord injury at birth: diagnostic and prognostic data in twenty-two patients. *J Pediatr* 122 (3):431–437.

Mateos F, J Esteban, JT Ramos et al. 1987. Fetal subdural hematoma: diagnosis in utero. Case report. *Pediatr Neurosci* 13 (3):125–128.

McQuivey RW. 2004. Vacuum-assisted delivery: a review. *J Matern Fetal Neonatal Med* 16 (3):171–180.

Menticoglou SM, M Perlman and FA Manning. 1995. High cervical spinal cord injury in neonates delivered with forceps: report of 15 cases. *Obstet Gynecol* 86 (4 Pt 1):589–594.

Michelow BJ, HM Clarke, CG Curtis et al. 1994. The natural history of obstetrical brachial plexus palsy. *Plast Reconstr Surg* 93 (4):675–680; discussion 81.

Miksovsky P and WJ Watson. 2001. Obstetric vacuum extraction: state of the art in the new millennium. *Obstet Gynecol Surv* 56 (11):736–751.

Mills JF, PA Dargaville, LT Coleman et al. 2001. Upper cervical spinal cord injury in neonates: the use of magnetic resonance imaging. *J Pediatr* 138 (1):105–108.

Morales R, CD Adair, L Sanchez-Ramos et al. 1995. Vacuum extraction of preterm infants with birth weights of 1,500–2,499 grams. *J Reprod Med* 40 (2):127–130.

Morgan C and SJ Newell. 2001. Cervical spinal cord injury following cephalic presentation and delivery by Caesarean section. *Dev Med Child Neurol* 43 (4):274–276.

Murphy DJ, RE Liebling, R Patel et al. 2003. Cohort study of operative delivery in the second stage of labour and standard of obstetric care. *Br J Obstet Gynaecol* 110 (6):610–615.

Negishi H, Y Lee, K Itoh et al. 1989. Nonsurgical management of epidural hematoma in neonates. *Pediatr Neurol* 5 (4):253–256.

Nygaard IE, SS Rao and JD Dawson. 1997. Anal incontinence after anal sphincter disruption: a 30-year retrospective cohort study. *Obstet Gynecol* 89 (6):896–901.

O'Mahony F, R Settatree, C Platt et al. 2005. Review of singleton fetal and neonatal deaths associated with cranial trauma and cephalic delivery during a national intrapartum-related confidential enquiry. *Br J Obstet Gynaecol* 112 (5):619–626.

Patel RR and DJ Murphy. 2004. Forceps delivery in modern obstetric practice. *Br Med J* 328 (7451):1302–1305.

Perlman JM. 2004. Brain injury in the term infant. *Semin Perinatol* 28 (6):415–424.

Perlow JH, T Wigton, J Hart et al. 1996. Birth trauma. A five-year review of incidence and associated perinatal factors. *J Reprod Med* 41 (10):754–760.

Piatt JH Jr. 2005. Birth injuries of the brachial plexus. *Clin Perinatol* 32 (1):39–59, v–vi.

Pollina J, MS Dias, V Li et al. 2001. Cranial birth injuries in term newborn infants. *Pediatr Neurosurg* 35 (3):113–119.

RCOG. 2005. Operative vaginal delivery. London: Royal College of Obstetricians and Gynaecologists.

Rieger N, A Schloithe, G Saccone et al. 1997. The effect of a normal vaginal delivery on anal function. *Acta Obstet Gynecol Scand* 76 (8):769–772.

Roshan DF, B Petrikovsky, L Sichinava et al. 2005. Soft forceps. *Int J Gynaecol Obstet* 88 (3):249–252.
Sachs BP, D Acker, R Tuomala et al. 1987. The incidence of symptomatic intracranial hemorrhage in term appropriate-for-gestation-age infants. *Clin Pediatr (Phila)* 26 (7):355–358.
Sadan O, S Ginath, A Gomel et al. 2003. What to do after a failed attempt of vacuum delivery? *Eur J Obstet Gynecol Reprod Biol* 107 (2):151–155.
Sandmire HF and RK DeMott. 2000. Erb's palsy: concepts of causation. *Obstet Gynecol* 95 (6 Pt 1):941–942.
Shenaq SM, E Berzin, R Lee et al. 1998. Brachial plexus birth injuries and current management. *Clin Plast Surg* 25 (4):527–536.
SOGC. 2004. Guidelines for Operative Vaginal Birth Society of Obstetricians and Gynaecologists of Canada. *Report No.: Guideline No 148*.
Tavani F, RA Zimmerman, RR Clancy et al. 2003. Incidental intracranial hemorrhage after uncomplicated birth: MRI before and after neonatal heart surgery. *Neuroradiology* 45 (4):253–258.
Towner D, MA Castro, E Eby-Wilkens et al. 1999. Effect of mode of delivery in nulliparous women on neonatal intracranial injury. *N Engl J Med* 341 (23):1709–1714.
Uchil D and S Arulkumaran. 2003. Neonatal subgaleal hemorrhage and its relationship to delivery by vacuum extraction. *Obstet Gynecol Surv* 58 (10):687–693.
Uhing MR. 2005. Management of birth injuries. *Clin Perinatol* 32 (1):19–38v.
Vacca A. 2002. Vacuum-assisted delivery. *Best Pract Res Clin Obstet Gynaecol* 16 (1):17–30.
Walle T and AL Hartikainen-Sorri. 1993. Obstetric shoulder injury. Associated risk factors, prediction and prognosis. *Acta Obstet Gynecol Scand* 72 (6):450–454.
Wen SW, S Liu, MS Kramer et al. 2001. Comparison of maternal and infant outcomes between vacuum extraction and forceps deliveries. *Am J Epidemiol* 153 (2):103–107.
Whitby EH, PD Griffiths, S Rutter et al. 2004. Frequency and natural history of subdural haemorrhages in babies and relation to obstetric factors. *Lancet* 363 (9412):846–851.
Whitlow BJ, O Tamizian, J Ashworth et al. 2005. Validation of traction force indicator in ventouse devices. *Int J Gynaecol Obstet* 90 (1):35–38.
Williams MC, RA Knuppel, WF O'Brien et al. 1993. Obstetric correlates of neonatal retinal hemorrhage. *Obstet Gynecol* 81 (5 (Pt 1)):688–694.
Wu JM, KS Williams, AF Hundley et al. 2005. Occiput posterior fetal head position increases the risk of anal sphincter injury in vacuum-assisted deliveries. *Am J Obstet Gynecol* 193 (2):525–528; discussion 8–9.

31

Obstructed Labour

Shashikala K Bhat

The case of Princess Charlotte of England is perhaps one of the famous accounts of obstructed labour. In 1817, the only eligible heir to the British throne went into labour after 42 weeks of gestation. Fifty hours later, after 24 hours of second stage and 6 hours of perineal pressure, she delivered a nine pound stillborn. About 5 hours after delivery, the Princess also died, presumably from hypovolemic shock as a result of uterine atony and post-partum hemorrhage. This was very likely connected to her obstructed labour. Three months later, Sir Richard Crofts, Princess Charlotte's obstetrician committed suicide, unable to bear the burden of responsibility for the death of the only heir to the throne. This event sometimes is historically referred to as the "Triple Obstetric Tragedy", as it resulted in the death of the infant, the patient and the obstetrician (Cron 2003).

The story is an example of the consequences of obstructed labour. The advances in obstetric care have made this complication obsolete in the developed world, but it continues to be a major problem affecting thousands of women in the less developed countries. Obstructed labour is one of the most common preventable causes of maternal and perinatal morbidity and mortality in the developing countries (Konje et al 2000). It is an important cause of maternal death in communities where undernutrition in childhood is common resulting in small pelvis in women, and there is also no easy access to health facilities capable of carrying out operative deliveries (Neilson et al 2003).

Nature and Magnitude of the Problem

Obstructed labour is the leading cause of hospitalisation comprising up to 39% of all obstetric patients in low resource countries (Mekbib et al 2003). Obstructed labour is the single most important cause of maternal death and is one of the three leading causes of perinatal mortality (Weeks et al 2005) with the case fatality rate of 87–100% (Berhan 2004). Maternal mortality ranges between 1% and 13%, and perinatal mortality between 74% and 92% (Rahman et al 2002, WHO Bulletin 2005). It is found to be directly or indirectly responsible for about half of all maternal deaths affecting mainly primigravida and grand multipara (Cox 1963, Gaym 2000). Maternal deaths occur as a result of ruptured uterus as well as genital sepsis in women having undergone cesarean section done for obstructed labour (WHO 2005, Rajaram et al 1995). Reports from India, Nigeria, Ghana, Ethiopia and Bangladesh indicate that up to 75% of cases of uterine rupture are seen with unscarred uterus and obstructed labour is one of the top five causes of maternal mortality (Kumar et al 1989; Tonks et al 1994; Dumont et al 2001; Geelhoed et al 2003; Bartlett et al 2005; Ebeigbe et al 2005; Onah et al 2005).

In countries where many women die from childbirth, many more suffer from significant morbidity from childbirth. Compared to the maternal mortality rate of 21 per 100,000 live births in developed countries, the rate is 1000 per 100,000 live births in the developing world (Cron 2003).

Definition Obstructed labour is seen when the progressive descent of the presenting part is arrested due to mechanical obstruction despite good uterine contractions (Philpott 1982; Adhikari et al 2005) . It is due to a mismatch between fetal size, more precisely, the presenting part of fetus, and the mother's pelvis (Neilson et al 2003). The mismatch may be due to genuine disproportion as when the vertex is in the occipitoanterior position, or relative disproportion due to deflexion and malposition (El-Hamamy 2005). It is a condition where further progress of labour is not possible without assistance (Lawson 1967; Konje et al 1992).

Contributory factors for absolute disproportion (Neilson et al 2003; Hayman 2004; El-Hamamy 2005)

Maternal factors

Bony abnormalities
- Severe kyphosis
- Severe scoliosis
- Poliomyelitis
- Maternal dwarfism
- Rickets
- Osteomalacia
- Impaired growth due to malnutrition
- Pelvic fracture

Soft tissue abnormalities
- Cervical fibroids (Hasan et al 1991)
- Ovarian tumour
- Pelvic kidney
- Excessive fat
- Cervical cancer
- Vaginal/vulval atresia
- Vaginal septum
- Gartner's duct cysts
- Tight perineum

Fetal factors
- Macrosomia (Diabetes, post-date)
- Hydrocephalus
- Iniencephaly
- Anencephaly
- Conjoined twins
- Fetal ascites or tumours
- Impacted shoulders
- Locked twins

Malpresentation
- Face-mentoposterior
- Brow
- Shoulder
- Compound presentations
- Impacted /Aftercoming head of breech

Contributory factors for relative disproportion

Malposition
- Occipitoposterior
- Occipitolateral
- Deflexion

Differences in behavior of the uterus in primigravid and multigravid women

There are fundamental differences in behaviour of the uterus in a primigravida and multigravid woman. In the presence of cephalopelvic disproportion, a primigravid woman may have premature rupture of membranes and delayed labour (Rao

2001). The uterine contractions gradually weaken and then stop, probably because of myometrial acidification which results from local myometrial energy depletion, anerobic metabolism and systemic ketosis. Hence, rupture of the uterus in a primi is rare. In a parous woman however, the uterus responds with powerful contractions to overcome the obstruction. As labour advances, contractions become more frequent and more intense with hardly any relaxation in between. This is perhaps because the myometrium becomes tolerant to the effects of acidification by an unknown mechanism (Neilson et al 2003). The powerful uterine contractions push the fetus into the lower uterine segment which stretches markedly both longitudinally and circumferentially. The demarcation between the extremely thinned out lower uterine segment and the contracted and retracted upper uterine segment becomes obvious and is called the pathological ring of Bandl. The junction ring begins to rise progressively, often up to the level of the umbilicus. Without relief of obstruction, the fetus will suffer from progressive hypoxia and will eventually die (Rao 2001). Continued contractions in the mother in the presence of hypoxia and myometrial energy depletion leads to myometrial edema and necrosis, thus contributing to uterine rupture. Rupture is more common when the woman is more than 35 years old or is a grand multipara (Kafkas 1991).

Clinical features Clinical features depend on the duration of labour, integrity of the uterus and the parity of the patient. The patient may give history of severe pain in the abdomen for a few hours after rupture of membranes. She may be tired, look anxious, exhausted and be dehydrated. Metabolic acidosis develops from the accumulation of lactic acid produced by contracting uterine and skeletal muscles. The acidosis is increased by ketones that are produced with the shift in metabolism from carbohydrate to fat due to reduced intake. Potassium may be mobilised from the cells to restore the acid-base equilibrium, which in turn diminishes the activity of the uterine muscle. There is a rise in temperature and pulse. The chance of intrauterine infection is increased if the membranes have been ruptured for a long time. Extreme pallor and shock may be present, especially if the complication of rupture uterus has already set in.

Abdominal examination reveals a uterus which is contracting. The Bandl's ring will be seen as an oblique demarcation between the well-contracting upper segment and the stretched out lower segment moving higher up as time elapses (Figure 31.1). The presence of uterine contour is very reassuring as it indicates that the uterus has still not ruptured. Round ligaments will be tense and palpable per abdomen (Oxorn 1986). The bladder is also drawn up into the abdomen and with continuing pressure of the fetus against the pubis, the bladder becomes edematous. Extreme compression may make catheterisation difficult. Blood-stained urine may be a feature. The bowel is distended and is very evident in the later stages. There may be a 'three tumour abdomen' with an edematous bladder, a distended, tender lower uterine segment, and a tonically contracted upper uterine segment above the Bandl's ring. It may be difficult to palpate the fetus as the liquor has drained away. Fetal distress may be present with the compromised blood supply due to tonic uterine contractions. And if the woman presents late, fetal heart sounds may be absent. Excessive moulding may give rise to tentorial tears and intracranial hemorrhage. These findings suggest a threatened rupture of the uterus.

On vaginal examination, there is vulval edema. The vagina may be dry and hot; the cervix if not fully dilated may be thick, edematous and loosely applied to the presenting part. There will be evidence of severe moulding and huge caput succedaneum. Meconium stained liquor may be present.

In the multigravid, clinical features are different depending on whether the rupture has taken place or not. If a rupture has occurred, the patient may give a history of continuous abdominal pain with the patient hardly able to move. The rent in the uterus starts in the lower uterine segment and often extends laterally on one side into the vagina or upwards into the fundus of the uterus. The presenting part of the fetus may be jammed in the pelvis and may prevent severe bleeding from the torn vessels because of the tamponade effect or may be expelled into the peritoneal cavity with massive bleeding, intra-peritoneally as well as per-vaginum, with resultant shock.

Presentation like this to the hospital is a rare phenomenon in the developed countries, but it is, nevertheless frequently encountered in the less developed world.

In centers where the partogram is routinely used, the classic pattern attributable to cephalopelvic disproportion, especially in a primi, is secondary arrest of dilatation with a normal initial rate of dilatation followed by cessation of dilatation. In a parous woman, there could be arrest of descent, usually in the second stage of labour. The situation is more complex because relative disproportion can be exarcebated by occipitoposterior positions or secondary failure of the power can occur as a result of prolonged labour (Philpott 1982; Neilson et al 2003). Unrecognised positional disproportion is commonly associated with obstructed labour (Konje et al 1992).

Complications of obstructed labour

Immediate complications Uterine rupture is a serious obstetric complication, with high maternal and perinatal morbidity and mortality, particularly in less resource countries. With ready access to obstetric care, including cesarean section for obstructed labour, rupture of the unscarred uterus should be rare (Ezegwui 1986; WHO 2005).

Rupture of the uterus is seen more in parous women, but in some less developed countries it is also a complication in a primigravid woman. Postpartum hemorrhage and subsequent shock are also commonly associated complications which further compromise the situation. With prolonged obstructed labour and rupture of the uterus, there is an increase in the development of sepsis, both intrapartum and postpartum.

Delayed complications Obstructed labour plays an important role not only in contributing to maternal mortality but also maternal morbidity. These complications are seen when the patient has not received proper obstetric care and differs in a primigravid and mutigravid patient.

The 'obstructed labour complex' represents a syndrome that involves multiple organ systems as a result of injuries from prolonged obstructed labour. It encompasses a wide range of gynecologic, skeletal, neurologic, psychosocial and dermatologic injuries in addition to its effect on the fetus.

The most common of all injuries is the obstetric fistula formation (Cook et al 2005; Khan et al 2005; Miller et al 2005). When obstructed labour is not relieved, the presenting part of the fetus is impacted against the soft tissues of the pelvis. A widespread ischemic vascular injury results in tissue necrosis and subsequent fistula formation. This obstetric fistula is the result of a 'field injury' to a large area. In addition to the vesicovaginal fistula, other injuries like total urethral loss, stress incontinence, hydroureteronephrosis, renal failure, recto-vaginal fistula formation, rectal atresia, anal sphincter incompetence are known to occur (Arrowsmith et al 1996). Postpartum stress urinary incontinence is sometimes seen and has similar prevalence when the station is above or below zero (Rimon et al 2003). Gynecologic sequelae are scarring of the genital tract (Ezegwui 2005), with possible pituitary and hypothalamic dysfunction that frequently leads to amenorrhea (Beiler 1976). Pelvic inflammatory disease also increases with obstructed labour. There is a high rate of secondary infertility in these patients owing to the combined effects of amenorrhea, pelvic inflammatory disease and genital tract scarring.

Women who have suffered from obstructed labour may experience bony abnormalities demonstrable on X-ray like bone resorption, fractures, bone spurs, obliteration of symphysis and symphyseal separation (Cockshott 1973).

Some women have symptoms of footdrop resulting from excessive compression of the sacral nerve plexus by the fetal head (Waaldjik 1994). It could result in perineal nerve damage and nerve damage to the bladder resulting in complex bladder dysfunction. Dermatological injuries like vulvar excoriation and ammoniacal dermatitis result from continuous leakage from the vesicovaginal fistulae.

As a result of excessive pressure on the placenta from prolonged uterine activity, fetal asphyxia and stillbirth are common. It is particularly distressing in societies that lay emphasis on childbirth. Women who have experienced obstructed labour, in addition to their physical injuries, suffer from serious social problems, including divorce, exclusion from religious activities and separation from their families and are the most dispossessed, outcast, powerless group of women in the world (Wall 1996).

Management of obstructed labour

PREDICTING OBSTRUCTED LABOUR Short stature is generally associated with a flattening of the pelvis and can indicate obstructed labour (Joud et al 2001). It varies due to genetic factors and is also an index of general health and nutritional status from childhood. Heights of < 150–153 cm in Ghana, < 155 cm in Burkina Faso, < 156 cm in Denmark, < 150 cm in Kenya, < 146 cm in Tanzania, < 140 cm in India, < 160 cm in Zimbabwe, < 157 cm in the United States are associated with increased risk of obstructed labour (Konje 2000).

Factors increasing the likelihood of difficult labour includes maternal body-mass index greater than 30, neonatal birth weight greater than 4 kg. Maternal pre-pregnancy is a strong marker for babies' weight and heavy women have bigger babies (Brost et al 1997). Increasing body mass index is associated with increasing requirement for Cesarean section (Cnattinguis et al 1998).

Increase in weight gain during pregnancy in women with normal pre-pregnant weight increases fetal birth weight. The presence of occipitoposterior position also enhances the chances of problems encountered in labour.

The head-fitting test of Munrokerr can be used, pushing the head into the pelvic brim with an abdominal hand assessing descent with two fingers of the right hand in the vagina and the thumb above the symphysis pubis (Lawson 1967).

The use of x-ray pelvimetry for predicting fetopelvic disproportion is discouraged

(Hofmeyr 2004).

Preventing Obstructed Labour

Community based strategies Community health education can be offered highlighting the effects of pregnancy soon after menarche during which the girls may not have attained their maximal growth potential. Safe motherhood requires large numbers of clinical staff including some trained in surgical techniques. Hence, community mobilisation with enhanced training for traditional birth attendants is required to ensure that more pregnant women in labour are taken care of. More primary care centres, better access to comprehensive emergency health services with skills to provide basic emergency obstetric care and availability of skilled attendance at delivery can decrease the number of women ending up with obstructed labour. The need for better equipment, improved supplies of drugs and utilisation of transport also merits great consideration (IMMPACT Review 2005, Rosenfield 2005).

Absent prenatal care and poor intrapartum care are major factors contributing to obstructed labour. If basic obstetric care is adequately established, obstructed labour can be averted to a large extent (Gottvall et al 2004; Ronsmans et al 2004). There are several organisations targeting different phases including pre-pregnancy, antenatal, delivery and the postpartum periods. Some of the strategies comprise programmes like the World Health Organization's Making Pregnancy Safer (MPS) Initiative, Mother Baby Package and the World Bank's Safe Motherhood Initiative (Herz 1987; WHO 1994; UNICEF 1999; WHO 2000).

Service quality improvements can take from criterion-based clinical audit of life-threatening complications like obstructed labour. Implementation of necessary changes can then be taken by programme planners and programme managers of larger organisations (Wagaarachchi et al 2001).

Specific interventions The consideration of family planning as a strategy is exemplified in the primary prevention of maternal mortality (IMMPACT Review 2005). Some studies have shown that family planning decreases the incidence of maternal mortality (Gaym 2000).

As the risk of obstructed labour is closely related to physical size, particularly the pelvic size of the mother (Rush 2000), micro-nutrient supplementation for the chronically malnourished populations appears to be an attractive intervention to reduce maternal and fetal mortality. It is believed to be cheap, safe and easier than the more fundamental societal changes that is otherwise required. Nutritional deficiencies such as calcium, vitamin D, folic acid, iron and zinc deficiencies which interact in combination with biological and biosocial factors can be prevented with adequate supplementation (Konje 2000).

Since nutritional strategies for increasing adult stature are rare, these interventions must be targeted at the younger age groups. First, babies and young children must be properly fed and protected from disease to aid good growth in early childhood, since that will determine ultimate adult height (Murphy et al 2001).

External cephalic version for breech presentation and transverse lie can be initiated. The use of early induction of labour to confer the benefits of delivering smaller babies is debatable (Hofmeyr 2004).

Use of hands and knees position for 10 minutes, twice daily, may aid in correcting the occipito posterior position of the fetus in the later weeks of pregnancy, but currently it is not recommended as an intervention (Hofmeyr 2005).

PROMOTING EFFICIENT MANAGEMENT OF FIRST STAGE OF LABOUR

If the woman is taken care of in a primary health center, it is wise to look for the presence of risk factors to facilitate early referral to a center with adequate facilities for performing emergency procedures.

Patients may present with primary dysfunctional labour (PDL), that is, poor progress during active phase of labour. This affects up to 26% of nulliparas and 8% of multiparas. It may be difficult to point to a single etiological factor responsible for these cases. However, it should be borne that this could culminate in obstructed labour and is associated with higher rates of maternal infection, rupture and postpartum hemorrhage.

Secondary arrest of dilatation defined as cessation of cervical dilatation following a normal period of dilatation affects about 6% of nulliparas. It is likely to be associated with an underlying pathological process with cephalopelvic disproportion, both absolute and relative being encountered frequently. Fetal occiput position can be accurately determined by ultrasonography in early labour and this can warn about increasing risk of cesarean section due to obstructed labour (Akaml et al 2004).

Assessment of maternal condition and fetal condition must be started once the patient is diagnosed to be in labour. Progress of labour is assessed by abdominal and pelvic examination. Use of WHO partogram helps in recognising the dystocia in labour. Though there seems to be an increased rate of referral with partogram, its use reduces the incidence of obstructed labour (Bosse 2002; Fahdhy 2004).

The definite diagnosis of CPD in a primi should be made if there is delay in the active phase and when the head is high (three- to four fifths above the brim). Increasing moulding is noted.

In multigravid women, there is normal progress in cervical dilatation to full dilatation and CPD is diagnosed mainly by failure of descent with increasing moulding. If there is no descent of the presenting part in the first half an hour of the second stage of labour, CPD must be suspected.

Prompt referral must be initiated in all labours lasting more than 12 hours in a primary care unit and patients sent to a higher center with facilities for performing surgery.

DIAGNOSING A PATIENT GOING INTO OBSTRUCTED LABOUR

Monitoring of labour is done by noting the changes in cervical effacement and dilatation along with descent of the presenting part against time in a chronological manner. Frequency and duration of contractions are observed. When the dilatation of the cervix is slower than the expected progress of labour, on to the right of the alert line in the WHO partogram, primary dysfunctional labour is diagnosed. At this juncture, it is better to review the diagnosis before the next intervention is considered. Causes due to power, passage or the passenger should be thought of. The progress of labour should be assessed both abdominally as well as vaginally. The options of amniotomy and augmentation of labour will only be possible if mechanical factors hindering further progress of labour are ruled out. Ineffective labour may be one of

Box 31.1: Checklist for clinical assessment in poor progression of labour (El-Hamamy 2005, Hayman 2004):

- Estimated fetal weight: Symphysio-fundal height >40 cm at this stage increases the likelihood of a large baby
- Degree of engagement in fifths per abdomen
- Position of presenting part
- Degree of cervical dilatation
- Presence of pelvic masses
- Descent of presenting part with contractions
- Frequency of contractions
- Fetal wellbeing: a normal pH with variable decelerations and a rising baseline are common features in obstructed labour

the warning signs of fetopelvic disproportion (Cunningham et al 2001). If the secondary arrest of dilatation is in the deceleration phase, clinically assess the parameters in box 31.1 carefully.

If the progress of labour remains unsatisfactory despite adequate augmentation of uterine contractions, mechanical factors like malposition and deflexion of the head should be considered. In a patient with an adequate pelvis, the presentation of larger occipitofrontal diameter (11 cm) rather than suboccipito-bregmatic diameter (9.5 cm) results in relative CPD. Usually, the dimensions of the presenting part is continuously altered through flexion, rotation and moulding in relation to the pelvis. It may therefore be difficult to evaluate the combinations of passenger and the passages to the delay. Hence, the progress of labour in cases of malposition should be assessed not only with dilatation, but also with rotation and descent. To do this, it is important to state the accurate position while monitoring the progress of labour. If there is absolute CPD or fetopelvic disproportion, with time, the characteristic clinical features of obstructed labour will be present.

Managing prolonged labour and facilitating delivery

Initial Resuscitation

- Assess maternal general condition.
- Set up intravenous access and correct dehydration, electrolyte imbalance and acidosis. If the patient is in shock, a central venous access may be required.
- Maintain an observational chart consisting of urine output, pulse, blood pressure and temperature.
- Empty the urinary bladder before any operative procedure. If there is any problem while passing the catheter, relieve compression of the urethra by inserting two fingers on either side of urethra, between the presenting part and the symphysis.
- Use a nasogastric tube to empty the stomach before general anesthesia is given.
- Measure serum electrolytes and arterial blood gases in the woman and arrange for blood transfusion depending on severity at presentation.
- Vaginal cleansing to reduce the risk of sepsis before any operative procedure is debatable (Lumbiganon et al 2005).

Mode of Delivery

Accurate assessment of the level of the head by abdominal examination, degree of moulding and cervical dilatation by pelvic examination must be made before embarking on the mode of delivery. The choice of the mode of delivery depends on the stage of labour, level of the presenting part and the associated maternal and fetal complications present at the time of presentation to the hospital. Accordingly, any of the procedures like cesarean section, symphysiotomy or destructive operation can be considered.

Cesarean Section

The operation should not be embarked upon lightly as there is a serious operative risk. It should be done by an experienced surgeon after initial resuscitation. It is indicated when the fetus is alive; if the cervix is not fully dilated and delivery is urgent for maternal indications, whether the baby is alive or dead; when there is evidence of imminent rupture even if the fetus is dead.

After incising the abdomen, preferably through a midline sub-umbilical incision, the peritoneal cavity is entered high up, to avoid injury to the bladder. To ensure the exact directions of opening of the lower uterine segment, scissors can be used. An assistant can help to disimpact the fetal head per-vaginum. Forceps can be used to deliver the fetal head after disimpaction. The fetus can also be delivered by pulling the feet through the uterine incision (Blickstein 2004). Care must be taken to avoid lateral tears if the head is jammed in the pelvis as they can compromise the blood supply to the already bruised myometrium and also attempts at securing hemostasis could endanger the ureters.

Women undergoing cesarean section are more likely to have a major hemorrhage and extended hospital stay than those with vaginal delivery. Babies delivered by cesarean section are more likely to require admission for intensive care but less likely to have trauma than babies delivered by forceps.

Symphysiotomy

Symphysiotomy seems to have no place in the obstetric arsenal in the developed world, as a cesarean section is a better option due to better facilities like good anesthetic cover and well-equipped operating theatres. It is a good alternative when facilities for cesarean are not available and in women with poor surgical and anesthetic risks (Engelkes 1992). It is a minimally invasive surgical procedure wherein the fibres and the supporting ligaments at the symphysis pubis are incised and cut by pivoting movements after insertion through the skin using a scalpel. This has to be done after passing the urinary catheter and pushing aside the urethra. A 2 cm symphyseal gap increases the area by about 12%, and a separation of 3.5 cm by about 22%. There is a permanent widening of the symphyseal joint of 1–1.5 cm.

Specific indications for symphysiotomy include engaged head arrested by mid-pelvic or outlet contraction, arrested abnormal presentation like brow or face, especially so when the disproportion does not permit the safe application of forceps or when forceps has failed, and as an emergency procedure when the aftercoming head has been trapped. Spontaneous delivery follows, but vacuum extraction may sometimes be necessary. It is a life-saving operation for the child, if not reserved for the desperate cases when the fetus is dead.

Complications like symphyseal hematoma and fistulas and walking difficulty do occur. Maternal mortality was higher with cesarean compared to symphysiotomy, while there was no difference in the perinatal mortality (Bjorklund 2002).

Destructive operations Destructive operations like craniotomy, decapitation may be the choice if the fetus is dead and the cervix is fully dilated (Gupta 1994) and performing cesarean section may be hazardous to the woman, especially in developing countries (Singhal et al 2005). Cephalocentesis can be performed if hydrocephalus is causing the obstruction. It is contraindicated in the presence of imminent rupture or when rupture of the uterus has already taken place.

The aim in resource-poor countries may be to deliver women vaginally, unless there are clear signs of absolute cephalopelvic disproportion and imminent rupture of the uterus. One must bear in mind that these women presenting with obstructed labour may not have access to a healthcare facility during the next pregnancy, in which case it could be detrimental to the life of the mother. It is also important that skilled obstetricians supervise complex operative deliveries.

Continuous bladder drainage for about two weeks is often recommended after obstructed labour to prevent obstetric fistulas.

Preventing and managing infection It is very important to use antibiotics to combat sepsis in all patients with obstructed labour as most of these women have been in labour for a long time (Smaill 2005). Both ampicillin and first generation cephalosporins have similar efficacy in reducing sepsis. There has been a systematic review showing a reduction of endometritis up to two-thirds to three-quarters with antibiotic use for a cesarean section (Hopkins 2005).

Preventing and managing postpartum hemorrhage The patients are at risk of developing both atonic and traumatic postpartum hemorrhage due to modified uterine contractility in prolonged obstructed labour and difficult delivery. Prompt action with oxytocics, surgical correction and blood transfusion needs to be taken to combat the morbidity and mortality in patients who have developed this complication.

References

Adhikari S, M Dasgupta, M Sanghamita. 2005. Management of obstructed labour: a retrospective study. *The Journal of Obstetrics and Gynecology of India* 55(1): 48–51

Akaml S, N Kametas, E Tsoi, R Howard, KH Nicolaides. 2004. Ultrasonographic occiput in early labour in the prediction of cesarean section. *BJOG* 111(6):532–536.

Arrowsmith S, E Hamlin, LL Wall. 1996. Obstructed labor injury complex: obstetric fistula formation and the multifaceted morbidity of maternal birth trauma in the developing world. *Obstet Gynecol Surv.* 51(9):568 LL 574

Bartlett LA, S Mawji, S Whitehead, C Crouse et al. 2005. Where giving birth is a forecast of death: maternal mortality in four districts of Afghanistan, 1999-2002. *Lancet* 365:864–870.

Beiler EU and T Schnabel. 1976. Pitutary and ovarian function in women with vesico-vaginal fistulae after obstructed and prolonged labor. *South African Med J* 50:257–266

Berhan Y and A Ahmed. 2004. Emergency obstetric performance with emphasis on operative delivery outcome: does it reflect quality of care? *Ethiopian Journal of health development.* 18(2):96–106

Bjorklund K. 2002. Minimally invasive surgery for obstructed labour: a review of symphysiotomy during the twentieth century (including cases). *Br J Obstet Gynecol* 109: 236–248

Blickstein I. 2004. Difficult delivery of the impacted fetal head during caesarian section: intraoperative disengagement dystocia. *J Perinat Med.* 32(6):465–469

Bosse G, S Massawe, A Jahn. 2002. The partograph in daily practice: its quality that matters. *Int J Gynecol Obstet.* 77:243–244

Brost BC, RC Goldenberg , BM Mercer , et al. 1997. The pre-term prediction study: association of Cesarean delivery with increases of maternal weight and body mass index. *Am J Obstet Gynecol.* 177: 333–341

Bulletin World Health Organization. June 2005. 83(6): 409–417. ISSN 0042-9686

Cnattinguis R, S Cnattinguis, FC Notzon. 1998. Obstacles to reducing Cesarean rates in a low Cesarean setting: the effect of maternal age height and weight. *Obstet Gynecol.* 92: 501–506

Cockshott PW. 1973. Pubic changes associated with obstetric vesicovaginal fistulae. *Clinical Radiology.* 24: 241–247

Cook RJ, BM Dickens, S Syed. 2004. Obstetric fistula: the challenge to human rights. *Int J Gynecol Obstet* 87(1): 72–77

Cox ML. 1963. Contracted pelvis in Nigeria. *J Obstet Gynaecol Br Emp.* 70:487–494.

Cron J. 2003. Lessons from the developing world: Obstructed labor and the vesico-vaginal fistula. *Ob/ Gyn and Women's Health, Medscape General Medicine*, 2003. 5(3), posted 08/14/2003

Cunningham FG, NF Gant, KJ Leveno, LC Gilstrap et al. 2001. Dystocia: Abnormal Labor and Fetopelvic Disproportion In *Williams Obstetrics* 21st edn. McGraw Hill International, 425–450.

Dumont A, LD Bernis, MH Bouvier-olle, G Breart. 2001. Caesarian section rate for maternal indication in sub Saharan Africa: A systematic review. *Lancet.* 358:1328–1333

Ebeigbe PN, E Enabudoso, AB Ande. 2005. Ruptured uterus in a Nigerian community: a study of sociodemographic and obstetric risk factors. *Acta Obstet Gynecol Scand.* 84(12):1172–1174.

El-Hamamy E and S Arulkumaran. 2005. Poor progress of labour. *Current Obstet Gynecol.* 15:1–8

Engelkes E and Van Roosmalen. 1992. The value of symphyseotomy compared with Caesarian section in cases of obstructed labour. *Soc Sci Med.* 35(6):789–793

Ezegwui HU and EE Nwogu-Ikojo. 2005. Trends in uterine rupture in Enugu, Nigeria. *J Obstet Gynaecol* 25(3):260–262.

Ezegwui HU and EE Nwogu-Ikojo. 2005. Vesico-vaginal fistula in Eastern Nigeria. *J Obstet Gynaecol* 25(6):589–591.

Fahdhy M and V Chongsuvivatwong. 2005. Evaluation of World Health Organization partograph implementation by midwives for maternity home birth in Medan, Indonesia. *Midwifery.* 21(4): 301–310

Gaym A. 2000. A review of maternal mortality at Jimma Hospital, Southwestern Ethiopia. *The Ethiopian Journal of Health Development.* 14(2):215–223

Geelhoed DW, LE Visser, K Asare, JHS Leeuwen, JV Roosmalen. 2003. Trends in maternal mortality: a 13 year hospital-based study in rural Ghana. *Eur J Obstet Gynecol and Reprod Biol.* 107(2):135-139

Gottvall K, Grunewald C, Waldenström U. 2004. Safety of birth centre care: perinatal mortality over a 10-year period *Br J Obstet Gynaecol* 111: 71–78

Gupta U and R Chitra. 1994. Destructive operations still have a place in developing countries. *Int J Gynecol Obstet.* 44(1): 15–19

Hasan F, K Arumugam, V Sivanesaratnam. 1991. Uterine leiomyomata in pregnancy. *Int J Gynecol and Obstet.* 34(1): 45–48

Hayman R. 2004. Poor progress in labour. In *Obstetrics and Gynecology an evidence-based text for MRCOG* ed DM Luesley and PN Baker. Arnold Publishers. 347–356

Herz B and AR Measham. 1987. The Safe Motherhood Initiative: proposals for action. Washington

(DC): The World Bank.

Hofmeyr GJ and R Kulier. 2005. Hands and knees posture in late pregnancy or labour for fetal malposition (lateral or posterior). Cochrane Library. Issue 4. Oxford: Update Software.

Hofmeyr GJ. 2004. Obstructed labor: using better technologies to reduce mortality. *Int J Gynecol Obstet.* 85: S62–S72.

Hopkins L and F Smaill. 2005. Antibiotic prophylaxis regimens and drugs for cesarean section. *The Cochrane Library*, Issue 4. Oxford: Update Software.

IMMPACT Review. 2005. Current strategies for reduction of maternal mortality. *Br J Obstet Gynaecol* 112: 1180–1188

Joud DOE, MH Bouvier-colle, MOMA Group. 2001. Dystocia: a study of its frequency and risk factors in seven cities of West Africa. Int J Gynecol Obstet. 74:171–178

Kafkas S and CE Taner. 1991. Ruptured uterus. *Int J Gynecol and Obstet.* 34(1): 41–44

Khan RM, N Raza, M Jehanzaib, R Sultana. 2005. Vesicovaginal fistula: an experience of 30 cases at Ayub Teaching Hospital Abbottabad. *J Ayub Med Coll Abbottabad.* 17(3):48–50.

Konje JC and OA Ladipo. 2000. Nutrition and Obstructed Labor. *Am J Clin Nutrition.* 72(1): 291S–297s

Konje JC, KA Obisesan, OA Ladipo. 1992. Obstructed labor in Ibadan. *Int J Gynecol and Obstet.* 39: 17–21

Kumar R, K Sharma, S Barik, V Kumar. 1989. Maternal mortality inquiry in a rural community in Northern India. *Int J Gynecol Obstet.* 29(4):313–319

Lawson JB. Obstructed labour. In *Obstetrics and gynecology in the tropics and developing countries*. London: Edward Arnold Press, 1967:172–202

Lumbiganon P, J Thinkhamrop, B Thinkhamrop, JE Tolosa. 2005. Vaginal chlorhexidine during labour for preventing maternal and neonatal infections (excluding Group B Streptococcal and HIV) *The Cochrane Library, Issue 4*.

Mekbib T, E Kassaye, A Getachew, T Tadasse, A Debebe. 2003. FIGO Save the Mothers Initiative: the Ethiopia-Sweden Collaboration. *Int J Gynecol Obstet.* 81(1): 93–102

Miller S, F Lester, M Webster, B Cowan. 2005. Obstetric fistula: a preventable tragedy. *J Midwifery Womens Health.* 50(4):286–294.

Murphy DJ, RE Liebling, L Verity, R Swingler, R Patel. 2001. Early maternal and neonatal morbidity associated with operative delivery in second stage of labour: a cohort study. *Lancet.* 358: 1203–1207

Neilson JP, T Lavender, S Quenby and S Wray. 2003. Obstructed Labour. *British Medical Bulletin.* 67(1): 191–204

Onah HE, JM Okaro, U Umeh, CO Chigbu. 2005. Maternal mortality in health institutions with emergency obstetric care facilities in Enugu State, Nigeria. *J Obstet Gynaecol.* 25(6):569–574.

Oxorn H. 1986. Normal and abnormal uterine action In. *Oxorn-Foote Human labour and birth* 5th edn. McGraw Hill International 655–671

Philpott RH. 1982. Obstructed Labour In. *Clinics in Obstetrics and Gynecology*. 9(3): 625–640

Rahman MH, HH Akter, ME Khan Chowdury, HR Yusuf et al. 2002 Obstetric deaths in Bangladesh 1996–1997. *Int J Gynecol Obstet.* 77(2):161–169

Rajaram P, A Agarwal, S Swain. 1995. Determinants of maternal mortality: a hospital based study from South India. *Indian J Matern Child. Health.* 6(1):7–10

Rao KB. 2001. Obstructed Labour In. *Obstetrics and Gynecology for Postgraduates* 2nd edn, ed SS Ratnam, K Bhasker Rao, S Arulkumaran. 1:139–144

Rimon E, A Grutz, S Peled, D Pauzner et al. 2003. Does the station of the fetal head in obstructed labour affect the risk of persistant postpartum stress urinary incontinence? A prospective study of 100 women one year after first delivery. *Am J Obstet Gynecol.* SMFM Abstracts: S124

Ronsmans C, V De Brouwere, D Dubourg, G Dieltiens. 2004. Measuring the need for life-saving obstetric surgery in developing countries *Br J Obstet Gynaecol* 111: 1027–1030

Rosenfield A and K Schwartz. 2005. Improving the health of women in developing countries: the time is now. *J Midwif Women's Health* 50(4) 272–274

Rush D. 2000. Nutrition and maternal mortality in the developing world. *Am J Clin Nutr.* 72: 2125–2405

Singhal SR, P Chaudhry, K Sangwan, SK Singhal. 2005. Destructive operations in modern obstetrics. *Arch Gynecol Obstet.* 273(2):107–109.

Smaill F and GJ Hofmeyr. 2005. Antibiotic prophylaxis for cesarean section. *The Cochrane Library, Issue 4*. Oxford: Update Software.

Tonks A. 1994. Pregnancy's toll in the developing world. *Br Med J.* 308:353-54.

UNICEF. 1999. Programming for Safe Motherhood: Guidelines for Maternal and Neonatal Survival. New York: UNICEF.

Waaldjik K and TE Elkins. 1994. The obstetric fistula and peroneal nerve injury: an analysis of 947 patients. *Int Urogynecol J* 5: 12–14

Wagaarachchi PT, WJ Graham, GC Penney et al. 2001. Holding up a mirror: changing obstetric practice through criterion-based clinical audit in developing countries. *Int J Gynecol Obstet.* 74: 119–130.

Wall LL. 1996. Obstetric fistulas in Africa and the developing world: new efforts to solve an age-old problem. *Womens Health Issues.* 6:229–234

Weeks A, T Lavender, E Nazziwa, F Mirembe. 2005 . Personal accounts of 'near-miss' maternal mortalities in Kampala, Uganda. *Br J Obstet Gynaecol* 112(9):1302–1307.

WHO systematic review of maternal mortality and morbidity: the prevalence of uterine rupture. 2005. *Br J Obstet Gynaecol* 112:1221–1228

WHO. 1994. The mother baby package: implementing safe motherhood in countries. Geneva: WHO. [WHO/FHE/MSM/94.11].

WHO. 2000. Making Pregnancy Safer: a health sector strategy for reducing Maternal and perinatal morbidity and mortality. Geneva: World Health Organization, [WHO/RHR/00.6].

32

Postpartum Hemorrhage

Rani Akhil Bhat

Postpartum hemorrhage (PPH) has been defined as blood loss greater than 500 ml in a vaginal delivery and greater than 1000 ml in a cesarean delivery.

Studies have shown that uncomplicated vaginal delivery often results in blood loss of more than 500 ml, without any maternal compromise, and that the incidence of PPH is being under-reported by 30–50%.

Based on these findings, PPH has been broadly defined as any bleeding that results in signs and symptoms of hemodynamic instability, or bleeding that could result in hemodynamic instability if untreated. Blood loss of greater than 1000 ml in a vaginal delivery, a decrease in postpartum hematocrit level greater than 10% of the prenatal value or that which requires a transfusion of red blood cells can also be considered as PPH (ACOG 2001).

Blood loss of these amounts within 24 hours of delivery is termed early or primary PPH, whereas such losses are termed late or secondary PPH if they occur 24 hours after delivery.

Incidence and Causes

Based on these definitions, the incidence of PPH has been estimated at 4% for vaginal deliveries and 6% for cesarean deliveries.

In the developing world, several countries have maternal mortality rates in excess of 1000 women per 100,000 live births, and World Health Organization (WHO) statistics suggest that 25% of maternal deaths are caused by PPH—this accounts for more than 100,000 maternal deaths per year (AbouZahr 1998).

The common causes of hemorrhage are tone, tissue, trauma and thrombosis. The risk factors of PPH are listed in Table 32.1.

Prevention

Active management of the third stage of labour is the most effective means of preventing PPH (Keirse Marc 1998; Prendiville et al 2002). Compared to physiological (or expectant) management, active management has been shown to reduce the risk of PPH, low hemoglobin levels postpartum and the use of blood transfusion, by more than 50%. Active management combines administration of a prophylactic oxytocic drug as the anterior shoulder delivers, with early cord clamping and cutting, and controlled cord traction with uterine stabilisation.

Stepwise Approach to Management of PPH

Step 1: Initial Assessment and Treatment (Table 32.2)

Step 2: Directed Therapy

Table 32.1: Antenatal and intrapartum risk factors (Combs et al 1991; SOGC 2000; Hostetler et al 2000)		
Causes	***Etiological Process***	***Clinical Risk Factors***
Abnormalities of uterine contraction (Tone) (70%)	• Atonic uterus	• Physiological management of 3rd stage • Prolonged 3rd stage (more than 30 minutes)
	• Over-distended uterus	• Polyhydramnios • Multiple gestation • Macrosomia
	• Uterine muscle exhaustion	• Rapid or incoordinate labour • Prolonged labour (1st or 2nd stage) • Labour dystocia • High parity • Labour augmented with oxytocin
	• Intra-amniotic infection	• Pyrexia • Prolonged ROM (>24 hours)
	• Drug-induced hypotonic	• Magnesium sulphate, nifedipine, salbutamol • General anaesthesia
	• Functional or anatomic dissertation of the uterus	• Fibroid uterus • Uterine anomaly
Genital tract trauma (20%)	• Episiotomy or lacerations (cervix, vagina or perineum)	• Labour induced • Labour augmented with oxytocin • Labour dystocia • Malposition • Precipitous delivery • Operative delivery (vacuum or forceps)
	• Extensions, lacerations at cesarean section	• Malposition • Deep engagement
	• Uterine rupture	• Previous uterine surgery
	• Uterine inversion	• Strong cord traction in 3rd stage, especially with fundal placenta • Short umbilical cord • High parity • Relaxed uterus, lower segment and cervix • Placenta accreta, especially fundal • Congenital uterine weakness or anomalies • Antepartum use of magnesium sulphate or oxytocin

Retained products of conception (Tissue) (9%)	• Retained products • Abnormal placenta • Retained cotyledon or succenturiate lobe	• Incomplete placenta at delivery • Placenta accreta or percreta • Previous cesarean or other uterine surgery • High parity • Abnormal placenta on U/S
Abnormalities of coagulation (Thrombin) (1%)	• Retained blood clot	• Atonic uterus
	• Coagulation disorders acquired in pregnancy • Idiopathic thrombocytopenic purpura (ITP) • Von Willebrand's disease • Hemophilia or carrier • Thrombocytopenia with pre-eclampsia • Disseminated intravascular coagulopathy (DIC) • Pre-eclampsia • Dead fetus *in utero* • Severe infection • Abruption • Amniotic fluid embolus	• Bruising • Elevated BP, HELLP • Fetal death • Pyrexia, WBC • Antepartum hemorrhage (current or previous) • Sudden collapse
	• Therapeutic anti-coagulation	• History of blood clot

I. 'Tone' – incidence of PPH due to atonic uterus is 70%.

Prompt recognition and intervention are the cornerstones of successful management of uterine atony. Reassure the woman and insert an indwelling catheter to keep the bladder empty, not only to monitor urine output, but also because a full bladder can precipitate PPH.

Management of atonic PPH is by uterine massage with simultaneous use of oxytocics.

Non-surgical emergency measure

A. Uterine massage:

External compression (Fig. 32.1)

- Put one hand above and behind the uterus and push it forward and press it against the other hand. Grasp it firmly for at least 10 minutes.
- Compress the uterus just above the symphysis pubis (at the uterine insertion) and with the other hand gently massage the fundus of the uterus, while simultaneously

TABLE 32.2: EARLY RECOGNITION, PROMPT RESUSCITATION, IDENTIFICATION OF CAUSE OF BLEEDING AND BASELINE LAB TESTS

Resuscitation	Assess Etiology	Laboratory Tests
- CALL FOR HELP - Have two large bore IV (16G) at hand - Give oxygen by mask - Monitor BP, pulse, respiration, urine output, other symptoms (for example, pain)	- Perform abdominal assessment of uterus (tone, tissue) - Explore lower genital tract (trauma) - Review history (thrombin) - Observe clots	- FBC - Coagulation screen - ABO group and cross match

pressing it against the spine to obliterate the aorta (Fig. 32.2).

Aortic compression (Riley 1995) (Fig. 32.3)

- Clench your left fist and keep the index finger at the level of the umbilicus and knuckles in the line of her spine. Then press firmly with your clenched left fist. Feel for her right femoral pulse with your right hand. Pulse should be obliterated. If her legs become numb, allow a little blood to flow through them, by releasing pressure on the aorta.

Bimanual/Internal compression

- Wear sterile or clean gloves.
- Introduce the right hand into the vagina. Clench the fist, with the back of the hand directed posteriorly and the knuckles in the anterior fornix.
- Place the other hand on the abdomen behind the uterus and squeeze the uterus firmly between the two hands.

B. DRUG THERAPY IN ATONIC PPH (THIS IS DESCRIBED IN TABLE 32.3)

C. UTERINE TAMPONADE Before uterine tamponade, exclude retained placental tissue and rule out or repair genital tract laceration. Where coagulation has been excluded or corrected, but intractable hemorrhage remains a problem despite all pharmacological means, uterine tamponade can be performed.

Uterine packing: This modality is useful in controlling hemorrhage from uterine atony and placental site bleeding caused by placenta previa or placenta accreta. Uterine atony unresponsive to oxytocics is the most common indication for its use. Uterovaginal packing has also been used to gain time to stabilise the patient while arranging for a surgical procedure. In some of these situations, packing itself proved successful, thereby obviating the need for surgery.

Its foremost advantage is that it is very simple and quick to perform and requires

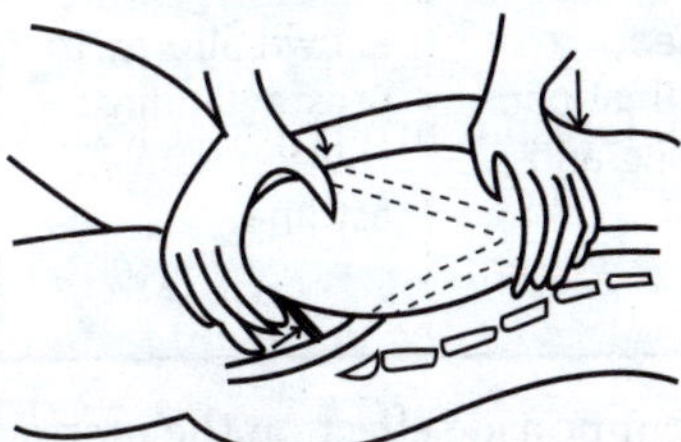

FIGURE 32.1: EXTERNAL COMPRESSION

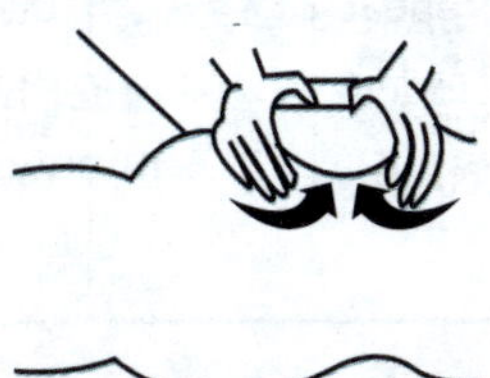

FIGURE 32.2: AORTIC COMPRESSION

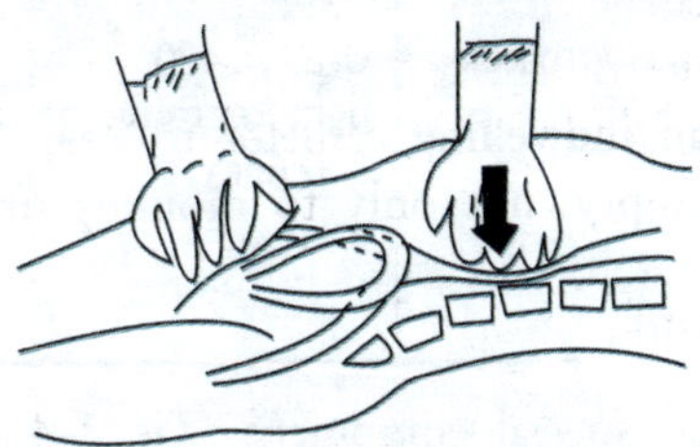

FIGURE 32.3: BIMANUAL/INTERNAL COMPRESSION

Table 32.3: Drugs used in atonic PPH

Drug	*Initial Dose*	*Continuing Dose*	*Action Time*	*Side Effects*	*Contra-indications*
Oxytocin	IM/IV 10 IU IV infusion: 20 IU in 1 litre at 60 drops/minute	IM/IV repeat 10 IU after 20 minutes if heavy bleeding persists. IV infusion: 10 IU in 1 litre at 30 drops/ minute	IM – 3 min; IV – 30 sec.	Usually none Pain, full contractions Nausea, vomiting Transient vasodilatation and hypotension if undiluted IV bolus High dose or prolonged administration in electrolyte-free fluids can cause water intoxication from antidiuretic effect	Hyper-sensitivity to the drug
Methyl-ergonovine maleate	IV/IM 0.2 mg slowly	Can repeat every 10-15 minutes, maximum dose 1.0 mg (five doses)	IM – 8 min. IV – 45 sec.	Nausea, vomiting Peripheral vasospasm Hypertension	Hypertension Hyper-sensitivity to the drug
Carboprost (Hemabate)	IM 250 μgm	Can repeat every 15 minutes, maximum eight doses	IM – 5 min	Acute hypotension, bronchospasm, nausea, vomiting, angina, headache, vertigo, death with IV injection	Caution in women with asthma, hypertension, renal or hepatic disease. Coronary artery disease Hyper-sensitivity to the drug
Misoprostol (PGE_1)	Orally: 400 μgm Rectally: 800 μgm	Orally repeat after 4 hours maximum dose 800 μg.		Diarrhea, abdominal pain, shivering and fever	Known allergy to prostaglandins; caution with asthma.

no special equipment. Tie 3–4 gauze rolls together, soak in an iodine solution and pack all areas of the uterine cavity up to the introitus to maintain a tamponade effect on the uterine sinuses and prevent concealed hemorrhage. Remove 24 hours later (Druzin 1989).

15 methyl derivative of prosta-glandin $F_{2\alpha}$	5 mg/ml diluted in 9 ml normal saline, inject 1 ml trans-abdominally into the myometrium on each side of the fundus			Nausea, vomiting diarrhea, headache, flushing, cardiac arrest, uterine rupture	Caution in women with asthma, hypertension, active cardiac, renal or hepatic disease hyper-sensitivity

Other methods of uterine tamponade can also be used:

Foley catheter procedure (Marcovici 1999): Guide the tip of a No. 24F Foley catheter into the uterine cavity and inflate with 60–80 mL of saline. Additional Foley catheters can be inserted if necessary. If bleeding stops, the patient can be observed with the catheters in place and then removed after 12–24 hours.

Sengstaken–Blakemore tube (Chan et al 1997): Like the Foley catheter, the Sengstaken–Blakemore tube has an open tip that permits continuous drainage. However, this device may be more difficult to obtain in an emergency setting because it is not routinely stored in labour and delivery suites. Like the Foley catheter, the Sengstaken–Blakemore tube should be guided through the cervix into the uterus and the esophageal balloon is then filled with 75–150 ml of warm saline until it just becomes visible at the cervical canal. The warm saline may speed up the rate of the clotting cascade.

To maintain uterine contraction over the balloon, a slow oxytocin infusion is run over the next 12–24 hours. Broad-spectrum antibiotics should be administered to minimise the risk of sepsis. The patient is then closely monitored, including vital signs, fluid input/output, fundal height and vaginal bleeding. After 12–24 hours, once the patient is stable, the balloon can be slowly deflated and observed for active bleeding. If there is no bleeding, infusion of oxytocin may be stopped after 30 minutes.

An alternative to the Sengstaken–Blakemore tube is a urological hydrostatic balloon catheter (Rusch balloon catheter). Around 400–500 ml of warm saline is used to inflate the balloon through the drainage port.

Condom with red rubber catheter: Recently, tamponade with a condom catheter, inflated with 250–500 ml of saline, has been demonstrated to be helpful in controlling atonic PPH.

Surgical management of PPH

A. Conservative *Under-suturing the placental bed for PPH during cesarean delivery:* Where PPH follows placenta previa or low-lying placenta, the large sinuses that are responsible for the bleeding must be under-sewn. Difficulty with under-sewing may arise due to narrowing of the isthmic portion and thinness of the lower segment, which may tear every time suturing is attempted. If faced with these difficulties, full thickness suture, entering the uterine cavity from outside below the bleeding point, and then exiting the cavity to the outside, such that a horizontal suture is placed across and below the bleeding point, may be done.

Hemostatic 'multiple square' suturing technique for PPH during cesarean delivery (Cho's Square Suture 2000): Hemostatic multiple square suturing using a straight number 7 or number 8 needle and number 1 chromic catgut is a new surgical technique to approximate anterior and posterior uterine walls, especially in areas where there is heavy bleeding (Fig. 32.4). It controls PPH by attachment and compression of the hemorrhage site of the endometrium or myometrium.

B-Lynch suture (Lynch et al *1997):* The objective of this technique is to compress the uterus without occluding either the uterine arteries or the uterine cavity (Fig. 32.5). Key points in the technique are:

- Done under GA, with patient in the Lloyd–Davies position to enable access to the vagina to facilitate objective assessment of bleeding control.
- Abdomen is opened through a Pfannensteil or midline or, if PPH follows a cesarean section, the same incision is re-opened.
- Uterus is exteriorised and bimanual compression is applied to check that this arrests bleeding before the suturing is performed.
- A lower segment uterine incision is made following downward reflection of the bladder or the uterine incision is re-opened.
- A number 2 Vicryl or Dexon on a round body needle is used to puncture the uterus about 3 cm below the right hand corner of the lower segment incision and brought about 3 cm above the same corner (as the first suture would be placed when closing this corner of the incision). From this point, the suture is passed over the right hand cornu of the uterus, approximately 3–4 cm from the right corneal border, where it may be fixed to prevent it from slipping off the fundus, and then fed posteriorly and vertically down to the same level where the suture has previously left the uterine cavity from the anterior. The suture is then placed through the posterior uterine wall into the cavity under the direct vision of the surgeon and back through the posterior wall about 4–5 cm left of the previous entry site. With the suture outside and posterior of the uterine cavity at this stage, it is now passed over the left hand cornu, approximately 3–4 cm from the left corneal border, where it may be again fixed to the fundus, then fed anteriorly and vertically down to the level of the left corner of the lower segment incision. The needle is then passed through the left corner in the same fashion as on the right hand side, to emerge below the incision margin on the left side. With the suture now in place, the assistant bimanually compresses the uterus while the surgeon pulls the chromic suture taut. If a third person confirms that the bleeding is controlled (as observed vaginally), the surgeon ties the suture to keep it in position and closes the lower segment uterine incision.

Modified B-Lynch technique (Hayman et al 2002): This technique is used to avoid opening of the uterine cavity (Fig. 32.6). A number 2 Vicryl or Dexon suture on a straight, blunt needle is used to transfix the uterus from front to back, just above the reflection of the bladder, and is then tied at the fundus of the uterus. This can be done as one suture on each side of the uterus, or more than one suture if the uterus is particularly broad. To prevent the sutures from slipping off, tie the knots at the top of the uterus and then tie the loose ends together.

Ligation of vessels: **A) Uterine and utero-ovarian artery (O'Leary 1995):** Uterine artery ligation has been shown to have a success rate of 92% and a complication rate of 1% (Fig. 32.7).

The procedure is as follows:

- Open the abdomen in layers.
- Pull on the uterus to expose the lower part of the broad ligament.

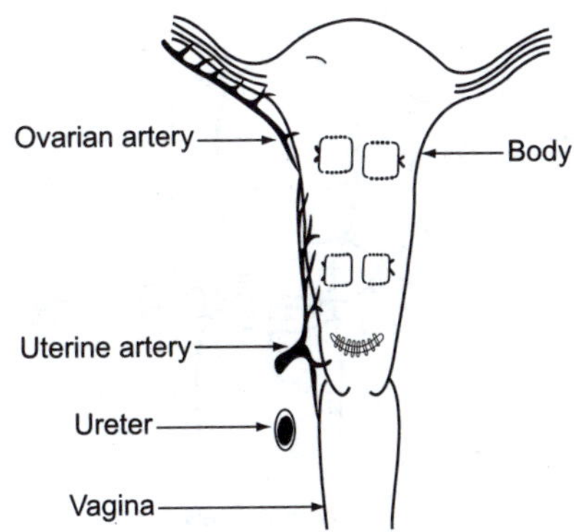

FIGURE 32.4: HEMOSTATIC 'MULTIPLE SQUARE' SUTURING

- Feel for pulsations of the uterine artery near the junction of the uterus and cervix.
- The uterine artery is ligated at the upper part of the lower uterine segment. If a cesarean section has been performed, the ligation is done 2–3 cm below the level of the uterine incision. To do this, it may be necessary to advance the bladder.
- The uterine artery and vein are ligated by passing the needle 2–3 cm medial to the vessels, including almost the full thickness of the myometrium, and then bringing it through a broad ligament in the avascular area, lateral to the vessel. Tie the suture securely.
- Place the sutures as close to the uterus as possible, as the ureter is generally only 1 cm lateral to the uterine artery.
- Repeat on the other side. If the artery has been torn, clamp and tie the bleeding ends.
- A second stitch can be placed if the above step is ineffective and for cases with continued lower uterine segment hemorrhage. With the bladder well mobilised, a second lower bilateral uterine vessel ligation is performed, 3–5 cm below the upper ligatures. This ligature would obliterate most of the branches of the uterine artery to the lower segment and a branch that extends to the cervix.
- If there is continued bleeding, unilateral or bilateral ovarian vessel ligation may be performed.
- Ligate the utero-ovarian artery just below the point where the ovarian suspensory ligament joins the uterus.
- Observe for continued bleeding or formation of hematoma.

B) INTERNAL ILIAC ARTERY LIGATION: (BURCHELL 1968; EVANS 1985): The technique involves identifying the bifurcation of the common iliac artery, where the ureter crosses it. To do this, an incision of 5–8 cm is made in the peritoneum, lateral and parallel to the line of the ureter. The ureter is retracted medially, and the artery is ligated 2.5 cm distal to the bifurcation of the internal and external iliac artery. Two ligatures are placed 1.5–2 cm apart, but the vessel is not divided. Care must be taken to avoid trauma to the internal iliac veins. External iliac artery and femoral pulse must be identified before and after tying the ligature.

The mechanism responsible for controlling pelvic hemorrhage with internal iliac ligation has been explained as follows—the ligation of internal iliacs greatly dampened the pulse pressure and transformed the pelvic arterial system into a venous-like system with slow and sluggish blood flow. The 'trip hammer effect' of the arterial pulsation was lost. The blood clots, which were formed distal to the ligation, therefore remained in place. It also allowed for identification of remaining individual bleeders for ligation, which would otherwise have been difficult. With bilateral ligation, the drop in pulse pressure was 85%, whereas with unilateral ligation it was 77% on the same side and 14% on the opposite side. The mean arterial pressure decreased to

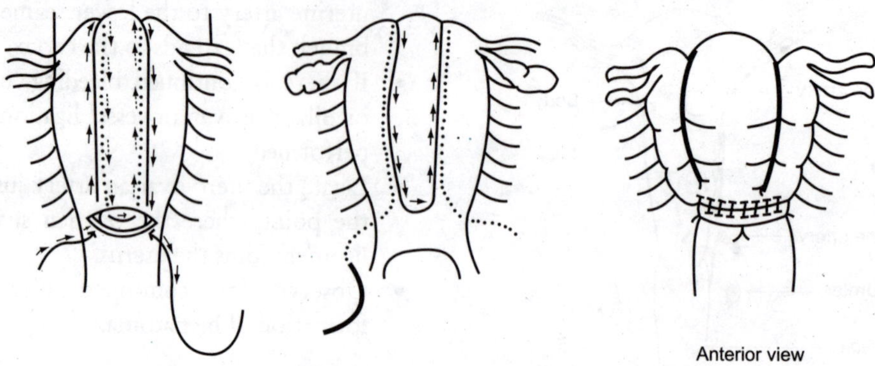

FIGURE 32.5: B-LYNCH SUTURE

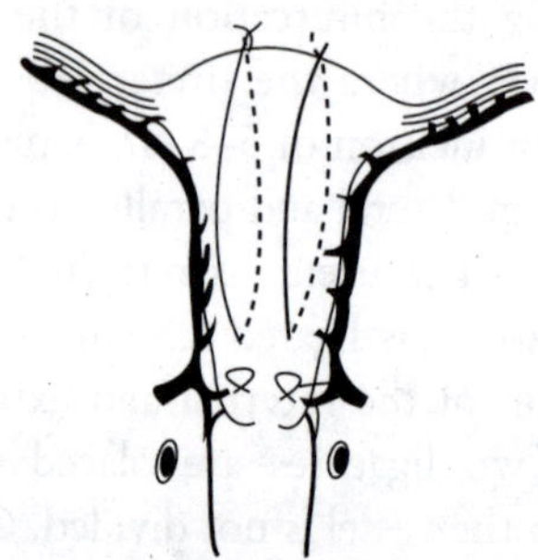

FIGURE 32.6: MODIFIED B-LYNCH TECHNIQUE

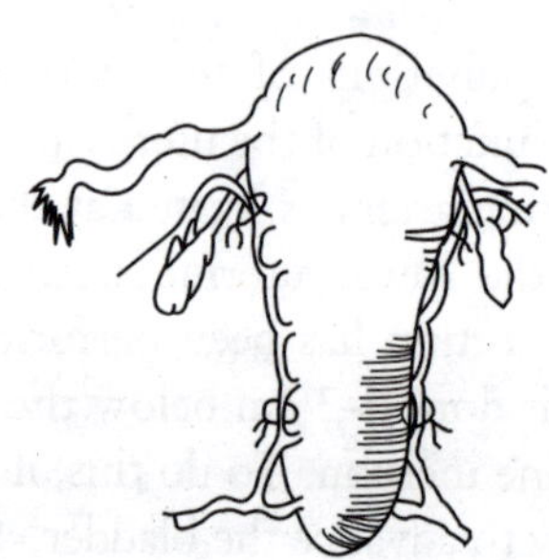

FIGURE 32:7: SITES FOR LIGATING UTERINE AND UTERO-OVARIAN ARTERIES

24% with bilateral ligation and with unilateral ligation the decrease was 22% on the same side and 10% on the opposite side. The rate of blood flow dropped to about 48% on the same side after ligation.

C) BILATERAL HYPOGASTRIC ARTERY LIGATION (CLARK 1985; CHATTOPADHYAY ET AL 1990):

- The hypogastric artery is exposed by ligating and cutting the round ligament and incising the pelvic sidewall peritoneum cephalad, parallel to the infundibulopelvic ligament.
- The ureter should be visualised and left attached to the medial peritoneal reflection to prevent compromising its blood supply.
- The hypogastric artery should be completely visualised.
- A blunt-tipped, right-angle clamp is gently placed around the hypogastric artery, 2.5–3.0 cm distal to the bifurcation of the common iliac artery.
- Passing the tips of the clamp from lateral to medial under the artery is crucial in preventing injuries to the underlying hypogastric vein.
- The artery is double-ligated with a non-absorbable suture, with 1-0 silk, but not divided.
- The ligation is then performed on the contralateral side in the same manner.
- The success rate ranges between 40–100%.

D) STEPWISE UTERINE DEVASCULARISATION (ABDRABBO 1994): This technique entails five successive steps; so if bleeding is not controlled by one step the next step is taken until bleeding stops. The steps are (1) unilateral uterine vessel ligation, (2) bilateral uterine vessel ligation, (3) low uterine vessel ligation, (4) unilateral ovarian vessel ligation and (5) bilateral ovarian vessel ligation.

E) Embolisation of internal iliac/uterine artery: (Vedantham et al 1997, Badaway et al 2001): In some settings, interventional radiology may provide another alternative. Using x-ray guidance, small catheters can be placed through the blood vessels in the leg and into the blood vessels supplying the uterus. The blood vessels can then be injected with gelatin sponge particles or spring coils to obstruct blood flow to the uterus. Although successful control of hemorrhage has been reported with this technique, it may not be available in emergency situations. Complications of pelvic embolisation for PPH occur at a rate of 8.7%. The commonest complication is low-grade fever, while rarer ones include pelvic infection, groin hematoma, iliac artery perforation, transient buttock ischemia, transient foot ischemia and bladder gangrene

Uterine artery embolisation and uterine artery ligation both have reported success rates of greater than 90% with low complication rates. If both techniques are available, embolisation is the preferred first choice as it obviates laparotomy, and ligation can be attempted subsequently if embolisation is unsuccessful. In contrast, after an unsuccessful uterine artery ligation, embolisation may be extremely difficult or even impossible, leaving hysterectomy as the only remaining option.

Emergency peripartum hysterectomy: Hysterectomy is another option for patients who failed to respond to more conservative measures. If the bleeding is caused by uterine atony and the patient is unstable, perform subtotal hysterectomy; but if bleeding is in the low uterine segment, total hysterectomy has to be performed.

II. Tissue

Retained placenta Retained placenta is defined in various ways. The most common definition is retention of the placenta in utero for more than 30 minutes. This is an arbitrary definition, and management is greatly influenced by the clinical assessment of whether significant bleeding is occurring. This bleeding may be visible or may manifest only by the increasing size of the uterus. In the absence of any evidence of placental detachment, consider the diagnosis of complete placenta accreta or a variant.

A number of trials have evaluated the role of injection of oxytocin (commonly 10 IU) or saline (20 ml) into the umbilical cord in the management of retained placenta in women not experiencing significant bleeding (Carroli and Bergel 2002). This intervention seems reasonable in stable women with minimal bleeding while preparations for manual removal are being made.

Manual removal of the placenta is warranted if the above manoeuvres have failed to deliver the placenta or if significant bleeding occurs. The retained or partially detached placenta interferes with uterine contraction and retraction and leads to bleeding. Perform manual removal with a level of analgesia that matches the clinical urgency of the situation. The cessation of oxytocin infusion or administration of uterine relaxants to promote uterine exploration and manual removal is of questionable value and may lead to increased bleeding. Ultrasound may be useful in select cases.

When possible, an elbow-length glove is worn and attention is paid to asepsis. The hand is passed into the vagina through the cervix and into the lower segment following the umbilical cord. Care is taken to minimise the profile of the hand as it enters, keeping the thumb and fingers together in the shape of a cone to avoid damage.

Holding the uterine fundus with the left hand is essential. If the placenta is encountered in the lower segment, it is removed. If the placenta is not encountered, the placental edge is sought. Once found, the fingers gently develop the space between the placenta and uterus and shear off the placenta. The placenta is pushed to the palmar aspect of the hand and wrist; when it is entirely separated, the hand is withdrawn.

Ensure that an oxytocin infusion is running rapidly as the hand is withdrawn, in order to encourage strong uterine contraction, and then perform uterine massage. Care must be taken to tease out the membranes. Once uterine contraction is established, examine the placenta and membranes to determine whether further exploration or curettage is necessary. The administration of antibiotics following manual removal is advocated.

Retained placental fragments When a portion of the placenta—one or more lobes—is retained, it prevents the uterus from contracting effectively. Feel inside the uterus for placental fragments. Manual exploration of the uterus is similar to the technique described for removal of the retained placenta. Remove placental fragment by hand, ovum forceps or large curette.

III. Trauma

Repair of cervical tears Anesthesia is not required for most cervical tears. For tears that are high and extensive, give pethidine and diazepam IV slowly (do not mix in the same syringe).

Ask an assistant to massage the uterus and provide fundal pressure. Gently grasp the cervix with ring or sponge forceps. Apply the forceps on both sides of the tear and gently pull in various directions to see the entire cervix. There may be several tears. Close the cervical tears with continuous 0 chromic catgut (or polyglycolic) suture starting at the apex (upper edge of tear), which is often the source of bleeding.

A laparotomy may be required to repair a cervical tear that has extended deep beyond the vaginal vault.

Repair of tears If first- or second-degree tear and heavy bleeding persists after applying pressure over the wound:

- Suture the tear using universal precautions, aseptic technique and sterile equipment.
- Use absorbable polyglycon suture material.
- Make sure that the apex of the tear is reached before you begin suturing.
- Ensure that the edges of the tear match up well.

Uterine inversion This condition is rare. The risk of uterine inversion is increased in abnormalities of placentation, such as accreta, and is more likely with fundal cord insertions and any condition that predisposes patients to uterine atony and prolapse. Cord traction should never occur without countertraction or in the absence of uterine contraction. Leave the placenta attached and focus management on maternal resuscitation and rapid return of the uterus to the abdominal cavity.

The fingers are formed into a single cone-shaped unit and placed at the most dependent portion of the protruding mass, which represents the inverted uterine fundus. Gentle upward pressure is exerted in the axis of the birth canal with the fingers and thumb together to minimise the risk of uterine perforation, using the other hand to support the uterus. Following uterine replacement, vigorous massage and uterotonic administration should be undertaken. If the placenta is still attached, perform manual removal after correction. Manual removal of the placenta may be performed when the mother's vital signs are stable, unless concern exists regarding abnormal placentation.

It is important that the part of the uterus that came out last (the part closest to the cervix) goes in first.

Uterine rupture Open the abdomen in layers through midline vertical incision. Lift the uterus out of the pelvis in order to note the extent of the injury. Examine both the front and the back of the uterus. Hold the bleeding edges of the uterus with Green–Armytage clamps (or Ring forceps). Separate the bladder from the lower uterine segment by sharp or blunt dissection. If the bladder is scarred to the uterus, use fine scissors.

a) Rupture through cervix and vagina: If the uterus is torn through the cervix and vagina, mobilise the bladder at least 2 cm below the tear. If possible, place a suture 1 cm below the upper end of the cervical tear and keep traction on the suture to bring the lower end of the tear into view as the repair continues.

b) Rupture laterally through uterine artery: If the rupture extends laterally to damage one or both uterine arteries, ligate the injured artery. Identify the arteries and ureter prior to ligating the uterine vessels.

c) Rupture with broad ligament hematoma: If the rupture has created a broad ligament hematoma, clamp, cut and tie off the round ligament. Open the anterior leaf of the broad ligament. Drain off the hematoma manually, if necessary. Inspect the area carefully for injury to the uterine artery or its branches. Ligate any bleeding vessels.

d) Repairing the uterine tear: Repair the tear with a continuous locking stitch of 0 chromic catgut (or polyglycolic) suture. If bleeding is not controlled or if the rupture is through a previous classical or vertical incision, place a second layer of suture.

Ensure that the ureter is identified and exposed, to avoid including it in a stitch.

If the patient has requested tubal ligation, perform the procedure at this time. If the rupture is too extensive for repair, proceed with hysterectomy. Control bleeding by clamping with long artery forceps and ligating. If the bleeding points are deep, use figure-of-eight sutures. Place an abdominal drain. Ensure that there is no bleeding. Remove clots using a sponge. In all cases, check for injury to the bladder. If a bladder injury is identified, repair the injury.

IV. Abnormalities of Coagulation (Thrombin)

Reverse anticoagulation and replace factors.

Secondary PPH Secondary postpartum hemorrhage is the presence of any excess, frank bleeding 24 hours after delivery. It usually occurs 8–10 days after this time. It occurs after approximately 1% of all deliveries.

The causes include:

- Retained products of conception
- Displacement of blood clot
- Infection
- Abnormal involution of the placental site
- Choriocarcinoma

If there are signs of infection (fever, foul-smelling vaginal discharge), give antibiotics as for metritis. Conservative management may be appropriate if the vaginal loss is slight and there is no sign of infection. Heavy vaginal bleeding, a tender uterus with an open os, or the suggestion of retained products on ultrasound examination requires obstetric exploration. Give oxytocic drugs. If the cervix is dilated,

TABLE 32.4: COMPARISON OF VARIOUS PPH MANAGEMENT OPTIONS

Management Options	*Quality of Evidence*	*Strength of Recommendation*
Bimanual compression is a temporary measure	-	✓
Commence intravenous oxytocin infusion	III	B
Give further intravenous bolus of oxytocin	-	✓
Uterine packing or balloon tamponade	III	B
Prostaglandin options:		
• $PGF_{2\alpha}$ (0.5-1.0 mg) into uterine muscle	III	B
• 15-methyl-PGF_{α} (0.25 mg)	III	B
• Rectal misoprostal	Ib	A
B-Lynch sutures	III	B
Arterial embolisation if units have resources and experience	III	B
Bilateral uterine artery ligation	III	B
Bilateral internal iliac artery ligation	III	B
Bilateral ovarian artery ligation	III	B
Hysterectomy	III	B

explore by hand to remove large clots and placental fragments. Manual exploration of the uterus is similar to the technique described for removal of the retained placenta. If the cervix is not dilated, evacuate the uterus to remove placental fragments.

If bleeding continues, consider selective arterial embolisation (Pelage et al 1999), uterine and utero-ovarian artery ligation or hysterectomy. Perform histologic examination of curettings or hysterectomy specimen, if possible, to rule out trophoblastic tumour.

POST-HYSTERECTOMY BLEEDING

Bleeding may persist from the pelvic surface because of decreased coagulation combined with the trauma from prolonged manipulation. These small sites may be difficult to isolate and ligate.

a) Abdominal packing: In this situation, large packs are inserted into the pelvis. These packs can be removed 24 hours later, after correction of the coagulopathy.
b) Uterine/Internal iliac artery embolisation.

REFERENCES

AbdRabbo SA. 1994. Stepwise uterine devascularization: a novel technique for management of uncontrolled postpartum hemorrhage with preservation of the uterus. *Am J Obstet Gynecol* 171(3): 694–700.

AbouZahr CL. 1998. Lessons on safe motherhood. *World Health Forum*; 19(3):253–260.

American College of Obstetricians and Gynecologists. 1998. Postpartum hemorrhage. In *2001 Compendium of Selected Publications*, ACOG Educational Bulletin Number 243. Washington DC: ACOG.

Badaway SZA, A Etman, M Singh, K Murphy, T Mayelli and M Philadelphia. 2001. Uterine artery embolization: The role in obstetrics and gynecology. *J Clin Imag* 25:288–295.

Burchell RC. 1968. Physiology of internal iliac ligation. *J Obstet Gynaecol Br Commonwealth* 75:642–651.

Carroli G and E Bergel. 2002. Umbilical vein injection for management of retained placenta (Cochrane Review). In *The Cochrane Library*, Issue 2. Oxford, UK: Update Software.

Chaltopadhyay SK, B Deb Roy and YB Edrees. 1990. Surgical control of obstetric hemorrhage; hypogastric artery ligation or hysterectomy? *Int J Gynecol Obstet* 32:345–351.

Chan C, K Razvi and K Tham. 1997. The use of Sengstaken-Blakemore tube to control postpartum hemorrhage. *Int J Gynaecol Obstet* 58:251–252.

Cho J, H Jun and C Lee. 2000. Hemostatic suturing technique for uterine bleeding during cesarean delivery. *Obstetrics & Gynecology* 96:129–131

Clark SL, JP Phelan, S Yeh, SR Bruce and RH Paul. 1985. Hypogastric artery ligation for obstetric hemorrhage. *Obstet Gynecol* 66: 353–356.

Combs CA, EL Murphy and RK Laros Jr. 1991. Factors associated with postpartum hemorrhage with vaginal birth. *Obstet Gynecol* 77:69–76.

Druzin ML. 1989. Packing of lower uterine segment for control of post cesarean bleeding in instances of placenta previa. *Surg Gynecol Obstet* 169:543–545.

Evans S and P McShane. 1985. The efficacy of internal iliac artery ligation in obstetric hemorrhage. *Surg Gynecol Obstet* 160:250–253.

Hayman RG, S Arulkumaran and PJ Steer. 2002. Uterine compression sutures: surgical management of postpartum hemorrhage. *Obstet Gynecol* 99(3):502–506.

Hostetler RD and FM Bosworth. 2000. Uterine inversion: A life-threatening obstetric emergency. *J Am Board Fam Prac* 13(2):120–123.

Keirse Marc JNC. 1998. What does prevent postpartum haemorrhage? *Lancet* 351:690–692.

Lynch C, A Coker and A Laval. 1997. The B-Lynch surgical technique for control of massive postpartum haemorrhage: an alternative to hysterectomy? Five cases reported. *Br J Obstet Gynaecol* 104:372–376.

Marcovici I and B Scoccia. 1999. Postpartum haemorrhage and intrauterine balloon tamponade: a report of three cases. *J Reprod Med* 44:122–126.

O'Leary JA. 1995. Uterine artery ligation in the control of post-Cesarean hemorrhage. *J Reprod Med* 40:1989–2193.

Pelage JP, P Soyer et al. 1999. Secondary postpartum hemorrhage: treatment with selective arterial embolization. *Radiology* 212:385–389.

Prendiville WJ, D Elbourne and S McDonald. 2002. Active versus expectant management in the third stage of labour (Cochrane Review). In *The Cochrane Library*, Issue 1. Oxford: Update Software.

Riley DP and RW Burgess. 1995. External abdominal aortic compression: a study of a resuscitation manouver for postpartum hemorrhage. *Obstet Gynecol Surv* 50:426

SOGC. 2000. Prevention and management of postpartum haemorrhage: SOGC Clinical Practice Guidelines No 88. *J Soc Obstet Gynaecol Can* 22(4):271–281.

Vedantham S, SC Goddwin, B McLucas and G Mohr. 1997. Uterine artery embolization: an underused method of controlling pelvic hemorrhage. *Am J Obstet Gynecol* 176:938–948.

33

Anesthesia and Analgesia in Obstetrics

Ramkumar Venkateswaran | Vani Ramkumar

Pregnancy is a physiological condition associated with changes in maternal physiology that influence the administration of anesthesia. The presence of the fetus complicates the situation. The anesthesiologist caring for a pregnant woman needs to keep these maternal physiological changes in mind to provide anesthesia that is safe, not only for the mother but also for the unborn fetus.

Labour pains have been described as one of the most excruciating pains that a human being can experience. Though relief from labour pain has not been the main focus of attention of medical personnel caring for the parturient, there is no doubt that such relief is not only humane but also necessary, if not mandatory. This is where anesthetics and analgesics come into play.

Obstetric Analgesia

Stages and Progress of Labour Labour is the term used to describe the physiological process by which the products of conception are expelled from the uterus through the vagina. This process requires coordinated uterine contractions and progressive dilatation of the uterine cervix. The preservation of muscle tone is important not only to aid rotation of the fetal head during descent but also to provide the secondary powers for expulsion of the fetus.

Labour is traditionally divided into three stages—the first stage commences with regular uterine contractions and lasts till effacement and full dilatation of the uterine cervix; the second stage starts at full dilatation of the cervix and continues till the fetus is delivered; and the third stage begins with the delivery of the fetus and ends with the complete expulsion of the placenta and membranes.

Several techniques have been used to relieve the pain experienced during the first and second stages of labour. The choice of technique, as also the timing of its initiation, has a bearing on successful relief from labour pain.

At times, labour may not progress normally through these three stages. Abnormal progress of labour (or prolonged labour) can result from obstetric and non-obstetric causes, which can be classified as indicated in Table 33.1.

Labour Pain Pathways Pain during the first stage of labour is caused by stretching and thinning of the uterine cervix. This occurs as a result of regular uterine contractions, which are infrequent and of low intensity during the early stages of labour. Once

Table 33.1: Diagnostic features of prolonged labour

Feature	*Primipara*	*Multipara*
Slow latent phase	>20 hours	>14 hours
Slow-slope active phase	<1.2 cm/hour	<1.5 cm/hour
Active phase arrest	No cervical dilatation for 2 hours	
Slow descent of fetus	<1 cm/hour	<2 cm/hour
Arrest of descent	No descent for 1 hour	
Prolonged second stage without regional analgesia	>2 hours	>1 hour
Prolonged second stage with regional analgesia	>3 hours	>2 hours

Adapted from Glosten 2000.

active labour has been established, these contractions increase in frequency, strength and duration.

In active labour, uterine contractions occur once every three minutes, last for about one minute and produce intrauterine pressures in the range of 50–70 mmHg. Pain produced during the first stage of labour arises from the uterine cervix, which is richly supplied by nociceptive nerve endings. As this pain is visceral in nature, it is poorly localised and dull in character.

The pain impulses travel through the visceral afferents accompanying the sympathetic nerves and enter the spinal cord at the T_{10}, T_{11}, T_{12} and L_1 segments. Pain during the first stage of labour is usually observed in the lower back.

In the second stage of labour, the descending fetal head stretches the perineum. Pain associated with stretching of the perineum produces somatic pain, which, in contrast, is sharp and localised. Pain of the second stage of labour is carried by the pudendal nerves to the S_2, S_3 and S_4 spinal segments.

Techniques of Labour Analgesia The perception of labour pain depends on the physical and psychological makeup of the individual. Labour and delivery encompass a highly emotional period in a woman's life. The presence of sympathetic and encouraging medical staff during this period can go a long way in making the whole experience tolerable. Labour pain can be relieved by non-pharmacological and pharmacological methods as listed below:

- Non-pharmacological
  Psychological techniques (hypnosis and psychoprophylaxis)
  Transcutaneous electrical nerve stimulation
  Acupuncture
- Pharmacological
  Systemic opioids
  Inhaled analgesics
  Regional techniques

Non-pharmacological interventions are those that require the participation and cooperation of a highly motivated parturient. The parturient who wishes to experience 'natural' childbirth finds the relative empowerment afforded by non-pharmacological methods attractive. In comparison with the pharmacological techniques, non-pharmacological techniques do not provide complete relief from labour pain. The advantage, however, is that the parturient remains fully involved in the entire process of labour.

Psychological Techniques (Hypnosis and Psychoprophylaxis) Psychological techniques act mainly through suggestion. Though the subject appears to be asleep, she is actually in a trance under which she is very receptive to suggestions.

Hypnosis is believed to reduce pain and the need for analgesic drugs. There is a wide variation in its efficacy, ranging from no effect at all to virtually pain-free labour. The technique needs long periods of antenatal training. However, because of the associated amnesia, the parturient may feel deprived of the sense of active participation in the process of labour.

The psychoprophylactic method of Lamaze is the most popular form of psychological analgesia. The technique involves antenatal training over several sessions, wherein the pregnant lady receives instructions on the anatomy and physiology of pregnancy and delivery. This knowledge helps her to prepare her body and mind for the physiological process of labour.

She is taught to focus on a specific object or location away from herself, concentrate on releasing muscle tension, maintain a learned breathing rhythm and listen to positive reinforcement from her 'coach'. The need to concentrate on specific behavioural patterns helps to distract the mind from the pain of labour. There has been no scientific evidence to prove that psychoprophylactic techniques provide significant relief from labour pain.

Transcutaneous Electrical Nerve Stimulation (TENS) In this technique repetitive currents of small strength are applied to specific points over the skin to provide modulation of pain. The TENS stimulator is a dual output pulse generator that provides biphasic, asymmetrical square-wave current through two channels.

The amplitude and frequency of the delivered current can be individually varied. The leads from one channel are connected to a pair of electrodes that are placed on either side of the vertebral column over the posterior rami of T_{10} to L_1 for control of pain during the first stage of labour. The other pair of electrodes is placed on either side of the midline, opposite the 3rd sacral vertebra, for control of pain during the second stage of labour.

Electrical impulses of 0.1–0.5 MS duration are generated at frequencies ranging between 0 Hz and 200 Hz. The amplitude of the stimulus is gradually increased until a tingling sensation is appreciated over the skin. The frequency of stimulus is then increased until the parturient is comfortable. A current strength of 5–10 mA is used as a background stimulus and the strength increased to 25–40 mA during uterine contraction. The low frequency stimulation increases endorphin production. This causes analgesia and produces a feeling of well-being. High frequency stimulation closes the 'gate' in the spinal cord and inhibits transmission of pain impulses along the pain pathway.

TENS works best for low-level pain and is therefore more effective in early labour. It does not effectively control abdominal, suprapubic or perineal pain. TENS can take up to 40 minutes to become effective. It has the advantage of being non-invasive. In addition is does not interfere with fetal heart rate monitoring and does not produce any harmful effects on the mother or the fetus. This technique has at best been used as an adjunct to other methods of pain relief.

Acupuncture This technique, based on a traditional form of Chinese medicine, involves stimulating specific points on the body with needles inserted to a depth of 2.5–3 cm. The needles are manipulated until a feeling of warmth, numbness, distension and heaviness are experienced by the parturient, and a feeling of tightness is apparent in the operator. At this point, the needle is left undisturbed for a period of 10–30 minutes for the effect to be manifest. Alternatively, low voltage electrical stimulation at 2–3 Hz may be applied to the acupuncture needles (electroacupuncture).

As with the psychological techniques, acupuncture also produces inconsistent, incomplete and unpredictable pain relief. It has no adverse effects on the mother or fetus. In addition, it needs the constant attendance of personnel trained in this form of therapy. It can, therefore, at best be recommended as an adjunct to other forms of pain relief. Electroacupuncture can interfere with electronic fetal heart rate monitoring.

SYSTEMIC OPIOIDS Parenteral opioids are commonly used to relieve labour pains. Though they provide some degree of pain relief, the technique is less popular because of the frequency of maternal complications and potential for neonatal depression. Opioids such as pethidine, morphine and fentanyl can be used for labour analgesia. Opioids are administered as intermittent boluses through the intramuscular (IM) or intravenous (IV) routes.

Pethidine is used at a dose of 50–100 mg IM or 25–50 mg IV. The peak analgesic effect occurs within 40–50 minutes of IM administration or 5–10 minutes of IV administration. The duration of action is 3–4 hours. Infants delivered between one and four hours after IM administration of pethidine are likely to be depressed.

The peak analgesic effect of morphine occurs 1–2 hours after IM administration and 20 minutes after IV administration. Given its long duration of action of 4–6 hours, morphine produces depression of the newborn for longer than pethidine. The advent of shorter acting opioids such as fentanyl, sufentanil and remifentanil has made the use of opioids for labour analgesia more predictable and controllable.

Opioids can also be administered as patient-controlled intravenous analgesia, where the parturient can herself participate in titrating the dose to her requirements. Patient-controlled intravenous analgesia is reserved for situations where regional anesthesia is either contraindicated (as in severe pre-eclampsia with profound platelet deficiency) or is technically difficult (as with musculoskeletal deformities or previous spinal surgery). Fentanyl (loading dose of 50–100 μg, demand bolus of 20–25 μg, lockout time of five minutes) is more popular than pethidine, as it has a more rapid onset with lower incidence of nausea and sedation. Fentanyl has also been found to be better than alfentanil (Morley-Forster et al 2000).

The introduction of remifentanil, which has a better pharmacokinetic and pharmacodynamic profile, has renewed interest in the technique of patient-controlled intravenous analgesia (Kan 1998). As analgesic concentrations are achieved in 1–2 minutes, the drug can be delivered to coincide with the onset of uterine contractions.

Rapid esterase metabolism and fetal redistribution result in a short neonatal elimination half life. As the 3-minute, context-sensitive, half life is independent of the duration of infusion, maternal recovery is also rapid.

Remifentanil can be suitably administered as a bolus dose of 0.25–0.5 μg/kg with a 2-minute lockout and no concurrent infusion (Blair et al 2001). Maternal drowsiness can occur if the boluses exceed 0.5 μg/kg and apnea may occur in between uterine contractions. Naloxone should be readily available to antagonise these adverse effects.

In view of the potentially dangerous adverse effects on both the mother and the neonate, patient-controlled intravenous analgesia should be used only in special situations where a high level of vigilance can be ensured.

Inhaled Anesthetics Inhaled anesthetic agents administered in a controlled manner at appropriately low concentrations can provide effective relief from labour pain. Nitrous oxide is the commonest inhaled agent used either with oxygen or in combination with volatile anesthetics.

The earliest report of the use of nitrous oxide for relief of labour pain was in 1880 when 80% nitrous oxide was administered with 20% oxygen from an anesthetic machine. This technique had two inherent drawbacks—the possibility of inadvertently producing unconsciousness due to high concentration of nitrous oxide and an increased risk of maternal and fetal hypoxemia due to the relatively low concentrations of oxygen.

Subsequent availability of premixed cylinders of 50% nitrous oxide in 50% oxygen as entonox has partially overcome this problem. The use of entonox for the relief of labour pains was first described in 1961 (Tunstall 1961). A system for administering labour analgesia using entonox consists of a single, premixed cylinder of entonox, a demand valve that allows the gas to flow only when triggered by the inspiratory effort of the parturient, a corrugated tubing with a one-way expiratory valve and a facemask or mouthpiece to carry this gas to the parturient.

The parturient applies the facemask firmly over the mouth and nose and begins inhaling as soon as she feels a uterine contraction. As the levels of nitrous oxide build up in the blood, the parturient experiences pain relief. This technique, where the parturient herself holds the facemask and controls the inhalation of agents, is called patient-controlled intermittent inhalational analgesia (PCIIA).

The technique is simple to use and is effective in 50% of parturients. The physical properties of nitrous oxide are such that it needs to be inhaled for around 45 seconds for analgesia to become evident. It takes up to 90 seconds for the maximum analgesic effect of nitrous oxide. Thus, individuals with a high pain threshold may not get satisfactory pain relief unless the inhalation is begun early along with the onset of uterine contractions.

The addition of low concentrations of volatile agents such as isoflurane can provide more complete analgesia in these parturients but at the expense of significant sedative effects. It must be remembered that sedation abolishes protective pharyngeal and laryngeal reflexes, predisposing the parturient to the risk of aspiration of gastric contents.

In addition, the ability of the parturient to actively participate in the process of labour is also lost. Isoflurane, in a concentration of 0.75% in oxygen, produces analgesia that is comparable to entonox in the first stage of labour. Addition of 0.2–0.25% isoflurane or 1–4.5% desflurane can also improve the quality of analgesia but at the expense of more sedation and amnesia (Abboud et al 1995; Ross et al 1999). A premixed cylinder of 50% nitrous oxide and 0.25% isoflurane in oxygen is available as a stable mixture in the United Kingdom (Ross et al 1999).

The technique of PCIIA has the advantage of being safe, because its success depends on the ability of the parturient to maintain an airtight seal with the mask. The demand valve that permits the gas mixture to flow can be opened only when a negative pressure is created during inspiration. Should the level of consciousness be depressed by inhalational agents, the parturient will be unable to maintain an airtight seal. The demand valve then cannot be opened, inhaled agents will not be delivered in proper concentrations and room air will be inhaled instead, resulting in rapid return to consciousness. This inherent safety of PCIIA is defeated if the mask is reapplied by any individual other than the parturient, such as the husband or the attending nurse.

The use of a demand valve permits intermittent flow of inhaled agents only when these are needed. In contrast, a continuous flow such as that provided by an anesthetic machine results in build up of high concentrations of anesthetics in the environment of the labour suite, exposing all personnel working in the area to the hazards of inhaling such agents. The equipment used to provide labour analgesia usually comprises intermittent flow machines.

Regional Techniques Systemic analgesics and inhaled anesthetics cannot provide satisfactory analgesia in more than 50% of primipara. Regional techniques are possibly the only method of providing complete relief of labour pain. Techniques used include epidural analgesia, subarachnoid analgesia, paracervical block and pudendal block.

Epidural Analgesia Epidural analgesia should be initiated only after assessing maternal fitness, fetal status and progress of labour. Consent should be obtained for the procedure and maternal heart rate, blood pressure and oxygen saturation, continuous fetal heart rate and uterine contractions should be monitored throughout labour.

Epidural analgesia should be initiated only after the parturient has started complaining of pain and onset of labour has been confirmed by a cervical dilatation of 4–5 cm in primipara and 3–4 cm in multipara. The epidural catheter is inserted through either the L_2–L_3 or L_3–L_4 lumbar interspace and threaded cephalad, until at least 3–4 cm of the catheter lies in the epidural space.

Inadvertent intrathecal or intravenous placement of the epidural catheter can be ruled out by the administration of an epidural test dose consisting of 3 ml of 2% lignocaine hydrochloride with 5 μg/ml of adrenaline. Accidental intrathecal injection of this test dose will produce evidence of sensory or motor block within five minutes. Intravenous injection of 15 μg of adrenaline results in a transient increase in heart rate of 20–30 beats per minute within 30 seconds. Continuous recording of the maternal electrocardiogram is essential to detect this increase. During active labour, the use of adrenaline is neither sensitive nor specific, as the spontaneous increases in heart rate that accompany uterine contractions can obscure an increase produced by adrenaline, resulting in false-negative results.

While adrenaline is commonly added to the epidural test dose for detecting accidental intravenous injection in the USA, anesthesiologists practising in other regions might avoid its use for the above-mentioned reasons. In addition, intravenous injection of adrenaline can cause an increase in uterine tone.

Anesthesiologists who do not favour the use of adrenaline as a marker in the epidural test dose for detecting accidental intravenous placement usually rely on constant vigilance and a high index of suspicion to avoid this possible complication. As blood cannot be consistently aspirated in the event of an intravenous placement of the catheter, the additional precaution of administering therapeutic doses in fractional amounts of 3–4 ml should be taken, observing the parturient carefully for 2–3 minutes between each injection. In addition, the attending staff should maintain verbal contact with the parturient throughout labour to ensure that all is well.

Continuous lumbar epidural analgesia through a catheter inserted at a single level has been the commonest technique for providing epidural labour analgesia. Other modifications used include a segmental epidural, double-catheter technique and combined spinal-epidural technique.

Bupivacaine (0.25%) has been the local anesthetic of choice through the lumbar epidural route for providing labour analgesia. However, the significant motor block produced by this concentration is unacceptable, as it results in loss of muscle tone required to aid rotation of the fetal head during descent and also for the expulsion of the fetus. Addition of preservative-free opioids, such as fentanyl 0.0002%, sufentanil 0.0001% or diamorphine 0.0025%, to a more dilute solution of bupivacaine (0.0625–0.125%) offers the advantage of improving analgesia while causing minimal motor block. This results in better expulsive efforts during delivery.

Once the lumbar epidural catheter is appropriately sited, an initial dose of 8–12 ml of 0.125–0.25% bupivacaine is administered at a cervical dilatation of 4–5 cm in a primipara (or 3–4 cm in a multipara). Alternatively, 8–12 ml of 0.0625–0.125% bupivacaine with 50 μg fentanyl can be used.

An epidural infusion of 5 ml/hour of 0.125% bupivacaine with 0.0002% fentanyl is then started and the rate of administration titrated to achieve adequate pain relief. A sensory level of block of up to T_{10} is aimed for. The rate of infusion is decreased to 4 ml/hour if the sensory level goes above T_{10}. If the level is inadequate, a bolus of 5 ml is administered and the same rate of infusion continued.

When the parturient complains of perineal pain indicative of onset of second stage of labour, an additional dose of 8–12 ml of epidural solution (0.25% bupivacaine or 0.125% bupivacaine with 0.0002% fentanyl) can be administered in the sitting position to aid in spread of the drug to the sacral segments.

If more intense anesthesia is needed for instrumental vaginal delivery, a top-up can be provided using a rapidly-acting local anesthetic such as 10 ml of 2–3% chloroprocaine or 2% lignocaine. The added advantage of having an ongoing epidural is that should the obstetrician decide to take up the parturient for a cesarean section, the block can be extended from T_{10} to T_4 within 10–15 minutes using 10–12 ml of 0.5% bupivacaine (or an equal volume of 2–3% chloroprocaine or 2% lignocaine).

A segmental epidural analgesia obtained by placing an epidural catheter at the T_{10}–T_{11} space and injecting small doses of local anesthetic such as 4 ml of 0.5% bupivacaine can be used to relieve pain during the first stage of labour. However, this technique has the drawback that perineal pain induced by the second stage of labour, which is often more distressing, is not relieved.

A double-catheter technique involves the use of an epidural catheter at the T_{10}–T_{12} level to relieve the pain of first stage of labour, while a second caudal catheter is used to relieve the pain of the second stage of labour. The administration of drugs is timed to provide rapid, intense analgesia in a sequential manner. However, the discomfort associated with the two needle and catheter insertions makes this technique less popular. The technique may find special use in a parturient with co-existent cardiac disease, as it can provide relief from labour pain with minimal sympathetic block (and therefore the least changes in hemodynamics).

In the technique of patient-controlled epidural analgesia, the patient can dial the administration of additional top-ups of epidural solution. A baseline infusion provides basal levels of analgesia. As individual pain thresholds vary, the parturient is given partial control over titrating the administration of drugs to her own level of comfort. Patient-controlled analgesia pumps can be set to control the maximum number of top-ups delivered on patient demand in a given time interval, thereby making the technique safe.

The combined spinal-epidural technique has become popular because it combines the advantages of both the techniques. The epidural space is identified at the L_3–L_4 level using a Tuohy needle and a long 29-gauge needle is passed through this needle into the subarachnoid space. The pain of the first stage of labour can be relieved for 60–120 minutes by injecting an opioid (25 μg of fentanyl or 5–10 μg of sufentanil) and the epidural catheter is then introduced. Local anesthetic solution is then injected through the epidural catheter at a later stage, when it is unlikely to impede the progress of labour. Use of intrathecal opioids provides early pain relief without affecting the progress of labour.

Several local anesthetics have been tried but the most popular has been bupivacaine. A concentration of 0.035–0.125% bupivacaine produces good analgesia with minimal motor block. Addition of an opioid such as fentanyl (1–2 μg/ml) improves the quality of analgesia without worsening the motor block. However, bupivacaine is cardiotoxic. Accidental intravenous injection of even 25 mg of bupivacaine can produce cardiac arrest. Hence, it is advisable that bupivacaine be administered by slow intravenous injection in fractions of no more than 20 mg at a time.

Ropivacaine (0.2%) has similar properties but has the advantage of being less cardiotoxic. It is currently a popular alternative to bupivacaine. Lignocaine in a concentration of 1–1.5% rapidly produces a sensory and motor block that lasts for up to 90 minutes. Chloroprocaine (2%) is another drug that produces rapid and intense sensory and motor blockade that lasts for a short duration.

The addition of opioids improves the quality of analgesia without increasing motor block, which is a desirable situation as it retains the ability of the parturient to actively participate in the process of labour. However, opioids are more effective in relieving pain during the first stage of labour than in relieving somatic pain that is characteristic of the second stage of labour.

Epidural Analgesia and the Progress of Labour Epidural analgesia can potentially affect the progress of labour. While it has not been found to increase the rate of primary cesarean section, it does seem to increase the rate of oxytocin administration and operative vaginal delivery (Echt et al 2000; Howell 2000). It also increases the length of both the first and second stages of labour (Howell 2000; Alexander et al 2002).

The quality of pain relief offered by epidural analgesia more than offsets the need for augmentation of insufficient uterine contractions by oxytocin. Appropriate instructions by the obstetric caregiver to encourage pushing at the time of uterine contractions can also overcome some of the problems associated with epidural analgesia.

Indications and Contraindications for Epidural Analgesia Epidural analgesia is primarily indicated in high-risk parturients. Parturients with anticipated difficult intubation, obesity and co-existing cardiac and pulmonary disease are at an increased risk when scheduled for emergency cesarean section under general anesthesia. When epidural analgesia is already established, it can be easily extended to provide anesthesia for emergency cesarean section, thereby avoiding the problems associated with general anesthesia in these high-risk parturients.

Fetal indications for epidural analgesia include babies that are premature or small for gestational age. Good relief from labour pain allows more controlled delivery conditions where the mother does not bear down too forcibly, offering protection to such babies.

Contraindications to the use of epidural analgesia include patient refusal, infection at the proposed site of epidural puncture, septicemia and pre-eclampsia/eclampsia with altered coagulation.

Subarachnoid Analgesia Subarachnoid injection of hyperbaric local anesthetics such as 5–10 mg of bupivacaine (or 15–20 mg of lignocaine) in the sitting position rapidly provides predictable and intense analgesia of the sacral segments, but some motor blockade is unavoidable. Intrathecal opioids block pain sensation without producing sympathetic or motor block. The major drawback of intrathecal opioids is the problem associated with delayed ventilatory depression. Fentanyl (25 μg) or sufentanil (5–10 μg) administered in the subarachnoid space provides good analgesia lasting for between 60 and 120 minutes.

Paracervical Block Paracervical block can be given to block the pain of the first stage of labour by injecting local anesthetic submucosally, through a purpose-designed needle, into the vaginal fornix at the 3 and 9 o'clock positions. A paracervical block interrupts uterine sympathetic afferent activity through the posterior cervical and superior hypogastric plexuses, producing acceptable relief of first-stage pain in 50–70% of parturients.

The duration of the analgesia is 30–90 minutes and the injection can be repeated. The major drawback is the incidence of fetal bradycardia (5–50%) that occurs within 2–3 minutes of administration of the block and persists for 10 minutes. In more severe cases, fetal bradycardia can last for 20–30 minutes, resulting in intense neonatal depression. The unacceptably high incidence of neonatal depression has led to many centres abandoning this technique.

Pudendal Block The pudendal nerve provides sensory and motor supply to the perineum. This nerve is blocked by the transvaginal route by injecting 1% lignocaine between the sacrotuberous and sacrospinous ligaments. Pudendal nerve block can effectively relieve pain during the second stage of labour.

OBSTETRIC ANESTHESIA

Anesthesia for Cesarean Section The choice of anesthesia for cesarean section depends on the obstetric indication, maternal and fetal status and desires of the mother. Regional techniques are being increasingly preferred over general anesthesia, for cesarean section because of the advantages that such a technique offers. While the advantages of spinal anesthesia include simplicity, low failure rate and rapid onset of action, the disadvantages include a higher incidence of hypotension.

A regional technique is preferred for a scheduled *elective cesarean section*. A cesarean section that is not scheduled on an elective basis is termed an *emergency cesarean section*. These are further classified as *stable, urgent* or *stat* depending on the maternal and fetal condition (Harris 1990).

A *stable emergency cesarean section is* one wherein maternal and fetal physiology is stable but cesarean section is indicated before destabilisation occurs, that is, chronic placental insufficiency. An epidural or spinal anesthesia is the anesthetic of choice for a stable emergency cesarean section.

An *urgent emergency cesarean section* is indicated when maternal and/or fetal physiology is unstable but the condition is not an immediate threat to maternal or fetal survival; for example, dystocia, previous cesarean section in active labour and variable deceleration with prompt recovery. The anesthesiologist can consider extending an existing epidural or administer spinal anesthesia for an urgent emergency cesarean section.

A *stat* emergency cesarean section is indicated when the condition is immediately life-threatening to the mother and/or the fetus, for example, massive hemorrhage, cord prolapse with fetal bradycardia and ruptured uterus. The anesthetic of choice is general anesthesia (unless an existing epidural can be satisfactorily extended without delay).

Spinal Anesthesia Once a decision is taken for cesarean section, 15–30 ml of a non-particulate antacid such as 0.3 molar sodium citrate is administered orally. The parturient is transferred to the operating room in the lateral position to prevent or minimise the effects of aortocaval compression by the gravid uterus. In the operating room, essential monitoring is set up. This comprises electrocardiography (Lead II), non-invasive blood pressure and pulse oximetry. The mother is positioned on the operating table with a wedge under the buttock and upper thigh to move the gravid uterus away from the aorta and inferior vena cava. Oxygen is administered at a rate of 2–3 l/min through nasal prongs. A large-bore (18 or 16 SWG) intravenous access is established and 500–750 ml of a dextrose-free balanced salt solution is administered over 10 minutes while the team prepares for regional anesthesia. Equipment such as oropharyngeal airways, tracheal tubes and laryngoscopes must be kept ready, as also drugs such as ephedrine and oxytocin.

The spinal anesthetic can be administered with the parturient in the lateral or sitting position according to the convenience of the parturient and the anesthesiologist. A 25 or 27 SWG spinal needle with a non-cutting point (Whitacre or Sprotte) is used to minimise the incidence of postdural puncture headache.

A dose of 9–12 mg (1.8–2.4 ml of 0.5% hyperbaric bupivacaine) is administered in the L_3–L_4 lumbar interspace to achieve a sensory level of T_4. Addition of 12.5–25 μg of fentanyl improves the quality of analgesia and provides good postoperative analgesia. Once the baby is delivered, the mother is given 10 IU of oxytocin IV followed by an infusion of 15–20 IU in a drip to promote uterine contraction.

Any hypotension that occurs is treated with intravenous fluids along with 3–6 mg boluses of ephedrine. Phenylephrine can also be used as an alternative.

General Anesthesia General anesthesia may be indicated for cesarean delivery in severe fetal compromise, maternal hemorrhage, overt coagulopathy or patient preference. General anesthesia has the advantages of rapid induction, better cardiovascular stability and better control of the airway and ventilation. However, it is also associated with higher incidence of maternal morbidity and mortality because of the risks of pulmonary aspiration of gastric contents, failed intubation, maternal awareness and uterine atony. Further, increased incidence of neonatal depression has been observed.

Parturients who are likely to be scheduled for cesarean section are allowed only clear fluids so that the chances of regurgitation and pulmonary aspiration can be minimised. In addition, as described earlier, 15–30 ml of a non-particulate antacid such as 0.3 molar sodium citrate should be administered orally as soon as the decision is taken for cesarean section, preferably within one hour of anesthetic induction. A histamine-2 receptor blocker such as ranitidine, along with metoclopramide, can also be administered to reduce gastric acidity and residual gastric volume.

The obstetrician can alert the anesthesiologist to some of the potential complications that can arise during general anesthesia such as a difficult intubation due to alteration in airway anatomy. A quick examination of the airway can be performed by the obstetrician using the simple '1-2-3 rule'. The ability to insinuate a finger into the temporomandibular joint space by placing a finger in front of the tragus and asking the parturient to open her mouth; checking whether two fingers can be placed between the upper and lower incisors with the mouth wide open; and clearance of at least three fingers between the chin and the thyroid notch (the thyromental distance) should indicate that the upper airway is grossly normal.

If this simple 1-2-3 rule is not satisfied, the obstetrician should alert the anesthesiologist to perform a preliminary examination in the labour suite so that the necessary preparations can be made by the anesthesiology team in anticipation of a difficult intubation. The anesthesiologist will, in addition, check the structures that are visible inside the oral cavity with the mouth wide open (Samsoon and Young's modification of the Mallampati classification of the airway), and movements of the head and neck, both of which will give additional information regarding possible airway difficulties.

The parturient is shifted to the operating room in the lateral position. Supplemental oxygen is administered, especially in the presence of a non-reassuring fetal status. Once inside the operating room, basic monitoring is established and intravenous access obtained as described earlier. Preoxygenation is begun with 6 l/min of oxygen for at least three to five minutes.

A rapid-sequence induction is performed in cesarean section to prevent the chances of regurgitation and pulmonary aspiration. The technique implies the rapid injection of 4–5 mg/kg of thiopentone sodium and 1.5 mg/kg of succinylcholine hydrochloride and performance of tracheal intubation within 60 seconds. The chances of pulmonary aspiration exist from the time consciousness is lost until isolation of the airway by inflation of the tracheal tube cuff. This critical period is taken care of by an anesthetic assistant who applies cricoid pressure from the time anesthetic induction is begun until the tracheal tube cuff is inflated after confirmation of the proper position. Cricoid pressure, which implies direct posterior pressure over the cricoid cartilage, helps to occlude the esophagus between the flat portion of the cricoid cartilage and the cervical spine, thereby preventing regurgitation of gastric contents.

Anesthesia is maintained with 0.5% halothane in 50% nitrous oxide and 50% oxygen. Alternatively, 0.75% isoflurane can be used. Muscle relaxants are administered as required. Maternal hyperventilation is avoided. Once the neonate is delivered and the umbilical cord has been clamped, the anesthetic is deepened with higher concentrations of nitrous oxide (up to 66%) and intravenous opioids (50–75 μg of fentanyl or 25 mg of pethidine). Oxytocics are administered as outlined earlier. At the end of the procedure, tracheal extubation is performed only when the mother is awake and responding to commands.

Failed Endotracheal Intubation A report of anesthesia-related maternal mortality in the United States during the period 1979–1990 revealed that 82% (106/179) occurred during anesthesia for cesarean delivery (Hawkins et al 1997). More than half these deaths occurred under general anesthesia, and an airway-related problem was the leading cause for anesthesia-related mortality. Reports of Confidential Enquiries into Maternal Deaths in the United

Kingdom also identified the inability to secure the airway as the leading cause of anesthesia-related mortality (Hibbard et al 1994, 1997).

Because airway difficulties cannot always be predicted by a preoperative airway assessment, the anesthesiologist should always be prepared to handle an unexpected difficulty in tracheal intubation. Equipment that should be available include two working laryngoscopes with a variety of laryngoscope blades, several sizes of tracheal tubes with stylets, laryngeal mask airway, Combitube, fibreoptic bronchoscope and a means of transtracheal administration of oxygen.

Should intubation prove difficult at the first attempt, the anesthesiologist should alert the theatre personnel, call for help and obtain difficult airway equipment. A pre-rehearsed drill, the failed intubation drill, should then guide the anesthesiologist through various decision-making steps that give top priority to maternal safety while at the same time safeguarding fetal welfare. Hypoxia can occur rapidly in a parturient. Hence, application of cricoid pressure is continued and gentle mask ventilation is provided, keeping the expiratory valve of the circuit partly open. Laryngoscopy is repeated using a different laryngoscope blade after optimising the position of the head and neck.

It is important to remember that patients develop hypoxia not because of failure to intubate but because of failure to ventilate. Therefore, in non-emergent situations, where ventilation proves difficult, oxygenation is continued, the muscle relaxant is allowed to wear off and the parturient allowed to awaken. The surgery is then performed either under regional anesthesia or after securing the airway in the awake state under topical anesthesia.

In emergency situations where the surgery cannot be postponed, the anesthesiologist must give top priority to maternal oxygenation. When mask ventilation is possible, surgery should be continued with anesthesia maintained using the face mask. The parturient is allowed to maintain spontaneous breathing of 100% oxygen with low concentrations of inhaled anaesthetics and intermittent IV ketamine.

When mask ventilation proves difficult in an emergency situation, maternal oxygenation must continue to receive top priority. The laryngeal mask airway (LMA) can be used to facilitate ventilation even though it does not protect the airway. The LMA can also be used to maintain spontaneous ventilation while intubation is attempted through it under fibreoptic guidance. If oxygenation still cannot be maintained, more invasive alternatives, such as transtracheal jet ventilation or tracheostomy, should be considered.

Neonatal depression is likely to occur as frequently in mothers receiving general anesthesia as in those receiving regional techniques. However, neonatal depression following general anesthesia can be minimised by limiting the time from induction to delivery (induction–delivery interval) to less than 10 minutes (Warren et al 1983).

This can be accomplished if anesthesia is induced only after the obstetrician has prepared and draped the parturient. Another important interval is the uterine incision–delivery interval, which, if kept below three minutes, provides better neonatal outcome (Datta et al 1981).

Anesthesia for Complicated Obstetrics

Emergency cesarean section may be indicated for complications that can occur unexpectedly during late pregnancy or labour. These include conditions such as pre-eclampsia/eclampsia, prolapsed umbilical cord and antepartum hemorrhage. When there is immediate danger to the mother or fetus, general anesthesia is often the technique of choice. However, in selected cases, extension of an existing epidural placed for labour analgesia or administration of a spinal anesthetic may also be acceptable.

Patients with pre-eclampsia/eclampsia have additional problems such as uncontrolled hypertension (with rapid swings of blood pressure during anesthesia), altered coagulation (influencing the choice of spinal or epidural anesthesia), hepatic dysfunction with low proteins (needing judicious use of intravenous fluids to prevent pulmonary edema), altered consciousness (needing protection of airway and elective postoperative ventilation) and possible drug interactions (magnesium sulphate can alter response to neuromuscular blocking agents).

Prolapse of the umbilical cord is often associated with breech presentations. If emergency cesarean section is scheduled for prolapsed umbilical cord, a general anesthetic would be the technique of choice.

Obstetric hemorrhage can occur due to placenta previa or placental abruption. The choice of anesthetic (general versus spinal) is dictated by the maternal and fetal condition. Retained placenta is one of the causes of postpartum hemorrhage. Removal of an adherent placenta can be facilitated by the administration of general anesthesia using inhalation agents such as halothane.

Summary Pregnancy is a physiological condition that has its natural culmination in labour. The anesthesiologist dealing with the pregnant woman needs to be aware of the changes in maternal physiology brought about by pregnancy to provide safe anesthesia for cesarean delivery.

The anesthesiologist also plays a role in making normal vaginal delivery painless. This chapter has outlined the principles that guide the anesthesiologist in providing safe analgesia and anesthesia to the parturient. Anesthetic concerns in selected situations of complicated obstetrics have also been described.

References

Abboud TK, F Swart, J Zhu et al. 1995. Desflurane analgesia for vaginal delivery. *Acta Anaesthesiol Scand* 39:259–261.

Alexander JM, SK Sharma, DD McIntire et al. 2002. Epidural analgesia lengthens the Friedman active phase of labor. *Obstet Gynecol* 100:46–50.

Blair JM, DA Hill and JPH Fee. 2001. Patient-controlled analgesia for labour using remifentanil: a feasibility study. *Br J Anaesth* 87:415–420.

Datta S, GW Ostheimer, JB Weiss et al. 1981. Neonatal effect of prolonged anesthetic induction for cesarean section. *Obstet Gynecol* 58:331.

Echt M, W Begneaud and D Montgomery. 2000. Effect of epidural analgesia on the primary cesarean section and forceps delivery rates. *J Reprod Med* 45:557–561.

Glosten B. 2000. Anesthesia for Obstetrics. In *Anesthesia*, ed Miller RD, 2024–68. New York: Churchill Livingstone.

Harris AP. 1990. Emergency cesarean section. In *Current Practice in Anesthesiology*, ed MC Rogers, 361–366. Toronto BC Decker.

Hawkins JL, LM Koonin, SK Palmer et al. 1997. Anesthesia-related deaths during obstetric delivery in the United States, 1979–1990. *Anesthesiology* 86:77.

Hibbard BM, MM Anderson, JO Drife et al. 1994. Deaths associated with anaesthesia. *Report on Confidential Enquiries into Maternal Deaths in the United Kingdom, 1988–1990, 80*. London: HMSO.

Hibbard BM, MM Anderson, JO Drife et al. 1997. Deaths associated with anaesthesia. *Report on Confidential Enquiries into Maternal Deaths in the United Kingdom, 1991–1993*. London: HMSO.

Howell CJ. 2000. Epidural versus non-epidural analgesia for pain relief in labour. *Cochrane Database Syst Rev*; 2:CD000331.

Kan RE, SC Hughes, MA Rosen et al. 1998. Intravenous remifentanil: placental transfer, maternal and neonatal effects. *Anesthesiology* 88:1467–1474.

Morley-Forster PK, D Reid and H Vanderberghe. 2000. A comparison of patient-controlled analgesia with fentanyl and alfentanil for labour analgesia. *Can J Anaesth* 47:113–119.

Ross JAS, ME Tunstall, DM Campbell et al. 1999. The use of 0.25% isoflurane premixed in 50% nitrous oxide and oxygen for pain relief in labour. *Anaesthesia* 54:1166–1172.

Samsoon GL and JR Young. 1987. Difficult tracheal intubation: a retrospective study. *Anaesthesia* 42:487.

Tunstall ME. 1961. Use of a fixed nitrous oxide and oxygen mixture from one cylinder. *Lancet* 2:964.

Warren TM, S Datta, GW Osthemer et al. 1983. Comparison of the maternal and neonatal effects of halothane, enflurane and isoflurane for cesarean delivery. *Anesth Analg* 62:516.

34

Perinatal Asphyxia

Narayan Jana | Nalini Arora

Perinatal asphyxia remains an important cause of perinatal mortality, and long-term neurological morbidity worldwide. Its consequences are multifaceted—medical, social, economic and medicolegal. Although the introduction of new techniques of fetal surveillance has given some cause for optimism, for several decades now, perinatal deaths related to fetal asphyxia have remained relatively constant. Neonatal brain damage related to perinatal asphyxia has been considered an important cause of cerebral palsy and mental retardation. Despite advancement of obstetric and neonatal technologies, the rate of cerebral palsy in term infants (one to two cases per 1000 births) has changed very little in the last decade in developed countries (ACOG 1994; Blair 2001). The lack of change in the incidence has prompted a more critical look at the antecedents and causes of cerebral palsy. Epidemiological studies have suggested that nearly 10% of cerebral palsy and a smaller proportion of mental retardation in term infants are associated with evidence of intrapartum asphyxia, and in some cases, there may have been an antenatal component (Blair and Stanley 1988; RCOG 2001). Therefore, effective intervention aiming at the reduction of perinatal asphyxia, and its consequences such as cerebral palsy and neurological disability, should involve both antepartum and intrapartum care along with advanced neonatal support.

Incidence Clinical studies have shown that asphyxial exposure with significant metabolic acidosis occurs in approximately 20 per 1000 births in developed countries (Low 1998). Neonatal encehalopathy, a severe complication of perinatal asphyxia has been reported in 7 per 1000 births in Western Australia (Spencer et al 1997). The diagnostic criteria for perinatal asphyxia are so stringent that it is hard to obtain reliable community-based data, particularly in developing countries. In India, approximately 40% of all perinatal deaths have been associated with fetal-neonatal hypoxia/asphyxia although current data remains inadequate. Both prematurity and intrauterine growth restriction (IUGR) are the leading contributors to perinatal asphyxia (Mehta and Jayant 1981; Mehta 1983).

Terminology The term 'asphyxia' indicates impairment of respiratory gas exchange leading to depletion of oxygen in blood and tissues, accompanied by metabolic acidosis. The hypoxic event can occur before, during or after birth, although the timing of onset and progression of these changes can be difficult or impossible to ascertain in many clinical scenarios. In clinical practice, 'fetal asphyxia' includes progressive hypoxemia, hypercapnia and metabolic acidosis that started either before the onset of labour (termed 'antenatal asphyxia') or during labour ('intrapartum asphyxia'). Asphyxia should be termed as 'neonatal' if it occurs after birth. However, such strict division may not be possible because of insidious onset of hypoxic process, and technical difficulties in confirming the diagnosis before or during labour. In a clinical context, hypoxia can be 'acute' or 'chronic' or 'acute on chronic,' and hypoxic events can be 'continuous' or 'intermittent.' Therefore, if uncertainty exists relating to the onset of the hypoxic event/process, the term 'perinatal asphyxia' may be used (MacLennan 1999). In obstetric practice, two terms, 'fetal distress' and 'birth asphyxia' are commonly used to indicate perinatal asphyxia. It has been suggested that these terms are inappropriate, and their use be avoided (ACOG 2005).

Pathophysiology Understanding fetal response to hypoxia is central to the diagnosis and management of perinatal asphyxia. Experimental studies suggest that a normally grown fetus is very able to compensate for hypoxic episodes with cardiovascular, hormonal, metabolic and behavioural changes. In mild to moderate hypoxia, the fetus resorts to a series of protective mechanism by redistribution of more blood to the vital organs such as the brain, heart and adrenal glands at the expense of less essential organs such as subcutaneous tissue, muscles, kidneys and liver (Luzietti et al 2002; Low 2004). This 'centralisation' of fetal circulation response is important to the integrity of the central nervous system during the 'compensatory' phase (Fig. 34.1).

However, with progressive fetal hypoxia there is anerobic metabolism causing lactic acidemia and energy depletion leading to

FIGURE 34.1: PATHOPHYSIOLOGY OF FETAL HYPOXIA

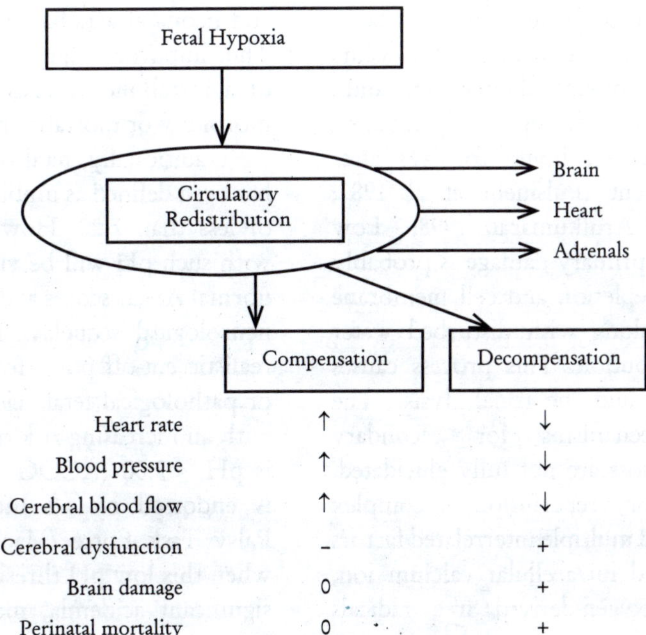

poor myocardial contractility, hypotension and decreased cerebral blood flow. Thus 'decompensation' sets in, resulting in cerebral dysfunction and brain damage (Low 1998).

The fetal circulatory responses and tolerance to hypoxia depend on the severity, acuteness and duration of the hypoxic events, and the condition of fetal reserve. A growth-restricted fetus has less energy reserve compared to a well grown one, and is prone to enter the stage of 'decompensation' early. This may be due to differences in metabolic adaptation between fetuses with normal and restricted intrauterine growth (Nicolini et al 1990). Each hypoxic stress produces a series of fetal heart rate (FHR) patterns that are important, but they are an imprecise clinical indicator of fetal condition in utero. In mild to moderate hypoxia, the window of opportunity to intervene can be in hours, whereas in severe acute hypoxia (for example, severe placental abruption, cord prolapse or uterine rupture), it may be extremely short or virtually absent.

At the cellular level, neuronal loss takes place in two phases. A primary loss occurs during an initial hypoxic/ischemic event, and a secondary loss occurs during the reperfusion/reoxygenation phase, hours to days after the primary event (Pulsinelli et al 1982; Nordstrom and Arulkumaran 1998; Low el al 2004). The primary damage is probably due to energy depletion and cell membrane depolarisation, along with disturbed water and ionic distribution. This process causes cellular edema and neuronal lysis. The underlying mechanisms for secondary phase neuronal loss are not fully elucidated. During circulatory reperfusion, a complex process starts and multiple interrelated factors such as increased intracellular calcium ion, nitric oxide, oxygen-derived free radicals and excitatory amino acids act in concert producing brain injury (Hagberg et al 2001). Oxygen-derived free radicals are produced during normal aerobic metabolism, but are effectively inactivated by naturally occurring scavenger systems (enzymes and antioxidants). However, after significant hypoxia, these protective mechanisms are impaired causing concomitant damage to the cell membrane and destruction of cellular DNA. In recent years, better understanding of the cellular mechanism of perinatal hypoxia opens up the scope for newer modalities in its treatment—scavengers for oxygen-derived free radicals, magnesium or calcium antagonists, lipid peroxidation inhibitors, superoxide dismutase and catalase (Rosenberg et al 1989).

Diagnostic criteria Asphyxia implies hypoxia severe enough to cause metabolic acidosis. Thus, clinical assessment such as Apgar score alone cannot be used to define or classify asphyxia. An appropriate method for defining this condition is assessment of fetal and neonatal acid-base status (ACOG 1995). The important question is the threshold of a metabolic acidosis beyond which fetal morbidity or mortality may occur.

Traditionally, fetal or newborn academia has been defined as umbilical artery blood pH of less than 7.20. However, most neonates with such pH will be vigorous at birth with normal Apgar scores and manifest no obvious neurological sequelae. Therefore, the more realistic cut-off point for defining significant or pathological fetal acidemia that correlates with an increasing risk of neurological deficit is pH <7.00 (ACOG 1995), and this view is endorsed by an International Cerebral Palsy Task Force (MacLennan 1999). Even when this low pH threshold is used to define significant acidemia, most neonates in this category will be neurologically normal, with no long-term morbidity (Goodwin et al 1992; Fee et al 1990).

Another biochemical method of determining metabolic acidosis is estimation of base deficit. Moderate and severe newborn complications occur only in newborns with umbilical artery base deficits >12 mmol/l. Thereafter, increasing metabolic acidosis is associated with a progression of severity of newborn complications (Low et al 1997). However, an international task force (MacLennan 1999) has suggested a higher cut-off point (>16 mmol/l).

On the basis of the current evidence, it seems reasonable to diagnose asphyxia as cord pH <7.0 and a base deficit >12 mmol/l. However, as a large majority of the neonates with asphyxia, by this definition, have no long-term deficit, it has been suggested that the term 'birth asphyxia' should be reserved to indicate more severe neonatal condition in which, in addition to acidosis, evidence of generalised multi-organ dysfunction is present. Thus, Thorp (1990) suggested the inclusion of neonatal depression as measured by the Apgar score, along with evidence of hypoxic damage manifested by neonatal seizures and end-organ dysfunction. The ACOG (1994) definition for intrapartum asphyxia has included both biochemical and clinical criteria (Table 34.1).

Clinical prediction All pregnancies are at risk of perinatal asphyxia. Several antepartum and intrapartum factors are associated with modest increase of perinatal asphyxia (Table 34.2).

The term 'low risk' based on clinical assessment cannot be applied to predict fetal exposure to asphyxia in labour. Clinical risk scoring has major limitations because of two reasons. First, fetal exposure to asphyxia does occur in a significant proportion of pregnancies with no risk factor. Approximately 40% of all perinatal deaths due to asphyxia had no clinical risk factors before or during labour (Low et al 1995). Second, in those cases where a clinical risk factor was present, risk was determined by the presence of a wide range of pregnancy complications. There was no single risk factor showing strong association with perinatal asphyxia. The positive predictive value for both antepartum and intrapartum risk factors for perinatal asphyxia was only 3%. Therefore, clinical risk scoring is fraught with high false-positives requiring further fetal assessment (Low et al 1992, 1995).

Screening For Fetal Hypoxia

Fetal surveillance has primarily evolved as a method of screening pregnant women at risk for intrauterine fetal death and identifying fetuses in a hypoxic condition, so that measures might be taken in time to avert permanent damage or death. A secondary objective of antepartum testing is to confirm the well being of an uncompromised fetus so that unnecessary intervention might be avoided. Fetal surveillance should begin at a gestational age that maximises the benefits and minimises the potential risks of iatrogenic prematurity due to false-positive test results. Once initiated, tests should be repeated at regular intervals, and the time interval depends on severity, duration and impact of hypoxia on the fetus. The threshold of viability depends on the level of neonatal facilities available in a particular set-up. In the Indian context, it may not be prudent to start antepartum testing before 26 weeks gestation, except in rare situations.

Hypoxic events may affect a fetus antepartum, intrapartum or both; thus, the screening methods also vary. Currently,

TABLE 34.1: AMERICAN COLLEGE OF OBSTETRICIANS AND GYNECOLOGISTS, 1994: CRITERIA FOR INTRAPARTUM ASPHYXIA

Severe intrapartum hypoxia sufficient to cause neonatal hypoxic encehalopathy

- Profound metabolic or mixed acidosis (umbilical arterial pH <7.0)
- Apgar score of 0-3 at 5 minutes
- Moderate to severe neonatal encehalopathy (e.g., seizures, coma or prolonged hypotonia)
- Multiorgan dysfunction (e.g., cardiovascular, gastro-intestinal, hematological, pulmonary or renal system)

ACOG Committee Opinion. Number 138. 1994. Utility of umbilical cord blood acid-base assessment. Washington DC: American College of Obstetricians and Gynecologists.

TABLE 34.2: RISK FACTORS FOR PERINATAL ASPHYXIA

Antepartum

Maternal medical complications

Hypertension, renal disease, heart disease, diabetes, collagen disease, respiratory disease, chronic infection, and acute severe infection

Maternal obstetric complications

Gestational hypertension/pre-eclampsia, eclampsia and diabetes with vasculopathy

Fetal complications

Intrauterine growth restriction, major fetal anomalies, oligohydramnios and polyhydramnios

Placental abnormalities

Placental insufficiency/dysfunction, placental abruption and placenta previa

Intrapartum

Preterm or post-term labour, meconium in amniotic fluid, malpresentation, and induced or prolonged or slow progress of labour

several fetal monitoring tests are used in isolation, or in combination, or in succession (Table 34.3).

However, precision of these tools remains a major source of comment in perinatal medicine. It is extremely important to understand that hypoxia has a global impact on fetal organ systems. Most of the antepartum surveillance tests (except biophysical profile) are responsible for assessing a small part of the fetal organ system; such 'focal' approach to a 'global' pathology is scientifically incomplete and imprecise. Therefore, a combination of tests (integrated fetal testing) will yield better results (Harman and Baschat 2003). To prevent the consequences of perinatal asphyxia, not only advanced technology and sophisticated gadgets, but also adequate knowledge, training and skill are essential for its prudent application.

Antepartum screening

DAILY FETAL MOVEMENT COUNT Fetal movement count as an indicator of fetal well being was introduced almost three decades ago. A hypoxic fetus conserves its energy expenditure by curtailing biophysical activities such as gross body movements or breathing movements. Documentation of four movements in 30 minutes or 10 movements in 12 hours, although arbitrary, has been shown to correlate with good perinatal outcome

TABLE 34.3: SCREENING TESTS/METHODS USED IN CLINICAL PRACTICE FOR IDENTIFICATION OF FETAL HYPOXIA

Antepartum Screening

- Daily fetal movements count
- Antepartum cardiotocography (non-stress test)
- Biophysical profile score
- Doppler velocimetry

Uterine artery Doppler
Umbilical artery Doppler
Middle cerebral artery Doppler

Intrapartum Screening

- Fetal heart rate auscultation
- Meconium staining of amniotic fluid
- Intrapartum cardiotocography (electronic fetal monitoring)
- Fetal ECG and ST waveform analysis
- Fetal pulse oximetry

(Sadovsky 1985). Formal counting of fetal movements by the pregnant women could possibly identify the fetuses, which are at risk of compromise, thus allowing for appropriate action (Olsen and Svare 2004). In practice, there are two commonly used methods of fetal movement count:

1) Time taken to complete 10 movements – 'count to ten'
2) Fetal movement counts for one hour, usually after a meal, three times a day.

These methods are designed to take care of the sleep–awake/rest–activity cycles of the fetus.

A reduction or cessation of fetal movements causes concern and anxiety to the pregnant women. Although cardiotocography (CTG), ultrasonography, and umbilical/uterine Doppler studies are being used for antepartum fetal assessment in such situations, the evidence of a clinical benefit is limited. The effects of fetal vibroacoustic stimulation (VAST) and biophysical profile (BPP) for assessing these fetuses are also not well documented (Olsen and Svare 2004). There is a need for further well-designed studies in order to provide evidence-based guidelines in the future. Currently, the evidence does not support the routine use of fetal movement count in all pregnancies.

ANTEPARTUM CARDIOTOCOGRAPH (NON-STRESS TEST)

The basic objective of non-stress test (NST) is to assess coordination between the central nervous system (CNS) and the cardiovascular system. This is based on the premise that a well oxygenated healthy fetus with functionally intact CNS-cardiac axis will show acceleration (rise of fetal heart rate 15 beats per minute for 15 seconds above baseline) with the fetal movements. A reactive NST characterised by two accelerations in 20 minutes is considered normal. In addition, good fetal heart rate variability (≥ 5 beats per min) suggests normal balance of sympathetic and parasympathetic activity, an indirect evidence of adequate oxygenation of fetal regulatory centres. Indeed, normal fetal heart rate variability is the hallmark of fetal well being.

However, there are two pitfalls with such an interpretation. First, a very premature

Table 34.4: Biophysical profile assessment with Manning score is a global assessment of antepartum hypoxia, and is equivalent to Apgar score in the newborns

Neonate (Apgar score)	*Fetus (Manning score)*
Respiration	Fetal breathing movement
Heart rate	Non-stress test
Colour (circulation)	Amniotic fluid pocket (renal circulation)
Reflex	Gross body movement
Tone	Fetal tone

fetus (<32 weeks) may not qualify for the criteria of reactivity, primarily because of immaturity of the nervous system. Therefore, different criteria have been suggested for them, which are still not widely accepted. Second, a normal fetus, similar to its newborn state, demonstrates sleep–wake or rest–activity cycles, which must be appreciated while performing CTG interpretations. Fetal sleep cycle can last 40–90 min, and this can lead to misclassification and misinterpretation of CTG. Such problems occur daily in the busy labour ward, and often cause undue anxiety and unnecessary intervention. A detailed discussion can be found in a contemporary publication of the RCOG (2001).

Due to the above factors, high false-positive results (non-reactive trace in a otherwise healthy fetus) leading to anxiety and subsequent intervention, are major concerns. This can be overcome in a significant proportion of cases by a fetal vibro acoustic stimulation test (VAST), to which a healthy fetus usually responds with accelerations and increased variability of heart rate (Smith 1995). In contrast, a hypoxic fetus with depressed CNS, usually fails to respond to VAST. This is a condition, where more detailed and global assessment of fetus by BPP and Doppler studies is indicated. The Cochrane meta-analysis of randomised controlled trials involving 1588 high/intermediate-risk pregnancies (combined sample size is too small) suggests antepartum CTG alone has no significant impact on perinatal outcome (Pattison and McCowan 1999).

Biophysical Profile Fetal biophysical profile (BPP) scoring is based upon the principle that fetal hypoxemia, ischemia and acidemia either alone or in combination will elicit protective adaptive compensatory responses, which can manifest as a change in biophysical activities and in dynamics of amniotic fluid circulation (Manning 1997). This is a logical extension of neonatal Apgar score performed in utero: it includes five variables (Table 34. 4).

Of these, four acute variables (fetal breathing, gross body movement and tone, and NST) become abnormal during an acute hypoxic event, whereas chronic variable (amniotic fluid pocket) is an indicator of long standing progressive placental insufficiency. If an acute component such as NST is abnormal along with reduced amniotic fluid pocket, the condition can be more ominous because of the presence of acute on chronic hypoxia. Such features are often observed in fetal growth restriction and pre-eclampsia.

To facilitate test reporting, each of the five variables was assigned a score of 2 if normal and 0 if abnormal. The cumulative BPP score ranged from a maximum of 10 (all variables normal) to a minimum of 0 (all variables abnormal). With progressive fetal hypoxemia, fetal adaptation involves gradual reduction and subsequent deletion of biophysical activities in order to reduce oxygen consumption (Manning 1997). As long as these protective adaptational changes are effective, the fetus can avoid metabolic acidosis due to anaerobic glycolysis. At a BPP score of 4/10, the risk of metabolic acidemia (pH ≤7.20) is around 10%; it increases to 20% with scores of 2/10, and is almost 100% with scores 0/10 (Manning et al 1993). It is therefore evident that the predictive accuracy of BPP in affirming or excluding acidemia reaches 100% only in both extremes (negative predictive value of 100%, that is,, no acidemia with BPP score 10/10; positive predictive value of 100% if score is 0/10).

A highly significant inverse relationship exists between the last test score and adverse perinatal outcome. As compared to the normal score of 10/10, a score of 0 yielded a 40-fold increase in risk of intrapartum fetal distress, and 400-fold increase of antepartum stillbirth (Manning 1997). Several reports stressed the practical importance of BPP in management of high-risk pregnancies—the corrected perinatal mortality (excluding fetal malformation) is 2–5 per 1000 deliveries; and false-negative rate (fetal death within one week of normal BPP score) is around 1 per 1,000. Intermediate abnormal scores (4/10 or 6/10) are associated with relatively high false-positive rate, and it requires serial monitoring to decide most appropriate timing of delivery by evaluating the risks of intrauterine life against those of prematurity (Harman and Baschat 2003). This balancing act needs statistical support of neonatal survival data in a particular set-up.

In the management of high-risk pregnancies, where the incidence of perinatal asphyxia is high, the BPP score plays a very important role. If BPP scores remain normal, conservative management can be performed with considerable confidence in the presence of traditional risk factors, with concomitant reduction of iatrogenic prematurity (Manning 1997). Also, appropriately timed delivery has also reduced stillbirth rate. Thus, BPP scoring has dramatically improved high-risk pregnancy care.

Doppler Velocimetry

Cardiovascular changes are central to fetal adaptation to perinatal hypoxia. Fetal asphyxia, real or impending, causes a series of circulatory changes, which have been studied by assessing Doppler velocimetry of three compartments—uteroplacental circulation (uterine artery Doppler), fetoplacental circulation (umbilical vessels Doppler) and fetal circulation (fetal vascular and cardiac Doppler). Detailed description of these changes is beyond the scope of this chapter and an excellent review can be found elsewhere (Tekay and Campbell 2000). From the practical point of view, Doppler velocimetry of uterine, umbilical and middle cerebral arteries are commonly assessed in prediction, screening and management of intrauterine hypoxia.

1. Uterine artery Doppler: Increased resistance to uteroplacental blood flow because of an inadequate invasion of trophoblast into spiral arteries is responsible for increased pulsatility or resistance index, and/or early diastolic notch in the uterine artery velocimetry (Harman and Baschat 2003). In late pregnancy, the persistence of bilateral notches in the uterine artery Doppler identifies pregnancies at risk of developing IUGR and pre-eclampsia, possibly leading to fetal hypoxia/asphyxia (Divon and Ferber 2002). Such findings should alert the obstetrician to intensify fetal surveillance. However, as there is a lack of randomised controlled trials regarding the utility of uterine artery Doppler studies in screening pregnancy complications, it should not be recommended as a general screening modality (Divon and Ferber 2002).

2. Umbilical artery Doppler. In intrauterine life, the fetus gets its oxygen from the placenta. Umbilical artery circulation is primarily influenced by low resistance in the placental vascular bed, which is a prerequisite for an undisturbed flow of fetal blood through the placenta, thus ensuring adequate transport of oxygen and nutrition. The umbilical arteries show a forward flow throughout the heart cycle (Divon and Ferber 2002).

Longitudinal Doppler studies of the umbilical artery show that the S/D ratio decreases as gestation progresses; this is an indirect evidence of decreasing placental resistance with advancing gestation (Divon and Ferber 2002). Increased resistance in umbilical arteries is observed with specific morphological lesions of the placenta, which are often associated with IUGR and pre-eclampsia and adverse perinatal outcome. However, there is no definite agreement as to what constitutes an abnormal Doppler study. Most authors have accepted an S/D ratio >3.0 as the cut-off beyond 30 weeks gestation. Gradual increase in the umbilical artery resistance leads to absent, and subsequently reversed end-diastolic flow, which is associated with progressively worse perinatal outcome. Further, follow-up studies (Valcamonico et al 1994; Wienerroither et al 2001) have shown that the long-term neurological sequelae, especially impaired neuromotor functions, are also increased as the umbilical artery end-diastolic flow decreases (35% with absent or reversed end-diastolic flow, 12% with reduced flow, and 0% with normal flow).

Several prospective studies have convincingly shown that abnormal umbilical artery Doppler is invaluable in identifying the IUGR fetuses at increased risk of perinatal hypoxia. It is also associated with increased operative delivery for fetal distress, low Apgar score with metabolic acidosis, and perinatal mortality. A Cochrane review of 11 trials consisting of nearly 7000 high-risk pregnancies has found that Doppler assessment is associated with a trend towards a reduction in perinatal death (OR 0.71, 95% CI 0.50–1.01). In addition, use of Doppler assessment has led to fewer induction of labour (OR 0.83, 95% CI 0.74–0.93) and fewer hospital antenatal admissions (OR 0.56, 95% CI 0.43–0.72), without reports of adverse perinatal effects (Nelson and Alfirevic 2006).

3. Middle cerebral artery Doppler. The developing fetal brain is an area of low vascular impendence and receives continuous forward flow throughout the cardiac cycle. Fetal hypoxia is likely to cause redistribution of blood flow in favour of the fetal brain--the so-called brain-sparing effect (Divon and Ferber 2002). Middle cerebral artery pulsatility index and cerebroplacental ratio (cerebral to umbilical artery Doppler ratio) have been used to predict adverse perinatal outcome in fetal hypoxia (Jain et al 2004). In the absence of randomised controlled trials, it seems that the addition of cerebral artery Doppler to umbilical artery Doppler studies is of little or no clinical benefit (Divon and Ferber 2002).

Although a large number of other fetal Doppler assessment such as Doppler of renal artery, descending aorta, ductus venosus and umbilical vein are carried out, its practical application in management of fetal/perinatal asphyxia is of limited value.

Intrapartum Screening The labour and delivery process is one of the most physiologically stressful events a human being ever faces. Although most fetuses tolerate this stress without adverse consequences, a few may sustain hypoxic damages resulting from uterine contractions. The response of a fetus to intrapartum stress depends on several factors, most important of which are the pre-existing fetal status before onset of labour, the intensity and duration of the stress, and the ability of the obstetric team to assess the fetal condition accurately and to respond appropriately (Huddleston 1999). A healthy term fetus has greater capacity to handle hypoxia than a preterm or growth restricted one. Therefore, careful evaluation of each woman in early labour is essential for identifying evidence of impending or established asphyxia.

At the time of admission to the labour ward, an initial evaluation should include review of all obstetric records, assessment of gestational age, and a thorough general physical and obstetric examination. This evaluation may be supplemented with an 'admission test' CTG. Following this assessment, the labour ward team should decide the best method of fetal monitoring. Current evidence suggests that low-risk pregnancies can be adequately monitored with intermittent auscultation. High-risk pregnancies or labours (induced or augmented or prolonged labour), where fetuses are at increased risk of hypoxia, should be monitored with electronic fetal monitoring (EFM) (RCOG 2001). All obstetric units, which deal with high-risk pregnancies or labours, must be equipped with EFM.

Fetal heart rate auscultation Listening to fetal heart by applying the ear to the maternal abdomen is the most primitive way to diagnose fetal health. Pinard's version of the fetal stethoscope that appeared in 1876 set the criteria for fetal heart rate variation in health, and in stress/distress. For many years, the only methods of fetal surveillance were auscultation of FHR and identification of meconium in the amniotic fluid. For a woman who is healthy and has an otherwise uncomplicated pregnancy, intermittent auscultation should be recommended to monitor fetal well being. In the active labour, intermittent auscultation should be carried out after a contraction, for ≥60 sec at an interval of 15 min and 5 min in the first stage and second stages, respectively (RCOG 2001). However, one needs to switch over to continuous EFM if there are abnormalities in FHR or intrapartum risk factors develop.

Meconium staining of amniotic fluid In most cases, passage of meconium is a reflection of fetal gestational maturity. The presence of moderate to thick meconium in the amniotic fluid is associated with increased incidence of meconium aspiration syndrome—a potentially fatal hypoxic condition develops because of mechanical obstruction of the bronchioles and chemical pneumonitis. Thick meconium with oligohydramnios may be due to reduced renal perfusion, an indicator of fetal circulatory adaptation to longstanding hypoxia. This is an indication for continuous EFM (Steer and Danielian 2006).

Intrapartum cardiotocography (Electronic fetal monitoring) Advances in the techniques and technology to detect the fetal heart beat came in the 1960s, when the Doppler principle was used to instantaneously record fetal heart rate; uterine contractions were also simultaneously recorded to detect any temporal changes of fetal heart rate in response to uterine contractions. The term 'electronic fetal monitoring' (EFM) is often substituted by 'cardiotocography' (CTG) to indicate the underlying principle. Since its introduction, continuous EFM has been used increasingly in clinical practice even before its effectiveness was fully evaluated scientifically.

EFM provides much information regarding fetal heart rate—the baseline rate, baseline variability, the periodic and temporal changes, which help us to categorise CTG traces into three subgroups—normal, suspicious and pathological (RCOG 2001). In normal fetus, accelerations of FHR occur with 90% of fetal movements as early as the second trimester, probably as a result of increased catecholamine release; it reflects adequate oxygenation of the CNS–cardiac axis. Although a normal trace indicates a healthy fetus because of 'reassuring' features, a suspicious or pathological trace deserves more attention and/or intervention. Therefore, more information has led to more anxiety as well as more interventions, but not necessarily a better outcome. A large proportion of suspicious and pathological traces are associated with delivery of perfectly healthy infants. This suggests that intrapartum EFM as a test of fetal well being is inaccurate because of high false-positive results. However, one can argue that the interventions prompted by EFM have a desirable effect to prevent fetal damage or death. As EFM cannot quantitate hypoxia, it is considered a screening test for fetal hypoxia.

The effectiveness of EFM has been evaluated in a landmark study, the Dublin randomised trial (MacDonald et al 1985). A recent Cochrane review has included nine controlled trials involving 18,561 pregnant women and their 18,695 infants in both high-risk and low-risk pregnancies from seven clinical centers in developed countries (Thaker et al 2002). When compared with intermittent auscultation, the use of continuous EFM is associated with increased rate of both caesarean delivery (RR 1.41, 95 per cent CI 1.23–1.61) and operative vaginal delivery (RR 1.20, 95% CI 1.11–1.30). The cesarean delivery rate was further increased in the absence of fetal scalp blood sampling (RR 1.72, 95% CI 1.38-2.51), and the rate was slightly reduced (RR 1.24, 95% CI 1.05–1.48) where fetal blood pH was estimated with fetal scalp blood sampling (Thaker et al 2002).

EFM was introduced with the aim of reducing perinatal mortality and cerebral palsy, two important adverse outcomes of fetal asphyxia. Meta-analysis of clinical trials shows a statistically significant decrease of neonatal seizures (RR 0.51, 95% CI 0.32–0.82) in continuous EFM group (Thacker et al 2002). No significant differences are observed in 1-min Apgar scores below four, rate of admissions to neonatal intensive care units, or perinatal deaths. In one review, a subgroup analysis has shown that the use of EFM is associated with a significant reduction of a perinatal death due to hypoxia (Vintzileos et al 1993). However, this type of posthoc analysis should be treated with caution because of potential bias. As the studies were carried out in the United States, Europe and Australia, where perinatal mortality is very low (8 per 1000 live births), a larger sample size (of around 56,000) would be required to address this issue (RCOG 2001). Type II error because of small sample size, is a major problem if any valid conclusions are to be drawn regarding effectiveness of EFM on perinatal mortality. Further, the trials have included a mix of low- and high-risk populations. It is not possible to quantify the real effect of EFM on perinatal mortality in these specific populations. Finally, in developing countries the background situation is very much different, and perinatal mortality is high (Mehta and Jayant 1981). Therefore, external validity of the trials conducted in developed countries remains debatable in the context of developing countries.

Epidemiological data suggest that only 10% of cases of cerebral palsy have potential intrapartum causes, and, even in some of these cases there may have been an antenatal component (MacLennan 1999). Three follow-up cohorts of babies included in EFM trials found contradictory outcome. The overall results have shown no significant difference in the development of cerebral palsy.

Continuous EFM is more expensive than intermittent auscultation because of two reasons—the first and most important is increased cesarean section rate; the second is the capital and maintenance cost of the equipment. These resource implications must be carefully balanced against potential benefits in high-risk and low-risk population.

FIGO (1987) has stipulated that 'For the monitoring (EFM) to be effective, the test must be performed correctly; its results must then be interpreted satisfactorily; and finally, this interpretation must provoke an appropriate response.' The problem in the interpretation remains despite its widespread use. Human errors in interpretation of the traces (both inter- and intra-observer error) cannot be eliminated by computer analysis. Regular training programmes on EFM for trainees and medical and nursing staff should be mandatory: it will improve their knowledge and skill, and prevent misuse and misinterpretation.

Fetal ECG and ST waveform analysis Fetal ECG is another way of assessing fetal hypoxia in labour. Evidence from experimental work indicates that ST waveform elevation reflects compensated myocardial stress and switch to myocardial anerobic metabolism. An elevation of ST segment and T wave, quantified by the ratio between the T wave and QRS amplitude (T/QRS) represents continuing anerobic metabolism with a risk of eventual decompensation due to gradual depletion of myocardial glycogen stores and progressive metabolic acidosis. Persistently biphasic and negative ST waveform changes indicate myocardial decompensation as a result of direct myocardial ischemic hypoxia (Luzietti et al 2002). The STAN recorder has an expert system (ST log) to make automatic assessment of ST changes over a period, by digital signal processing. A unipolar fetal ECG lead on the scalp with an active skin electrode placed on the maternal thigh is required to obtain ECG signals from the fetus. Fetal ECG waveform analysis improves the specificity of detecting intrapartum fetal hypoxia when the CTG shows an abnormal FHR pattern. It is suggested that ST changes usually appear in parallel with an abnormal CTG pattern, and an appropriate action can be taken on the basis of CTG plus ST analysis; a scalp pH will add no significant information but may cause delay in obstetric intervention.

Randomised control trials have suggested several benefits of fetal ECG with ST analysis. The Plymouth trial showed a 46% reduction of operative interventions for fetal distress in the CTG plus ST analysis compared to CTG alone (Westgate et al 1993). The Swedish trial showed a significantly lower rate of metabolic acidosis and less chance of developing moderate to severe neonatal encephalopathy if ST analysis is incorporated with conventional CTG monitoring (Amer-Wåhlin et al 2001). However, the trials emphasised the need for training, educational efforts and local experience (Amer-Wåhlin et al 2001; Ojala et al 2006).

Fetal pulse oximetry Fetal pulse oximetry monitoring provides a quantitative, direct and real-time measurement of fetal arterial oxygen saturation (SpO_2). The pulse oximeter sensor is placed on the fetal cheek or temple by sliding it along the examiner's fingers through the cervix, after the membranes have ruptured. It is based on an established, safe and non-invasive technology, widely used in operation theatres and intensive care units. It is used in labour if CTG is non-reassuring, or when conventional monitoring is unreliable, such as with fetal arrhythmias (East et al 2002). Based on both animal and human data, fetal oxygen saturation values ≥30% can be considered reassuring, and values < 30% may be associated with fetal acidosis and warrant further assessment and/or intervention, if persisting for >10 min (East et al 2002). Multicentre randomised trials have suggested better accuracy of fetal pulse oximetry in predicting perinatal asphyxia compared to conventional fetal monitoring technique (Garite et al 2000; East et al 2006). Fetal oxygen saturation is still not used as a primary modality for intrapartum fetal monitoring, and it should not form the sole basis of obstetric management; the total clinical picture should be considered in the decision making process.

Diagnosis

Fetal scalp blood sampling and acid-base assessment Fetal/neonatal acid–base assessment is the mainstay of diagnosis of intrapartum/perinatal asphyxia. During labour, a fetal scalp blood sampling is performed if the CTG arouses suspicions, and immediate delivery is not indicated. A fetal scalp blood pH less than 7.2 is often considered fetal acidosis, and at this point immediate delivery is indicated, although a large proportion of these fetuses remain vigorous at birth and will show no evidence of brain damage (Nordstrom and Arulkumaran 1998). The limitations of fetal scalp blood sampling and acid–base assessment are well known. This test provides a measurement at one point in the continuum of labour and delivery. Therefore, repeated sampling may be required to clarify fetal condition if CTG abnormalities persist for a while. Moreover, this invasive procedure is technically challenging, requires rupture of the membranes and cervical dilatation >2 cm, and access to the presenting part (Greene 1999). Maternal infections such as HIV, hepatitis B and genital herpes are contraindications for the procedure because of increased risk of transmission to the fetus.

Hypoxia lasting over 10 minutes leads to an increase in lactate production in the fetus, and a level >4.8 mmol/l is considered abnormal (Kruger et al 1999). Compared to pH estimation, lactate measurement requires less amount of blood (5 µl compared with 25 µl for pH estimation), fewer scalp incisions, less chance of sampling failure and quicker results (Nordstrom and Arulkumaran 1998). A randomised controlled trial comparing these two techniques found lactate to be more favourable because of fewer instances of sampling failure and the reduced time for generating reports (Westgren et al 1998). Results of a multicentre trial from Sweden are awaited, and as of now, estimation of pH and base deficit remains the gold standard for diagnosis of perinatal asphyxia.

A neonate who has had severe hypoxia proximate to delivery should have an umbilical artery pH measured to document significant acidosis. Following resuscitation and stabilisation, each neonate requires close observation for evidence of hypoxic-ischemic encephalopathy and multi-organ dysfunction.

Management

Management of perinatal asphyxia poses a major challenge to obstetricians and neonatologists alike. This condition may be diagnosed during the antenatal period or labour, or immediately after birth. Therefore, the management will differ according to the timing of diagnosis. Here, we propose to discuss the management of perinatal hypoxia from the obstetrical point of view; for details of neonatal management, published guidelines on neonatal resuscitation may be consulted (Chawla and Deorari 2005).

The mainstay of antepartum management includes appropriate screening for fetal jeopardy by fetal surveillance, referral to a higher centre, where better perinatal care can be provided, and decision regarding optimum timing and mode of delivery. In a hypoxic fetus, balancing the risks such as iatrogenic prematurity because of early delivery versus continuing pregnancy with potential chance of intrauterine fetal death could be a daunting task. There are no effective means for reversing chronic fetal hypoxemia/acidemia. As in the foreseeable future, we do not expect many changes in the current scenario, delivery of the baby from a hostile uterine environment into supportive neonatal care remains the mainstay of improving perinatal outcome (Manning 1997).

A term fetus (>37 weeks) which is potentially hypoxic should be delivered; however, if gestation is between 32 to 36 weeks, careful monitoring with fetal biometry, AFI, umbilical artery Doppler, BPP and NST should be done to select optimum time for delivery. If the gestation is less than 32 weeks, delivery should be considered if there are gross abnormalities in BPP score (<6), pathological CTG, or reversed end-diastolic flow in the umbilical artery. Corticosteroid for fetal lung maturation should be given if the gestation is less than 36 weeks. Each step of care should be based on knowledge, skill, experience and judgment. A regional perinatal centre can provide significant inputs in the management of these cases.

The basic principles of management of fetal hypoxia in labour are:

- Assessment of the entire clinical situation
- Measures to correct probable causes of hypoxia
- Delivery of the baby if hypoxia persists
- Neonatal resuscitation

A systematic approach can prevent many errors because of inadvertent omission of important factors, which can influence management and outcome. The authors follow a simple checklist, which is divided into five components:

a. Is there an antepartum factor? This may affect fetal reserve for compensation.
b. Is there an intrapartum factor? This may have precipitated hypoxia. How can it be corrected?
c. Is the overall FHR pattern improving, persisting or deteriorating?
d. Does it require further assessment?
e. Is immediate delivery indicated, and is assisted delivery possible?
f. Is the neonatal resuscitation team available immediately?

a. Antepartum factor: It is important to look for risk factors such as IUGR, maternal hypertension, anemia, diabetes, smoking, post-term pregnancy and meconium stained liquor. In these conditions, fetal reserve is usually compromised for some duration. This can adversely affect the ability of the fetus to respond to hypoxic events. As these fetuses develop hypoxic decompensation rapidly, corrective measures should be prompt.

b. Intrapartum factor: Precipitating factors such as uterine hyperstimulation due to oxytocin, maternal hypotension as with supine hypotension and epidural analgesia, evidence of placental abruption or cord prolapse should be managed at the earliest. In certain cases 'intrauterine resuscitation' may be effective—to discontinue oxytocin infusion if in use, to change maternal position, to administer oxygen at 5–10 l/min, and to correct hypotension. In the event of uterine hyperstimulation, administration of tocolytics such as terbutaline may help tide over the crisis. These measures are no substitute for conditions where delivery of the fetus is indicated (that is, cord prolapse and placental abruption).

Meconium staining of amniotic fluid, a clinical marker of fetal hypoxia, deserves special attention because of high perinatal morbidity and mortality related to meconium aspiration syndrome. Transcervical intrapartum amnioinfusion is found to be beneficial in the presence of variable decelerations/ or meconium staining of amniotic fluid in widely varying obstetric and neonatal set-up (Hofmeyr 2003; Fraser et al 2005; Patil et al 2006). Amnioinfusion provides multiple benefits by increasing amniotic fluid volume—cushioning effects on the umbilical cord and thus, improvement of variable deceleration; dilution of meconium leading to less mechanical obstruction at the bronchioles and reduction of chemical pneumonitis. Systematic review of randomised controlled trials suggested beneficial effects of amnioinfusion on the frequency of meconium aspiration syndrome, cesarean section and perinatal death (Hofmeyr 2003). In contrast, a recent multicentre trial has failed to reproduce these benefits (Fraser et al 2005). However, pooled data from several controlled trials carried out in the developing countries with limited intrapartum surveillance facilities have shown substantial benefit of amnioinfusion on reduction of meconium aspiration syndrome, perinatal deaths and cesarean section rate (Khosla et al 1997; Hofmeyr et al 1998; Das et al 2001; Rathore et al 2002).

c. *Overall FHR pattern:* Continuous assessment of the fetal condition and its response to the above measures are essential for judging fetal 'compensation'. A careful review of cardiotocographic trace over a period (usually 40–60 min), and comparing it with the preceding trace may be extremely helpful. When there is no improvement of the overall pattern, further assessment or delivery is essential to avoid fetal damage or death.

d. *Further assessment:* In the event of continuing FHR abnormality, scalp blood sampling may be useful. A pH level less than 7.20 requires immediate delivery, while one between 7.2–7.25 requires the test to be repeated within 30 min. A pH greater than 7.25 needs observation; the procedure may be repeated if the FHR pattern fails to improve.

e. *Immediate delivery or Assisted delivery:* A fetus with evidence of metabolic acidosis must be delivered. In cases where there are persistent FHR abnormalities in early labour, when the prospect of vaginal delivery is remote, cesarean delivery is preferable. In certain cases, forceps or ventouse delivery is an option, but it depends on several factors such as parity, past obstetric history, cervical dilatation, presentation, position and station of the presenting part. At this stage, procrastination in decision-making and intervention can lead to disaster.

f. *Neonatal resuscitation:* Even with prompt intervention, many newborns would be depressed at birth. A well-prepared neonatal team can resuscitate a large proportion of asphyxiated newborns. There are both national and international guidelines for neonatal resuscitation, and the obstetric/ neonatal team must be well versed with the current changes (Chawla and Deorari 2005). In order to avoid time lapse, the neonatal team must be present during delivery. To bridge the communication gap and to achieve the best perinatal outcome, the obstetric and the neonatal team must act in tandem while managing high-risk fetuses.

Management of perinatal asphyxia is a stressful challenge, which taxes the obstetrician's ability of clinical judgment and technical skills. Balancing an adequate measure and excessive intervention is often difficult. In the developing countries, this problem may be further compounded with inadequate facilities available for antepartum/intrapartum fetal surveillance and provision of immediate operative delivery.

Conclusion Perinatal asphyxia is a major challenge in obstetric and neonatal practice. Its prediction by clinical risk scoring still remains an unfulfilled goal. There are no effective means for reversing chronic fetal hypoxemia/acidemia. As in the foreseeable future, we do not expect many changes in the current scenario, its screening by antepartun and intrapartum surveillance, and appropriate timing of delivery are the mainstay of improving perinatal outcome. Integrated screening by NST, BPP and Doppler studies plays a crucial role in antepartum screening of fetal hypoxia, while intermittent auscultation and EFM play a pivotal role during labour. Although fetal pulse oximetry and ECG are promising reduction of false-positive results related to EFM, more evidence is required for its widespread application. Fetal/neonatal acid–base assessment (pH and base deficit) is the gold standard to confirm diagnosis of perinatal asphyxia. A significant proportion of intrapartum hypoxia is unpredictable, but a prepared and well-equipped neonatal team can play a crucial role to make a difference in the outcome of the babies affected by perinatal asphyxia.

References

ACOG Committee Opinion. Number 138. 1994. Utility of umbilical cord blood acid–base assessment. Washington DC: American College of Obstetricians and Gynecologists.

ACOG Committee Opinion. Number 326. 2005. Inappropriate use of the terms fetal distress and birth asphyxia. Washington DC: American College of Obstetricians and Gynecologists.

ACOG Technical Bulletin. Number 216. 1995. Umbilical artery blood acid-base analysis. Washington DC: American College of Obstetricians and Gynecologists.

Amer-Wåhlin I, C Hellsten, H Norén et al. 2001. Cardiotocography only versus cardiotocography plus ST analysis of fetal electrocardiogram for intrapartum fetal monitoring: a Swedish randomised control trial. *Lancet* 358: 534–538.

Blair E and FJ Stanley. 1988. Intrapartum asphyxia: a rare cause of cerebral palsy. *J Pediatr* 112: 515–519.

Blair E. 2001.Trends in cerebral palsy. *Indian J Pediatr* 68:433–438.

Chawla D and A Deorari. 2005. Neonatal resuscitation guidelines 2005: Salient changes. *J Neonatol* 19:371–375.

Clerici G, Luzietti R and Di Renzo. 2001. Monitoring of antepartum and intrapartum fetal hypoxemia: Pathophysiological basis and available techniques. *Biol Neonate* 79:246–253.

Das V, S Srivastava, P Kumar, GK Malik and M Kumar. 2001. Amnioinfusion during labour complicated by meconium. *J Obstet Gynaecol India*.51:105–107.

Divon MY and A Ferber. 2002. Doppler evaluation of the fetus. *Clin Obstet Gynecol* 45:1015–1025.

East CE, PB Colditz, LM Begg and S Brennecke. 2002. Update on intrapartum fetal pulse oximetry. *Aust NZ J Obstet Gynaecol* 42:119–124.

East CE, SP Brennecke, JF King, FY Chan and PB Colditz; FORMOST Study Group. 2006. The effect of intrapartum fetal pulse oximetry, in the presence of a nonreassuring fetal heart rate pattern, on operative delivery rates: a multicenter, randomized, controlled trial (the FORMOST trial). *Am J Obstet Gynecol* 194:606–616.

Fee SC, K Malee, R Deddish, JP Minogue and ML Sokol. 1990. Severe acidosis and subsequent neurologic status. *Am J Obstet Gynecol* 162:802–806.

FIGO Subcommittee on standards in Perinatal Medicine. 1987. Guidelines for the use of fetal monitoring. *Int J Gynecol Obstet* 25:159–167.

Fraser WD, GJ Hofmeyr, R Lede et al. 2005. Amnioinfusion for the prevention of the meconium aspiration syndrome. *N Engl J Med* 353:909–917.

Garite TJ, GA Dildy, H McNamara et al. 2000. A multicenter controlled trial of fetal pulse oximetry in the intrapartum management of nonreassuring fetal heart patterns. *Am J Obstet Gynecol* 183:1049–1058.

Goodwin TM, Belai I, P Hernandez, M Durand and RH Paul. 1992. Asphyxial complications in the term newborn with severe umbilical academia. *Am J Obstet Gynecol* 167:1506–1512.

Greene KR. 1999. Scalp blood gas analysis. *Obstet Gynecol Clin North Am* 26:641–657.

Hagberg H, K Blomgren and C Mallard. 2001. Neuroprotection of fetal and neonatal brain. In *Fetal and Neonatal Neurology and Neurosurgery*, 3rd ed, ed MI Levene, FA Chervenak, MJ Whittle, 505–520. London: Churchill Livingstone.

Harman CR and AA Baschat. 2003. Arterial and venous Dopplers in IUGR. *Clin Obstet Gynecol* 46:931–946.

Hofmeyr GJ, AM Gülmezoğlu, E Buchmann et al. 1998. The Collaborative Randomised Amnioinfusion for Meconium Project (CRAMP): 1.South Africa. *Br J Obstet Gynaecol* 105:304–308.

Hofmeyr GJ. 2003. Amnioinfusion for meconium-stained liquor in labour. In *The Cochrane Library*, Issue 4. Chester: UK: John Wiley & Sons Ltd.

Huddleston JF. 1999. Intrapartum fetal assessment: a review. *Clin Perinatol* 26:549–567.

Jain M, T Farooq and RC Sukla. 2004. Doppler cerebroplacental ratio for the prediction of adverse perinatal outcome. *Int J Gynecol Obstet* 86:384–385.

Khosla AH, K Sangwan and SD Ahuja. 1997. Prophylactic amnioinfusion during labour complicated by meconium. *Aust NZ J Obstet Gynaecol* 37:294–296.

Kruger K, B Hallberg, M Blennow, M Kublickas and M Westgren. 1999. Predictive value of fetal scalp blood lactate concentration and pH as markers of neurological disability. *Am J Obstet Gynecol* 181:1072–1078.

Low JA, BG Lindsay and EJ Derrick. 1997. Threshold of metabolic acidosis associated with newborn complications. *Am J Obstet Gynecol* 177:1391–1394.

Low JA, LL Simpson and DA Ramsey. 1992. The clinical diagnosis of asphyxia responsible for brain damage in the human fetus. *Am J Obstet Gynecol* 167:11–15.

Low JA, LL Simpson, G Tonni and S Chamberlain. 1995. Limitation in the clinical prediction of intrapartum fetal asphyxia. *Am J Obstet Gynecol* 172:801–804.

Low JA, R Victory and EJ Derrick. 1999. Predictive value of electronic fetal heart monitoring for intrapartum fetal asphyxia with metabolic acidosis. *Obstet Gynecol* 93:285–291.

Low JA. 1998. Intrapartum fetal asphyxia: prediction and diagnosis. In *Textbook of Perinatal Medicine,* ed A Kurjak, vol. 2, pp 1414–1423. London: Parthenon Publishing Group.

Low JA. 2004. Determining the contribution of asphyxia to brain damage in the neonate. *J Obstet Gynecol Res* 30:276–286.

Luzietti R, G Clerici, KG Rosén and GC Di Renzo. 2002. Advances in the diagnosis of intrapatum asphyxia In *The Fetus as a Patient – Evolving Challenge,* ed FA Chervenak, A Kurjak and Z Papp, 235–247. Bocaraton: The Parthenon Publishing Group.

MacDonald D, A Grant, M Sheridan-Pereira, P Boylan and I Chalmers. 1985. The Dublin randomized trial of intrapartum fetal heart rate monitoring. *Am J Obstet Gynecol* 152:524–539.

MacLennan A for the International Cerebral Palsy Task Force. 1999. A template for defining a causal relation between acute intrapartum events and cerebral palsy: international consensus statement. *BMJ* 319:1054–1059.

Manning FA, RJM Snijders, CR Harman, KH Nicolaides, S Menticoglou and I Morrison. 1993. Fetal biophysical profile scoring. VI. Correlation with antepartum umbilical venous fetal pH. *Am J Obstet Gynecol* 169:755–763.

Manning FA.1997. Fetal biophysical profile: a critical appraisal. *Fetal Maternal Med Rev* 9:103–123.

Mehta A and K Jayant. 1981. Perinatal mortality survey in India. *J Obstet Gynaecol India.* 31:183–215.

Mehta A. 1983. Strategies for reduction of perinatal mortality in India. *J Obstet Gynaecol India.* 33:721–733.

Nelson JP and Z Alfirevic. 2006. Doppler ultrasound for fetal assessment in high risk pregnancies. *The Cochrane Database of Systematic Reviews,* issue 2. Art. no.: CD000063.

Nordström L and S Arulkumaran. 1998. Intrapartum fetal hypoxia and biochemical markers: a review. *Obstet Gynecol Surv* 53:645–657.

Ojala K, M Vaarasmaki, K Makikkalio, M Valkama and A Tekay. 2006. Acomparison of intrapartum automated fetal electrocardiography and conventional cardiotocography – a randomised controlled study. *Br J Obstet Gynaecol* 113:419–423.

Olsen AG and JA Svare. 2004. Decreased fetal movements: background,assessment, and clinical management. *Acta Obstet Gynecol Scad* 83:818–826.

Patil KP, MK Swamy and K Samatha. 2006. A one year cross-sectional study of management practices of meconium stained amniotic fluid and perinatal outcome. *J Obstet Gynaecol India.* 56:128–130.

Pattison N and L McCowan. 1999 Cardiotocography for antepartum fetal assessment. *The Cochrane Database of Systematic Reviews,* issue 1. CD001068.

Pulsinelli W, JB Brierly and F Plum. 1982. Temporal profile of neuronal damage in a model of transient forebrain ischemia. *Ann Neurol* 11:491–498.

Rathore AM, R Singh, S Ramji and R Tripathi. 2002. Randomised trial of amnioinfusion during labour with meconium stained amniotic fluid. *Br J Obstet Gynaecol* 109:17–20.

Rosenberg AA, E Murdaugh and CW White. 1989. The role of oxygen free radicals in post-asphyxia cerebral hypoperfusion in new-born lambs. *Pediatr Res* 26:215–219.

Royal College of Obstetricians and Gynaecologists: Clinical Effectiveness Support Unit. 2001. *The use of electronic fetal monitoring.* The use and interpretation of cardiotocography in intrapartum fetal surveillance. Evidence based clinical guideline number 8. London: RCOG Press.

Sadovsky E. 1985. Monitoring fetal movements: A useful screening test. *Cont Obstet Gynecol* 25: 123–127.

Smith CV. 1995. Vibroacoustic stimulation. *Clin Obstet Gynecol* 38:68–77.

Spencer JA, N Badawi, P Burton, J Keogh, P Pemberton and F Stanley. 1997. The intrapartum CTG prior to neonatal encephalopathy at term. A case control study. *Br J Obstet Gynaecol* 104:25–28.

Steer PJ and P Danielian. 2006. Fetal distress in labour. In *High Risk Pregnancy: Management options,* 3rd ed, ed DK James, PJ Steer, CP Weiner, B Gonik, 1450–1472. Philadelphia: W.B. Saunders Company.

Tekay A and S Campbell. 2000. Doppler ultrasonography in obstetrics. In *Ultrasonography in Obstetrics and Gynecology,* 4th ed, ed PW Callen, 677–723. Philadelphia: WB Saunders Company.

Thacker SB, D Stroup, M Chang. 2002. Continuous fetal heart monitoring for fetal assessment in labor. In *Cochrane Library*, Issue 1. Oxford:Update Software.

Thorp JA. What is birth asphyxia. 1990. Reply. *Am J Obstet Gynecol* 163:1368.

Valcomonico A, L Danti, T Frusca, M Soregaroli, S Zucca, F Abrami and A Tiberti. 1994 Absent end-diastolic velocity in umbilical artery: risk of neonatal morbidity and brain damage. *Am J Obstet Gynecol*; 170(3):796–801.

Vintzileos AM, A Antsaklis, I Varvarigos, C Papas, I Sofatzis, JT Montgomery. 1993. A randomized trial of intrapartum electronic fetal heart rate monitoring versus intermittent auscultation. *Obstet Gynecol* 81:899–907.

Westgate J, M Harris, JSH Curnow, KR Greene. 1993. Plymouth randomized trial of cardiotocogram only versus ST waveform plus cardiotocogram for intrapartum monitoring: 2400 cases. *Am J Obstet Gynecol* 169:1151–1160.

Westgren M, K Kruger, S Ek, et al. 1998. Lactate compared with pH analysis at fetal scalp blood sampling: a prospective randomised study. *Br J Obstet Gynaecol* 105:29–33.

Wienerroither H, H Steiner, J Tomasselli et al. 2001. Intrauterine blood flow and long-term intellectual, neurologic and social development. *Obstet Gynecol* 97:449–453.

35

Thromboembolic Disorders

Amita Suneja

Pregnant women are about 5–6 times more likely to develop venous thromboembolism (VTE) than non-pregnant women (ACOG Practice Bulletin 2001). The current data, using objective tests for diagnosis, indicates the frequency of VTE in pregnancy and puerperium as 1 in a 1000, VTE occurs with similar frequency in all trimesters and an equal number is identified in pregnancy and puerperium. About two-thirds of these events manifest as deep venous thrombosis (DVT) and a third as pulmonary embolism (PE). The rate of mortality from PE remains about 1 in every 100,000 pregnancies (McPhedran 2005).

Epidemiology

Virchow's triad favours VTE in pregnancy. Hemodynamic changes, causing venous stasis and hypercoagulability, contribute to the increased risk of VTE during pregnancy (Macklon et al 1997). The risk factors for VTE in pregnancy are listed in Table 35.1 (Weiss 2000). It is estimated that nearly half of the patients with TE have identifiable underlying genetic disorders. The risk of VTE in pregnancy is increased in women with thrombophilia (Cunningham et al 2005).

Thrombophilias

Inherited or acquired deficiencies of the inhibitory proteins of coagulation are collectively referred to as thrombophilias. A few aspects of their nature, thrombogenic potential and site of action are summarised in Fig. 35.1 (Lockwood 2002; Jordan et al 2005).

Thrombin, on binding to endothelial cells, forms thrombodulin and loses its procoagulant activity. This further activates Protein C, a natural anticoagulant, that in the presence of Protein S controls thrombin generation by inactivating factors Va and VIIIa (Fig. 35.1) (Clarke et al 1998). The most prevalent of known thrombophilic syndromes is the factor V Leiden mutation. It is characterised by resistance of plasma to the anticoagulant effects of activated Protein C. Resistance to Protein C (factor V Leiden) is measured by bioassay. The estimated prevalence among people of European ancestry is 5% but it is rarely found in Asians and Africans (Raes et al 1995). Protein C and Protein S deficiencies result in a loss of inactivation of factors Va and VIIIa (Lindqvist et al 1999). Prothrombin G20210A mutation is a G-to-A mutation at nucleotide 20210 in the prothrombin gene and results in excessive production of

Table 35.1: Causes of thromboembolism in pregnancy

1	Virchow's triad—stasis, hypercoagulability, trauma	
2	Independent risk factors	RR of PE
	Pregnancy related	
	Severe pre-eclampsia	4.8
	Multiple gestation	2.3
	Diabetes mellitus	2.7
	Instrumental vaginal delivery	—
	Cesarean delivery	3.8
	Others	
	Age >35 yrs	
	Parity >4	
	Smoking	
	Obesity	
	Prior VTE	
	Oral contraceptive pill (OCP) use	
	Inflammatory and infective illness	
	Immobility—long distance air travel, prolonged bed rest	
3	Thrombophilic disorders	
	Inherited	
	AT deficiency *Protein C deficiency* *Protein S deficiency*	Uncommon, strongly thrombogenic, diagnosed by functional assays and requires treatment during pregnancy
	*Factor V Leiden mutation (APCR)** *Prothrombin gene (G20210A) mutation* *Deficiency of antithrombin* *Hyperhomocysteinemia (serum level >18.5 μmol/l)*	Common, weakly thrombogenic, gene testing available, treatment on individual basis
	Acquired	
	Antiphospholipid antibodies	

*APCR-activated Protein C resistance

prothrombin. This mutation is extremely uncommon in the non-white population.

Antithrombin deficiency is the most thrombogenic disorder but is rare (De Stetanov, 1994). Hyperhomocysteinemia has been described in association with inherited polymorphism of the methylenetetrahydrofolate reductase (MTHR) gene, as well as the environmental deficiencies of folates and vitamin B_{12}. Homocysteine, an intermediate by-product formed during the metabolism of methionine, is toxic to endothelial cells and inhibits activation of Protein C. All genetic thrombophilias are autosomal dominant except hyperhomocysteinemia, which is autosomal recessive.

Antiphospholipid antibodies (a PL Abs) are detected in 2% of patients with non-traumatic VTE. A PL Abs are also a predisposing factor

FIGURE 35.1: SITE OF ACTION OF INHERITED THROMBOPHILIA (SHOWN IN RECTANGLES)

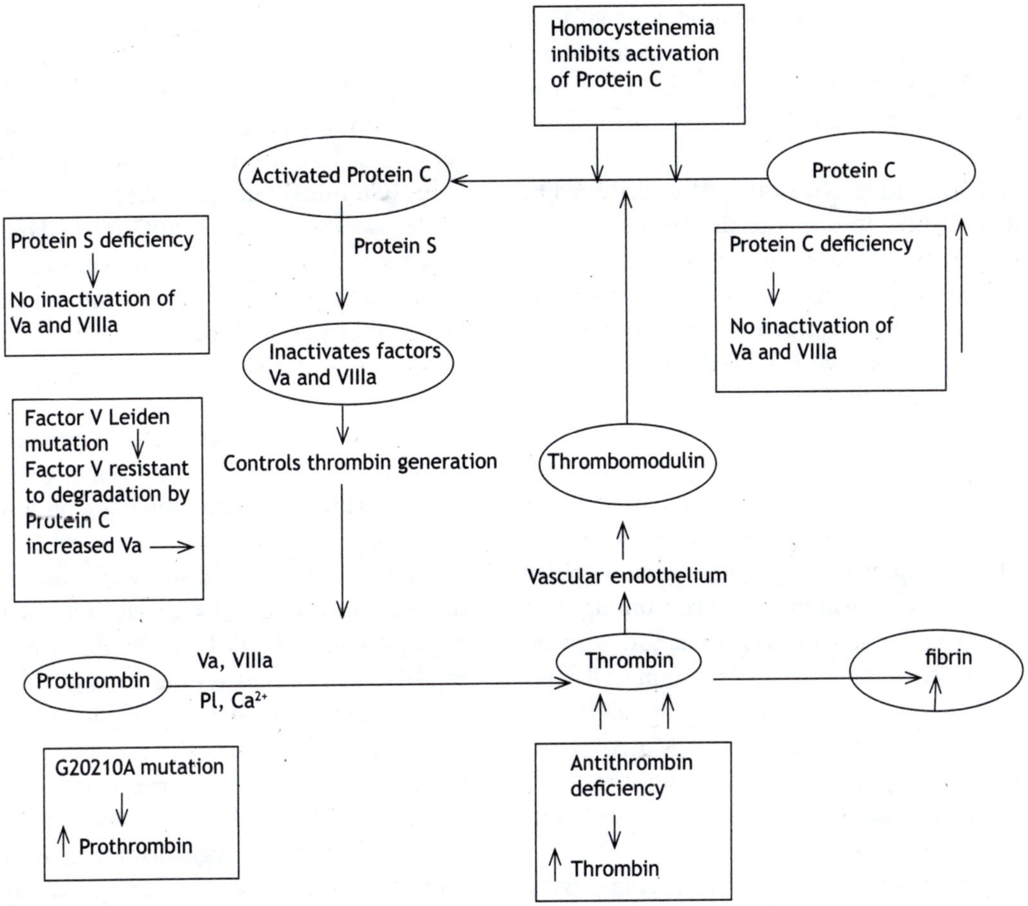

for arterial thrombosis. In fact, they account for up to 5% of arterial strokes in otherwise healthy young women, and thrombosis may occur in relatively unusual locations such as the retinal, subclavian, brachial or digital arteries (Ginsberg et al 1995, Higgins and Said 2005).

DEEP VENOUS THROMBOSIS

Clinical Features Most cases of DVT during pregnancy are confined to the deep veins of the lower extremities. The clinical methods of detecting DVT are insensitive; clinical suspicion forms the basis of further evaluation. Therefore, high index of suspicion is the key to diagnosis.

The characteristic symptoms of DVT are pain, swelling, tenderness, warmth and colour change in the legs. There is a striking propensity for venous thrombi during pregnancy to occur in the left leg, possibly due, in part, to compression of the left iliac vein by the right iliac artery as they cross. Occasionally, reflex arterial spasm may result in a pale, cool, painful extremity with diminished pulsations—the so-called *phlegmasia alba dolens* or *milk leg*. By itself, the clinical diagnosis of DVT is unreliable (Kearon et al 1998). Pain in the calf or Homans sign (calf pain in response to squeezing or to stretching the Achilles tendon) may be due to muscle strain or contusion.

Investigations In suspected cases of VTE, it is essential to diagnose the disease when it is present and to exclude it when it is not, because anticoagulant treatment of pregnant women carries significant risks, whereas not treating patients with VTE can result in fatal and nonfatal PE (Ginseberg, 1996).

Venography remains the gold standard test for the diagnosis of DVT of the lower extremities, and a normal test excludes calf and proximal DVT. Despite this, the performance of venography during pregnancy is unpopular because it is painful, time-consuming and cumbersome and ionising radiation may be absorbed by the fetus—300 mrad in unilateral venography without shielding the abdomen (Doll and Wakefield 1997). Moreover, it may induce thrombosis in some cases. This technique has largely been replaced by non-invasive methods.

Compression ultrasound (CUS) along with colour Doppler is the first investigation to be used. The diagnosis is based on the non-compressibility and typical echo pattern of a thrombosed vein. It is sensitive and specific for the diagnosis of proximal DVT—femoral, popliteal and calf trifurcation (Heijboer et al 1993; Kearon et al 1998)—but less sensitive for detecting a calf vein thrombosis that may extend proximally. Positive CUS calls for treatment; however, negative CUS is followed by Doppler of the iliac vein if iliac vein thrombosis is suspected. In case of positive Doppler for iliac vein, treatment is instituted, while a negative test is followed by magnetic resonance venography (MRV) or venography, if there is strong suspicion of DVT. If there is no strong suspicion of DVT, negative CUS can be followed by serial CUS on Days 2, 3, 6 and 8 to detect any extension of the calf thrombus (undetected at initial CUS) into proximal veins (Cunningham et al 2005).

Impedance plethysmography (IPG) is based on the observation that alteration in venous return in the calf, produced by the inflation and deflation of the thigh cuff, results in changes in the electrical resistance detected at the skin surface (Huisman et al 1986). However, IPG has largely been abandoned because the test is less accurate than CUS in women who are not pregnant and the machines are no longer being manufactured.

High levels of *D-dimer*, a specific fibrin degradation product, have been reported in most patients with DVT and PE (Bounameaux et al 1994). D-dimer testing has assumed an increasingly prominent role in the exclusion of acute DVT in the non-pregnant population, but it is not specific to pregnancy. D-dimer levels increase with gestational age and during complicated pregnancies such as those associated with preterm labour, abruptio placentae or gestational hypertension (Nolan et al 1993). However, normal levels of D-dimer do rule out thromboembolism. (Bates et al 2001).

Computed tomography (CT) with lead shielding can be useful for detecting lower extremity DVT. *Magnetic resonance venography (MRV)* of the lower extremities appears to be accurate for DVT. It has the potential to be useful in pregnancy because it appears to be sensitive for all lower extremity DVTs, including calf and ileofemoral DVT, and is not associated with radiation exposure. MRI also rules out nonspecific causes simulating

DVT such as cellulite, myositis, edema, hematoma and superficial phlebitis (Fraser et al 2002).

Management Once the diagnosis of DVT is established, prompt anticoagulation is necessary to i) diminish the severity and duration of symptoms and prevent thrombus growth ii) reduce the risk of pulmonary embolism, iii) minimise the risk of recurrent TE iv) prevent post-thrombotic syndrome (Augustinos and Ouriel 2004). At present, rapid anticoagulation can be effected by parenteral agents. Low molecular weight heparin (LMWH) is rapidly replacing unfractionated heparin (UFH) as the drug of choice for initial treatment as well as for the rest of the pregnancy because of its obvious advantages—more predictable therapeutic response, increased bioavailability, longer half life, reduced incidence of heparin-induced thrombocytopenia and osteoporosis and much less need for laboratory monitoring (Suneja et al 2001).

For acute treatment of VTE, therapy is initiated with LMWH on a weight-adjusted dose as shown in Table 35.2 (Higgins and Said 2005). As the pregnancy progresses, the volume of distribution of LMWH changes. It is prudent to periodically (for example, every 1–3 months) check the heparin (antifactor Xa) levels, 4–6 hours after the morning dose, and adjust the dose of LMWH to achieve an antifactor Xa level of approximately 0.5–1.2 U/ml for a twice-daily LMWH regimen and 1.0–2.0 U/ml for a once-daily dose. LMWH should not be given to patients with prosthetic heart valves because of reports of valvular thrombosis (Shiach CR, 2003; McRae and Ginsberg 2004; McColl and Greer 2004).

Alternatively, UFH initiated by either an intravenous bolus followed by a continuous infusion to maintain the activated partial thromboplastin (aPTT) levels in the therapeutic range or adjusted-dose subcutaneous UFH for at least five days, followed by adjusted-dose subcutaneous UFH for the remainder of the pregnancy, can be used. Injections are given every eight hours to prolong the aPTT levels to at least 1.5–2.5 times that of the control level throughout the dosing interval (Table 36.3). The mid-interval aPTT

Table 35.2: Low molecular weight heparin (LMWH) dosage schedule

LMWH	Therapeutic Dose	Prophylactic Dose
Dalteparin (Fragmin)	100 U/Kg twice daily	5000 U daily
Enoxaparin (Clexane)	1 mg/kg twice daily or 1.5 mg/g daily	40 mg daily
Tinzaparin (innohep)	175 IU/kg daily	4500 IU daily or 75 IU/kg

Table 35.3: Anticoagulation with UFH for VTE during pregnancy

Initial heparin dose	80 U/kg IV push (maximum 10,000 U) then 18 U/kg/hr infusion adjusted by PTT or heparin assay (maximum 2200/hr) for 5–7 days
Maintenance dose	10,000-20,000 U SC q12h, push to PTT 1.5–2 x control PTT or to heparin assay level of 0.5–0.8 u/ml 4h after dose
Duration of treatment	From diagnosis of VTE to 6–8 weeks postpartum, withheld during labour, resumed or replaced by warfarin postpartum

should be monitored every 1–2 weeks because UFH requirements often vary as pregnancy progresses (Prandoni et al 1992; Chunilal et al 2002). Heparin resistance is arbitrarily defined as the need for more than 40,000 units per day. It mainly occurs in patients with large venous thromboemboli because of inherited or acquired decrease in AT III levels, increased plasma levels of factor VIII and/or increased plasma levels of heparin-binding proteins. In such patients, monitoring with the aPTT is not recommended; instead, monitoring with antifactor Xa assay can be used and the dose adjusted to attain a 6-hour postdose anti-Xa level of 0.3–0.7 U/ml (McPhedran 2005). Alternatively, LMWH appears to be effective because it has less protein-binding properties.

FETAL COMPLICATIONS OF ANTICOAGULANTS UFH, LMWH and danaparoid do not cross the placenta and therefore do not have the potential to cause fetal bleeding or teratogenicity, although bleeding at the uteroplacental junction is possible (Ginsberg et al 2001). Coumarin derivatives cross the placenta and may be harmful. It is probable that oral anticoagulants are safe during the first 6 weeks of gestation, but there is a risk of embryopathy, consisting of nasal hypoplasia and/or stippled epiphyses, if coumarin derivatives are taken between 6 and 12 weeks of gestation. Central nervous system abnormalities can occur after exposure to these drugs during any trimester. In addition, oral anticoagulants produce an anticoagulant effect in the fetus. This is a concern, particularly at the time of delivery, when the combination of the anticoagulant effect and trauma of delivery can lead to bleeding in the neonate (Wong et al 1993; Herlocker 1994; Ginseberg 1996; Greer 1999).

MATERNAL COMPLICATIONS OF ANTICOAGULANTS The rate of major bleeding with various doses of UFH was found to be 2% (Levine et al 2001). Therapeutic doses of subcutaneous UFH can cause a persistent anticoagulant effect at the time of delivery, which can complicate its use prior to labour. Bleeding complications appear to be uncommon with LMWH (Sanson et al 1998).

Heparin-induced thrombocytopenia (HIT). Approximately 3% of non-pregnant patients receiving UFH develop immune, immunoglobulin G (IgG)-mediated thrombocytopenia (HIT), which is frequently complicated by the extension of pre-existing VTE or the development of new arterial thrombosis (Workentin, 1995). This should be differentiated from an early, benign, transient thrombocytopenia that can occur with initiation of UFH. The incidence of HIT is much lower with LMWH than UFH. HIT should be suspected when the platelet count falls to less than 100 × 10^9/l or to 50% of the baseline value, 5–15 days after commencing heparin (sooner with recent heparin exposure).

Heparin-induced osteoporosis. Symptomatic vertebral fractures have been reported in 2–3% of cases and significant reductions in bone density in up to 30% of patients receiving long-term UFH (Ginseberg, 2001). UFH causes bone loss by the decreasing rates of bone formation, while at the same time, increasing the rates of bone resorption (Douketis et al 1996; Muir et al 1997; Shaughnessy et al 1999; Pettila et al 2002).

MANAGEMENT OF ANTICOAGULANT THERAPY AT THE TIME OF DELIVERY Discontinuing LMWH or UFH 24 hours prior to elective induction of labour is recommended. An interval of more than 20 hours from the last dose should allow the insertion of a regional block without significant increased risk (Hague et al 2001). An epidural catheter can be removed 12–20 hours after placement, and the next injection can be delayed until 4 hours after removal. A prophylactic dose can be recommenced within 6 hours of the delivery. If the woman is deemed to have a very high risk of recurrent VTE (for example, proximal DVT or PE within four weeks), therapeutic doses of intravenous UFH can be initiated and discontinued 4–6 hours prior to the expected time of delivery. If spontaneous labour occurs in women receiving heparin, judicious use of protamine sulphate should be considered.

Use of anticoagulants in the nursing mother UFH and LMWH are not secreted into breast milk and can be safely given to nursing mothers. (Ginsberg et al 2001). Warfarin is safe when ingested while breastfeeding (American Academy of Pediatrics and ACOG 2002). Heparin and warfarin can be started simultaneously, and heparin can usually be discontinued after 5 days. Postpartum women require larger dose of warfarin (45 mg versus 24 mg) and for a longer time (7 versus 4 days) to achieve the target international normalised ratio (INR) of 2.0 or greater. The mean maintenance dose is also more in postpartum women—4.9 mg versus 4.3 mg (Brooks et al 2002).

Duration of treatment Pain disappears in 7–10 days, and graded ambulation is then started. Elastic stockings are fitted and anticoagulation continued for at least for 3 months after the acute event. If the woman is still pregnant at this juncture, anticoagulation should cover 6 weeks after delivery; however, it is not known whether it is better to continue with a therapeutic or a lower dose of heparin throughout pregnancy. For antenatal anticoagulation, warfarin was recommended for use after the period of greatest risk of congenital abnormalities—weeks 6–12 of pregnancy—to be continued until 36 weeks, when a switch back to heparin is suggested to decrease the risk of bleeding at delivery. This is because heparin dosing can conveniently be reduced or withheld at the time of delivery. An alternative, preferred protocol is to use LMWH throughout pregnancy (Nelson Piercy 1994; Kearon 2004).

New Anticoagulants Recently, three new anticoagulants have been introduced in an attempt to overcome the limitations of heparin and vitamin K antagonists. These include fondaparinux and indraparinux, synthetic analogs of the pentasaccharide sequence that mediates the interaction of heparin and LMWH with antithrombin and ximelagatran, an orally active inhibitor of thrombin. However, their safety in pregnancy is yet to be proven (Weitz 2004).

Inferior vena cava filters are indicated in women with contraindications to anticoagulants; predominantly those who develop clinically significant bleeding while receiving anticoagulants or who have a high risk of major bleeding if given anticoagulants. Removable filters are a reasonable approach to women who have a transient contraindication (Augustinos and Ouriel 2004).

Pulmonary Embolism

Diagnosis Clinical presentations such as chest pain, tachypnea, dyspnea, hypoxia and hypocapnia and routine laboratory testing such as for arterial blood gases, electrocardiography (sinus tachycardia, right axis deviation, right bundle branch block, peak P waves in lead II or classical S,Q3,T3 pattern) and chest radiography (rules out other lesions or may show hypoperfused transluscent segment) are often the first indications that PE is present. However, taken alone, they are insufficient to diagnose PE and therefore, objective testing is necessary. It is reasonable to start with bilateral lower extremity ultrasound, and if this is positive, treatment can be started. In the face of negative ultrasonography, further testing is warranted for evaluation of suspected PE (Stone and Morris 2004).

Ventilation/Perfusion scanning (V/Q scan) remains the first imaging modality for diagnosis of PE (PIOPED study 1990). The amount of radiation exposure depends on the isotope used, but it can be performed safely during pregnancy (Chan et al 2002). This technique entails locating one or more ventilated areas of lung that are non-perfused (a V/Q 'mismatch'), together with a chest film free of infiltrate in the non-perfused area. Such a result is a 'high probability scan' and is considered sufficient proof for anticoagulation treatment. A less conclusive V/Q scan in a patient, clinically suspected of PE, might lead to *pulmonary angiography* (a more invasive but more sensitive and specific test), in which a large non-perfused segment of the lung is sought. *CT of chest—'helical' or 'spiral' CT*—has been used instead of V/Q scans with perhaps less sensitivity but good specificity; sensitivity of the CT is said to be improving (Mullins et al 2000; Winer-Muram et al 2002).

Treatment The aim of treatment is to dissolve the pulmonary clots and prevent recurrent embolisation. This is achieved by rapid anticoagulation in a dosage schedule similar to that for DVT (Tables 35.2 and 35.3). Most authors recommend continuation of therapeutic anticoagulation for months. Warfarin can be used for maintenance anticoagulation in the postpartum period. However, a woman with recent PE who must undergo cesarean section presents a grave problem. Reversal of anticoagulation may be followed by recurrent embolus, while surgery in a fully anticoagulated woman may result in life-threatening hemorrhage or hematoma. In this situation, an inferior vena caval filter should be placed before surgery (Augustinos and Ouriel 2004).

For a pregnant patient with a large PE, treatment should probably begin with a fibrinolytic agent such as streptokinase, urokinase, tissue plasminogen activator (tPA) or, if fibrinolytics are contraindicated, surgical embolectomy. The postpartum state is a contraindication to fibrinolytic agents, as is any recent surgery and any serious bleeding tendency. Most clinical experiences indicate use of streptokinase, and the success rate is high. If any fibrinolytic agent is used, full dose heparinisation is done after therapeutic fibrinolysis (Stone and Morris 2004).

THROMBOPROPHYLAXIS

Women with previous VTE should be screened for inherited and acquired thrombophilia, ideally before pregnancy. Regardless of their risk of VTE, immobilisation of women during pregnancy, labour and the puerperium should be minimised and dehydration should be avoided. Women should be reassessed before or during labour for risk factors for VTE. Age over 35 years and BMI greater than 30/ body weight greater than 90 kg are important independent risk factors for postpartum VTE even after vaginal delivery. The combination of either of these risk factors with any other risk factor for VTE (such as pre-eclampsia or immobility), or the presence of two other persisting risk factors should lead the clinician to consider the use of LMWH for 3–5 days postpartum. The thromboprophylaxis protocol for women with previous VTE or thrombophilia is given in Table 35.4 (RCOG guidelines 2004).

These women require joint specialist management by obstetricians and experts in hemostasis and pregnancy.

TABLE 35.4: SUMMARY OF PROTOCOL FOR THROMBOPROPHYLAXIS IN WOMEN WITH PREVIOUS VTE AND/OR THROMBOPHILIA

Risk	*Previous VTE and/or Thrombophilia Status*	*Prophylaxis*
Very high	Previous VTE (± thrombophilia) on long-term warfarin	Antenatal high prophylactic or therapeutic dose and at least 6 weeks of postnatal warfarin
High	Previous recurrent VTE not on long-term warfarin Previous VTE + thrombophilia Previous VTE + family history of VTE Asymptomatic thrombophilia (antithrombin deficiency, combined defects, homozygous factor V Leiden or prothrombin gene defect)	Antenatal and six weeks postnatal prophylactic LMWH
Moderate	Single, previous, provoked VTE without thrombophilia, family history or other risk factors Asymptomatic thrombophilia (except antithrombin deficiency, combined defects, homozygous FVL or prothrombin gene defect)	Six weeks of postnatal prophylactic LMWH ± antenatal low-dose aspirin

TABLE 35.5: GUIDELINES FOR RISK ASSESSMENT IN GYNECOLOGIC SURGERY

Major gynecologic surgery with age >60 or major surgery for cancer	High Risk = 3
Major gynecologic surgery with age 40-60 or minor surgery and age >60	Moderate Risk = 2
Minor gynecologic surgery and age 40-60	Low Risk = 1
PREDISPOSING RISK (S):	
History of DVT /PE	1.5
Age >70 years	1.5
(Heriditary or acquired) Thrombophilia	1.5
Malignancy	1.5
Age >60 years	1.0
Obesity	0.5
Major varicosities	0.5
Estrogens/HRT	0.5
OCP	0.5
Inflammation/Infection	0.5

THROMBOEMBOLIC DISORDERS IN GYNECOLOGY

The risk factors for VTE in non-pregnant women are listed in Table 35.5 (Bick and Haas 2004). Ovarian stimulation for the purpose of in vitro fertilisation has occasionally resulted in venous or arterial thrombosis because of acquired activated Protein C resistance, thought to be caused by increased estrogen levels (Curvers et al 2001).

THROMBOSIS PROPHYLAXIS IN SURGICAL PATIENTS

Thrombosis prophylaxis should be administered based on the risk category of each patient. Besides early ambulation, the use of graduated elastic stockings should be considered even in patients undergoing low-risk surgery, and their use should be continued throughout the postoperative period in the hospital. This practice has become common in Europe; although to date, no general recommendations for thrombosis prophylaxis in addition to the use of elastic stockings or intermittent pneumatic compression (IPC) during major surgery have been made. The use of low-dose heparin prophylaxis (5000 IU three times/day) has been effective in these patients. This regimen should be started two hours before surgery and continued throughout the time of hospitalisation. It has been shown that in gynecologic patients, especially cancer patients, LMWH is as effective as, and may carry a lower bleeding risk than, UFH. In addition to women who undergo gynecologic cancer surgery (including breast cancer surgery), patients with extensive pelvic surgery or a history of idiopathic thrombosis belong to the high-risk group, the use of graduated compression stockings combined with LMWH (or UFH) prophylaxis is strongly recommended. Because some studies have found a high incidence of late postoperative VT in ovarian cancer patients, even after discharge from hospital, these authors recommend prolonged thrombosis prophylaxis for 3 months after surgery, including the time of adjuvant chemotherapy. Dextran or adjusted-dose warfarin may be an alternative treatment for patients for whom heparin is contraindicated (von Tempelhoff and Heilmann 2000). These agents should not, however, be routinely used for prophylaxis in gynecologic surgery.

References

ACOG Practice Bulletin. 2001. Thromboembolism in pregnancy. *Int J Gynaecol Obstet* 203–212.

American Academy of Paediatrics and American College of Obstetricians and Gynecologists. 2002. *Guidelines for Perinatal Care*, 5th ed.

Augustinos P and K Ouriel. 2004. Invasive approaches to treatment of venous thromboembolism. *Circulation* 110 (supple I): I-27–I-34.

Bates SM and JS Ginsberg. 2001. Pregnancy and deep vein thrombosis. *Semin Vasc Med* 1:97–104.

Bates SM, A Grand'Maison, M Johnston et al. 2001. A latex D-dimer reliably excludes venous thromboembolism. *Arch Intern Med* 161:447–453.

Bick RL and S Haas. 2003. Thromboprophylaxis and thrombosis in medical, surgical, trauma and obstetric gynecologic patients. *Hematol Oncol Clin N Am* (17): 217–258.

Bounameaux H, P de Moerloose, A Perrier and G Raber. 1994. Plasma measurement of D-dimer as a diagnostic aid in suspected venous thromboembolism: an overview. *Thromb Haemos* 71:1–6.

Brooks C, JM Rutherfold, J Gould et al. 2002. Safety of wafarin dosage in postpartum women: a case-control study. *Br J Obstet Gynecol* 109:187.

Chan WS, JG Ray, S Murray et al. 2002. Suspected pulmonary embolism in pregnancy. *Arch Intern med* 162:1170–1172.

Chunilal SD, E Young, MA Johnston et al. 2002. The APPT response of pregnant plasma to unfractionated heparin. *Thromb Haemost* 87:92–97.

Clark P, J Brennand, JA Conkie et al. 1998. Activated protein C sensitivity, protein C, protein S, and coagulation in normal pregnancy. *Thromb Haemost* 79:1166–1170.

Cunningham FG, KJ Leveno, SL Bloom et al. 2005. Thromboembolic disorders. In *William's Obstetrics*, eds. FG Cunningham, KJ Leveno, SL Bloom et al; 22nd edn, McGraw Hill, 1073–1092.

Curvers J, AW Nap, MC Thomasson et al. 2001. Effect of in vitro fertilization treatment and subsequent pregnancy on the protein C pathway. *Br J Hamatol* 115:400.

Doll R and R Wakefield. 1997. Risk of childhood cancer from fetal radiation. *Br J Radiol* 70:130–139.

Douketis JD, JS Ginsberg, RF Burrows et al. 1996. The effects of long-term heparin therapy during pregnancy on bone density: a prospective matched cohort study. *Thromb Haemost* 75:254–257 [Medline] [Order article via Infotrieve].

Fraser DGW, AR Moody. PS Morgan et al. 2002. Diagnosis of lower-limb deep venous thrombosis: a prospective blinded study of magnetic resonance direct thrombus imaging. *Ann Intern Med* 136: 89–98.

Ginsberg JS, I Greer and J Hirsh. 2001. Use of antithrombotic agents during pregnancy. *Chest* 119:122s–131s.

Ginsberg JS, PS Wells, P Brill-Edwards et al. 1995. Antiphospholipid antibodies and venous thromboembolism. *Blood* 86:3685–3691.

Greer IA. 1999. Thrombosis in pregnancy: maternal and fetal issues. *Lancet* 353(9160): 1258–1265.

Hague WM, RA Norh and AS Gallus et al. 2001. A working group on behalf of the Obstetric Medicine Group of Ausralasia. Anticoagulation in pregnancy & puerperium. *Med J Aus* 175:258–263.

Heijboer H, HR Buller, AWA Lensing et al. 1993. A comparison of real-time compression ultrasonography with impedance plethysmography for the diagnosis of deep-vein thrombosis in symptomatic outpatients. *N Engl J Med* 329:1365–1369.

Herlocker TT. 1994. Central neural blockage for patients receiving anticoagulants. *Clin Anaesthesia Update* 5:1–9.

Huisman MV, HR Buller, JW Cate and J Vreeken. 1986. Serial impedance plethysmography for suspected deep venous thrombosis in outpatients: the Amsterdam General Practioner Study. *N Engl J Med* 314:823–828.

Higgins JR and J Said. 2005. The clinical implications of thrombophilia in pregnancy. In *Recent Advances in Obstetrics and Gynaecology,* eds. J Bonnar and W Dunlop. The Royal Society of Medicine Press Ltd; 13–29.

Jordan DJ, MG Schoon and PN Badenhorst. 2005. Thrombophilia screening in pregnancy - CME review article. *Obstet Gynecol Surv* Vol 60 (6); 394–404.

Kearon C, JA Julian, JS Ginsberg et al. 1998. Noninvasive diagnosis of deep venous thrombosis. *Ann Intern Med* 128:663–677.

Kearon C. 2004. Long term management of patients after venous thromboembolism. *Circulation* 110 (supple I): I-10–I-18.

Levine MN, G Raskob, S Landefeld and C Kearon. 2001. Hemorrhagic complications of anticoagulant treatment. *Chest* 119:108s–121s.

Lindqvist PG, PJ Svensson, K Marsaal et al. 1999. Activated protein C resistance (FV:Q506) and pregnancy. *Thromb Hemost* 81:532–537.

Lockwood CJ. 2002. Inherited thrombophilia in pregnant patients: detection and treatment paradigm. *Obstet Gynecol* 99:333.

Macklon NC, IA Greer and AW Bowman. 1997. An ultrasound study of gestational and postural changes in the deep venous system of the leg in pregnancy. *Br J Obstet Gynecol* 104:191–197.

McColl and IA Greer. 2004. Low molecular weight heparin for the prevention and treatment of venous thromboembolism in pregnancy. *Clin Pulm Med* 10:371–375.

McPhedran P. 2005. Venous thrombo embolism during pregnancy. In *Medical complications during pregnancy*, eds. GN Burow, JP Duffy and JA Copel. 6th ed. Elsevier Saunders; 87–101.

McRae SJ and Ginsberg JS. 2004. Initial treatment of venous thromboembolism. *Circulation* 110 (supple I): I-3–I-9.

Muir JM, J Hirsh, JI Weitz et al. 1997. A histomorphometric comparison of the effects of heparin and low-molecular-weight heparin on cancellous bone in rats. *Blood* 89:3236–3242.

Mullins MD, DM Becker, KD Hagspiel and JT Philbrick. 2000. The role of spiral volumetric computed tomography in the diagnosis of pulmonary embolism. *Arch Intern Med* 160:293–298.

Nelson Piercy C. 1994. LMWH for obstetric thromboprophylaxis. *Br J Obstet Gynaecol* 101:6–8.

Nolan TE, RP Smith and LD Devoe. 1993. Maternal plasma D-dimer levels in normal and complicated pregnancies. *Obstet Gynecol* 81:235–238 [Abstract].

Pettila V, P Leinonen, A Markkola et al. 2002. Postpartum bone mineral density in women treated for thromboprophylaxis with unfractionated heparin or LMW heparin. *Thromb Haemost* 87: 182–186.

PIOPED study. 1990. Value of the ventilation/perfusion scan in acute pulmonary embolism. Results of the prospective investigation of pulmonary embolism diagnosis (PIOPED). The PIOPED Investigators. *JAMA* 263:2753–2759.

Prandoni P, AW Lensing et al. 1992. Comparison of subcutaneous LMWH with i/v standard heparin in proximal vein thrombosis. *Lancet* 339: 441–45.

Raes DC, M Cox and JB Clegg. 1995. World distribution of factor V Leiden. *Lancet* 346:1133–34.

RCOG guidelines No. 37. 2004. Thromboprophylaxis during Pregnancy, Labour and after Vaginal Delivery (37). Clinical Green Top Guidelines.

Sanson BJ, AWA Lensing, MH Prins et al. 1998. Safety of low molecular weight heparin in pregnancy: a systematic review. *Thromb Haemost* 81:668–672.

Shaughnessy SG, J Hirsh, M Bhandari et al. 1999. A histomorphometric evaluation of heparin-induced bone loss after discontinuation of heparin treatment in rats. *Blood* 93:1231–1236.

Stone SE and TA Morris. 2004. Pulmonary embolism and pregnancy. *Crit Care Clin* vol 20: 661–677.

Suneja AR, M Arora and N Agarwal. 2001. Deep vein thrombosis in pregnancy. *J Indian Academy of Clin Med* No. 4(2): 260–269.

von Tempelhoff GF and L Heilmann. 2000. Anti-thrombotic therapy in gynecologic surgery and gynecologic oncology. *Hematol Oncol Clin N Am* 14 (5): 1151–1169.

Weiss N and PS Bernstein. 2000. Risk scoring system for predicting venous thromboembolism in obstetric patients. *Am J Obstet Gynecol* 182:1073.

Weitz JI. 2004. New anticoagulants for treatment of venous thromboembolism. *Circulation* 110 (suppl I): I-19–I-26.

Winer-Muram HT, JM Boone, HL Brown et al. 2002. Pulmonary embolism in pregnant patients: Fetal radiation dose with helical CT. *Radiology* 224–487.

Wong V, CH Cheng and KC Chan. 1993. Fetal and neonatal outcome of exposure to anticoagulants during pregnancy. *Am J Med Genet* 145:17–21.

36

Doppler Sonography

S Suresh | Indrani Suresh

Doppler ultrasound has become an integral part of obstetric imaging. Fitzgerald and Drumm reported the use of Doppler in assessing blood flow in the umbilical artery in 1977. Since then, numerous studies to assess the value of Doppler as a screening test in pregnancy and the relationship of abnormal Doppler waveforms to adverse fetal outcome have been published. In 1983, Campbell and co-workers demonstrated the use of Doppler in the assessment of uteroplacental flow using continuous wave Doppler equipment. The advent of colour Doppler paved the way for a more precise imaging of the uterine arteries and fetal vessels, as it provided a 'road map' of even the smaller fetal vessels. Today, Doppler is used in pregnancy to identify placental dysfunction, fetal hypoxia and its sequelae, fetal anemia and markers for chromosomal abnormalities. A combination of umbilical artery Doppler, middle cerebral artery Doppler and Doppler of the ductus venosus is helpful in identifying fetal adaptation in IUGR due to placental dysfunction. Colour Doppler is also a useful adjunct in the diagnosis of certain anomalies such as vein of Galen aneurysm, placental chorioangiomas, renal agenesis and other vascular lesions in the fetus. Applications in gynecology include identification of neo-angiogenesis in pelvic malignancy and the study of endometrial flow in infertility.

DOPPLER FUNDAMENTALS

When a source of sound interrogates a moving reflector, there is a small change in the reflected frequency when compared to the transmitted frequency. This difference is called the Doppler shift. In ultrasound, the Doppler shift frequency falls in the audible range and hence can be heard as an audio signal. Using the fast Fourier transform technique, Doppler signals are processed to provide a visual display on the screen. This is called the flow velocity waveform or spectral waveform. The spectral waveform consists of a continuous display of Doppler shift frequencies throughout the cardiac cycle. Several cycles can be displayed on one screen, thus providing hemodynamic information over a period of time. From the spectral waveform, it is possible to measure the Doppler shift information as a frequency (khz) or as a velocity (cm/second). Velocity measurements are used more often as they are easier to understand. Two types of Doppler are available, namely, continuous wave and pulsed wave. Continuous wave Doppler is not currently used in obstetric and gynecological imaging due to its inherent limitations. It is used only in fetal monitors and pocket fetal Dopplers to listen to fetal heart sounds. With the pulsed wave technique, it is possible to sample a specific point in the blood vessel using a 'gate' or 'sample volume' which can be adjusted.

The Doppler shift represents the change in velocity of movement of blood cells over a period of time (cardiac cycle). Hence, the Doppler waveform may be used to detect blood flow velocities at specific points in the cardiac cycle. In clinical practice, the peak systolic velocity (A) and the end diastolic velocity (B) are measured for a semi-quantitative analysis of blood flow. In addition, the mean velocity during a single cardiac cycle can also be measured. The pattern of the waveform is influenced by both upstream and downstream events. While the peak systolic flow depends on cardiac contractility, the diastolic flow alters with downstream resistance. For the uterine and umbilical arteries, the downstream vascular bed is the placental vascular bed. Hence, changes in the placenta will be reflected in the diastolic flow pattern in both these vessels.

Several Doppler indices are used to describe the ratio of systolic and diastolic flow. The simplest index is the ratio of the peak systolic velocity and end diastolic velocity (the maximum and minimum velocities in a cardiac cycle). The resistance index and pulsatility index are two other indices. The pulsatility index is now more widely used as it takes into consideration the systolic velocity, diastolic velocity and mean velocity in the cardiac cycle. The Doppler indices and their formulae are shown in Fig. 36.1.

PLACENTAL VASCULAR BED

Since Doppler waveforms alter with changes in vascular resistance, it is essential to have a

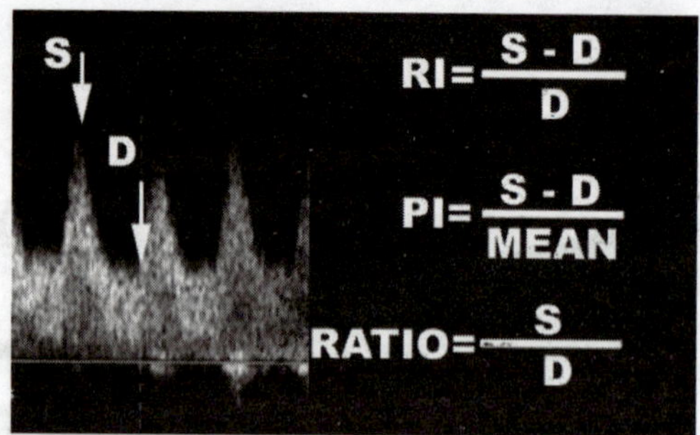

Figure 36.1: Doppler waveform showing calculation of Doppler indices

thorough understanding of the vascular beds in the fetus. The uterine arteries give rise to about eight arcuate arteries. These arteries encircle the uterus and give rise to the radial arteries, which in turn give rise to about 200 spiral arteries after penetrating the middle-third of the myometrium. The spiral arteries course into the decidua. The developing trophoblastic cells penetrate into the spiral arteries and, in the process, the spiral vessels lose their muscular coat and are converted into uteroplacental arteries (Rotmensh et al 1995), which are in a state of maximal vasodilatation. Thus, the placental vasculature forms a 'dynamic' vascular bed, with decreasing resistance to flow as gestational age advances.

It is interesting to note that this trophoblastic invasion occurs in two phases. The first wave of invasion occurs between 6 and 12 weeks and the second wave at 16–22 weeks. During the second phase of invasion, the trophoblast reaches the portion of the spiral artery in the myometrium. From then on, the invasion continues throughout pregnancy. The increasing trophoblastic proliferation and loss of elasiticity of the spiral arteries help accommodate the increasing uterine blood flow, from about 50 ml/min in early pregnancy to about 500 ml/min near term (Maini 1985).

Doppler Technique Obtaining an optimal Doppler waveform is essential for proper interpretation. The vessel is first located on B-mode and colour Doppler. The spectral waveform is then obtained by choosing an optimal angle to the vessel. It is important that the angle between the axis of the blood flow and the Doppler beam should not be 90° as it will result in poor Doppler signals. Care should be taken to record uniform waveforms for at least four consecutive cardiac cycles.

Using colour Doppler, the uterine arteries on either side can be located by imaging the iliac vessels and angulating the probe towards the uterus at the level of the cervix and lower part of the uterus. The uterine artery is identified as the only vessel that crosses the iliac vessels to reach the uterus. The spectral waveforms are obtained after imaging the vessel on B-mode and colour. The main stem of the uterine artery in its proximal portion, prior to the iliac crossing, is an ideal site for sampling. The optimal angle is assessed by obtaining a good audio signal.

Applications of Doppler in Early Pregnancy Applications of Doppler in early pregnancy are limited. In selected cases, Doppler serves as an adjunct to B-mode diagnosis.

The initial enthusiasm of the possibility of detecting poor placental vascularisation and relating it to early pregnancy failure has given way to cautious optimism in this regard. In a study of 19 patients with early pregnancy failure, Arduini et al (1991) have shown normal values in the spiral arteries. These results tallied with the study of Stabile et al (1990) in similar circumstances. From the evidence available, it may be inferred that most early pregnancy failures are not due to a failure of vascularisation. However, some patients with early pregnancy failure may show abnormal Doppler indices, allowing for some speculation. Larger studies will be required to throw more light in this regard. Increased peritrophoblastic venous flow may be seen in failed intrauterine pregnancies.

Ectopic pregnancy may be suspected on B-mode by visualising an empty uterine cavity and an adnexal 'ring' representing the gestational sac. The presence of echogenic fluid in the POD is strongly suggestive of ectopic pregnancy. Transvaginal colour Doppler shows a vascular ring, demonstrating flow in the trophoblast. Spectral Doppler shows varying impedances, depending on the viability of the trophoblast. With treatment, it is possible to demonstrate reduced vascularity in the adnexal ring by serial ultrasound and this can be used in the follow-up of ectopic pregnancies, medically treated with methotrexate in addition to serial β-hCG. Colour Doppler is also used to differentiate between a true and a 'pseudo' gestational sac in the uterine cavity. The presence of peritrophoblastic flow and increased myometrial flow suggests intrauterine gestation. Poor myometrial vascularity and the absence of peritrophoblastic flow suggests a 'pseudo' gestational sac.

The absence of peritrophoblastic flow may represent a recent complete abortion, but this diagnosis is easily made on B-mode and hence Doppler is not essential. In trophoblastic disease, a low impedance pattern is seen in the myometrium because of increased uterine flow (Aoki 1989). This finding is useful in the follow-up of patients treated by curettage to check for residual trophoblastic tissue. The efficacy of treatment can be assessed by serial Doppler examinations, in addition to serial β-hCG.

Colour Doppler in the Second and Third Trimesters Fetal growth in the second trimester allows better visualisation of fetal anatomy and vasculature. In the second trimester, imaging of fetal vessels aids in the diagnosis of certain malformations. The most widely used application of Doppler is for evaluation of placental dysfunction by studying the uterine and umbilical circulation. Flow in both uterine arteries and the umbilical artery aids the study of placental vascular bed impedance, thereby indicating that a Doppler of these vessels can be used to predict placental function. The fetal middle cerebral artery is sampled to understand fetal adaptation to reduced fetal perfusion. Changes in Doppler are correlated with adverse perinatal outcome.

Uteroplacental Circulation The uterine artery is imaged as it crosses the iliac vessels to pierce the myometrium. A Doppler sample close to the 'crossing over' is chosen and the Doppler beam adjusted to obtain maximal flow velocities (Colour plate 4). The uterine artery waveform has a sharp systolic peak and forward flow in diastole. Up to about 16 weeks of gestation, an early diastolic notch can be noticed; this indicates the presence of the elastic coat in the spiral arteries. Beyond this period, the diastolic notch gradually disappears and is not seen during the targeted scan (18–23 weeks). This corresponds to the second wave of trophoblastic invasion. The RI of the uterine arteries shows a gradual decrease with advancing gestational age (Fig. 36.2).

Differences in Doppler impedance may be seen between the right and left uterine arteries depending on the placental implantation site—lower impedances being present on the side of the placenta. These differences reduce with advanced gestational age, implying the contribution of both uterine arteries to the placental vascular bed. Therefore, it is essential to sample both uterine arteries in every patient.

The role of uterine artery Doppler as a screening test in low-risk patients has been extensively studied. Varying results have

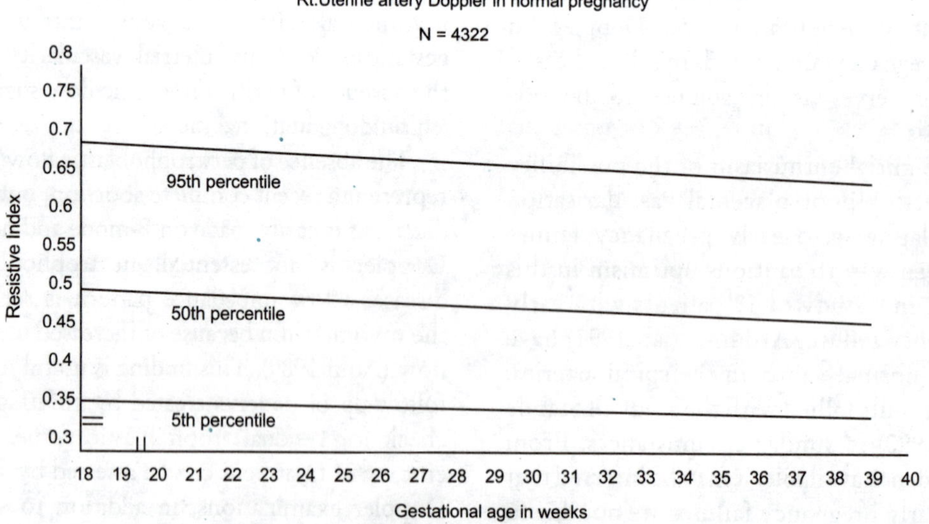

FIGURE 36.2: RI OF RIGHT UTERINE ARTERY IN NORMAL PREGNANCIES AT 18–40 WEEKS' GESTATION

been reported, presumably due to varying techniques of sampling adopted to obtain the waveforms. Campbell et al (1986) in a study of 149 low-risk women between 16 and 18 weeks of gestation have shown an overall sensitivity and specificity of 68% and 69% in predicting development of pregnancy-induced hypertension. In a larger study of 2058 women, Bower et al in 1993 reported that 16% had abnormal uterine artery waveforms with elevated RI and an early diastolic notch. In this group, the sensitivity and specificity of prediction of development of moderate pre-eclampsia was 87% and 85%, respectively. An abnormal waveform had increased the relative risk of pre-eclampsia by 24-fold. In a subsequent study (Bower 1993), the same authors have shown that if a second Doppler examination is done after 24 weeks, the positive predictive value of Doppler increases from 4.3 to 28%. From these studies, it may be inferred that the persistence of a diastolic notch beyond 24 weeks signifies increased risk of pre-eclampsia. The Cochrane Collaboration Systematic Review (Bricker and Neilson 2000) on the use of routine Doppler ultrasound in pregnancy, based on five trials on a total of 14,338 women, came to the conclusion that 'based on existing evidence, routine Doppler ultrasound in low-risk or unselected populations does not confer benefit on mother or baby. Future research should be powerful enough to address small changes in perinatal outcome, and should include evaluation of maternal psychological effects, long-term outcomes such as neurodevelopment, and issues of safety.'

Fetoplacental Circulation The umbilical arteries can be sampled near the placental insertion, free loop or fetal abdomen. The normal flow velocity waveform of the umbilical artery has a low resistance pattern (Colour plate 5). The resistance decreases with advancing gestational age, which can be explained by the increasing size of the placenta and the number of villous arteries. The RI decreases with advancing gestational age as depicted in Fig.36.3. In placental insufficiency, increased placental vascular resistance causes reduced diastolic flow and increased resistance index in the umbilical artery. Further reduction in placental resistance causes absent end diastolic flow velocities or even a reversal of flow (Figs 36.4 and Colour plate 5). Diastolic flow reversal is considered as the worst presentation of an abnormal umbilical artery waveform.

The role of umbilical artery velocimetry in IUGR has been extensively studied. It should be emphasised that Doppler of the umbilical artery is a test of placental vascular bed resistance and not the fetus. Hence, umbilical artery Doppler cannot be used to predict or diagnose IUGR, which is best done by fetal biometry. Doppler changes in the umbilical artery have been correlated with adverse perinatal outcome in IUGR fetuses. Trudinger et al (1991) studied 2178 high-risk pregnancies with a 27% incidence of IUGR (birth weight less than the 10th centile). The sensitivity and specificity for diagnosis of IUGR based on abnormal umbilical artery waveform was 64% and 74%, respectively. The positive predictive value was 55% and the negative predictive value was 83%. They also observed that fetuses with abnormal S/D ratios and which were born preterm, spent twice as much time in the neonatal intensive care unit as preterm infants who had normal S/D ratios antenatally. Further, they studied the value of serial Doppler measurements of the umbilical artery. About 794 patients with serial umbilical artery Doppler waveforms

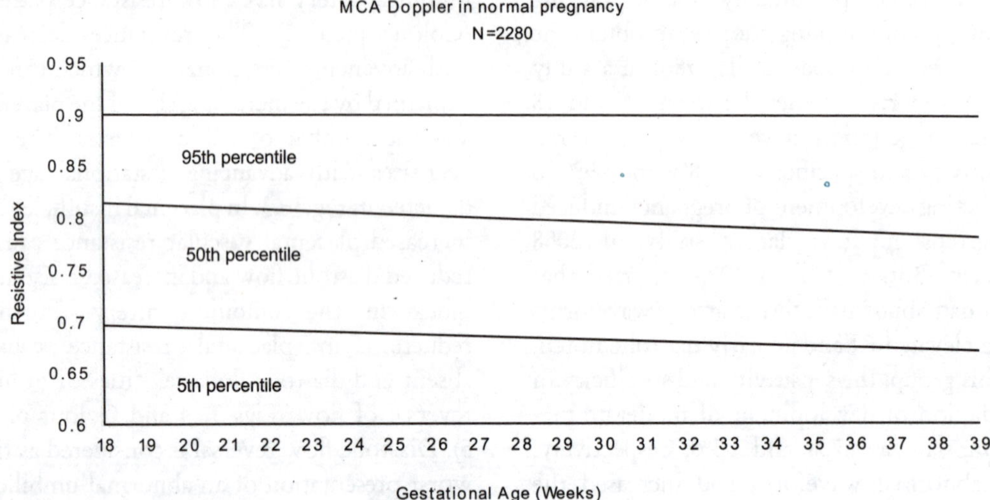

FIGURE 36.3: RI OF UMBILICAL ARTERY IN NORMAL PREGNANCIES AT 18–40 WEEKS' GESTATION

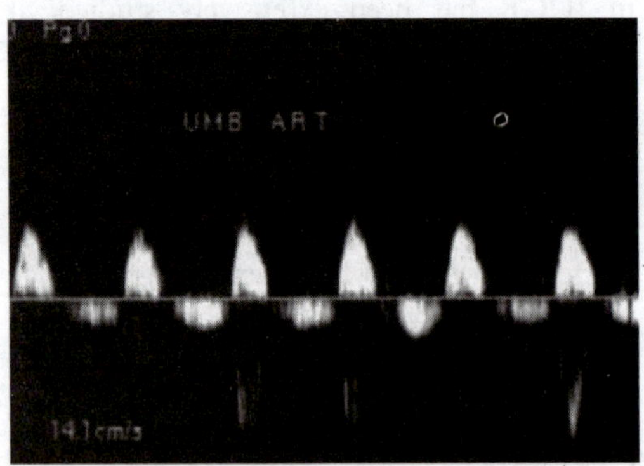

FIGURES 36.4: UMBILICAL ARTERY DOPPLER SHOWING ABSENT END DIASTOLIC FLOW

were examined. Of these, 567 had normal Doppler indices. In this group, the incidence of IUGR was 17%. In another group of 117 patients, the Doppler was abnormal at the first examination but normal on subsequent examination. The incidence of IUGR was 40% in this group. The third group of 110 patients were those with progressive abnormality of the Doppler indices. In this group, the incidence of IUGR was 71%. This group had the worst perinatal outcome, with a perinatal mortality of 63.6/1000. In another study, Burke et al (1990) studied 179 IUGR fetuses and reported a perinatal mortality of 54.5/1000 in those with abnormal Doppler indices, as compared with no perinatal mortality in those with normal indices.

This data suggests that umbilical artery Doppler is a good test to predict adverse perinatal outcome in IUGR fetuses. These fetuses should be subjected to intensive surveillance. A normal umbilical artery waveform indicates decreased risk of adverse perinatal outcome.

Doppler of the umbilical artery may be useful in differentiating between placental and non-placental causes of IUGR. This may help determine further investigation and management of pregnancy.

Fetal Middle Cerebral Artery The middle cerebral artery (MCA) indicates intracerebral flow through the internal carotid artery. It can be identified at the base of the brain as it courses through the lateral sulcus over the anterior perforator substance. In normal

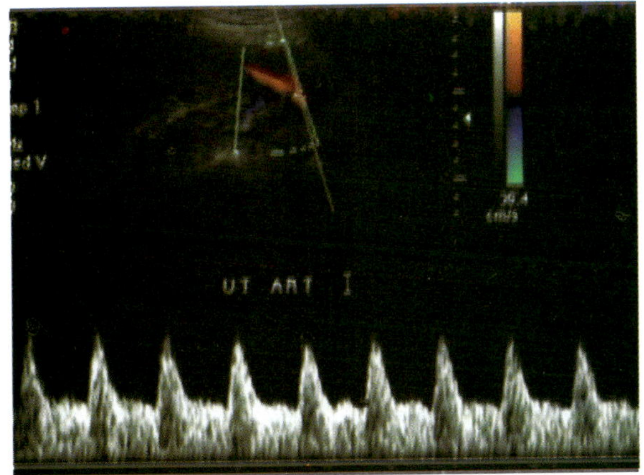

Colour plate 4: Uterine artery Doppler at 20 weeks in a low-risk pregnancy

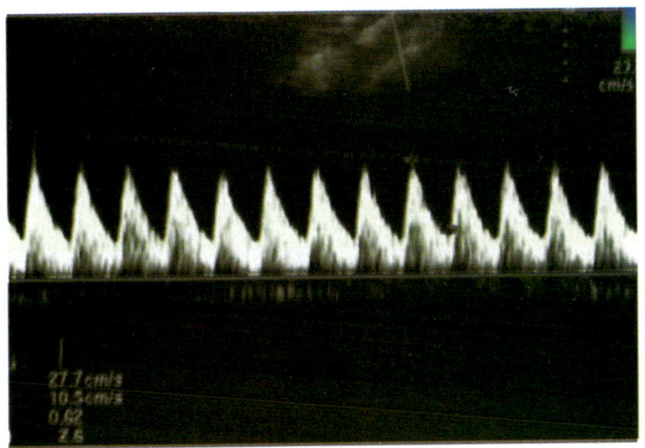

Colour plate 5: Normal umbilical artery waveform at 22 weeks.

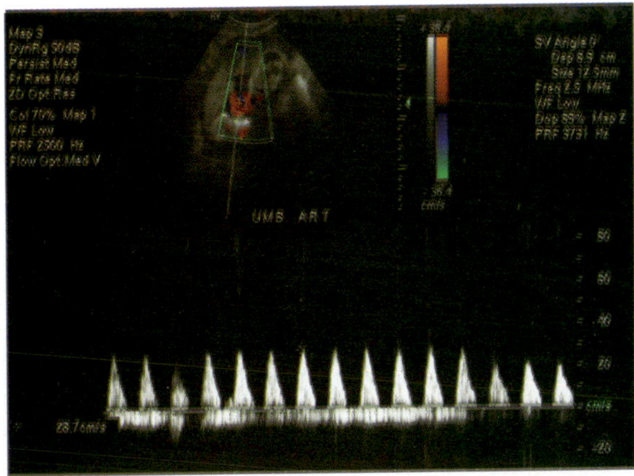

Colour plate 6: Umbilical artery Doppler showing reversal of flow in diastole

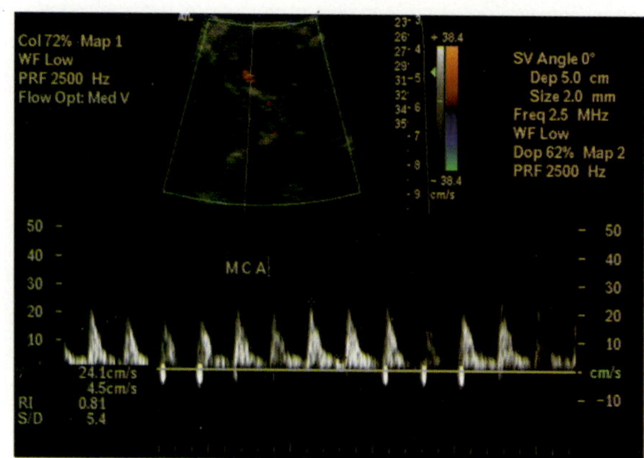

Colour plate 7: Normal middle cerebral artery waveform

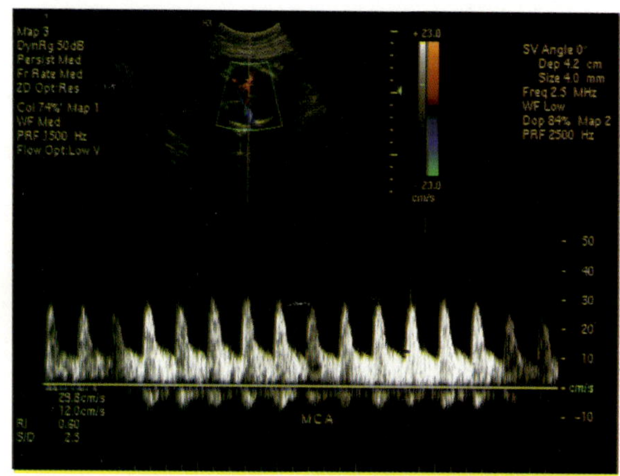

Colour plate 8: Middle cerebral artery showing increased diastolic flow in IUGR

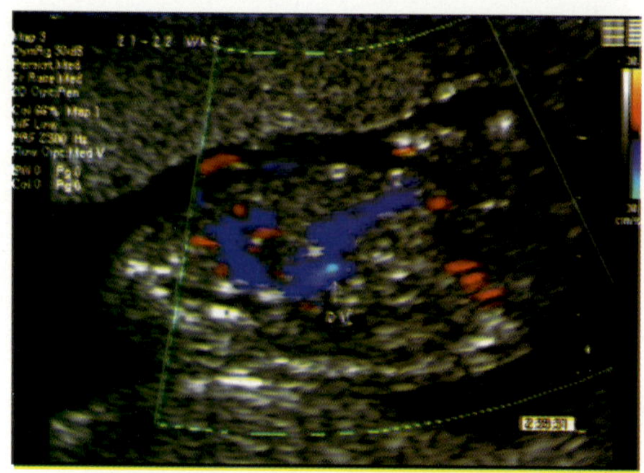

Colour plate 9: Ductus venosus B mode and colour Doppler

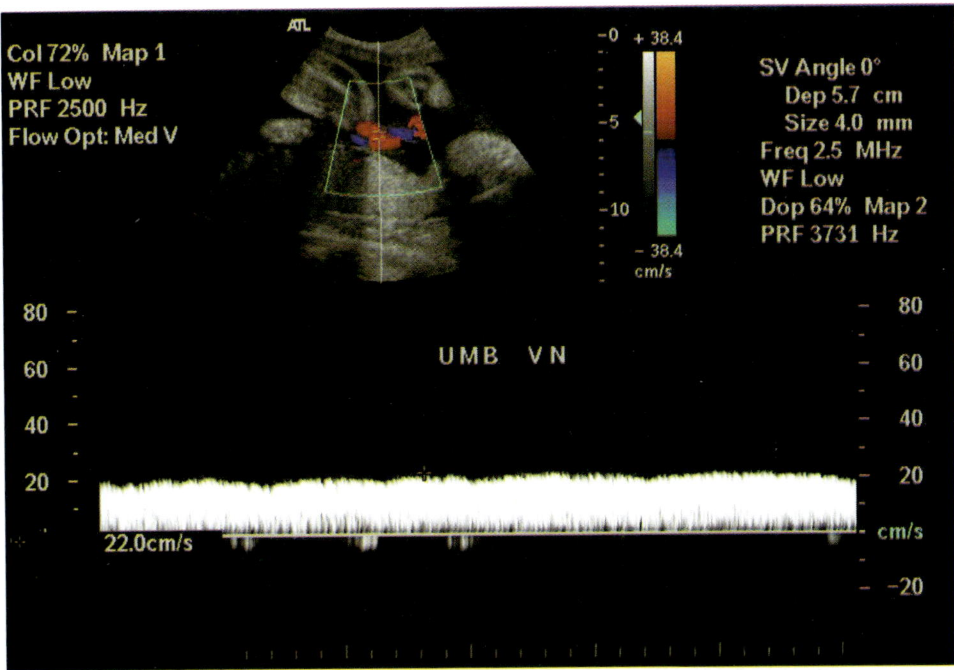

COLOUR PLATE 10: NORMAL VENOUS WAVEFORMS

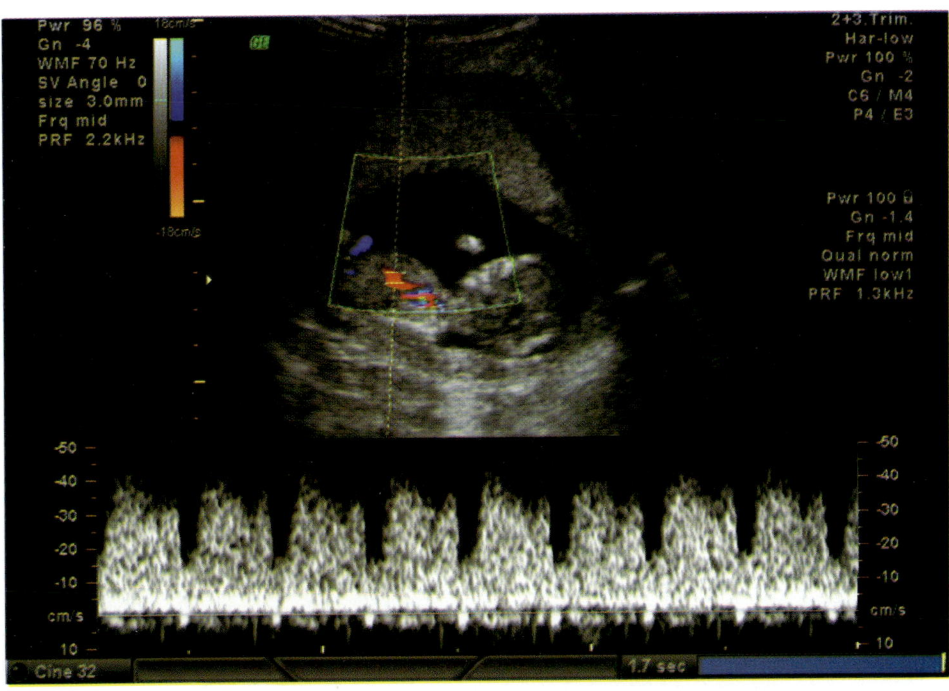

COLOUR PLATE 11: SAW TOOTHED PATTERN IN PORTAL VEIN IN FETAL ANEMIA

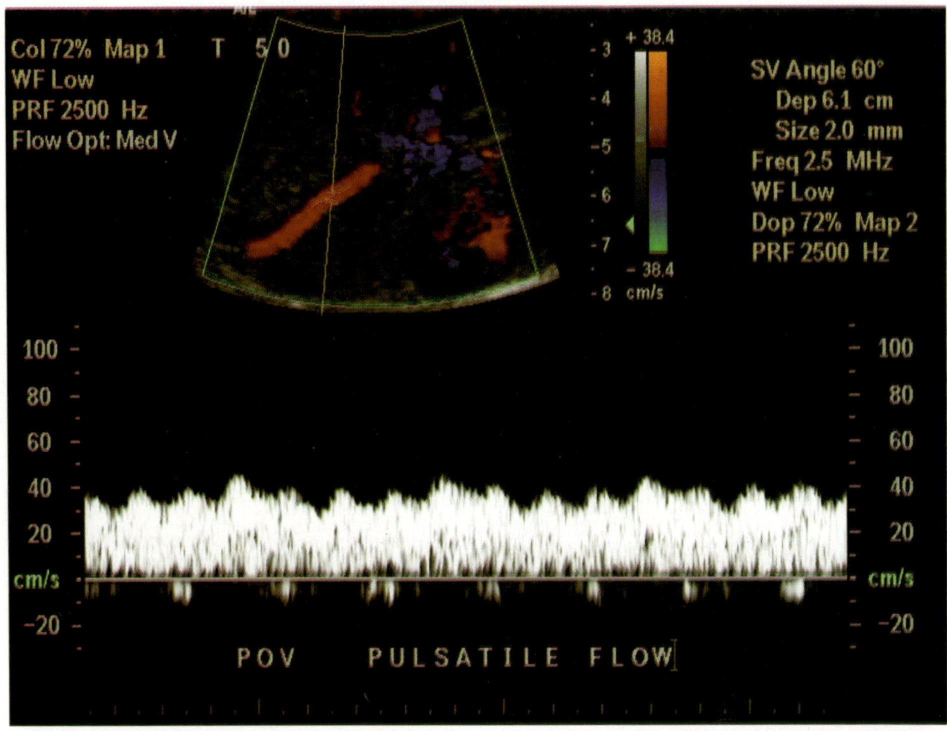

COLOUR PLATE 12: REVERSAL OF FLOW IN THE IVC IN CARDIAC FAILURE

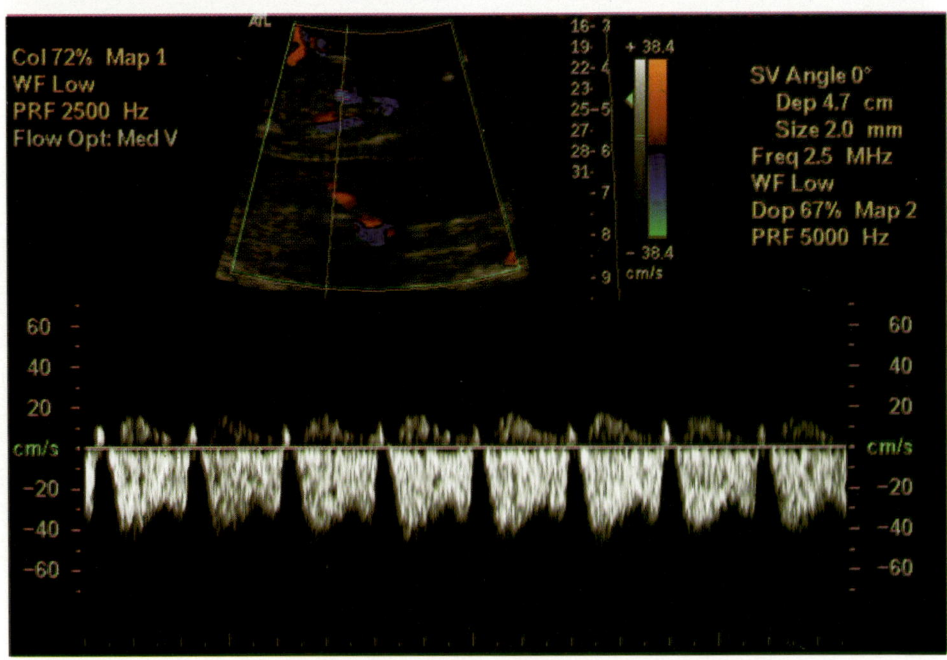

COLOUR PLATE 13: REVERSAL OF FLOW IN DUCTUS VENOSUS

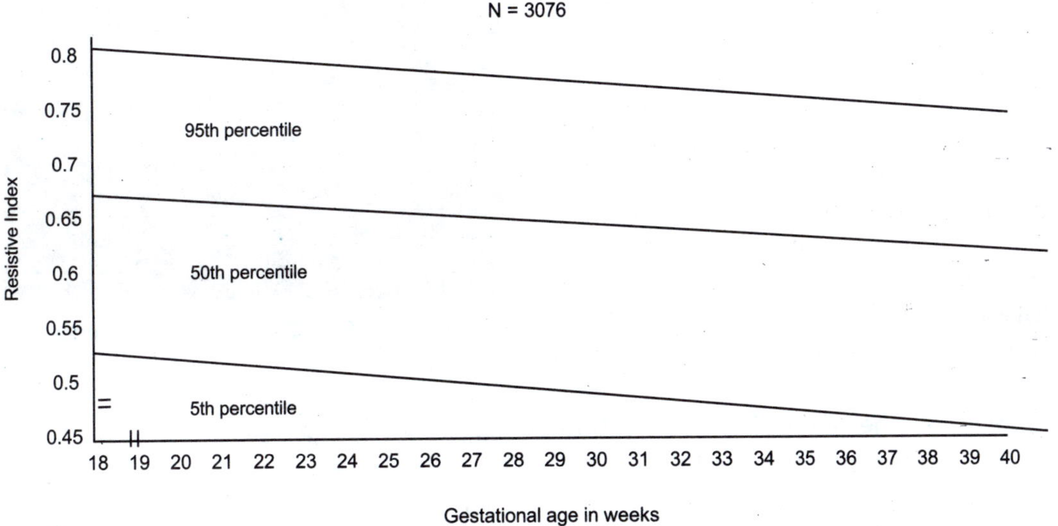

FIGURE 36.5: RI OF MIDDLE CEREBRAL ARTERY IN NORMAL PREGNANCIES AT 18–40 WEEKS GESTATION

fetuses, there is minimal diastolic flow in the MCA and diastolic flow velocity increases minimally during gestation (Colour plate 7 and Fig 36.5). Colour Doppler sonography permits easy visualisation of the Circle of Willis to identify MCA. Fetal compromise can be assessed by an increase in diastolic flow indicating fetal redistribution in the presence of placental insufficiency. IUGR fetuses that show redistribution and increased diastolic flow in the MCA (Fig. 36.8) are at greater risk of adverse perinatal outcome. When maximum redistribution occurs, the fetal PO2 is 2–4 SD below the normal for the gestational age. With prolonged hypoxemia, MCA diastolic flow begins to lessen and may even become absent. This stage possibly indicates fetal brain edema (Mari and Copel 1996).

Cerebroplacental Ratio The resistance in the middle cerebral artery is higher than that of the umbilical artery in normal pregnancies at any period of gestation. The ratio of the RI in the MCA and the RI in the umbilical artery is termed the cerebro-placental ratio (CPR) and it helps in the understanding of the vascular beds of the placenta and the brain. This ratio is >1 in normal pregnancies and <1 in IUGR with redistribution of cerebral flow. This ratio helps identify fetuses with increased cerebral blood flow.

Peak Systolic Velocity of MCA as a Marker for Fetal Anemia Mari et al in 1995 made a significant observation that the peak systolic velocities in the fetal middle cerebral artery can be correlated with fetal hemoglobin levels. This landmark observation paved the way for accurate non-invasive diagnosis of fetal anemia. The antenatal management of Rh alloimmunised pregnancies has changed, with fewer interventions being required now. A threshold value for the peak systolic velocity of 1.50 MoM for the gestational age had 100% sensitivity (95% CI, 86–100%) for the detection of moderate to severe anemia.

Subsequently, Moise (2008) observed that the timing of the second transfusion in an alloimmunised pregnancy can be done when the MCA peak systolic velocities reaches 1.32 MoM. MCA Doppler, however, was not useful to time further transfusions. MCA Doppler can also be used to predict fetal anemia due to other causes such as Kell alloimmunisation, fetal parvovirus infection, fetomaternal hemorrhage, alpha thalassemia and after laser therapy for twin-twin transfusions.

Doppler of the Fetal Venous System

The fetal venous system has attracted much attention in recent years. Whereas umbilical artery Doppler is a test of the placental vascular bed, venous flow, which is towards the fetus, should logically give information about fetal well-being. Oxygenated blood from the placenta enters the umbilical vein; 55% of this blood is shunted through the ductus venosus to reach the IVC. The remaining 45% enters the portal vein and reaches the IVC through the hepatic veins. Venous Doppler flow patterns change with proximity of the vein to the heart—the veins closer to the heart reflecting right atrial events.

The umbilical vein can be sampled at any point in the cord, while the portal vein can be sampled in its straight portion inside the fetal abdomen. The ductus venosus is visualised in both longitudinal and transverse sections of the fetal abdomen and identified by a characteristic 'mosaic' colour between the portal vein and the IVC (Colour plate 9, and Fig. 36.6). It acts as a conduit between the peripheral circulation (umbilical vein) and the central vein. The blood ejected from the ductus venosus flows through the dorsal left vena cava through the foramen ovale directly into the left atrium, thus ensuring preferential shunting of oxygenated blood.

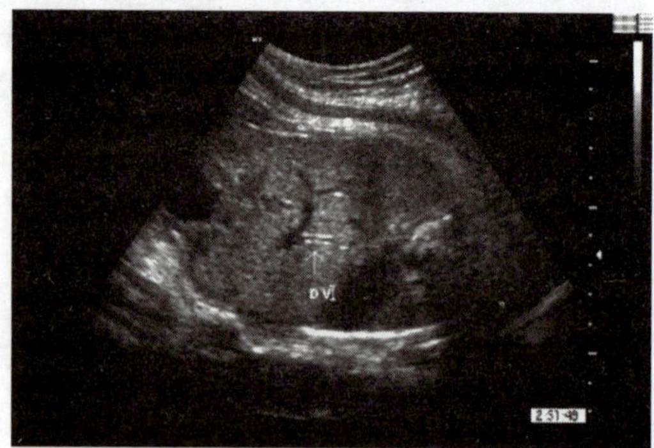

FIGURE 36.6: DUCTUS VENOSUS B MODE

The normal venous waveforms of the umbilical vein and ductus venosus are shown in Colour plate 10 and 11. The umbilical and portal veins show continuous low velocity flow whereas the ductus venosus has a characteristic 'biphasic' pattern which represents ventricular systole and diastole.

The venous wave patterns in the umbilical and portal veins are usually continuous and have a low velocity (about 10–30 cm/sec). High velocities are seen in hyperdynamic flow states like fetal anemia (Colour plate 12 and Fig 36.7). The presence of a pulsatile pattern or turbulent flow is usually associated with fetal anemia and occurs as a result of cardiac decompensation.

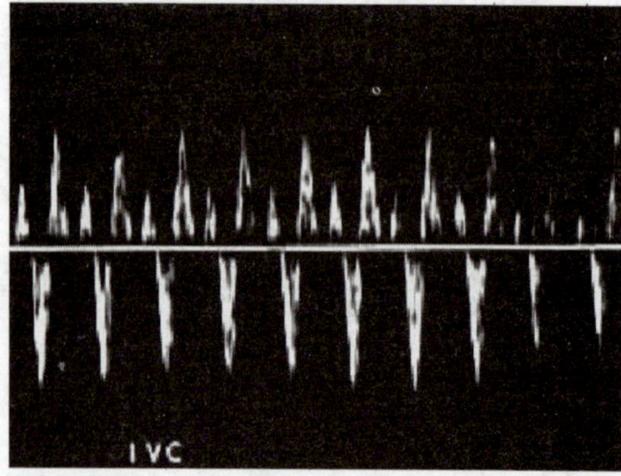

FIGURE 36.7 : REVERSAL OF FLOW IN THE IVC IN CARDIAC FAILURE

The ductus venosus waveform has a characteristic M shape or biphasic pattern. It has the highest flow velocity in the fetus. Low velocity flow can be seen in placental insufficiency, congestive cardiac failure (Colour plate 13), myocardial disease, hypoxia and fetal arrhythmia. High velocities in the ductus can be seen in fetal anemia and hemoglobinopathies. Reversal of flow in the ductus venosus signifies cardiac decompensation and can be seen in severe hypoxia, cardiac failure and in some cardiac malformations. Ductus venosus flow between 11 and 14 weeks has been shown to have significant association with trisomy 21 and has been described later in this chapter.

Colour Doppler in Anomalies Colour flow imaging plays an invaluable role in enhancing the prenatal diagnosis of congenital cardiac anomalies. In a study conducted by Copel et al (1991) on the role of colour Doppler on cardiovascular system anomalies, it was concluded that it was absolutely essential in the diagnosis of 29% of the anomalies. In 47% of the anomalies, colour Doppler aided diagnosis but was not essential, and in about 24% of the anomalies it was not helpful. Colour flow mapping has its uses, both for studying the structural anatomy of the heart and the great vessels and also for identifying abnormal flow across the chambers and valves. Malposition of vessels, reversal of normal flow direction, absence of filling of cardiac chambers and valvular regurgitation are diagnosed with ease and enhance diagnostic confidence with the application of colour Doppler.

Recently, pulsed Doppler has been used in the characterisation of fetal arrhythmia. By placing the sample volume in the left ventricular outflow tract, it is possible to map and time the ventricular and atrial events. Doppler sampling can also be done across the aorta and SVC and the renal artery and vein.

Other anomalies where colour flow is used to establish diagnosis are diaphragmatic hernia, where the deviated portal vein can be identified with ease, and locating the cord attachment to differentiate between an omphalocele and gastroschisis. In suspected renal agenesis with severe oligohydramnios, colour Doppler helps identify the presence or absence of the renal arteries.

Abnormal fetal vasculature as in certain conditions such as hydranencephaly, vein of Galen aneurysm, hemangiomas, etc are better understood and analysed by colour flow and Doppler imaging. Colour flow has been used for distinguishing between a true uterine synechiae and a myometrial contraction simulating the appearance of a synechiae. Presence of colour within the membrane favours diagnosis of a true uterine synechiae and can be quite conclusive when in doubt.

Other uses of colour flow imaging include accurate estimation of the amniotic fluid index (AFI), as the colour flow highlights the umbilical cord which may appear echolucent on B-mode imaging and can be mistaken for a liquor pocket.

Nuchal Cord A nuchal cord is diagnosed when one or multiple loops of the cord encircle the neck. Though this can be demonstrated by colour Doppler, its clinical utility has not been proved. In a prospective study of 289 women in whom colour Doppler was done immediately prior to induction of labour, Peregrine et al (2005) concluded that the nuchal cord was present in 18% of deliveries and this incidence was not affected by parity, position or liquor volume. The sensitivity of ultrasound was only 37.5%, with specificity, positive and negative predictive values of 80%, 29% and 85%, respectively. The presence of the nuchal cord did not appear to increase the risk of cesarean section or of poor neonatal outcome. Oin et al have reported that tight and loose cords may not be distinguishable by ultrasound. A study using two-dimensional and three-dimensional ultrasound and colour Doppler for detection of nuchal cord has shown that 3D ultrasound did not provide more useful diagnostic information, compared to 2D and colour Doppler (Hanaoka et al 2002).

Multiple Pregnancy In dichorionic pregnancies, the application and interpretation of fetal Doppler is similar to that of singleton pregnancies. Monochorionic pregnancies may be complicated by twin–twin transfusion syndrome or twin-reversed arterial perfusion sequence. In twin–twin transfusion syndrome, abnormal Doppler in the umbilical artery of the donor twin is an indication of increasing severity of the condition. If the donor twin shows reversal of flow in the ductus venosus, early delivery should be planned.

In twin-reversed arterial perfusion sequence, the normal fetus is called the 'pump' twin and the other fetus, which is the acardiac twin, is called the 'perfused' twin. Colour Doppler can be used to demonstrate 'flow reversal' in the umbilical artery of the acardiac twin.

Doppler in the First Trimester The advent of the 11–14 weeks scan as a potential tool for diagnosis of chromosomal defects and structural abnormalities has led to a more detailed examination of the fetus during this period. Increased nuchal translucency has been shown to be a significant marker for Down syndrome. Abnormal flow velocity waveforms, that is, reversal of 'a' wave in the ductus venosus, have been observed in 80% of fetuses with Down syndrome and in about 5% of chromosomally normal fetuses. In chromosomally normal fetuses, an abnormal ductus venosus may point to the presence of a major cardiac anomaly (Nicolaides 2008). Hence, all these fetuses require a detailed fetal echocardiography in the second trimester. More recently, tricuspid regurgitation in this period has also been found to be associated with Down syndrome.

Doppler ultrasound has provided a safe, non-invasive and rapid method of assessing the physiology and pathophysiology of fetal and maternal uterine circulations. Although Doppler does not appear to be sensitive enough to be used as a screening test for intrauterine growth retardation, it helps to differentiate between placental and non-placental causes of IUGR. The reversal of flow in the ductus venosus suggests cardiac decompensation and is a terminal event. The use of fetal middle cerebral artery Doppler for detection of fetal anemia has revolutionised the diagnosis and management of fetal anemia. Abnormal ductus venosus Doppler in the 11–14 weeks scan is a marker for Trisomy 21 and structural cardiac anomalies.

References

Aoki S, T Hata, K Hata et al. 1989. Doppler colour flow mapping of an invasive mole. *Gynecol Obstet Invest* 27: 52–54.

Arduini D, G Rizzo and C Romanini. 1991. Doppler ultrasonography in early pregnancy does not predict adverse pregnancy outcome. *Ultrasound Obstet Gynaecol* 1:180–185.

Bower S, K Schuchter and S Campbell. 1993. Doppler ultrasound screening as part of routine antenatal scanning: prediction of pre-eclampsia and intrauterine growth retardation. *Eur J Obstet Gynaecol Reprod Biol* 100:989.

Bower S, S Bewley and S Campbell. 1993. Improved prediction of pre-eclampsia by two stage screening of uterine arteries using the early diastolic notch and colour Doppler imaging. *Obstet Gynaecol* 82:78–83.

Bricker L and JP Neilson. 2000. Routine Doppler ultrasound in pregnancy. *Cochrane Database Syst Rev* (2):CD001450.

Burke G, B Stewart, P Crowley, SN Scanaill and J Drumm. 1990. Is intrauterine growth retardation with normal umbilical artery blood flow a benign condition? *Br Med J* 300:1044–1045.

Campbell S et al. 1983. New Doppler technique for assessing uteroplacental blood flow. *Lancet* 1:675.

Campbell S, JM Pearce, G Hackett, T Cohen-Overbeek and C Hermandez. 1986. Qualitative assessment of uterine blood flow: early screening test for high risk pregnancy. *Obstet Gynecol* 68: 649–653.

Copel JA, R Morotti, JC Hobbins and CS Kleinman. 1991. The antenatal diagnosis of congenital heart disease using fetal echocardiography: Is colour flow mapping necessary? *Obstet Gynecol* 78:1–8.

Fitzgerald DE and JE Drumm. 1977. Non-invasive measurement of human fetal circulation using ultrasound: A new method. *Br Med J* 2:1450–1451.

Hanaoka U, T Yanagihara, H Tanak and T Hata. 2002. Comparison of three-dimensional, two-dimensional and colour Doppler ultrasound in predicting nuchal cord at birth. *Ultrasound Obstet Gynecol* 19(5): 471–474.

KH Nicolaides. 2008. The 11-13+6 weeks scan. The Fetal Medicine Foundation, 103.

Maini CL, P Rosati, G Galli, U Bellati, MG Bonetti and E Moneta. 1985. Non-invasive radioisotopic evaluation of the placental blood flow. *Gynaecol Obstet Invest* 19:196–206.

Mari G and JA Copel. 1996. Doppler ultrasound–Fetal physiology and clinical application. In *Sonography in Obstetrics and Gynaecology*: Principles and Practice, 5th ed, 251–283, ed AC Fleischer, FA Manning, P Jeanty and R Romero. Prentice Hall.

Mari G, A Adrignolo, AZ Abuhamad et al. 1995. The diagnosis of fetal anaemia with Doppler ultrasound in the pregnancy complicated by rhesus-immunisation. *Ultrasound Obstet Gynaecol* 5: 400–405.

Moise KJ Jr. 2008. The usefulness of middle cerebral artery Doppler assessment in the treatment of fetus at risk for fetal anemia. *Am J Obstet Gynecol* 198(2): 161.e1–4.

Peregrine E, P O'Brien and E Jauniaux. 2005. Ultrasound detection of nuchal cord prior to labor induction and the risk of Cesarean section. *Ultrasound Obstet Gynecol* 25(2): 160–164.

Rotmensh S, M Liberati, J Santolaya-Forgas and J Copel. 1995. Uteroplacental and intraplacental circulation. In *Doppler Ultrasound in Obstetrics and Gynaecology*, Chapter 11, ed. JA Copel and KL Reed. New York: Raven Press Ltd.

Stabile I, J Grudzinkas and S Campbell. 1990. Doppler ultrasonographic evaluation of abnormal pregnancies in the first trimester. *J Clin Ultrasound* 18:497–507.

Trudinger BJ, CM Cook, WB Giles et al. 1991. Fetal umbilical artery waveforms and subsequent neonatal outcome. *Br J Obstet Gynaecol* 98:378–384.

37

Malignancy and Premalignancy of Genital Tract in Pregnancy

V Sivanesaratnam

Introduction One of the commonest sites for malignancies is the female genital tract. However, the peak incidence of such malignancies does not correspond with the peak reproductive years. Thus, their association with pregnancy is unusual; such a combination is one involving a controlled growth (pregnancy) and an uncontrolled growth (carcinoma) in the same patient. A malignancy discovered during pregnancy raises a number of important issues:

- What effect will the malignancy or the therapy have on the fetus?
- Does the presence of pregnancy require deferment of therapy for the malignancy?
- Is the prognosis affected by the malignancy?
- Does the presence of the malignancy call for termination of pregnancy?

Because of the rarity of this combination, the experience of individual clinicians is often limited; clear therapeutic decisions are thus not readily available. In deciding the best therapeutic modality, the study of published reviewers (Koren et al 1990; Antonelli et al 1996; Sivanesaratnam 2001) and the experience from individual case reports should be assessed.

Pregnancy-Associated Breast Cancer

The obstetrician often forgets that the breasts are a part of the female reproductive system. However, as breast cancer is rare in women younger than 35 years of age, the occurrence of this malignancy is unusual.

Incidence About 15% of patients with cancer of the breast are of childbearing age. Incidences in pregnancy ranging from 0.2% to 3.8% have been reported (Wallach et al 1983; Barber 1992). Of all the patients with breast cancer, about 1–2% were found to be pregnant at the time of diagnosis (DiSaia and Creasman 1989).

Diagnosis Examination of the breast at the first antenatal visit is mandatory. If an abnormality is detected, diagnostic procedures such as ultrasound and mammogram may be used. Adequate shielding during mammography results in little risk of radiation exposure to the fetus (Barnavon and Wallach 1990); the radiation dose to the fetus using modern equipment is less than 50 mrad (500 μGy), which is well below the 10 rad (100 μGy) toxic level (Wagner et al 1985). However, radiological signs of malignant lesions are often obscured by the increased density of the breasts during pregnancy and lactation (Kitchen et al 1987), making mammography of questionable value.

Fine-needle aspiration or excisional biopsy under local anesthesia may be done to establish diagnosis; however, the former runs the risk of missing the mass (Petrek 1994), while the hyperproliferative cellular state of mammary tissue in pregnancy may result in misinterpretation of the histological findings (Novotny et al 1991).

Therapy Surgeons, gynecologists and radiotherapists hold widely differing views on the treatment of breast carcinoma during pregnancy. Interdisciplinary discussions on the best modality of treatment must be made on a patient-to-patient basis.

Termination of pregnancy does not confer any beneficial effect on the outcome of Pregnancy associated (PA) breast cancer (Barnavon and Wallach 1990; Hoover 1990). Thus, there does not appear to be any valid reason for recommending termination of pregnancy, unless the continuation of pregnancy significantly limits adjuvant chemotherapy and radiation.

Therapy of PA breast cancer should not be delayed, whatever the stage of the disease. For early-stage disease (Stages 1 and II), the treatment of choice is a modified radical mastectomy; it should be borne in mind that adjuvant radiation in therapeutic doses may harm the fetus. In view of the increased risk of local recurrence, breast conservation surgery is discouraged. Should the patient opt for breast conservation in the first or second trimester, to commence optimal doses of chemotherapy/radiation, a therapeutic abortion should be considered. It is worth noting that such adjuvant treatment in PA breast cancer is less effective (Petrek 1994).

If the diagnosis is made in the third trimester, management is individualised. Lumpectomy seems to be a reasonable option, adjuvant radiation being deferred till after delivery (DiFronzo and O'Connell 1996). The risk of cancer passing through the placenta and metastasising to the fetus is negligible; thus, continued gestation does not pose a risk to the fetus.

Patients with late-stage PA breast cancer (Stages III and IV) have a five-year survival rate of only 10% (Hoover 1990). Therefore, advanced, incurable tumours are best palliated, and the pregnancy allowed to continue or palliated depending on the wishes of the patient and the therapy required. A recent report suggests that 'standardised' therapy, including chemotherapy, could be given in the second or third trimester; no congenital fetal anomalies were observed in 24 patients who received chemotherapy (Berry et al 1999).

When the cancer is diagnosed in the puerperium, lactation should be suppressed to decrease the size and vascularity of the breasts, and definitive therapy of the cancer carried out. In general, breastfeeding by women receiving chemotherapy should be discouraged.

Prognosis Although the overall survival rate for breast cancer is about 50%, pregnancy-associated breast cancer has a poor prognosis, particularly for women aged 30 years or less (Guinee et al 1994; Anderson et al 1996). However, when matched for age and stage of disease, the outcome for PA breast cancer is similar to that of their non-pregnant counterparts (Tretli 1988; Petrek 1991). The reasons for such poor outlook in PA breast cancer are multifactorial:

- The main factor is delayed diagnosis. In some cases, this was by 5–15 months (Hoover 1990). Epidemiological studies show that diagnosis delayed for 3–6 months is associated with poor survival, whether the patient is pregnant or not. The lesions can be obscured by the engorged breasts, during pregnancy, and lactation for longer periods.

- In a high proportion of young patients (71%), the tumours are estrogen receptor-negative (Nugent et al 1985; Mercer et al 1984).
- Inflammatory breast cancer, which carries a poor prognosis, is the more common type during pregnancy (Bonnier et al 1977).
- The increased vascularity and lymphatic drainage of the breast in pregnancy and lactation helps easier drainage to the regional lymph nodes; thus, a high proportion (72%) have already metastasised (Robiero et al 1986) at presentation.
- Pregnancy itself is an independent risk factor in a multivariate analysis (Guinee et al 1994; Bonnier et al 1997).
- Treatment is often postponed for fetus management.
- Incidence of family history of breast cancer is three times higher in PA breast cancer (Ishide et al 1992); BRCA 1 and 2 are more common in young breast cancer patients (Langston et al 1996).
- Adjuvant therapy has been shown to be less effective in PA breast cancer (Bonnier et al 1997).

Subsequent Pregnancies

It is important to remember that breast cancer may recur any time after diagnosis. Should pregnancy, therefore, be avoided following mastectomy for breast cancer?

On the basis of limited retrospective data, pregnancy does not appear to compromise survival in those with a previous history of breast cancer. There is in fact evidence to show better survival in those who became pregnant after treatment of breast cancer (Clark and Reid 1978), suggesting a potential 'protective effect' of subsequent pregnancy.

One study reported a five-year survival rate of 80% (Harvey et al 1981); 10-year survival rates of 90% and 56% have been reported in node-negative and node-positive patients, respectively (Ariel et al 1989). Clark and Chua (1989) studied the effect of the interval between breast cancer therapy and subsequent pregnancy. They observed poorer survival among women who became pregnant within 6 months compared with those who deferred pregnancy for 6–24 months (53.8% versus 78%). Those who become pregnant 5 years or more after treatment had five-year survival rates similar to that of those who did not become pregnant. As younger women have significantly poorer survival rates and higher local and distant relapses than their older counterparts, de la Rochefordiere et al (1993) advise delaying pregnancies in women under 33 years of age for at least 3 years to reduce the risk of relapse.

Ovarian Cancer

Incidence and Diagnosis These tumours are relatively uncommon in pregnancy. The incidence of ovarian tumours in pregnancy varies from 1 in 81 to 1 in 591 pregnancies (Grimes et al 1954; Booth 1963; Sivanesaratnam et al 1976). More than 90% of functional ovarian cysts disappear as pregnancy advances. An ovarian mass, more than 5 cm in diameter, must be viewed with suspicion and requires an exploratory laparotomy; this procedure, if carried out between 12 and 14 weeks, has negligible fetal wastage.

Wang et al (1999) removed ovarian tumours greater than 10 cm or with a teratoma component after the seventh week without the risk of fetal loss, thus avoiding the unpredictable complications of the tumours.

Whitecar et al (1999) found significantly fewer adverse pregnancy outcomes in patients undergoing laparotomy before 23 weeks compared with those after 23 weeks (P = 0.005).

Recent case reports have described the laparoscopic management of adnexal masses in pregnancy. Moore and Smith (1999) described this technique on 14 patients with adnexal masses at an average gestational age of 16 weeks with no fetal loss. However, the fetus could be affected by carbon dioxide pneumoperitoneum, which could directly produce more pressure on the uterus or alter maternal hemodynamics and acid–base balance (Hunter et al 1995).

In the latter half of pregnancy, ovarian tumours are particularly difficult to diagnose as the tumour ascends into the abdominal cavity, often lying posterior to the enlarged gravid uterus. It is important that the ovaries of all women having a cesarean section or postpartum tubal sterilisation be inspected during the procedure.

The chance of malignant tumours in pregnancy is relatively low–malignancy rates of 2.4–7.4% have been reported (Beischer et al 1971; Sivanesaratnam et al 1976). The incidence of ovarian cancer in pregnancy has been reported to be 1 in 18,000 pregnancies (0.005%) by Munnell (1963). An incidence of 1:18,733 deliveries over a 23-year period has also been reported by the author (Sivanesaratnam 1998). Such a low incidence should not, however, make the clinician complacent as early diagnosis is the key to successful management.

The signs and symptoms of ovarian neoplasms in pregnancy are similar to those in the non-pregnant state. Torsion and incarceration are common with these tumours, and they often require emergency surgical intervention (Karlen et al 1979; Lee et al 1989).

Therapy The management of ovarian cancer in pregnancy is essentially similar to that in non-pregnant patients. At exploratory laparotomy, fluid from the pelvis and paracolic gutters is aspirated for cytology. If the tumour is well-encapsulated, unilateral and of low-grade malignancy, a unilateral salpingo-oophorectomy is performed; if wedge biopsy of the opposite ovary is negative, the treatment is considered to be adequate and the pregnancy allowed to go to term.

When the tumour has extended beyond the ovary, it would be necessary to undertake the more radical approach of total abdominal hysterectomy, bilateral salpingo-oophorectomy and appendicectomy. Tumour debulking procedures are carried out as in the non-pregnant state, taking into account fetal viability and the patient's wishes; if the tumour is diagnosed in the third trimester, surgery may be delayed until the fetus is viable. Adjuvant chemotherapy is then administered as in non-pregnant patients.

Prognosis In view of the generally favourable type of tumours and early stage of disease encountered in these young women, the overall five-year survival is good—76% (Novak et al 1975). A review of nine published reports (Table 38.1) reveals that germ cell tumours make up 46.2% of all primary ovarian tumours in pregnancy; the commonest tumour is ovarian dysgerminoma (33.9%). It is also important to note that epithelial ovarian malignancies are just as common.

Endometrial Carcinoma and Choriocarcinoma in Pregnancy

Endometrial cancer complicating pregnancy is

extremely rare. Several factors are responsible for this rarity:

- Endometrial carcinoma is a disease of postmenopausal women; only less than 8% of cases occur in women under the age of 40 years (Kempson and Pokorny 1968).
- The carcinomatous endometrium is unfavourable for successful implantation.
- The high levels of progesterone in pregnancy produce an unfavourable effect on tumour survival.

So far, only about 24 cases of endometrial cancer in pregnancy have been reported in the literature. Nearly all of these were associated with first trimester abortions and only five were associated with a live fetus (Ayhan et al 1999).

Of the four cases reported by Vaccarello et al (1999), the diagnosis was made four months postpartum in two cases. Thus, although a full-term pregnancy can have a protective effect against endometrial cancer (McPherson et al 1996), the importance of endometrial sampling for abnormal postpartum bleeding should not be overlooked.

Many argue that some of the reported cases may be misdiagnosed Arias–Stella phenomenon (DiSaia and Creasman 1989), and that adenocarcinoma of the endometrium does not occur in pregnancy. Endometrial carcinoma coexisting with pregnancy, and presumed to derive from adenomyosis, has also been reported (Ichikawa et al 2001).

The treatment is total abdominal hysterectomy and bilateral salpingo-oophorectomy; in 'high-risk' patients with poor prognostic features, adjuvant pelvic irradiation is administered as in non-pregnant patients.

Table 37.1: Types of Primary Ovarian Malignancies Reported in Pregnancy (nine published reports)

Histological type		Numbers reported (%)	%
Epithelial tumours		30	46.2
Serous	13 (20)		
Mucinous	8 (12.4)		
Endometriod	5 (7.7)		
Mesonephric	4 (6.2)		
Gonadal Stromal tumours		2	3.1
Granulosa cell	1 (1.5)		
Sertoli-Leydig	1 (1.5)		
Germ cell tumours		30	46.2
Dysgerminoma	22 (33.9)		
Malignant teratoma	3 (4.5)		
Endodermal sinus tumour	4 (6.2)		
Choriocarcinoma	1 (1.5)		
Others		3	4.5
Sarcoma	2 (3.1)		
Anaplastic carcinoma	1 (1.5)		
Total		65	100.0

(Beischer et al 1971; Novak et al 1975, Sivanesaratnam et al 1976; Kulenthran and Sivanesaratnam 1986; Malone et al 1986; Desel et al 1988, Lee et al 1989; Metz et al 1989; Sivanesaratnam 1991; van der Zee et al 1991)

Malignant Mixed Mullerian Tumour of Uterus

A case of malignant Mullerian tumour of the uterus in association with a viable pregnancy has been reported (Scioscia et al 1986). The patient was already in Stage III of the disease at the time of presentation; despite aggressive chemotherapy and irradiation, the patient succumbed 14 weeks later. However, no evidence of fetal or placental metastases was noted.

Uterine Choriocarcinoma in Pregnancy

Primary and secondary postpartum hemorrhage is rarely caused by choriocarcinoma. Nine cases caused by choriocarcinoma were reported by Dobson et al (1999); all were successfully treated using multiagent chemotherapy.

Carcinoma of the Cervix

Carcinoma of the cervix is the malignancy most commonly associated with pregnancy (Nieminen and Remas 1970; Barber and Brunschwig 1963).

Preinvasive Lesions of the Cervix

The incidence of carcinoma-in-situ of the cervix has been reported to be 1 in 770 pregnancies (Hacker et al 1982). Only routine screening will help identify patients with preinvasive or early invasive disease. Pregnancy provides an ideal situation for cervical screening. A routine speculum examination for inspection of the cervix and a pap smear test at booking should be done.

An abnormal smear in pregnancy often indicates the presence of a cervical intraepithelial neoplasia (CIN) lesion of the cervix in over 90% of cases (Lees and Singer 1982).

Colposcopic evaluation of the cervix is aided by the physiological changes that occur during pregnancy. Hypertrophy and eversion of the endocervical epithelium occurs from as early as the tenth week of pregnancy; the upper extent of the transformation zone thus becomes easily visible, allowing a full colposcopic evaluation of the abnormal transformation zone. However, the dynamic phase of metaplasia occurring in pregnancy, together with the increased vascularity and decidual changes in the cervix, can make interpretation of the colposcopic findings difficult, resulting in over-diagnosis.

A high degree of experience and expertise is required. Colposcopy alone, without directed biopsies, carries a significant risk of underestimating the lesion (Benedet et al 1987); 0.2% of patients with cytological evidence of mild/moderate dysplasia have been reported to have invasive cancer (LaPolla et al 1988). Thus, unless the colposcopist is very experienced, a directed biopsy should be performed in all pregnant women with colposcopic evidence of abnormality. Directed biopsies may help avoid an unnecessary cone biopsy. Vaginal bleeding may occur following directed biopsies, but this often ceases with pressure on a gauze. Bleeding that requires transfusion is exceedingly uncommon (Hacker et al 1982; Benedet et al 1987; Coppola et al 1997).

If the directed biopsy reveals normal lasitology, re-evaluation is deferred till after delivery. If the biopsy shows CIN, repeat cytology and colposcopy every 6–8 weeks is advisable. Should progression be noted, repeat directed biopsies need to be done. While current data suggests that if invasive carcinoma can be excluded, the definitive treatment of CIN can be safely deferred till 6–8 weeks after delivery, 75% of those with CIN diagnosed in pregnancy continued to have persistent or progressive disease at postpartum evaluation (Pallé et al 2000). In a series of 28 patients with CIN 3 in pregnancy,

Coppola et al (1997) reported a regression rate of only 12%, emphasising the importance of re-evaluation postpartum.

Cold-knife cervical conisation in pregnancy carries significant morbidity to the mother and the fetus; spontaneous abortions in up to 25% and excessive cervical bleeding in 5–15% of patients have been reported (Hanningan et al 1982; Coppola et al 1997). Similar results have been reported recently after loop excision during pregnancy (Robinson et al 1997). Further, conisation during pregnancy may not be therapeutic— even with cone biopsies performed under colposcopic guidance, persistent disease has been reported in up to 50% of cases (Hacker et al 1982; LaPolla et al 1988; Robinson et al 1997). A wedge biopsy would seem to be an accurate and relatively atraumatic alternative diagnostic procedure.

One of the patients in the care of the author was found to have microinvasive carcinoma of the cervix on colposcopically directed biopsy. She was para 3 and 24 weeks pregnant. As the transformation zone could be completely visualised, pregnancy was allowed to continue with careful colposcopic evaluation at six to eight weekly intervals. No progression of the lesion was noted. At 38 weeks, a classical cesarean section and an extrafascial Type 1 hysterectomy was performed. Such a conversation approach is feasible if expert colposcopic follow-up evaluation is available. If cone biopsy needs to be performed because of inadequate colposcopic evaluation, a 'modified' cone or limited resection as suggested by De Petrillo (1975) and Yoonesi (1982) would appear to be appropriate; the accompanying morbidity is directly proportional to the size of the cone.

Invasive Carcinoma in Pregnancy

The incidence varies from 1 in 2200 (Hacker et al 1982) to 1 in 4077 pregnancies (Sivanesaratnam et al 1993). Nineteen out of 20 patients studied had squamous cell carcinoma, the large cell non-keratinising variety being commonest (Sivanesaratnam et al 1993). The age of the patients varied from 33 to 38 years (Hacker et al 1982; Sivanesaratnam et al 1993).

It is important to note that 3–55% of these patients were asymtomatic (Baltzer et al 1990; Lee et al 1981; Sivanesaratnam et al 1993). Despite this, a significant number (15–87%) had bleeding in pregnancy (Stander and Lein 1960; Talehian et al 1976; Sivanesaratnam et al 1993). Often, this has been mistaken as being brought about by pregnancy and thus diagnosis is often delayed. Speculum examination and inspection of the cervix should be routine at early antenatal booking. Excessive discharge and vaginal bleeding during pregnancy requires investigation. In patients presenting with antepartum hemorrhage, gentle speculum examination will help rule out the presence of a concomitant cervical growth.

Therapy for invasive cervical cancer depends on:

- The stage of the disease
- The duration of pregnancy
- The institutional preference and expertise available
- The desire of the patient and her family

Although many physicians choose radiation therapy for invasive carcinoma in pregnancy (Sablinska et al 1977), surgery is preferred for early invasive cancer of the cervix in pregnancy.

Patients with a microinvasive lesion, <3 mm in depth without confluence or lymphatic/vascular channel permeation, can be closely followed up by an experienced colposcopist. If no colposcopic progression is seen, vaginal delivery is allowed and definitive therapy carried out subsequently. A cesarean hysterectomy may be performed, if cesarean section is indicated.

Patients presenting with Stage 1A lesions with lymphatic/vascular channel permeation, Stage 1B or early Stage 2A lesions diagnosed before 24 weeks of pregnancy are best treated by Type 3 radical *hysterectomy* and pelvic *lymphadenectomy.*

Those between the 24–32 weeks of pregnancy present a difficult problem; in such a situation, treatment may be delayed until the fetus has a better chance of survival. This would be governed by the neonatal facilities in each institution and the patient's understanding of the the risks involved. While no adverse maternal outcomes were observed when delays of 11–17 weeks were allowed (Lee et al 1981; Hacker et al 1982; Sivanesaratnam et al 1993), reports of progression of the clinical stage of the disease if therapy was delayed (Dudan et al 1973) are worth noting.

After 32 weeks, once the fetus has reached sufficient maturity, it is important that delivery be performed through a classical *cesarean section.* The lower segment, cervix and placenta are left undisturbed for detailed histopathological evaluation and to avoid tumour dissemination. The uterine wound is rapidly closed in one layer and radical hysterectomy is then carried out (Fig. 37.1). Lower segment cesarean section should be avoided at all times in these patients.

The tumour was seen to be eroding through the lower segment in the puerperium. (Fig 37.2). The patient subsequently developed abdominal wall metastases (Sivanesaratnam et al 1993).

Radical surgery offers a number of advantages:

- Ovarian conservation and maintenance of vaginal integrity and function in these young women (Sivanesaratnam 1991), thus avoiding the long-term complications of radiotherapy. Conserved ovaries are best transposed paracecally on the right and paracolically on the left to protect the ovaries should adjuvant pelvic irradiation become necessary.
- The softening of tissues in pregnancy gives the technical advantage of developing cleavage planes easily.
- Surgery also allows accurate assessment of the extent of the disease.
- Vaginal delivery in the presence of an invasive cancer of the cervix carries the risk of:
  (i) Dissemination of malignant cells into lymphatics or the vascular channels (Waldrop and Palmer 1963; Sood 2000)
  (ii) Hemorrhage, sepsis, obstructed labour and cervical laceration
  (iii) Metastases to episiotomy sites (Copeland et al 1987)

Increased vascularity in pregnancy is of some concern. However, with care, the blood loss can be minimised. In the author's experience, mean blood loss has been no different from that in non-pregnant patients undergoing radical hysterectomy. Major complications of uretero–vaginal fistulae, pelvic abscess and gram-negative septicemia have been reported by some (Thompson et al 1975). Several other studies have shown no major complications (Lash 1961; Barber and Brunschwig 1963; Pratt 1964; Creasman et al 1970; Dudan et al 1973; Sall et al 1974; Sivanesaratnam et al 1993). On the other hand, increased morbidity and mortality from primary radiotherapy during pregnancy is well documented (Dudan et al 1973; Thompson et al 1975; Saunders and Landon 1988).

Careful surgical technique (Sivanesaratnam 1993), use of prophylactic antibiotics and availability of modern anesthetic facilities make radical hysterectomy and pelvic lymphadenectomy safe in pregnancy.

In patients presenting in the *more advanced stages* (2B, 3 and 4), and those with poor surgical risk and early invasive disease, radiotherapy is the treatment of choice. In early pregnancy, external beam irradiation is begun, resulting in abortion of the fetus. Brachytherapy applications complete the treatment after the uterus is evacuated.

In later pregnancy, hysterotomy or classical section should be performed first. Sood et al (1997) found that the immediate and long-term complications of pelvic radiotherapy in pregnancy were similar to those in non-pregnant patients, and concluded that radiotherapy was a safe and effective therapy for cervical cancer in pregnancy.

Tewari et al (1998) treated two cases of invasive carcinoma of the cervix (Stages 2A and 1B, respectively) with chemotherapy (cisplatinum and vincristine) after the twentieth week, when organogenesis was completed. Dramatic tumour reduction at the time of cesarean section rendered radical hysterectomy feasible; recurrence occurred in one case five months later, whereas the other remained disease free after two years. Although this is a possible therapeutic option in women who want to continue their pregnancy, the potential adverse effects of chemotherapy during the second and third trimester, discussed later in this chapter, need to be considered.

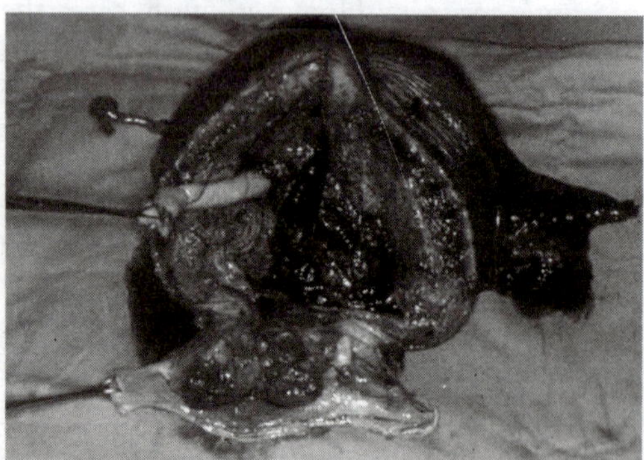

Figure 37.1: Uterus with placenta left attached in the fundus; a classical caesarean section had been performed prior to radical hysterectomy and pelvic lymphadenectomy at 34 weeks gestation. Notice the large exophytic cervical growth.

Prognosis An overall five-year survival rate of 77.7% was observed in patients with early invasive cancer of the cervix in pregnancy. However, the five-year survival in antenatally diagnosed patients was 92.8%; a significantly poorer survival rate in the postpartum patients has been reported in several studies (Baltzer et al 1990; Sivanesaratnam 1993; Sood 2000). This emphasises the importance of early diagnosis and institution of therapy in pregnancy rather than after delivery.

Carcinoma of the Fallopian Tube

The mean age of occurrence of primary adenocarcinoma of the fallopian tube is between 52 and 61 years (Benedet and Miller 1992); thus, the occurrence of this malignancy is extremely *rare*. Isolated cases of unilateral adenocarcinoma have been reported (DiSaia and Creasman 1989). The author has seen only one case over the past 32 years in the University of Malaya Medical Centre. The diagnosis in most cases was established at laparotomy. The treatment was total abdominal hysterectomy, bilateral salpingo-oophorectomy, omentectomy and adjuvant chemotherapy. This would depend on the operative findings and residual disease after surgery.

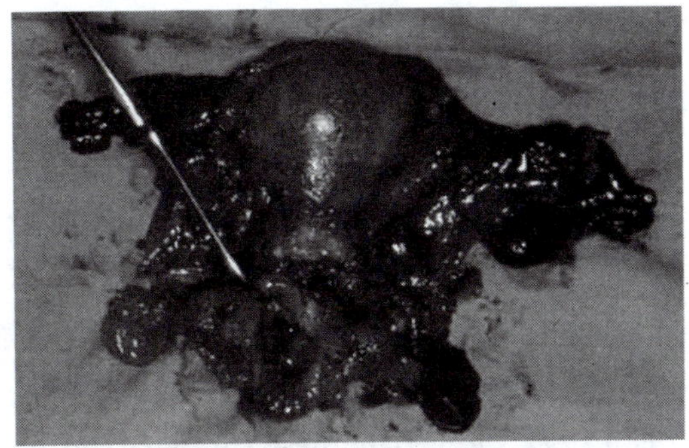

FIGURE 37.2: TUMOUR PERFORATING THROUGH THE LOWER SEGMENT OF THE UTERUS; PATIENT HAD A LOWER SEGMENT CESAREAN SECTION PERFORMED THREE WEEKS PRIOR TO REFERRAL FOR MANAGEMENT OF INVASIVE CANCER OF THE CERVIX. A CLASSICAL CESAREAN SECTION SHOULD HAVE BEEN PERFORMED INSTEAD.

CARCINOMA OF THE VAGINA

Vaginal Intraepithelial Neoplasia (VAIN)

The diagnosis is often made after colposcopic evaluation for an abnormal smear and directed biopsies. The average age at diagnosis is around 52 years; recent publications suggest that the mean age is falling (Stuart et al 1988; Woodman et al 1988). It is, therefore, likely that the clinician will encounter this increasingly common problem more often in pregnancy.

A well-demarcated lesion may be excised or treated with laser vapourisation. Alternatively, pregnancy may be allowed to continue with careful frequent colposcopic assessment, and definitive therapy carried out after delivery.

Invasive Carcinoma of the Vagina *Squamous cell carcinoma* of the vagina is found mainly in women over the age of 50 years. Thus, its occurrence in association with pregnancy is extremely *rare*. Up to 1986, only 12 cases have been reported in the literature (Collins and Barclay 1973; Lutz 1977; DiSaia and Creasman 1989). Among those followed up, the prognosis was reported as being unfavourable.

Management should, in general, be no different from that if the patient were not pregnant. The pregnancy is disregarded if the patient is in the first or early second trimester. Awaiting fetal viability between 24 and 32 weeks may be justified. In the presence of a viable fetus, a classic cesarean section followed by radiotherapy is generally acceptable. However, an early Stage 1 localised disease within the upper third of the vagina could be treated by radical hysterectomy, vaginectomy and pelvic lymphadenectomy.

Twenty-four patients with *clear cell adenocarcinoma,* 20 occurring in the vagina and 4 involving the cervix, have recently been reported by Senekjian et al (1985). The actuarial survival rates at five and 10 years were similar to those of the non-pregnant group analysed concomitantly, suggesting that pregnancy has no adverse effect on this type of carcinoma. The management is similar to that of squamous cell carcinoma of the vagina; radical surgery would appear to be appropriate for early lesions involving the upper vagina and/or cervix.

Isolated reports of *sarcoma bortryoides* involving the vagina and cervix have been reported. When these lesions involve the upper vagina and/or cervix, radical hysterectomy, upper vaginectomy and pelvic lymphadenectomy followed, if necessary, by adjuvant chemotherapy appear to be effective.

CARCINOMA VULVA

Vulval Intraepithelial Neoplasia (VIN) and Microinvasion In the West, in situ lesion of the vulva and marked condylomata has been encountered with increasing frequency in pregnant patients. The early age of coitus, sexual habits of both partners, human papilloma virus (HPV) and smoking are causative factors.

Localised lesions in pregnancy can be treated by excision. However, vulval intraepithelial neoplasia (VIN) tends to be multifocal and multicentric; laser surgery is ideally suited for treating this without mutilating the vulva. However, microinvasive lesions greater than 1 cm in diameter or 1 mm in depth should be considered for more aggressive surgery.

Invasive Vulval Carcinoma This is mainly a disease of perimenopausal and menopausal women with a peak incidence in the seventh decade of life. It is rare in the young and, hence, its occurrence in association with pregnancy is extremely rare. It is not surprising, therefore, that to date only 19 cases have been reported (Goff et al 2000).

The first case of squamous cell carcinoma of the vulva in Malaysia and possibly the second in Asia was recently reported by the author (Sivanesaratnam and Pathmanathan 1990). The commonest histological lesion is squamous cell carcinoma.

Therapy should be planned after careful individualised assessment. It would be influenced by the period of gestation at the time of presentation. Wide local excision, with or without ipsilateral or bilateral inguinal lymphadenectomy, is performed depending on the depth of invasion and location of the lesion on the vulva, as in non-pregnant patients (Sivanesaratnam and Pathmanathan 1990). Treatment, any time up to 36 weeks gestation, was advocated by some (Monaghan and Lindeque 1986), beyond which, delaying the treatment until delivery is advised.

Separate groin incisions for inguinal lymphadenectomy are advocated (Hacker et al 1981). These modifications allow closure without tension and decreased morbidity (Sivanesaratnam 1991).

Does pregnancy adversely affect prognosis in these patients? Pregnancy is said to have no adverse effects on the overall outcome, and termination of pregnancy is not indicated (Kempas and Symmonds 1985). However, the fairly rapid growth of the tumour from 2 cm at 16 weeks of pregnancy to 14 cm at delivery (Sivanesaratnam and Pathmanathan 1990) does show that these tumours can be aggressive and grow rapidly in pregnancy (Fig 37.3). Thus, definitive surgery should not be delayed.

In a young patient who has been successfully treated for carcinoma of the vulva, *future pregnancies are not contraindicated.* Recent reports of successful pregnancy and normal vaginal delivery among patients who had radical vulvectomy and inguinal lymphadenectomy would support such a view (Monaghan and Lindeque 1986). Cesarean section is only done if obstetrically indicated. The decision to allow vaginal delivery or perform a cesarean section would of course be influenced by the post-surgical vulva.

Adjuvant Chemotherapy in Pregnancy

Almost all cytotoxic drugs are capable of crossing the placenta, and are thus, theoretically teratogenic or mutagenic. Their effect on the fetus is influenced by *two simultaneous processes*—the physiological changes associated with pregnancy and the developmental stage of the fetus.

Pregnancy may markedly alter the absorption, distribution and excretion of various cytotoxic drugs (Cunningham et al 1993). The rate of renally excreted drugs may be increased by a rise in renal blood flow, glomerular filtration and creatinine clearance. The amniotic fluid, by acting as a physiological third space, may increase toxicity to the

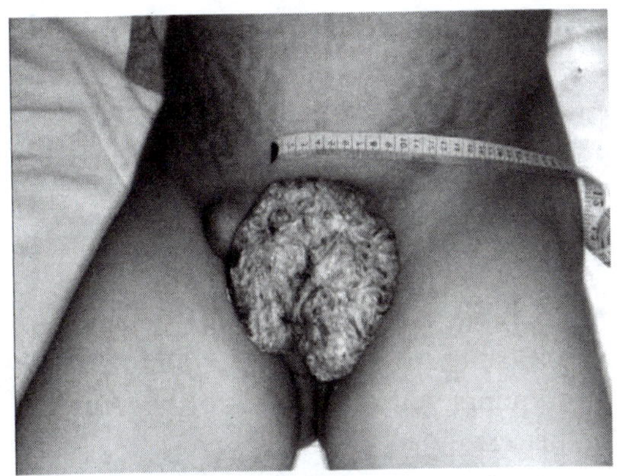

FIGURE 37.3: LARGE VULVAL CARCINOMA DISCOVERED IN PREGNANCY; RAPID GROWTH OF THE TUMOUR WAS SEEN IN PREGNANCY. SHE HAD A NORMAL VAGINAL DELIVERY PRIOR TO REFERRAL FOR SURGERY.

fetus by delayed elimination of the drugs administered. Further, the increase in plasma volume may reduce peak drug concentration (Doll et al 1989).

The first trimester, when organogenesis occurs, is the most crucial period. The blastocyst is resistant to teratogens for the first two weeks as its circulation is not established. Subsequent to this period, chemotherapy either induces severe damage resulting in spontaneous abortion or, if the fetus survives, it will not manifest any abnormality. The third to eighth week of development (5–10 weeks gestation) is the period of maximal susceptibility. During this period, the fetal stem cell population is limited; damage or destruction to a small number of these stem cells may result in anatomical defects.

The risk of major malformation during this period is 10% for single-agent chemotherapy (Nicholson 1968) and 25% for combination chemotherapy (Doll et al 1988) (cf. 3% in the general population). *Chemotherapy is, thus, best avoided in the first trimester of pregnancy. After 13 weeks of gestation,* organogenesis is completed, with the exception of the brain and gonads. After this period, the risk of fetal anomalies is low and *intrauterine growth restriction* is the predominant effect. However, as the central nervous system continues to develop thereafter, *cortical brain function could be affected* (Cunningham et al 1993).

In at least three recent case reports of advanced endodermal sinus tumour in the *second trimester* of pregnancy, adjuvant chemotherapy was administered after unilateral salpingo-oophorectomy and omentectomy. The pregnancies were allowed to continue and the babies delivered at 32, 33 and 37 weeks, respectively, with no adverse effects on the mother or fetus (Malone et al 1986; Metz et al 1989; van der Zee et al 1991). A recent report of a patient with Stage 3C papillary cystadenocarcinoma of the ovary, who was treated from 16 weeks of pregnancy with paclitaxel and carboplatin suggests that this combination causes no adverse outcome in the infant (Mendez et al 2003).

These isolated reports might suggest that the use of cytotoxic drugs after the first trimester of pregnancy is safe and without an increased teratogenic risk. Other reports, however, seem to indicate otherwise.

Elit et al (1999) recently reported one patient who underwent salpingo-oophoerectomy at 23 weeks gestation for an endodermal sinus tumour (Stage 3 disease) and two weeks later commenced adjuvant chemotherapy and delivered by cesarean section at 28 weeks. The infant developed significant ventriculomegaly with cerebral atrophy.

Of the 10 women treated by Tomlinson et al (1997) with cisplatinum in the second and third trimester of pregnancy, growth retardation was noted in half the infants, one had persistent bilateral hearing loss from birth and neonatal leucopenia was seen. There is also another report of congenital malformations in a child exposed to cyclophosphamide in utero for the treatment of maternal leukemia and who later developed neuroblastoma and thyroid carcinoma (Reynoso et al 1987). The possible delayed consequences of in utero exposure to cytotoxic chemotherapy are developmental and growth disturbances, gonadal disorders, immunosuppression and genetic and teratogenic disorders in future generations. About one-third of all babies exposed in utero to chemotherapy will have pancytopenia at birth (Reynoso et al 1987).

Thus, it is the author's view that because of these potential risks to the fetus, cytotoxic chemotherapy is best avoided in pregnancy complicated by gynecological malignancies.

Placental Transfer of Cancer to the Fetus

When cancer occurs in pregnancy, both the patient and her relatives always worry about the risk of it spreading to the fetus. Fortunately, such metastases to the fetus have not been encountered with most of the gynecological malignancies described above.

Of about fifty documented metastatic diseases in the placenta, the most common primary tumours have been melanoma, breast carcinoma and leukemia. In only 2 out of 35 cases reported by Rothmore et al (1973) was the tumour demonstrated on both the maternal and fetal sides of the placenta and fetus. Holland (1949) reported a case of melanoma that metastasised to the placenta and fetus. Recently, the simultaneous occurrence of choriocarcinoma in both the mother and the child has been reported (Tsukamoto et al 1986).

The reasons why the *placenta* appears to be *relatively resistant to metastases* remain obscure. A combination of factors may be responsible:

- The usual gross and histological evaluation may not be able to detect microscopic metastases.
- The trophoblast is actively resistant to these malignant cells.
- Foreign cells that cross the placental barrier face an unfavourable fetal environment and are rejected.
- Multiple factors, still to be defined, are probably involved in determining which tumours will metastasise to the fetus and placenta.

Conclusion Malignancies of the genital tract in pregnancy are uncommon. The current trend for women to delay childbearing will no doubt result in an increased association of these malignancies with pregnancy in the future.

When the diagnosis is confirmed, there is always a conflict between optimal maternal therapy and fetal well-being. In most instances, the cancer is best managed as though the patient is not pregnant. Surgery is the preferred therapy for various site-specific cancers; the timing and mode of delivery should be decided on individual case evaluation and after detailed and frank discussion with the patient and husband.

The overall prognosis in patients with breast cancer complicating pregnancy is poor. With cervical and vulval carcinoma, the prognosis is similar to that in non-pregnant patients. Ovarian cancer in pregnancy has a good prognosis; this is because of the early stage at the time of diagnosis and generally favourable histological type. Chemotherapeutic agents are highly teratogenic in the first trimester; other fetal problems can occur when these drugs are used after 12 weeks of pregnancy. Therefore, chemotherapy is best avoided in pregnancy, if possible.

References

Anderson BO, JA Petrek, DR Byrd et al. 1996. Pregnancy influences breast cancer stage at diagnosis in women 30 years of age and younger. *Ann Surgical Oncol* 3:204–211.

Antonelli NM, DJ Dotters, VL Katz and JA Kuller. 1996. Cancer in pregnancy: a review of the literature. *Obstet Gynecol Surv* 51:125–142.

Ariel I and R Kempner. 1989. The prognosis of patients who become pregnant after mastectomy for breast cancer. *Int Surg* 75:185–187.

Ayhan A, S Gunalp, C Karaer et al. 1999. Endometrial adenocarcinoma in pregnancy. *Gynecol Oncol* 75:298–299.

Baltzer J, ME Regenbrecht, W Kopoke and J Zander. 1990. Carcinoma of the cervix and pregnancy. *Int J Gynae Obst* 31:317–323.

Barber HRK and A Brunschwig. 1963. Gynaecologic cancer complicating pregnancy. *Am J Obstet Gynecol* 85:156–164.

Barber HRK. 1992. Malignant disease in pregnancy. In *Gynaecologic Oncology*, ed M Coppleson, 1076. London: Churchill Livingstone.

Barnavon Y and MK Wallach. 1990. Management of the pregnant patient with carcinoma of the breast. *Surg Gynecol Obstet* 171: 347–352.

Beischer NA, BW Buttery and DW Fortune. 1971. Growth and malignancy of ovarian tumours in pregnancy. *Ausst NZ Obstetrics Gynaecol* 11:208–220.

Benedet JL and DM Miller. 1992. Tumours of the fallopian tube: clinical features, staging and management. In *Gynaecologic Oncology* Vol. 2, ed M Coppleson, 853–860. London: Churchill Livingstone.

Benedet JL, PA Selke and KG Nickerson. 1987. Colposcopic evaluation of abnormal Papanicolaou smear in pregnancy. *Am J Obstet Gynecol* 157:932–937.

Berry DL, RL Therianlt, FA Holmes et al. 1999. Management of breast cancer during pregnancy using standardized protocol. *J Clin Oncol* 17:855–861.

Bonnier P, S Romain et al. 1997. Influence of pregnancy on the outcome of breast cancer: A case control study. *Int J Cancer* 72:720–727.

Booth RT. 1963. Ovarian tumours in pregnancy. *Obstet Gynecol* 21:189–195.

Clark RM and J Reid. 1978. Carcinoma of the breast in pregnancy and lactation. *Surg Chin North Am* 76:293–298.

Clark RM and T Chua. 1989. Breast cancer and pregnancy: the ultimate challenge. *Clin Oncol* R *Coll Radiology* 1:11–18.

Collins CG and DL Barclay. 1973. Cancer of the vulva and cancer of the vagina in pregnancy. *Clin Obstet Gynecol* 6:927–934.

Copeland LJ, PB Saul and N Sneige. 1987. Cervical adenocarcinoma: tumour implantation in the episiotomy sites of two patients. *Gynecol Oncol* 28:230–235.

Coppola A, J Sorosky, R Casper et al. 1997. The clinical course of cervical carcinoma in situ diagnosed during pregnancy. *Gynecol Oncol* 67:162–165.

Creasman WT, F Rutledge and G Fletcher. 1970. Carcinoma of the cervix associated with pregnancy. *Obstet Gynaecol* 36:495–501.

Cunningham FG, PC MacDonald, NF Gant et al. 1993. Neoplastic disease. In *William Obstetrics, ed* CT Norwalk; 19th ed, 1267–1269. Appleton and Lange.

de la Rochefordiere A, B Asselain, F Campana et al. 1993. Age as a prognostic factor in pre-menopausal breast carcinoma. *Lancet* 341:1039–1043.

De Petrillo AD, DE Townsend and CP Morrow. 1975. Colposcopy in evaluation of the abnormal Papanicolaou test in pregnancy. *Am J Obstet Gynecol* 121:441–445.

Desel TV, TM Hameeteman and SS Wagenaar. 1988. Mucinous cystadenocarcinoma in pregnancy: case report. *Br J Obstet Gynecol* 95:527–529.

DiFronzo LA and TX O'Connell. 1996. Breast cancer in pregnancy and lactation. *Surg Clin North Am* 76:267–268.

DiSaia PJ and WT Creasman. 1989. Cancer in pregnancy. In *Clinical Gynaecologic Oncology* 511–559. St. Louis: CV Mosby Co.

Dobson LS, AM Gillespie, RE Coleman and BW Hancock. 1999. The presentation and management of post-partum choriocarcinoma. *Br J Cancer* 79:1531–1533.

Doll DC, OS Ringesberg and DW Yarbro. 1988. Management of cancer during pregnancy. *Arch Intern Med* 148:2058–2064.

Doll RC, OS Ringesberg and JW Yarbo. 1989. Antineoplastic agents and pregnancy. *Semin Oncol* 16:337.

Dudan RC, JL Yon, JH Ford and HE Averette. 1973. Carcinoma of the cervix and pregnancy. *Gynecol Oncol* 1: 283–289.

Elit L, A Bocking, C Kenyon and R Natale. 1999. An endodermal sinus tumour diagnosed in pregnancy: case report and review of the literature. *Gynecol Oncol* 72:123–127.

Goff BA, PJ Paley, WJ Koh et al. 2000. Cancer in the pregnant women. In *Principles and practice of gynaecologic oncology*, 3rd ed, eds WJ Hoskins, CA

Grimes WA, RA Bartholomew and ED Golvin et al. 1954. Ovarian cysts complicating pregnancy. *Am J Obstet Gynec* 68:594.

Guinee VF, H Olsson, T Moller et al. 1994. Effect of pregnancy on prognosis for young women with breast cancer. *Lancet* 343:1587–1589.

Hacker NF, JS Berek, LD Lagasse et al. 1982. Carcinoma of the cervix associated with pregnancy. *Obstet Gynecol* 59:735–740.

Hacker NF, RS Lenchter, JS Berek et al. 1981. Radical vulvectomy and bilateral inguinal lymphadenectomy through separate groin incisions. *Obstet Gynecol* 58:574.

Hanningan EV, HH Whitehouse, WD Atkinson and St N Becker. 1982. Cone biopsy during pregnancy. *Obstet Gynecol* 60:450–455.

Harvey JC, PP Rosen, R Ashikari et al. 1981. The effect of pregnancy on the prognosis of carcinoma of the breast following radical mastectomy. *Surg Gynecol Obstet* 153:723–735.

Holland E. 1949. A case of trans-placental metastasis of malignant melanoma from mother to fetus. *J Obstet Gynecol Br Empire* 59:529–536.

Hoover HC. 1990. Breast cancer during pregnancy and lactation. *Surg Clin North Am* 70:1151–1162.

Hunter JG, L Swanstrom and K Thonburg. 1995. Carbon dioxide preumoperitoneum induces fetal acidosis in pregnant ewe model. *Surg Endosc* 9:272–279.

Ichikawa Y, Takano K, Higa S et al. 2001. Endometrial carcinoma co-existing with pregnancy presumed to derive from adenomyosis: A case report. *Int J Gyneal Oncol* 11:488–490.

Ishide T et al. 1992. Clinicopathologic characteristics and prognosis of breast cancer patients associated with pregnancy and lactation. Analysis of case-control study in Japan. *Jpn J Cancer Res* 83:1143–1149.

Karlen JR, A Akbari and WA Cook. 1979. Dysgerminoma associated with pregnancy. *Obstet Gynecol* 53:330–335.

Kempas RD and RE Symmonds. 1985. Invasive carcinoma of the vulva in pregnancy. *Obstet Gynecol* 26:749–751.

Kempson RL and GE Pokorny. 1968. Adenocarcinoma of the endometrium in women aged forty and younger. *Cancer* 21:650–654.

Kitchen PRB and R McLeannan. 1987. Breast cancer and pregnancy. *Med J Aust* 147:337–339.

Koren G, L Weiner, M Lishner et al. 1990. Cancer in pregnancy: Identification of unanswered questions on maternal and fetal risks. *Obstet Gynecol Surv* 45:509–514.

Kulenthran A and V Sivanesaratnam. 1986. Dysgerminoma of the ovary with pregnancy. *Asia-Oceania J Obstet Gynecol* 12:217–220.

Langston AA, KE Malone, JD Thomas et al. 1996. BRCA 1 mutations in a population-based sample of young women with breast cancer. *New Engl J Med* 334:1143–1149.

LaPolla JP, C O'Niel and D Wetrich. 1988. Colposcopic management of abnormal cervical cytology in pregnancy. *J Reprod Med* 33:301–306.

Lash AF. 1961. Management of carcinoma of the cervix in pregnancy. *Obstet Gynecol* 17:41–48.

Lee CH, S Raman and V Sivanesaratnam. 1989. Torsion of ovarian tumours: a clinico-pathological study. *Int J Gynecol Obstet* 28:21–25.

Lee RB, W Neglia and RC Park. 1981. Cervical carcinoma in pregnancy. *Obstet Gynecol* 58:584–589.

Lees D and A Singer. 1982. Management of abnormal smear in pregnancy. In *Colour atlas of gynaecological surgery*, eds D Lees and A Singer, 147. London: Wolfe Medical.

Lutz MH. 1977. Genital malignancy in pregnancy. *Am J Obstet Gynecol* 129:536–545.

Malone JM, DM Gershenson, RK Creasy et al. 1986. Endodermal sinus tumour of the ovary associated with pregnancy. *Obstet Gynecol* 68 (Suppl.):86–88.

McPherson CP, TA Sellers, JD Potter et al. 1996. Reproductive factors and risk of endometrial cancer: the Iowa Women's Health Study. *Am J Epidemiol* 143:1195–1202.

Mendez LE, A Mueller and E Salom Gonzalez-Quintero. 2003.. Paclitaxol and carboplatin chemotherapy administered during pregnancy for advanced epithelial ovarian cancer. *Obstet Gynaecol* 102:1200–2.

Mercer RJ, RM Bryan, RC Bennett et al. 1984. The prognostic value of oestrogen receptors in breast cancer. *Aust NZ J Surg* 54:7–10.

Metz SA, TG Day and SH Pursell. 1989. Adjuvant chemotherapy in a pregnant patient with endodermal sinus tumour of the ovary. *Gynecol Oncol* 32:371–374.

Monaghan JM and G Lindeque. 1986. Vulvar carcinoma in pregnancy. *Br J Obstet Gynecol* 93: 785–786.

Moor RD and WG Smith. 1999. Laparoscopic management of adnexal masses in pregnant women. *J Reprod Med* 44:97–100.

Munnell EW. 1963. Primary ovarian cancer associated with pregnancy. *Clin Obstet Gynecol* 6: 683–689.

Nicholson H. 1968. Cytotoxic drugs in pregnancy: review of reported cases. *J Obstet Gynecol Br Commonwealth* 75:307–312.

Nieminen U and N Remas. 1970. Malignancy during pregnancy. *Acta Obstet Gynecol Scand* 49: 315–319.

Novak ER, CD Lambron and JF Woodruff. 1975. Ovarian tumours in pregnancy: an ovarian tumour registry review. *Obstet Gynecol* 46:401–408.

Novotny DB, SJ Maygarden, RW Shermer et al. 1991. Fine needle aspiration of benign and malignant breast masses associated with pregnancy. *Acta Cytol* 35:656–686.

Nugent P and TX O'Conell. 1985. Breast cancer in pregnancy. *Arch Surg* 120:1221–4.

Palle C, S Bangeboll and B Andreasson. 2000. Cervical intraepithelial neoplasia in pregnancy. *Acta Obstet Gynecol Scand* 79:306–310.

Petrek JA, R Dukoff and A Rogatko. 1991. Prognosis of pregnancy-associated breast cancer. *Cancer* 67:869–872.

Petrek JA. 1994. Breast cancer during pregnancy. *Cancer* 74:518–527.

Pratt JR and GD Malkarsian. 1964. The treatment of invasive carcinoma of the cervix during pregnancy. *Am NY Acad Sci* 114:868–874.

Reynoso EE, FA Shepherd, HA Messner et al. 1987. Acute leukaemia during pregnancy: The Toronto Leukaemia Study Group experience with long-term follow-up of children exposed in utero to chemotherapeutic agents. *J Clin Oncol* 5:1098–1102.

Robiero G, DA Jones and M Jones. 1986. Carcinoma of the breast associated with pregnancy. *Br J Surg* 73:607–9.

Robinson WR, S Webb, J Tirpack et al. 1997. Management of cervical intraepithelial neoplasia during pregnancy with LOOP excision. *Gynecol Oncol* 64:153–155.

Rothmore LA, CJ Cohen and J Asterloa. 1973. Placental and fetal involvement by maternal malignancy. A report of rectal carcinoma and review of the literature. *Am J Obstet Gynecol* 116: 1023–1034.

Sablinska RE, L Tarlowska and J Stelmachew. 1977. Invasive carcinoma of the cervix associated with pregnancy. Correlation between patient age, advancement of cancer and gestation, and result of treatment. *Gynecol Oncol* 5:563–567.

Sall S, S Rini and A Pineda. 1974. Surgical management of invasive carcinoma of the cervix in pregnancy. *Am J Obstet Gynecol* 118:1–5.

Saunders N and CR London. 1988. Management problems associated with carcinoma of the cervix diagnosed in the second trimester of pregnancy. *Gynecol Oncol* 30:120–122.

Scioscia AL, MJ Merino, M Haas et al. 1986. Malignant mixed mullerian tumour of the uterus arising in association with a viable gestation. *Obstet Gynecol* 71: 1047–1050.

Senekjian EK, M Hubby, and AL Herbst. 1985. Clear cell adenocarcinoma (CCA) of the cervix and vagina associated with pregnancy. Gynecol Oncol 20:250.

Sivanesaratnam V and R Pathmanathan. 1990. Carcinoma of the vulva in pregnancy: a rare occurrence. *Asia-Oceanic J Obstet Gynecol* 16:207–210.

Sivanesaratnam V, LT Ang and TA Sinnathuray. 1976. Ovarian tumours complicating pregnancy in a Malaysian Study. *Med J Malaysia* 30:291–295.

Sivanesaratnam V, P Jayalaksmi and EC Loo. 1993. The surgical management of early invasive cancer of the cervix associated with pregnancy. *Gynecol Oncol* 48:68–75.

Sivanesaratnam V. 1991. Current strategies in the surgical management of early invasive carcinoma of the cervix. *Contemp Rev Obst Gynecol* 3:178–183.

Sivanesaratnam V. 1991. New directions in gynaecologic oncology (Editorial) *Med J Malaysia* 46: 205–211.

Sivanesaratnam V. 1998. Ovarian malignancy in pregnancy. *J Obstet Gynecol.Res* 24 (Suppl. 3):46.

Sivanesaratnam V. 2001. Management of the pregnant mother with malignant conditions. *Curr Opin Obstet Gynaecol* 13:121–125.

Sood AK, JI Sorosky, N Mayr et al. 1997. Radiotherapeutic management of cervical carcinoma that complicates pregnancy. *Cancer* 80:1073–1079.

Sood AK. 2000. Pregnant women with cervical cancer should deliver by Caesarean. *Obstet Gynecol* 95:832–838.

Stander RW and Lein JW. Carcinoma of the cervix and pregnancy. 1960. *Am J Obstet Gynecol* 79: 164–167.

Stuart GCE, EA Flagler, JG Nation, M Duggan and DI Robertson. 1988. Laser vapourisation of vaginal intraepithelial neoplasia. *Am J Obstet Gynecol* 158:240–243.

Talehian F, BA Krumholz and A Shayan. 1976. Colposcopic evaluation of patients with abnormal cytological smears during pregnancy. *Obstet Gynecol* 47:693–696.

Tewari K, F Cappuccini, A Gambino et al. 1998. Neoadjuvant chemotherapy in the treatment of locally advanced cervical carcinoma in pregnancy: a report of 2 cases and review of issues specific to the management of cervical carcinoma in pregnancy including planned delay of therapy. *Cancer* 82:1529–1534.

Thompson JD, TA Caputo and EW Franklin. 1975. The surgical management of invasive carcinoma of the cervix in pregnancy. *Am J Obstet Gynecol* 121:853–863.

Tretli S, G Kualheim, S Thoreson et al. 1988. Survival of breast cancer patients during pregnancy or lactation. *Br J Cancer* 58:382–384.

Tsukamoto N, M Matsumara, K Matsukuma et al. 1986. Choriocarcinoma in mother and fetus. *Gynecol Oncol* 24:113–119.

Vaccarello L, SM Apte, LJ Copeland et al. 1999. Endometrial carcinoma associated with pregnancy: a report of the cases and review of the literature. *Gynecol Oncol* 74:118–122.

van der Zee AGJ, HWA de Bruijin, J Bonna et al. 1991. Endodermal sinus tumour of the ovary during pregnancy: A case report. *Am J Obstet Gynecol* 164:504–506.

Wagner LK, RG Lester and L Saldana. 1985. Exposure of the pregnant patient to diagnostic radiation: a guide to medical management, 40–60. Philadelphia: Lippincott.

Waldrop GM and JP Palmer. 1963. Carcinoma of cervix associated with pregnancy. *Am J Obnstet Gynecol* 86:202–206.

Wallach MK, JA Wolf Jr, J Bedwinck et al. 1983. Gestational carcinoma of the female breast. *Curr Problems Cancer* 7:1–58.

Wang PH, HT Chao, CC Yuen et al. 1999. Ovarian tumours complicating pregnancy. Emergency and elective surgery. *J Reprod Med* 44:279–289.

Whitecar P, S Turner and K Higby. 1999. Adnexal masses in pregnancy: a review of 130 cases undergoing surgical management. *Am J Obstet Gynecol* 181:19–24.

Woodman CB, JJ Mould and JA Jordan. 1988. Radiotherapy in the management of VAIN after hysterectomy. *Br J Obstet Gynecol* 95:976–979.

Yoo Nessi M, W Wieckowska, D Marinello and J Antkowiak. 1982. Cervical intraepithelial neoplasia in pregnancy. *Int J Obstet Gynecol* 20:111–118.

38

Postpartum Maternal Collapse

Niraj Krishnamurthy Yanamandra | Sabaratnam Arulkumaran

Introduction Maternal collapse is one of the nightmare scenarios in the labour ward that an obstetrician hopes will never occur, though the threat is never completely absent. Collapse signifies an acute event that could take place because of inadequate cerebral perfusion or oxygenation, abnormal cerebral activity or major brainstem dysfunction. Loss of consciousness is the usual cause of collapse. The happiness of delivering a healthy baby at the end of an anxious wait during the antenatal period could easily turn into one of the scariest and most life-threatening conditions for the mother.

Postpartum maternal collapse may have a hemorrhagic cause such as postpartum hemorrhage (PPH). The non-hemorrhagic causes could be vascular, for example, pulmonary thromboembolism (PTE), or obstetric, such as amniotic fluid embolism (AFE), uterine inversion and sepsis. Anesthetic problems and conditions related to the central nervous system (CNS) and cardiovascular or respiratory system can also lead to maternal collapse. Though these are relatively uncommon conditions, they are responsible for the majority of maternal deaths in the developed world.

Other relatively non-serious causes include vasovagal attack, hypoglycemia and hyperventilation. These conditions are usually self-limiting and need patient reassurance along with close monitoring.

In this chapter, the immediate care required for a woman with postpartum collapse is discussed, followed by the management of the conditions responsible for the collapse.

Causes

The following conditions should be considered as probable causes leading to postpartum maternal collapse:

Cardiovascular event leading to decreased cardiac output

- Absolute decrease in circulating volume, for example, major hemorrhage—postpartum hemorrhage (PPH)
- Circulation blockage, for example, massive pulmonary embolism (PE)
- Relative decrease in effective circulating volume, for example, sepsis and amniotic fluid embolism (AFE)
- Cardiac conditions, for example, arrhythmia, myocardial infarction and cardiomyopathy

Primary cerebral event leading to loss of consciousness

- Intracerebral bleeding
- Hypoglycemia
- Profound hypoxia
- Anesthetic drugs or cerebral infarction

Acute Management Of Collapse

Prompt recognition and aggressive management is crucial for a successful outcome in a woman who has collapsed. The immediate management of a collapsed postnatal woman includes commencing Basic Life Support (BLS) and identifying the underlying cause so that definitive treatment can be carried out to correct it. Failure of circulation for 3–4 minutes (less if the patient is hypoxemic initially) will lead to irreversible cerebral damage. Management should follow the structured approach recommended by the Advanced Life Support Group (Advanced Life Support Course). This includes A - Airway, B - Breathing, C - Circulation, D - Disability and E - Exposure.

A—Airway A clear airway must be quickly established with the head tilt–jaw thrust or head tilt–chin maneuver and then maintained (Morris et al). To reduce the risk of aspiration of gastric contents, the airway should be cleared of secretion or vomit and an oropharyngeal or nasopharyngeal airway should be inserted. The gold standard in airway protection is intubation. An experienced anesthetist should carry out this procedure as laryngeal edema, which is likely to be present because of pregnancy changes, may complicate it.

B—Breathing Keeping the airway open, the obstetrician should assess breathing for 10 seconds, by looking for chest movement, listening for breath sounds at the victim's mouth and feeling for air on the cheek. In the presence of breathing, the woman should be put in the recovery position and further help should be sought while checking for continued breathing.

If the patient is not breathing adequately, intermittent positive pressure ventilation should be started. Mouth-to-mouth, mouth-to-nose, or mouth-to-airway ventilation should be carried out till a self-inflating bag and mask are available. High-flow supplementary oxygen should be administered in all cases of collapse at a flow rate of 12–15 litres/minute.

C—Circulation The 'gold standard' sign of cardiac arrest is an absent carotid (or other large artery) pulse. In the absence of carotid pulsation, resuscitation should commence with external chest compressions. A cardiac rhythm monitor should be attached and the defibrillator prepared. A ratio of 15 chest compressions to two breaths should be maintained until signs of circulation are established or defibrillation is advised by the Advanced Life Support team.

D—Disability Assessment of the level of consciousness and papillary function reflects the neurological status and cerebral tissue perfusion. The Glasgow coma scale (GCS) should be used to assess any woman with impaired consciousness, especially if a neurological cause is suspected.

E—Exposure Adequate exposure of the collapsed woman is essential for full assessment to avoid missing vital information and to make a definitive diagnosis. This should include a vaginal examination. Figure 39.1 shows an algorithm from the ALS Provider Manual that summarises the steps in BLS.

Postpartum Hemorrhage

In obstetric practice, the threat of massive blood loss should be recognised when the the loss is over 1500 ml, which represents around 25% of the blood volume (Bonnar 2000). Massive hemorrhage can lead to maternal cardiac arrest.

Figure 38.1: Adult BLS algorithm

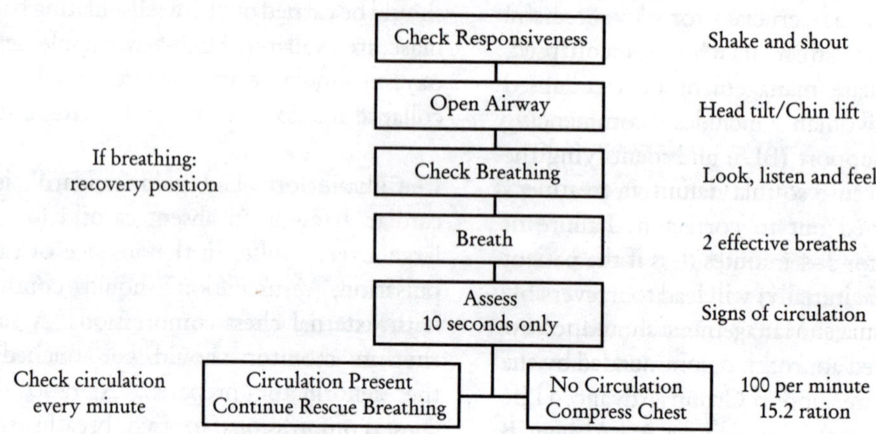

Send or go for help as soon as possible according to guidelines

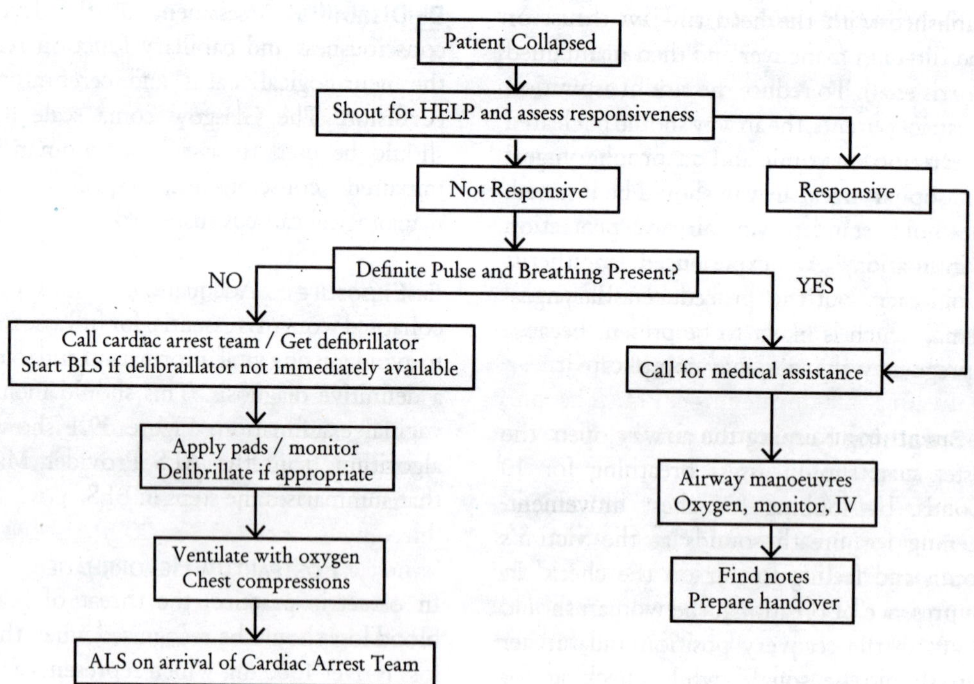

Management PPH is best managed using a multidisciplinary approach (also see Chapter 32). Achieving hemodynamic stability should be the goal while trying to identify the cause of bleeding. Hypovolemia should be corrected by infusing crystalloids. Adequacy of intravascular fluid replacement could be monitored by central venous pressure and pulmonary capillary wedge pressure, while mainting a urine output record. Whole blood, platelets, cryoprecipitate and fresh frozen plasma should be transfused depending on the estimated blood loss and associated coagulopathy.

Treating the Cause of Bleeding Uterine atony is the commonest cause of PPH. Bimanual compression of the uterus, along with administration of uterotonic drugs, is usually effective in controlling the bleeding. Carboprost, misoprostol and intramuscular carbetocin (Chong et al 2004) could be used in women who do not respond to oxytocin or ergometrine.

Retained placental tissue may need manual removal under anesthetic. Surgical causes including episiotomy, and vaginal/cervical tears should be promptly sutured. Intrauterine tamponade with a Sengstaken–Blakemore tube or Rush urological balloon is a simple, low-cost, readily available and effective means of treating life-threatening PPH. The only apparent contraindication is the discovery of an infection during delivery (Seror et al 2005).

Angiographic arterial embolisation has been reported as being successful in the control of PPH (Vedantham et al 1997; Pelage et al 1998; Hansch et al 1999). Transcatheter embolisation offers an effective means of controlling PPH while obviating much of the morbidity and mortality of open surgical procedures. Bloom et al noted that complications associated with uterine artery embolisation include fever, transient buttock and foot ischemia, iliac artery perforation and abscess. They recommend that in selected cases it should be incorporated into the treatment algorithm at an earlier stage (2004).

Failure to control bleeding despite using the abovementioned measures may require the use of laparotomy. Of the various surgical options available to control bleeding, the B-Lynch compression suture (Lynch et al 1997) has been proposed as a simple, first surgical step to control atonic uterine bleeding. It reduces blood flow to the uterus from its lateral margins and from the placental bed vessels by the apposition of the anterior and posterior uterine walls. The current trend is to use simple vertical compression sutures. Surgical ligation of the internal iliac artery (Floyd and Morrison 1992) is a relatively less effective method of controlling PPH. The reported success of this procedure is 42%. Uterine (Still 1999) and ovarian artery ligation (Plauche 1992) is also described but is not very widely practised.

Peripartum hysterectomy is undertaken, in approximately 1 in 2500 deliveries, as a last resort to control the bleeding. This figure varies between 1 in 1400 and 1 in 4000 based on studies reported from around the world (Park and Duff 1980).

The use of recombinant factor VIIa continues to be reported for all types of surgical bleeding including postpartum bleeding (Clarke and Butt 2005), though there is no clear consensus about the dosage or when it should be administered. It is expensive and not widely available.

Pulmonary Thromboembolism

One of the commonest causes of maternal collapse is pulmonary thromboembolism.

If not managed correctly, it could prove fatal. Although venous thrombosis and thromboembolism (VTE) remain the leading causes of direct death in the UK, the maternal death rate from thromboembolism continues to decline.

The most recent confidential enquiry has shown a reduction in deaths from pulmonary embolism (PE) in the antenatal period (Lewis and Drife 2002). However, successive reports of Confidential Enquiries into Maternal Deaths have highlighted a failure in recognising the risk factors of VTE and employing adequate prophylaxis. Therefore, all healthcare professionals looking after pregnant women must be aware that PE can present for the first time in the postnatal period.

Management The clinical picture of a woman with pulmonary embolism is that of sudden onset dyspnea, collapse, chest pain, hemoptysis, faintness, raised jugular venous pressure (JVP), focal signs in chest and symptoms and signs associated with deep vein thrombosis (DVT). Immediate management of the patient will be on similar lines for postpartum collapse.

The clinical diagnosis of PE is unreliable. Palla et al have shown that no more than one-third of emboli are diagnosed clinically (1995). It is critical to obtain an objective diagnosis so as to institute the most appropriate treatment and, more importantly, to avoid unnecessary anticoagulation in the absence of PE.

Certain bedside investigations such as ECG, arterial blood gas (ABG) analysis and chest x-ray should be performed. ECG may be normal except for a sinus tachycardia. In cases of large PE, right-axis deviation, right-bundle branch block and peaked P waves in lead II due to right atrial dilation may be seen. ABG reveals hypoxemia and hypocapnia (Nelson-Piercy 2006). Chest x-ray is often normal but is an essential part of investigation for ruling out other conditions such as pneumothorax and pneumonia. Common radiological findings include focal infiltrate, segmental collapse, raised diaphragm (normal feature of pregnancy) and pleural effusion (Thomson and Greer 2000).

While waiting for the objective confirmation of the diagnosis, if clinical suspicion of PE exists—especially in the presence of risk factors of VTE— unfractionated heparin or low molecular weight heparin (LMWH) should be started to reduce morbidity and mortality (Thomson and Greer 2000; RCOG 2001). In massive pulmonary embolism, when the risk of cardiac arrest is imminent, thrombolysis with 50 mg altepase is the first line of treatment (Clarke and Butt 2005).

Before anticoagulant treatment is initiated, blood should be collected for a full thrombophilia screen, full blood count and coagulation screen. Blood should also be sent for urea, electrolyte and liver function tests, to exclude renal or hepatic dysfunction, which are cautions for anticoagulant therapy.

Ventilation perfusion or (V/Q) scan, bilateral Doppler ultrasound of both legs and large pelvic veins studies should be performed (Clarke and Butt 2005). In the first instance, a perfusion scan alone is done, with ventilation scan being performed only if the perfusion scan is abnormal. Pulmonary angiography is considered to be the gold standard for the diagnosis of PE (Goodman 1984). However, it is rarely necessary.

Amniotic Fluid Embolism (AFE)

This rare obstetric condition is a catastrophic syndrome which causes sudden maternal collapse and is associated with high mortality rates. The rarity of this condition means that there is very little information about it in the literature and few centres are equipped with the facilities required to diagnose and manage the condition effectively. It therefore remains unpredictable, unpreventable and rapidly progressive.

The overall incidence of AFE has been reported to range from 1 in 20,000 to one in 80,000 deliveries (Mabie 1994). In the USA and Australia, it is responsible for 7.5–10% of maternal deaths (Atrash et al 1990; Burrows and Khoo 1995). Fortunately, in the UK, the number of maternal deaths due to AFE has fallen significantly over the last three triennia (Lewis and Drife 2002).

Management It is typified by maternal collapse, associated with breathlessness, cyanosis, cardiac dysrrhythymia and hypotension. Most cases eventually lead to maternal collapse (Tuffnell 2003). More than half the patients die within the first hour. Of the survivors, 40% develop disseminated intravascular coagulation (DIC) while 10–15% of patients develop grand mal seizures. These seizures may even be the initial sign of an amniotic fluid embolus (Martin and Rick 1996). PPH usually follows because of associated coagulation failure.

There is no single clinical or laboratory test to diagnose AFE. The diagnosis of AFE has traditionally been at post mortem, by identifying fetal squames and debris in the pulmonary vasculature.

Investigations such as ABG, ECG, chest x-ray and coagulation screening must be performed immediately. ABG may show metabolic acidosis. ECG may reveal right ventricular strain pattern and tachycardia, while chest x-ray may uncover changes consistent with pulmonary edema in the absence of any clinical evidence of left ventricular failure. Coagulation screen may show features of disseminated intravascular coagulation.

Use of zinc coproporphyrin and the monoclonal antibody TKAH-2 has been reported as a means of rapid diagnosis of AFE (Kanayama et al 1992; Kobayashi et al 1993). Early recognition with high index of suspicion and ruling out other possible causes for collapse remains the cornerstone of management. These patients are best managed using a multidisciplinary approach, by a team that includes a senior obstetrician, anesthetist and hematologist. BLS should be started.

The treatment of AFE is directed at the maintenance of left ventricular output (Clark 1990). The patient is best managed in the intensive care unit. In unconscious patients, endotracheal intubation must be performed and mechanical ventilation initiated. The highest concentration available of oxygen should be administered. Shock should be corrected using intravenous crystalloids, dopamine and vasopressors. Careful monitoring of fluids is essential to avoid fluid overload. Pulmonary capillary wedge pressure will aid in directing fluid resuscitation. DIC should be corrected using fresh frozen plasma, platelets and other component therapy.

High-dose corticosteroids and epinephrine have been suggested because of the similarities between anaphylactoid reactions and AFE (Clark 1995). Thrombectomy and cardiopulmonary bypass (Esposito et al 1990) have been used successfully to treat AFE. Among the newer treatment modalities reported in the management of AFE are recombinant factor VIIa (Lim et al 2004), extracorporeal membrane oxygenation and intra-aortic balloon counterpulsation (Hsieh et al 2000), uterine artery embolisation (Dorne et al 2002; Goldszmidt and Davies 2004), continuous hemofiltration (Kaneko et al 2001) and plasma exchange transfusion (Awad 2001). Other reported treatment methods, especially for refractory hypoxemia, include nitric oxide and inhaled aerosolised prostacyclin (Tanus-Santos and Moreno 1999; Capellier et al 1997; van Heerden et al 1996).

Septic Shock

Sepsis remains one of the most important causes of maternal mortality worldwide. It causes death by DIC, multiorgan failure and adult respiratory distress syndrome.

Recent confidential enquiries have shown a small decrease in the number of deaths due to genital tract sepsis. The main risk factors for development of sepsis are prolonged rupture of membranes with subsequent development of chorioamnionitis, postpartum endometritis (Lee et al 1988), emergency cesarean section or retained products of conceptions after delivery. Other causes of shock include pyelonephritis, chorioamnionitis, toxic shock, ruptured appendix, ruptured ovarian abscess, necrotising fascitis and bacterial endocarditis (Mabie at al 1997).

A wide variety of organisms has been associated with septic shock including *Escherichia coli*, Klebsiella, *Proteus mirabilis*, *Pseudomonas aeruginosa*, *Staphylococcus aureus* and bacteroides (Thomson and Greer 2000). Group B streptococcus may be responsible for puerperal septicemia with an incidence of approximately 1–2/1000 deliveries, and accounts for up to 15% of positive blood cultures from postpartum patients (Blanco et al 1981). Tewari et al reported a rare case of legionella infection in pregnancy complicated by sepsis and hemodynamic compromise (Tewari et al 1997).

Septic shock must be suspected in a woman who has predisposing factors and develops pyrexia and hypotension. Other signs would depend on the severity of systemic involvement. Advanced septic shock is associated with decreased cardiac output and continued low systemic vascular resistance.

Management The two main components of the management of septic shock are commencement of resuscitation and identification and eradicatation of the source of infection.

Resuscitation should be aimed at maintaining cardiorespiratory stability. One of the recommendations in managing this condition is a hemodynamic algorithm based on volume therapy, inotropic agents and peripheral vasoconstrictors (Lee et al 1988). Better treatment decisions could be aided by an aggressive and earlier central monitoring of hemodynamic status (Marcovici and Ferretti 1997).

Supportive care to control temperature should be provided with antipyretic agents and cooling blankets. Blood should be taken for blood culture (aerobic and anerobic), full blood count, coagulation screen, renal and liver function tests, along with vaginal swabs and midstream urine for microscopy, culture and sensitivity. While waiting for the reports, broad-spectrum antibiotics should be administered by the parenteral route after consulting with the microbiologist. If retained, placental tissue should be suspected and arrangements made for evacuation.

Associated coagulopathy should be treated after liaising with hematologists. Fresh frozen plasma and blood components may be administered as required. Despite volume replacement and ionotropic agents, if hypotension persists, peripheral vasoconstrictors should be considered. If the patient continues to deteriorate, laparotomy should be considered for septic foci. Hysterectomy may be required if the focus of infection is thought to be in the uterus.

Eclampsia

Eclampsia remains one of the life-threatening conditions in pregnancy. It is defined as the occurrence of convulsions, not caused by any coincidental neurological disease such as epilepsy, in a woman whose condition also meets the criteria for pre-eclampsia (ACOG 1986). The incidence of eclampsia in the UK is 4.9/10,000 maternities. About 44% of seizures occur postnatally, the remainder being antepartum (38%) or intrapartum (18%) (Douglas and Redman 1994). Postpartum eclampsia denotes convulsions appearing within 7 days after delivery of the fetus and placenta in a patient who had pre-eclampsia (Thomas 1998). Late postpartum eclampsia has been defined as seizures that occur 3 or 4 days to 4 weeks postpartum (Sibai et al 1990).

In many instances, it can present without pre-eclampsia. Since many of the patients develop neurological symptoms prior to the onset of pre-eclampsia/eclampsia, due attention to these symptoms and close follow-up can lead to early diagnosis (Mathew 2003).

Though a detailed discussion of etiopathology and management of eclampsia is beyond the scope of this chapter, the management of postpartum collapse due to eclampsia is discussed briefly.

The diagnosis of eclampsia is usually evident due to tonic-clonic convulsions in the presence of hypertension and protienuria. However, other conditions that can cause convulsions and coma should be taken into consideration. These include epilepsy, intracranial hemorrhage and thrombosis, rupture of a cerebral aneurysm, meningitis, encephalitis, cerebral tumours and hyperventilation syndrome (Cunningham et al 1989).

Management From a clinical standpoint, the immediate management of eclampsia should involve placing the patient in the recovery position, securing the airway and administering oxygen.

Further management involves three components:

i) controlling the fits and avoiding recurrence
ii) controlling the hypertension and
iii) fluid management

A. Controlling the convulsions Of the various drugs used for eclampsia, there is now compelling evidence in favour of magnesium sulphate, rather than diazepam or phenytoin (Collaborative Eclampsia Trial 1995). Magnesium sulphate should be given as a loading dose of 4 g intravenously over a period of 5–10 minutes followed by an infusion at a rate of 1 g per hour for at least 24 hours after the last seizure. Recurrent seizures should be treated by a further bolus of 2 g.

The therapy should be monitored by hourly assessment of patellar reflex, respiratory rate (and oxygen saturation by pulse oximetry when available) and urinary output. If toxicity is suspected, serum levels should be monitored. The therapeutic range is between 2 and 4 mmol/l. Any evident toxicity should be treated with 1 g intravenous calcium gluconate given over 10 minutes (RCOG 1999).

B. Control of hypertension Hydralazine, labetelol and nifedipine are the preferred drugs for controlling blood pressure. The aim of therapy is to gradually lower the blood pressure by 10 mmHg systolic and diastolic from pre-treatment levels and maintain mean arterial pressure below 125 mmHg (but not less than 105 mmHg) and diastolic pressure below 105 mmHg but not less than 90 mmHg (Gifford 1990; Paterson-Brown 1994).

The advocated dose for hydrallazine is 5 mg intravenously (IV), repeated every 20 minutes, up to a maximum of 20 mg. Labetalol can be given at 20 mg IV, escalating to 80 mg every 10 minutes, up to a maximum cumulative dose of 300 mg.

c. **Fluid management** To reduce the chances of iatrogenic complications, especially pulmonary edema, left ventricular failure and adult respiratory distress syndrome, both fluid input and output should be closely monitored (Osama and James 1999). Intravenous fluids should be given at a rate of 80 ml/hour (1 ml/kg/h) or the previous hour's urine output plus 30 ml (RCOG 1999). Fluid therapy should be limited to maintenance with the use of crystalloids.

Acute Uterine Inversion

Uterine inversion is a potentially life-threatening complication of childbirth that occurs in one in 2148–6407 births (Platt and Druzin 1981; Shah-Hosseini and Evrard 1989). It has also been known to occur at cesarean delivery. In a recent review, the incidence of acute inversion after vaginal delivery and cesarean section was found to be 1 in 3734 and 1 in 1860 patients, respectively (Baskett 2002). In a study period of 8 years, Hussain et al reported 36 acute uterine inversions following delivery, of which 75% were thought to be due to mismanagement of third stage of labour. Three of these patients died, while one needed a hysterectomy (Hussain et al 2004).

Management Acute uterine inversion may present with sudden collapse during the third stage of labour, with a degree of shock that is inconsistent with the visible blood loss. The classical presentation is of an obviously displaced uterus while delivering the placenta, usually in association with PPH and clinical shock (hypotension and inadequate tissue perfusion) (Beringer and Patteril 2004). The shock is thought to be neurogenic in origin, resulting from traction on the infundibulopelvic ligaments.

Management should be directed towards correcting hemorrhagic shock and uterine inversion. Manual reduction without anesthesia may be possible if inversion is recognised immediately.

Basic resuscitative measures such as maintaining the airway, breathing and circulation should be instituted. Hypovolemia should be corrected by administering intravenous crystalloids. An urgent request should be made for cross-matched blood. The amount of blood to be transfused should be determined by the estimated blood loss.

If the placenta is still adherent, it should be removed once the uterus is replaced back. The chances of immediate reduction is between 22% and 43% (Brar et al 1989; Abouliesh et al 1995). The methods for replacement include manual replacement, hydrostatic replacement and surgical correction.

Tocolysis and general anesthesia facilitate reduction, especially when the patient is severely hemodynamically compromised (Beringer and Patteril 2004). Various tocolytic agents have been advocated including magnesium sulphate, nitroglycerine and β_2-adrenergic agonists such as ritodrine or terbutaline. Terbutaline is recommended because of its rapid onset of action, short duration, simplicity, availability in the labour suite and familiarity to the obstetrician. General anesthesia with its inherent problems should be avoided in preference to regional anesthesia.

To prevent this potentially life-threatening condition, the personnel involved in caring for the pregnant women should be trained in managing the third stage of labour and recognising and managing uterine inversion.

Cardiac Arrest

Cardiac arrest occurs only once in every 30,000 late pregnancies, but survival from such an event is exceptional (Morris and Stacey 2003). Most units will thus only see a case once every 10–20 years and when it occurs, staff may be slow to respond (Clarke and Butt 2005).

Cardiac arrest during the postpartum period could result from a pre-existing cardiac condition, local anesthetic toxicity, total spinal anesthesia, electrocution or trauma. The woman should be tilted by 45° to avoid pressure on IVC and allow blood to return to the heart; ideally, the uterus should be emptied. This is the best chance of survival for the baby in the viable gestation period.

Morris et al have described the changes in pregnancy that weigh the balance against successful resuscitation. These include the anatomical and physiological changes peculiar to pregnancy. Early recognition and rapid response remains the key factors for a successful outcome. The Resuscitation Council (UK) has suggested that staff who come in contact with patients be given regular resuscitation training, appropriate to their expected abilities and care (Resuscitation Council 2004).

While BLS is being carried out, the cardiac team should be summoned and equipment and drugs for advanced life support should be assembled. Further management should involve the cardiac team with therapy directed towards the precipitating cause and probable management on the intensive therapy unit.

Women with known significant cardiac conditions should ideally have individualised care plans made during the antenatal period and are probably best managed in specialised centres with a multidisciplinary team approach.

Diabetic Ketoacidosis

Pregnancy is a diabetogenic condition. Diabetic ketoacidosis is a serious metabolic complication of diabetes that could prove fatal if not detected in time. With antepartum diabetes screening becoming routine and the availability of early and frequent prenatal care/surveillance, the incidence and outcome of diabetic ketoacidosis in pregnancy has vastly improved. However, it still remains a major clinical problem in pregnancy, since it tends to occur at lower blood glucose levels and more rapidly than in non-pregnant patients, often causing delay in the diagnosis (Kamalakannan et al 2003). A history of diabetes may be a clue to diagnosing the condition. Associated signs include hyperventilation, ketotic breath, tachycardia, hypotension, dry mucous membranes, disorientation and coma.

Management Women suspected of having diabetic ketoacidosis should be managed by a team consisting of an obstetrician and diabetologist. It needs prompt and vigorous treatment. Blood glucose levels should be measured along with arterial blood gases and electrolytes. Urine dipstick will reveal ketonuria and glycosuria.

The patient should be treated in an intensive therapy unit. Features in management include fluid replacement, insulin therapy and electrolyte replacement. A search for possible sources of infection should be performed. Urine and blood samples should be collected to diagnose any possible infective source (Chauhan and Perry 1995).

Prevention, early recognition and hospitalisation, and aggressive management remain the cornerstones for minimising the outcomes of this dreaded complication (Kamalakannan et al 2003).

Other Medical Conditions Leading To Collapse

Though rare, one should be aware of the neurological conditions for collapse. Prompt referral should be made to a neurologist for diagnosis and management where appropriate.

Ischemic Stroke and Transient Ischemic Attacks The incidence of pregnancy-associated ischemic stroke is approximately 3–4 cases/per 100,000 every year (Wiebers 1985). Internal carotid artery occlusions may be more common during the postpartum period, as opposed to middle cerebral artery occlusion during pregnancy (Carhuapoma et al 1999).

Cerebral Vein Thrombosis This condition usually occurs in the second or third week postpartum (Srinivasan 1983). The incidence is highest in developing countries where it is the most common cause of stroke associated with pregnancy. It has classically been associated with infection and dehydration.

The features of this condition include headache, vomiting, seizures, photophobia, impaired consciousness and signs of raised intracranial pressure. About 30–60% of patients display focal signs such as hemiparesis, which may be transient. It may cause fever and leukocytosis (Nelson-Piercy 2006).

Subarachnoid Hemorrhage Collapse may be preceded by severe, often occipital, headache of sudden onset associated with vomiting, neck stiffness, loss of (or impaired) consciousness and papilloedema. Focal neurological signs may also be present.

All of the abovementioned conditions will need to be investigated with computerised tomography (CT) scan or magnetic resonance imaging (MRI). These women should be managed by a team of obstetricians, neurologists and physiotherapists.

Key Features for Clinical Practice

- It is recommended that caregivers are trained in recognising and instituting BLS.
- Adequate training, including skills and drills sessions on a regular basis, should be conducted in all maternity departments. This should include communication to ensure a coordinated team approach.
- All maternity units should have protocols for maternal collapse which should be reviewed regularly.
- Active management of the third stage of labour could prevent significant blood loss during labour.
- Early recognition of PE and administering anticoagulants while awaiting objective confirmation of diagnosis is a good practice.
- A high index of suspicion of AFE should be entertained in the absence of other competing diagnoses.
- Appropriate management of the third stage of labour can help avoid uterine inversion.
- In cases with risk factors for septic shock, early commencement of broad-spectrum antibiotics and eradication of focus of infection should be given priority.
- Women with known cardiac conditions should have a plan of care made during the antenatal period and managed in specialised centres.
- Rare neurological conditions should be considered in the differential diagnosis and appropriate medical referral made.

References

American College of Obstetricians and Gynecologists. 1986. Management of preeclampsia. Am Coll of Obst and Gynecol, Technical Bulletin, no. 91

Abouliesh E, Ali V, Joumaa B, Lopez M and Gupta D. 1995. Anaesthetic management of acute puerperal uterine inversion. *Br J Anaesth* 75:486–7.

Atrash HK, LM Koonin, HW Lawson et al. 1990. Maternal mortality in the United States 1979–1986. *Obstet Gynecol* 76:1055–60.

Awad IT. 2001. Shorten GD: Amniotic fluid embolism and isolated coagulopathy: Atypical presentation of amniotic fluid embolism. *Eur J Anaesth* 18:410–413.

Baskett TF. 2002. Acute uterine inversion: a review of 40 cases. *J Obstet Gynaecol Can* 24:953–956.

Beringer RM and M Patteril. 2004. Puerperal uterine inversion and shock. *Br J Anaesth* 92 (3): 439–441.

Blanco JD, RS Gibbs and YS Costaneda. 1981. Bacteremia in obstetrics: clinical course. *Obstet Gynecol* 58:621–626.

Bloom AI, A Vertandig, Y Gielchinsky et al. 2004. Arterial embolisation for persistent primary postpartum haemorrhage: before or after hysterectomy? *Br J Obstet Gynaecol* 3:880–884.

Bonnar J. 2000. Massive Obstetric Haemorrhage. *Balliere's Clinical Obstetrics and Gynaecology* 14(1):1–18.

Brar HS, JS Greenspoon, LD Platt et al. 1989. Acute puerperal uterine inversion. New Approaches to Management. *J Repro Med* 34:173–177.

Burrows A and SK Khoo. 1995. The amniotic fluid embolism syndrome: 10 years experience at a major teaching hospital. *Aust NZ J Obstet Gynaecol* 35:245–250.

Capellier G, T Jacques, P Balvay, G Blasco, E Belle, F Barale F. 1997. Inhaled nitric oxide in patients with pulmonary embolism. *Intensive Care Med* 23: 1089–1092.

Cardiopulmonary Resuscitation. 2004. Standards for clinical practice and training. *Resuscitation Council (UK)*.

Carhuapoma JR, MW Tomlinson, SR Levine. 1999. Neurological diseases. In *High Risk Pregnancy Management Options*, 2nd ed, Philadelphia: WB Saunders, 809.

Chauhan SP and KG Perry Jr. 1995. Management of diabetic ketoacidosis in the obstetric patient. *Obstet Gynecol Clin North Am* 22:143–155.

Chong, Yap-Seng Su, Lin-Lin, S Arulkumaran. 2004. Current strategies for the prevention of postpartum haemorrhage in the third stage of labour *Curr Opin Obstet Gynaecol* 16(2)143–150.

Clark SL, GD Hankins, DA Dudley, GA Dildy and TF Porter. 1995. Amniotic fluid embolism: analysis of the national registry. *Am J Obstet Gynaecol* 172:1158–1169.

Clark SL. 1990. New concepts of amniotic fluid embolism: a review. *Obstet Gynecol Surv* 45:360–368.

Clarke J and M Butt. 2005. Maternal Collapse. *Curr Opin Obstet Gynecol* 17 (2):157–160.

Clinical green-top guidelines. 1999. Management of Eclampsia (10). London. *RCOG*

Cunningham FG, MacDonald PC and Gant NF. 1989. Hypertensive disorders in pregnancy. In *Williams Obstetrics,* 653–694

Dorne R, C Pommier, JC Emery et al. 2002. Amniotic fluid embolism: successful evolution course after uterine arteries embolization. *Ann Fr Anesth Reanim* 21:431–435.

Douglas KA and CWG Redman. 1994. Eclampsia in the United Kingdom. *Br Med J* 309:1395–1400.

Eclampsia Trial Collaborative Group. 1995. Which anticonvulsant for women with eclampsia?

Evidence from Collaborative Eclampsia Trial. *Lancet* 345: 1455–63.

Esposito RA, EA Grossi, G Coppa et al. 1990. Successful treatment of postpartum shock caused by amniotic fluid embolism with cardiopulmonary bypass and pulmonary artery thromboembolectomy. *Am J Obstet Gynecol* 163:572–574.

Floyd RC and JC Morrison. 1992. Postpartum haemorrhage. In, editors. *Surgical Obstetrics*, 373–382, eds WC Plauche, JC Morrison, MJ O'Sullivan. Philadelphia: WB Saunders.

Gifford RW, PA August, LC Chesley et al. 1990. National High Blood Pressure Education Program Working Group report on high blood pressure in pregnancy. *Am J Obstet Gynecol* 163:1689–1712.

Goldszmidt E and S Davies. 2004 Two cases of hemorrhage secondary to amniotic fluid embolism managed with uterine artery embolisation. *Can J Anaesth* 50:917–921.

Goodman PC. 1984. Pulmonary Angiography. *Clin Chest Med* 5:465–477.

Hansch E, U Chitkara, J McAlpine et al. 1999. Pelvic arterial embolisation for control of obstetric haemorrhage: a five year experience. *Am J Obstet Gynecol* 180:1454–1460.

Hsieh YY, CC Chang, PC Li et al. 2000. Successful application of extracorporeal membrane oxygenation and balloon counterpulsation as lifesaving therapy for a patient with amniotic fluid embolism. *Am J Obstet Gynecol* 183:496–497.

Hussain M, T Jabeen, N Liaquat, K Noorani, SZ Bhutta. 2004. Acute puerperal uterine inversion. *J Coll Physicians Surg Pak* 14(4):215–217.

Kamalakannan D, V Baskar, DM Barton et al. 2003. Diabetic ketoacidosis in pregnancy. *Postgrad Medical Journal* 79:454–457.

Kanayama N, T Yamazaki, H Naruse et al. 1992. Determining zinc coproporphyrin in maternal plasma—a new method for diagnosing amniotic fluid embolism. *Clin Chem* 38:526–529.

Kaneko Y, T Ogihara, H Tajima et al. 2001. Continuous hemodiafiltration for disseminated intravascular coagulation and shock due to amniotic fluid embolism: report of a dramatic response. *Intern Med* 40:945–947.

Kobayashi H, H Ohi, T Terao. 1993. A simple, noninvasive, sensitive method for diagnosis of amniotic fluid embolism by monoclonal antibody TKH-2 that recognizes NeuAc[alpha]2-6GalNAc. *Am J Obstet Gynecol* 168:848–853.

Lee W, SL Clark, DB Cotton, B Gonik, J Phelan, S Faro, R Giebel. 1988. Septic shock during pregnancy. *Am J of Obstet Gynecol* 159(2):410–416.

Why Mothers Die? 2000–2002. The Confidential Enquiries into Maternal Deaths in the United Kingdom. Lewis G and Drife J, ed. CEMACH.

Lim Y, CC Loo, V Chia et al. 2004. Recombinant factor VIIa after amniotic fluid embolism and disseminated intravascular coagulopathy. *Int J Gynaecol Obstet* 87(2):178–179.

Lynch CB, A Coker, AH Laval et al. 1997. The B-Lynch surgical technique for control of massive postpartum haemorrhage: an alternative to hysterectomy? Five cases reported. *Br J Obstet Gynaecol* 104:372–376.

Mabie WC, JR Barton, B Sibai. 1997. Septic shock in pregnancy. *Obstet Gynecol* 90:553–561.

Martin, W Rick. 1996. Amniotic fluid embolism. *Clin Obstet Gynecol* T39(1):101–106.

Mabie WC. 1994. Amniotic fluid embolism. In *Maternal-fetal Medicine: Principles and Practice* 3rd ed, 744–6, eds RK Creasy and R Resnik. Philadelphia: WB Saunders.

Marcovici I and JM Ferretti. 1997. Septic shock in pregnancy: a case report. *Am J Obstet Gynecol* 177(6):1556–1557.

Mathew R, RS Raj, P Sudha P. 2003. Late postpartum eclampsia without prodroma, 51:539–540.

Morris S and M Stacey. 2003. Resuscitaion in Pregnancy. *Br Med J* 327:1277–1279.

Nelson-Piercy C. 2006. Differential diagnoses of medical problems in pregnancy. In *Handbook of Obstetric Medicine,* 2nd ed, Martin Dunitz, 300.

Nolan J. 2001. Advanced Life Support Course Provider Manual, 4th ed (revised) 4:19–30, Elsevier.

Osama S and JW James. 1999. Modern management of eclampsia. *Postgrad Med J* 75:78–82.

Palla A, S Petruzzelli, V Donnamaria, C Giuntini. 1995. The role of suspicion in the diagnosis of pulmonary embolism. *Chest* (suppl)21S–24S: 107.

Park RC and WP Duff. 1980. Role of caesarean hysterectomy in modern obstetric practice. *Clin Obstet Gynecol* 23:601–620.

Paterson-Brown S, SC Robson, N Redfern et al. 1994. Hydralazine boluses for the treatment of severe hypertension in pre-eclampsia. *Br J Obstet Gynaecol* 101:409–413.

Pelage JP, O Le Dref, J Mateo et al. 1998. Life threatening primary postpartum haemorrhage: treatment with emergency selective arterial embolisation. *Radiology* 208:359–362.

RCOG 2001. Green-top Guideline. Thromboembolic disease in pregnancy and the puerperium: acute management (28). London: Royal College of Obstetricians and Gynaecologists.

Platt LD and ML Druzin. 1981. Acute puerperal inversion of the uterus. *Am J Obstet Gynecol* 141: 187–90.

Plauche WC. 1992. Peripartal hysterectomy. In *Surgical Obstetrics*, 447–65, eds WC Plauche, JC Morrison, MJ O'Sullivan. Philadelphia: WB Saunders.

Seror J, C Allouche, S Elhaik S. 2005. Use of Sengstaken-Blakemore tube in massive postpartum hemorrhage: a series of 17 cases. *Acta Obstet et Gynecol Scand* 84(7):660–664.

Shah-Hosseini R and JR Evrard. 1989. Puerperal uterine inversion. *Obstet Gynecol* 73:567–570.

Sibai BM, JM Schneider, JC Morrison et al. 1980. The late postpartum eclampsia controversy. *Obstet Gynecol* 55:74–78.

Srinivasan K. 1983. Cerebral venous and arterial thrombosis in pregnancy and peurperium: a study of 135 patients. *Angiology* 34:731–746.

Still DK. 1999. Postpartum haemorrhage and other third stage problems. In *High risk pregnancy management options*, eds DK James, PJ Steer, CP Weiner and B Gonik. London: WB Saunders.

Tanus-Santos JE and Moreno Jr H. 1999. Inhaled nitric oxide and amniotic fluid embolism. *Anesth Analg* 88:691.

Tewari K, SM Wold, T Asrat. 1997. Septic shock in pregnancy associated with legionella pneumonia: case report. *Am J Obstet Gynecol* 176(3):706–707.

Thomas SV. 1998. Neurological aspects of eclampsia. *J Neurol Sci* 155:37–43.

Thomson AJ and IA Greer. 2000. Non-haemorrhagic obstetric shock. *Balliere's Clinical Obstetrics and Gynaecology* 14 (I):19–41.

Tuffnell Derek J. 2003. Amniotic fluid embolism. *Curr Opin Obstet Gynecol* 15(2):119–122.

van Heerden PV, SAR Webb, G Hee, M Corkeron, WR Thompson WR. 1996. Inhaled aerosolized prostacylin as a selective pulmonary vasodilator for the treatment of severe hypoxaemia. *Anaesth Intensive Care* 24: 87–90.

Vedantham S, SC Goodwin, B McLucas, G Mohr. 1997. Uterine artery embolisation: an underused method of controlling pelvic haemorrhage. *Am J Obstet Gynecol* 176:938–948.

Wiebers D. 1985. Ischemic cerebrovascular complications of pregnancy. *Archives of Neurology* 42: 1106–1113.

39

Fetal Therapy

Soma Mukherjee | Shanthi Sairam | BaskaranThilaganathan | Amar Bhide

The ability to correct problems while the fetus is still in utero is the dream that fetal medicine is striving for, although it is far from being realised. The treatment of rhesus allo-immunisation using intrauterine transfusion in the 1960s could be seen as the beginning of invasive fetal therapy. Despite an increasing volume of literature advocating the use of fetal therapy, there is still a lack of high quality evidence from randomised controlled trials supporting fetal therapy. There is a need for more trials such as in the Eurofetus Twin to Twin Transfusion Study, so that data from them can be useful in management.

Fetal therapy should only be delivered in tertiary referral centres with a large patient base, so that experience and skills can be developed. Audit and research should produce progress within the field.

Ethical Considerations of Fetal Therapy

Fetal therapy can be broadly divided into four categories:

1. Transplacental drug treatment
2. Invasive procedures
3. Fetal surgery
4. Gene therapy

The key areas of ethical concern are balance of potential benefit and harm, autonomy and informed consent, duty of the doctor to the mother and duty of the doctor to the fetus.

Fetal therapy could be justified when:

- there is reasonable certainty that the fetus will suffer substantial harm without intervention
- the intervention has been shown to be effective
- the risk to the health and well-being of the mother is negligible
- the parents can give informed consent to the intervention

Fetal therapy should be provided in a multidisciplinary setting with clear strategies and good communication on diagnostic, therapeutic and care needs of the mother and the fetus. Some interventions such as administration of antenatal steroids to prevent hyaline membrane disease and zidovudine to prevent perinatal transmission of HIV infection are accepted practices of proven efficacy. Thus, invasive fetal therapy should be recommended only when it has a realistic chance of saving the life of the fetus or preventing serious and irreversible disease or disability. Clinicians should respect maternal choice and limitations with assessment of risk; which is not always easy to define or quantify relative to the perceived potential benefits. Counselling of parents should ensure that they understand possible outcomes and have the necessary support after the birth of their baby (Noble and Rodeck 2008).

Fetal Blood Sampling and Intravascular Therapy

Fetal blood sampling provides access to the fetal vascular compartment for both diagnostic and therapeutic purposes (Colour plate 14). The sampling is usually performed from the umbilical vein in the cord either at the placental or fetal end. Other sampling sites include the intra-hepatic part of the umbilical vein or the fetal heart.

Indications: The indications for fetal blood sampling include

Diagnostic Indications (Refer Chapter 3):

1. Chromosome abnormalities and single gene defects
2. Fetal anemia and thrombocytopenia
3. Hypoxia/acidosis
4. Fetal infection

Therapeutic Indications

1. Treatment of fetal anemia or thrombocytopenia
2. Treatment of fetal arrhythmia
3. Administration of drugs such as strong potassium chloride for fetocide, selective termination for abnormalities and multifetal pregnancy reduction.

Technique: Fetal blood sampling was originally carried out in the 1960s under fetoscopic guidance, but this was associated with 2% to 5% risk of pregnancy loss (Weiner 1998). More recently, it has been established that needling the umbilical vein under real time ultrasound guidance is much safer and is the preferred technique.

Cordocentesis is usually carried out after 18 weeks of gestation as the risk of fetal loss is higher prior to this gestation (Orlandi et al 1990; Buscaglia et al 1996; Ulm et al 1997). The preferred sampling site is at the placental cord insertion. A free loop of cord would be difficult to puncture, as the needle would push the cord away. Needling the umbilical vein at the umbilical end would be prone to failure without the use of fetal paralysis. The fetal heart is usually punctured for fetocide or for emergency transfusions. Some operators use the intra-hepatic portion of the umbilical vein for this purpose.

Cordocentesis may be carried out with either a needle guide mounted on the transducer or using a free-hand technique. In either case, a good length of umbilical vein is visualised and the needle is advanced with the entire needle in vision (Colour plate 16). Once in the vein, an assistant would be required to withdraw the needle stilet and fix a syringe and aspirate the required sample or attach the infusion line for transfusions.

After completing the procedure, it is important to observe for prolonged bleeding from the puncture site and for changes in the heart rate especially after fetal transfusions.

Complications: Transient bleeding from the puncture is commonly seen and settles spontaneously, within 10–15 seconds. Life-threatening complications like cord hematomas, prolonged bleeding and fetal bradycardia occur in about 1% to 2% of cases. These complications are more likely to be related to the indications for the procedure such as fetal transfusions, hydrops fetalis, severe growth restriction and multiple fetal abnormalities (Weiner 1991; Donne 1994).

Laboratory Analysis: The rapidly dividing white blood cells allow the analysis of the karyotype completely, including banding within 48–72 hours from the fetal blood sample. Transfusion of red blood cells in the setting of rhesus isoimmunisation in the fetus is the second common indication for cordocentesis. This procedure emerged from the finding that extrapolation of the amniotic fluid Δ OD 450 values from the original Liley charts for the second trimester resulted in false assessments of fetal anemia (Nicolaides 1986). Thus, the only way to determine fetal hemoglobin levels was to perform cordocentesis and plan a transfusion. More recently, middle cerebral artery Doppler indices are being used to ascertain the level of hemoglobin deviation from the median to time the transfusion (Delle et al 2001; Deren and Onderoglu 2002). Cordocentesis to assess the fetal platelet count is invaluable in the management of pregnancies complicated by idiopathic or alloimmune thrombocytopenia (Greaves and Letsky 1997). It helps in assessing the need for fetal platelet transfusion and also the mode and place of delivery.

Fetal and Neonatal Alloimmune Thrombocytopenia

Fetal and neonatal alloimmune thrombocytopenia (FNAIT) is one of the major causes of severe thrombocytopenia and intracranial hemorrhage (ICH) in fetuses and term neonates. The incidence is one in 1 in 2000 births. FNAIT is caused by maternal Ig G allo-antibodies, which cross the placenta and are directed against human platelet antigens (HPA) on fetal platelets.

The incidence of thrombocytopenia (platelet count <150 x 10^9/l) is 1% to 4%. The mechanism of FNAIT is the platelet equivalent of Rhesus disease but it can occur in a severe form in the first pregnancy.

As most countries do not have a screening programme, women are identified as at risk only after a previous pregnancy was affected with FNAIT. In 1984, Daffos et al published the successful use of FBS in obtaining the fetal platelet count at 34 weeks followed by an intrauterine platelet transfusion (IUPT) at 37 weeks, followed by a cesarean section (Daffos et al 1984). Complication rates of FBS and IUPT in FNAIT pregnancies was 1.6% fetal loss and 2.4% other complications (Radder et al 2003). Recent studies showed a 6% fetal loss rate directly related to IUPT (Overton et al 2002; Birchall et al 2003; Berkowitz et al 2006).

Bussel et al in 1988 were the first to report the use of maternal administration of intravenous gammaglobulin (IVIg) 1.0 g/kg/week in the treatment of FNAIT. The long-term side effects are still unknown as IVIG is known for its immuno-modulating properties. An international multicentre study (the NOICH study) is currently underway.

Though cesarean section is often the mode of delivery in FNAIT pregnancies, the optimal treatment strategy is unclear (Van den Akker and Oepkes 2008).

Fetoscopy

Fetoscopy is a technique that allows direct visualisation of the fetus and the intrauterine environment during pregnancy through small diameter endoscopes. Visual access to the fetus has allowed the development of fetoscopic surgical procedures. Obviously, fetoscopy should only be used in a selected number of pregnancy complications affecting the fetus which may benefit from the use of this technique. Fetoscopy can be used for diagnostic or therapeutic purposes.

Operative fetoscopy is used to perform operations on the fetus, the cord, placenta or membranes. In some very rare conditions, an operation on the fetus may save its life or prevent irreversible significant sequelae. Fetoscopic procedures allow operating on the fetus through minimally invasive access. One or more small diameter instruments can be introduced in the uterus and several procedures

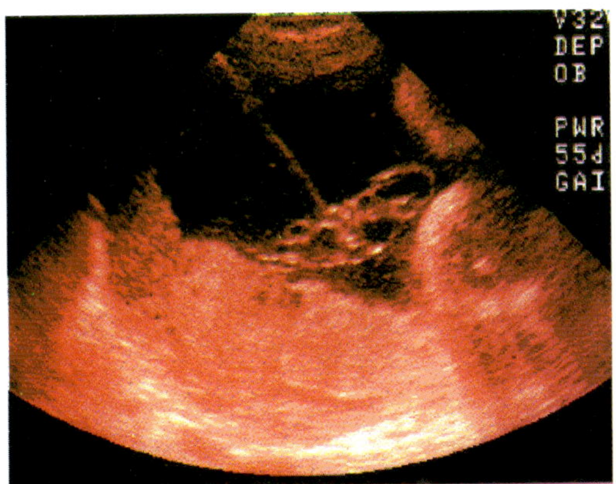

Colour plate 14: Cordocentesis with the needle in the umbilical vein at the placental insertion in a posterior placenta

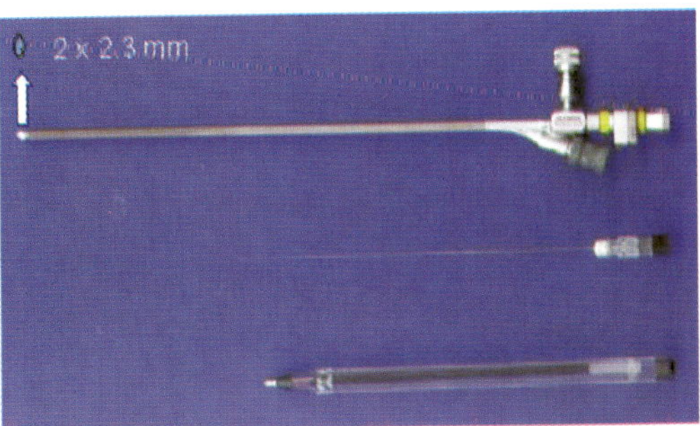

Colour plate 15: The fetoscope in comparison to the sizes of a spinal needle and a common pen. The diameter of the scope is included.

can be performed. The main indication for operative fetoscopy is laser ablation in twin to twin transfusion syndrome (TTTS). Other indications include cord occlusion in acardiac twins, lysis of bands in amniotic band syndrome, application of tracheal plugs/ clips in congenital diaphragmatic hernia, cord ligation in monoamniotic twins.

Technique: The fetoscope is introduced into the amniotic cavity under local anesthesia with the help of a trocar, under ultrasound guidance. Endoscopes with diameters ranging from 1.2 to 2.3 mm are available with fiber-optic lenses (Colour plate 15). The fetoscope is connected to a good quality light source and a video camera. Although diagnostic fetoscopy can be carried out in a natural amniotic fluid environment, operative procedures may require distension media such as normal saline for better visualisation of the operating area. The fetoscopes have additional channels that can be used for introducing laser fibres and also for use as irrigation systems. Additional ports may rarely be needed in some procedures and these are inserted as in a laparoscopy.

The advantages of operative fetoscopy over open fetal surgery would include:

- Minimal skin or uterine incision
- Minimal maternal blood loss
- Minimal discomfort
- Minimal uterine irritation
- Minimal disturbance to the pregnancy
- Does not affect mode of delivery (a cesarean section is not indicated because of having had the surgery)

Fetoscopic surgery for fetal tumours and hernias are currently research areas and are performed in selected centres. The position of the placenta and the fetus may sometimes pose a problem for a fetoscopic approach, although in most cases it can be overcome. The role of fetoscopy in TTTS will be discussed below as other procedures are performed less commonly or as experimental techniques.

Twin to Twin Transfusion Syndrome: The role of operative fetoscopy is well established in the treatment of complications of monochorionic twin pregnancies, in most fetal medicine centres. Severe TTTS complicates about 10% to 15% of monochorionic twin pregnancies and is associated with >90% risk of perinatal mortality. The diagnosis is usually made in monochorionic twins when there is ultrasound evidence of worsening poly-oligohydramnios sequence with significant differences in the size of the bladder between the donor and the recipient. The reduction in the liquor volume in the donor sac results in that twin being 'stuck'. Active management of TTTS has included aggressive therapeutic amnioreduction and laser photocoagulation of inter-twin vascular anastomoses. Fetoscopic laser ablation is a safe and effective form of treatment in the management of severe TTTS with significant advantages over aggressive serial amniodrainage. The fetal survival rate of pregnancies managed by serial aggressive amnioreduction has been reported to be 60% to 70% but serious neurologic handicap can occur in 15% to 50% of survivors (Pinette et al 1993; Trespidi et al 1997). Although fetoscopic laser ablation is associated with survival rates similar to serial amniodrainage, studies have reported significantly reduced neonatal neurologic morbidity (Ville et al 1998; Hecher et al 1999). The use of this technique has a reported overall survival rate of 60% to 70% with suspicious lesions on neonatal brain scans in 5% to 6% of infants (Hecher et al 1999; Thilaganathan et al 2000). A large randomised controlled trial has clearly shown that fetoscopic laser photocoagulation of the intercommunicating vessels is superior to serial amniodrainage in the treatment of TTTS with a higher survival rate and lower risk of neurological handicap (Senat et al 2004).

Complications: The most important complication is loss of one or both twins. Loss of both twins is usually caused by rupture of membranes or miscarriage. Other rare complications include incomplete ablation of intercommunicating vessels requiring a repeat procedure, placental abruption, maternal hemorrhage from the uterine puncture site, amniotic fluid embolism and amniotic bands following the procedure.

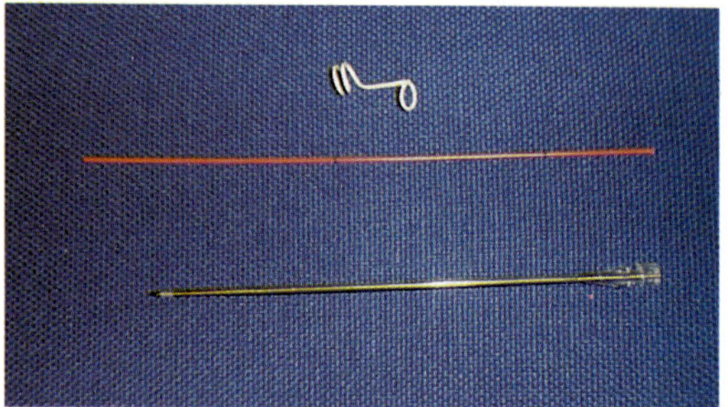

COLOUR PLATE 16: INSTRUMENTATION FOR FETAL SHUNT SHOWS THE TROCAR, THE PUSHER AND THE PIG-TAIL CATHETER.

Interstitial Laser

There have been sporadic case reports of the use of percutaneous ultrasound guided laser therapy for photocoagulation of vessels in an acardiac twin and also for ablation of congenital cystic adenomatoid malformation of the fetal lung. It has also been used anecdotally in placental chorioangiomas. The technique involves the introduction of a 17-gauge needle into the target transabdominally. The laser fibre is then introduced through its lumen to reach the tissue and photocoagulation carried out. Although the initial results are promising, the side effects and safety of this procedure remains to be determined (Bruner et al 2000; Jolly et al 2001).

Fetal Shunts

The introduction of ultrasound guided fetal shunting procedures in the 1980s appeared to enhance the profile of invasive fetal therapy initially. However, the relative lack of information about the natural history of the conditions and the poor selection criteria of cases resulted in disappointing results.

Hydrocephalus: The introduction of ventriculo-amniotic shunting for fetal hydrocephalus by Clewell in 1982 was based on the observations that shunting for hydrocephalus in the newborn period improved the neurologic outcome. However, it was disappointing to find that most studies in fact highlighted worse outcome in fetuses that underwent shunting (Manning et al 1986). This was due to the presence of unidentified associated CNS anomalies and also due to the underlying pathophysiology such as migration disorders that may not be reversed merely by shunting. Currently, shunting for hydrocephalus is not performed.

Fetal obstructive uropathy: Prenatal intervention for fetal urinary tract obstruction was first described in 1981 in San Francisco. Presence of amniotic fluid around the fetus between 16 and 26 weeks is essential for normal lung development. Fetuses with likely bladder outlet obstruction have a high fetal mortality rate in the absence of any intervention. Neonatal death due to severe pulmonary hypoplasia is a common sequel. Relieving the obstruction to the urinary bladder has the potential of allowing normal lung development and preventing further renal damage. Several authors have attempted to identify fetuses with relatively well-preserved renal function of prenatal intervention. The candidate tests included biochemical analysis of the fetal urine, measurement of urinary osmolality and beta-2 macroglobulin. None of these have emerged as reliable predictors.

Prenatal intervention by placement of vesico-amniotic shunt improves survival in the subgroup with predicted poor outcome (Clarke et al 2003). However, there are significant long-term problems in survivors. End-stage renal disease requiring renal transplant is necessary in 30% to 40% of survivors within the first two years of life. Moreover, significant proportions of children suffer from voiding difficulties and have to rely on intermittent self-catheterisation (Freedman et al 1999). Gender re-assignment may be necessary with associated cloacal abnormalities.

There is a reasonable incidence of chromosomal abnormalities with obstructive uropathy. Fetal karyotyping should be considered. Vesico-amniotic shunting and vesicocentesis was first reported by Golbus et al (1982) and is the commonest method used to relieve urinary tract obstruction. The procedure involves placing a double pig-tailed catheter into the fetal bladder percutaneously, under local anesthesia and ultrasound guidance (Colour plate 16). Postnatal management involves an ultrasound in the first week of life, repeated at 4–6 weeks of age and antibiotic prophylaxis.

PLUTO is a randomised controlled trial which is ongoing and designed to investigate the role of vesico-amniotic shunting in fetuses with moderate or severe lower urinary tract obstruction (Kilby 2007).

Hydrothorax: The management of fetal hydrothorax is based on the high perinatal mortality and morbidity associated with this finding, due to its adverse effect on lung development. Thoraco-amniotic shunting to relieve intrathoracic pressure was first reported by Rodeck et al in 1988 and appears to have promising results in isolated primary cases of fetal hydrothorax. However, current literature fails to differentiate the primary from secondary hydrothoraces and hence the results appear to be disappointing. Most authors agree that the presence of associated hydrops is indicative of a poor outcome. Eliminating cases of secondary hydrothoraces, survival rates of 92% may be achieved (Nicolaides and Azar 1990; Morin et al 1994). The successful management with thoraco-amniotic shunts depends as in most other situations, on the correct selection of patients. It would be prudent to exclude other possible underlying causes such as chromosomal abnormalities or fetal infections prior to considering a thoraco-amniotic shunt. Ahmad et al (1996) from their experience conclude that in appropriate cases, thoraco-amnitoic shunting may result in resolution of fetal hydrops and prevent intrauterine death. This is likely to be effective in isolated cases of chylothorax. An alternative option for fetuses with hydrothorax at an advanced gestation would be thoracocentesis with the possibility of delivery within the next few weeks. The likelihood of serial drainage and the associated increase in the risk of iatrogenic preterm prelabour rupture of membranes is to be borne in mind if thoracocentesis is chosen.

Technique: In general, the placement of a shunt involves the introduction of a trocar (Colour plate 16), under ultrasound guidance at the appropriate maternal abdominal site, under local anesthesia. Some operators prefer to paralyse the fetus prior to this to reduce fetal movements during the procedure. The trocar is then advanced into the fetal thorax or bladder. The stilet of the trocar is then withdrawn and the guide with the self-retaining pig-tail catheter and the pusher is then introduced into the target site. Gentle withdrawal of the guide wire alternating with the pusher allows correct placement of the shunt with the outer end of the shunt draining into the amniotic cavity (Figs 39.1, 39.2).

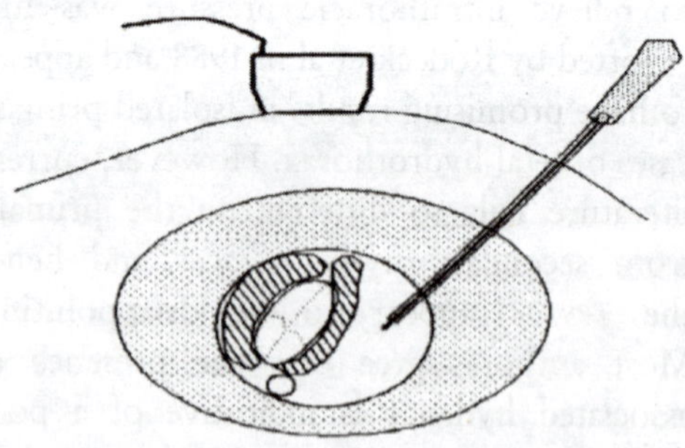

Figure 39.1: Schematic diagram showing the placement of the trocar in the pleural cavity in the fetal chest, under ultrasound guidance. The lung tissue is compressed due to the hydrothorax.

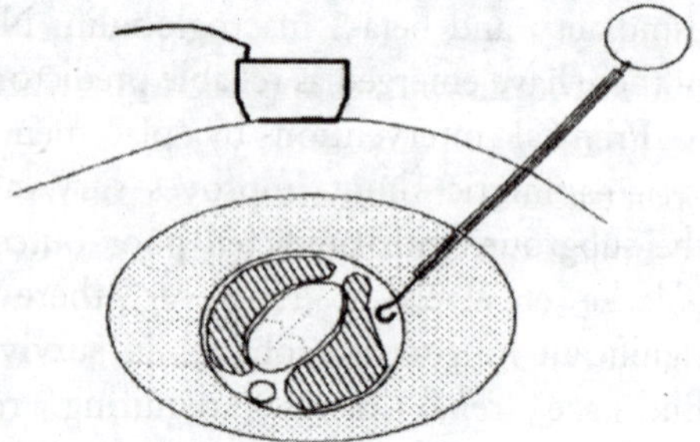

Figure 39.2: Schematic diagram showing the pigtail catheter being introduced into the pleural cavity. The lung has expanded as some of the fluid has been drained by the trocar.

AMNIO-INFUSION

Oligohydramnios is historically associated with increased incidence of adverse perinatal outcome (Sherer and Langer 2001). Amnioinfusion is a relatively recent technique in fetal medicine, used either intrapartum or antepartum. Intrapartum amnioinfusion is performed in cases with oligohydramnios to reduce the risk of cord compression. A recent meta-analysis by Pitt et al (2000) evaluated 35 randomised controlled trials and concluded that prophylactic intrapartum amnioinfusion significantly improved the neonatal outcome and reduced the rate of cesarean delivery without increasing the incidence of postpartum endometritis. However, the role of antepartum amnioinfusion remains unclear. Several authors have advocated the use of diagnostic amnioinfusion to enhance visualisation of fetal structures (Fisk et al 1991; Pryde et al 2000). The potential for antepartum amnioinfusion as a therapeutic technique to improve the outcome of pregnancies with oligohydramnios appears to be limited.

Fetal Surgery

Elaborate research on animal models to study the natural history and pathophysiology of some life-threatening congenital abnormalities has been carried out over the last two decades. This has resulted in open and endoscopic fetal surgery offering higher chances of survival for those conditions, which would otherwise have extremely poor prognosis. Fetal surgery has been attempted for a variety of congenital abnormalities and is currently recognised only as a research tool.

Congenital diaphragmatic hernia: Congenital diaphragmatic hernia (CDH) occurs in approximately 1:2200 births. In isolated CDH, mortality is 20% to 30%, mainly from lung hypoplasia. The prognostic indicators include gestational age at diagnosis, development of polyhydramnios, large defects with the liver in the chest, mediastinal shift and poor fetal cardiac function. Of these, the presence of liver in the chest (liver-up) confers the worst prognosis with a high mortality, primarily due to pulmonary hypoplasia. Based on the findings of Wilson et al in 1993 that pulmonary hypoplasia can be prevented by tracheal occlusion, two approaches for tracheal occlusion have emerged. The first involves open tracheal clipping after hysterotomy. The complications associated with hysterotomy and open surgery severely compromised the survival. The second approach was far less invasive with a tracheal clip or plug placed using a fetoscope. Obstructing the outflow of fetal lung fluid would accelerate the lung development, gradually reduce the herniation of abdominal structures (stomach and intestine) and prevent pulmonary hypoplasia. At birth, the clip or plug needs to be removed while the placental circulation is still operative. This involves 'EXIT' technique (ex utero intrapartum treatment), where removal of the clip/plug is carried out at cesarean section prior to complete extraction of the fetus from the uterine incision. The fetoscopic approach is preferred as it is less invasive. One trial had to be discontinued prematurely, because of unexpectedly high (77%) survival in the control (predicted 'poor survival') arm (Harrisson 2003). The interest in this approach still continues, and another European randomised controlled trail is underway.

Myelomeningocele: Myelomeningocele is a common birth defect that is associated with significant lifelong morbidity. Despite improvements in technology and overall patient care, little progress has been made in the postnatal surgical management of a child with spina bifida. Postnatal surgery is aimed at covering the exposed spinal cord and preventing infection. Although myelomeningocele is a non-lethal fetal anomaly, the limitations with current postnatal treatment strategies have led to extensive investigation of prenatal treatment options. Intrauterine closure of exposed spinal cord tissue has been shown to prevent secondary neurologic injury in animals with a surgically created spinal defect. It remains to be seen whether in utero repair of myelomeningocele actually improves outcome in infants with spina bifida. Bruner et al (2000) demonstrated that in their study, the requirement for ventriculoperitoneal shunt postnatally was significantly decreased in the group that underwent in utero surgery. However, treatment necessitated open fetal surgery, and the study group had a high risk of oligohydramnios and preterm delivery. Holmes et al (2001) concluded from their study of six patients that the urodynamic parameters and the urinary tract abnormalities were similar whether the spinal defect was corrected in utero or postnatally. The risk of preterm delivery was high in the study group. Fetal intervention for spinal defect is not justified at present (Cochrane et al 2001). A randomised prospective trial (the MOMS trial) is being conducted by three centres in the USA and is expected to be completed in 2009 (Sutton 2008).

MISCELLANEOUS

There are several fetal conditions such as cystic adenomatoid malformation of the lung, sacrococcygeal teratoma and complex cardiac malformations that have been managed with either open or endoscopic fetal surgery and have shown promising results. However, the risk–benefit ratio for the mother with an affected fetus and the long-term benefits remain to be determined.

Fetal dysrhythmias: Fetal dysrhythmias are common (2% of pregnancies); often due to ectopic beats which are benign and do not require treatment. But some fetal cardiac dysrhythmias are potentially life threatening conditions. Intermittent extrasystoles do not require treatment, but sustained forms of brady- and tachyarrhythmias might require intervention. Fetal echocardiography is essential to diagnosis, allows exclusion of any underlying CHD and also monitors fetal response to therapy.

The commonest form of supraventricular tachycardia (SVT) is caused by an atrioventricular re-entry circuit and should be differentiated from atrial flutter and atrial ectopic tachycardia. Sustained tachycardia may lead to the development of congestive cardiac failure and hydrops fetalis, particularly if the fetal heart rate is persistently over 220 bpm. Prompt treatment with anti-arrhythmic drugs or delivery should be considered.

Transplacental therapy is the preferred route and is often effective in treating heart failure. Flecainide, digoxin and sotalol are safe and are commonly used. Baseline maternal ECG should be performed and it is also advisable to check serum electrolytes, maternal serum levels of the drug and liver and renal function tests. Fetal mortality rate of < 10% has been reported in a large series of fetal tachy-arrhythmia (Gembrugh 2003).

Persistent fetal bradycardia with complete heart block can be associated with maternal anti-Ro/La autoantibodies. The use of steroids may be justified in cases of partial heart block but there is no firm evidence that they are an effective form of treatment. If hydrops develops, fetal morbidity and mortality are high. Sympathomimetics (terbutaline, salbutamol) have been used to increase heart rate with limited success. Direct fetal pacing has been attempted (Api and Carvalho 2008).

Management of Fetal Tumours

Fetal tumours are rare, with a prevalence of less than 1 in 10,000 live births. The majority have intrauterine surveillance as the primary form of management, but when hydrops develops, in utero therapy may be needed.

Sacrococcygeal teratomas require regular growth scans due to their potential for rapid growth and fetal echocardiograms to monitor cardiac output with large tumours. The majority require delivery after 33–34 weeks by cesarean section.

Chorioangiomas are benign vascular tumours of the placenta. They are encapsulated, round and intraplacental and the commonest primary tumour of the placenta. Ultrasound appearances are of a hyperechoic mass within the placenta, protruding into the amniotic cavity near the placental cord insertion site, seen after 20 weeks of gestation. They may act as an arteriovenous shunt, resulting in fetal anemia, hydrops and polyhydramnios. The fetus is usually structurally normal.

Doppler surveillance of the middle cerebral artery peak systolic velocity allows identification of fetal anemia with treatment by intrauterine transfusion, thus preventing fetal hydrops from developing (Wilson 2008).

Gene Therapy

Gene therapy uses the intracellular delivery of genetic material for the treatment of disease. As the fetus is immunologically immature, gene therapy in utero would make the fetus tolerant to the missing gene product and restore proper protein function. Research shows that gene transfer to the developing fetus targets rapidly expanding populations of stem cells, which are inaccessible after birth, and indicates that the use of integrating vector systems results in permanent gene transfer. Application of this therapy in the fetus must be shown to be safe, reliable and cost-effective. More research needs to be done before it can be introduced as therapy (David and Peebles 2008). A vector is used to deliver the genes into the appropriate cell, either somatic or germ cells.

Fetal gene therapy has been proposed to be appropriate for life-threatening disorders such as cystic fibrosis and Duchenne muscular dystrophy, in which prenatal gene delivery maintains a clear advantage over cell transplantation or postnatal gene therapy and for which there are currently no satisfactory treatments available (Wilson and Wivel 1999). The ideal vector for fetal gene therapy would introduce a transcriptionally regulated gene into all organs relevant to the genetic disorder by a single safe application. Minimally invasive techniques such as ultrasound-guided injection or even fetoscopy could be used to deliver gene therapy to the fetus with less morbidity and mortality.

In the human fetus, the immune system develops from 12 to 14 weeks. So, it would be necessary to deliver gene therapy before this gestational age, which limits the routes of application that can be used safely. Risks of fetal gene therapy include insertional mutagenesis, vector toxicity, fetal immune response, maternal and fetal morbidity and mortality. Germ-line transmission is another concern.

Fetal gene therapy could give parents another option when the prenatal diagnosis of inherited disease is given to them. Currently the choices available to them are either termination of the affected pregnancy or accepting the birth of an affected child. A prenatal gene-therapy procedure will have to be extremely safe, reliable and effective at treating the disease (Contelle and Rodeck 2002). Any such procedure poses the risks of infection, immune reactions and the onset of preterm labour for the fetus and the potential of harm to the mother.

Currently, fetal gene therapy remains an experimental procedure. There is a need for a better understanding of the development of genetic disease in the fetus and improved vector design before it is applied in clinical practice.

Fetal Stem-cell Transplantation

Stem cells are totipotent cells, capable of differentiating into any mature cell type. Fetal stem-cell transplantation is an attractive alternative in the treatment of hematological, metabolic and immunological diseases before birth. The first attempt was made by Davies in 1967 and the first success by Touraine in 1989.

Fetal tolerance is the inability to raise an immunological response against foreign antigens. The developing immune system in the fetus learns to distinguish between autologous and foreign antigens and, if introduced early enough, foreign antigens are recognised as 'self' and not rejected (Billingham et al 2003). Although successfully used in hemoglobinopathies after birth, the most successful group of patients transplanted in utero are fetuses with immunodeficiencies.

The ethical issues are complex and the possibility is raised only if the parents have decided not to terminate the pregnancy (Tiblad and Westgren 2008).

REFERENCES

Ahmad FK, SJ Sherman, KH Hagglund, MP Johnson and E Krivchenia. 1996. Isolated unilateral fetal pleural effusion: the role of sonographic surveillance and in utero therapy. *Fetal Diagn Ther* 11(6): 383–389.

Api O and JS Carvalho. 2008. Fetal dysrhythmias. *Best Prac Res Clin Obstet Gynaecol.* 22(1): 31–48.

Berkowitz RL, EA Kolb, JG McFarland et al. 2006. Parallel randomized trials of risk-based therapy for fetal alloimmune thrombocytopenia. *Obstet Gynecol* 107: 91–96.

Billingham RE, L Brent and PB Medawar. 2003. 'Actively acquired tolerance' of foreign cells. 1953. *Transplantation* 76: 1409–1412.

Birchall JE and MF Nurphy, C Kaplan et al. 2003. European collaborative study of the antenatal management of feto-maternal alloimmune thrombocytopenia. *Br J Haematol* 122: 275–288.

Bruner JP, BK Jarnagin and L Reinisch. 2000. Percutaneous laser ablation of fetal congenital cystic adenomatoid malformation: too little, too late? *Fetal Diagn Ther* 15(6): 359–363

Bruner JP, N Tulipan, RL Paschall, FH Boehm, WF Walsh et al. 1999. Fetal surgery for myelomeningocele and the incidence of shunt-dependent hydrocephalus. *JAMA* 282(19): 1819–1825.

Buscaglia M, L Ghisoni, M Bellotti, E Ferrazzi et al. 1996. Percutaneous umbilical blood sampling: indication changes and procedure loss rate in a nine years' experience. *Fetal Diagn Ther* 11(2): 106–113.

Bussel JB, MD Richard, L Berkowitz et al. 1988. Antenatal treatment of neonatal alloimmune thrombocytopenia. *N Engl J Med* 319: 1374–1378.

Clewell WH, ML Johnson, PR Meier, JB Newkirk et al. 1982. A surgical approach to the treatment of fetal hydrocephalus. *N Engl J Med* 306(22): 1320–1325.

Cochrane DD, B Irwin and K Chambers. 2001. Clinical Outcomes that fetal surgery for myelomeningocele needs to achieve. *Eur J Pediatr Surg* 11 Suppl 1:S18–20.

Contelle C and Rodeck C. on the scientific and ethical issues of fetal somatic gene therapy. *Gene Ther* 2002; 9; 670–673.

Daffos F, Forestier F, Muller JY et al. 1984. Prenatal treatment of alloimmune thrombocytopenia. *Lancet* 2: 632.

David AL and D Peebles. 2008. Gene therapy for the fetus: is there a future? *Best Prac Res Clin Obstet Gynaecol.* 22(1): 203–218.

Delle Chiaie L, Buck G, Grab D and Terinde R. 2001. Prediction of fetal anemia with Doppler measurement of the middle cerebral artery peak systolic velocity in pregnancies complicated by maternal blood group alloimmunization or parvovirus B19 infection. *Ultrasound Obstet Gynecol* 18(3): 232–236.

Deren OO and L Onderoglu. 2002. The value of middle cerebral artery systolic velocity for initial and subsequent management in fetal anemia. *Eur J Obstet Gynecol Reprod Biol* 101(1): 26–30.

Dommergues M, F Muller, S Ngo, P Hohlfeld et al. 2000. Fetal serum beta 2-microglobulin predicts postnatal renal function in bilateral uropathies. *Kidney Int* 58(1): 312–316.

Donner C, P Simon, A Karioun, F Avni and F Rodesch. 1994. Experience of a single team of operators in 891 diagnostic funipunctures. *Obstet Gynecol* 84(5): 827–831.

Elder JS, JP O'Grady, G Ashmead, JW Duckett and E Philipson. 1990. Evaluation of fetal renal function: unreliability of fetal urinary electrolytes. *J Urol* 144(2 Pt 2): 574–578.

Fisk NM, D Ronderos-Dumit, A Soliani, U Nicolini, J Vaughan and CH Rodeck. 1991. Diagnostic and therapeutic transabdominal amnioinfusion in oligohydramnios. *Obstet Gynecol* 78(2): 270–278.

Freedman AL, MP Johnson, CA Smith, R Gonzalez and MI Evans. 1999. Long-term outcome in children after antenatal intervention for obstructive uropathies. *Lancet* 354(9176): 374–377.

Gembruch U. 2003. Fetal tachyarrhythmia. In Yagel S, Silverman NH and Gembruch U eds, *Fetal cardiology*. London: Martin Dunitz, 355–371.

Golbus MS, MR Harrison and RA Filly. 1982. In utero treatment of urinary tract obstruction. *Am J Obstet Gynecol* 142(4): 383–388.

Greaves M and EA Letsky. 1997. Guidelines on the investigation and management of thrombocytopenia in pregnancy and neonatal alloimmune thrombocytopenia. *Br J Obstet Gynaecol* 104(10): 1108.

Guez S, BM Assael, ML Melzi, B Tassis and U Nicolini. 1996. Shortcomings in predicting postnatal renal function using prenatal urine biochemistry in fetuses with congenital hydronephrosis. *J Pediatr Surg* 31(10): 1401–1404.

Harrison MR, Keller RL, Hawgood SB et al. 2003. A randomized trial of fetal endoscopic tracheal occlusion for severe fetal congenital diaphragmatic hernia. *N Engl J Med* 349: 1916–1924.

Hecher K, H Plath, T Bregenzer, M Hansmann and BJ Hackeloer. 1999. Endoscopic laser surgery versus serial amniocenteses in the treatment of severe twin-twin transfusion syndrome. *Am J Obstet Gynecol* 180: 717–724.

Holmes N, Harrison MR and Baskin LS. 2001. Fetal surgery for posterior urethral valves: long-term postnatal outcomes. *Pediatrics* 108(1): E7.

Holmes NM, Nguyen HT, Harrison MR, Farmer DL and Baskin LS. 2001. Fetal intervention for myelomeningocele: effect on postnatal bladder function. *J Urol* 166(6): 2383–2386.

Jolly M, M Taylor, G Rose, L Govender and NM Fisk. 2001. Interstitial laser: a new surgical technique for twin reversed arterial perfusion sequence in early pregnancy. *Br J Obstet Gynaecol* 108(10): 1098–1102.

Kilby MD. 2008. Preface. *Best Prac Res Clinical Obstet Gynaecol*. 22(1): 1.

Lyerly AD, RC Cefalo, M Socol et al. 2001. Attitudes of maternal-fetal specialists concerning maternal-fetal surgery. *Am J Obstet Gynecol* 185: 1052–1058.

Manning FA, MR Harrison and C Rodeck. 1986. Catheter shunts for fetal hydronephrosis and hydrocephalus. Report of the International Fetal Surgery Registry. *N Engl J Med* 315(5): 336–340.

McLorie G, W Farhat, A Khoury, D Geary and G Ryan. 2001. Outcome analysis of vesicoamniotic shunting in a comprehensive population. *J Urol* 166(3): 1036–1040.

Morin L, Crombleholme TM and D'Alton ME. 1994. Prenatal diagnosis and management of fetal thoracic lesions. *Semin Perinatol* 18(3): 228–253.

Muller F, M Dommergues, L Mandelbrot, MC Aubry, C Nihoul-Fekete and Y Dumez. 1993. Fetal urinary biochemistry predicts postnatal renal function in children with bilateral obstructive uropathies. *Obstet Gynecol* 82(5): 813–820.

Noble R and CH Rodeck. 2008. Ethical considerations of fetal therapy. *Best Practice and Research Clinical Obstetrics and Gynaecology* 22(1): 219–231.

Nicolaides KH, GB Azar. 1990. Thoraco-amniotic shunting. *Fetal Diagn Ther* 5(3-4): 153–164.

Nicolaides KH, CH Rodeck, RS Mibashan, JR Kemp. 1986. Have Liley charts outlived their usefulness? *Am J Obstet Gynecol* 155(1): 90–94.

Nicolini U, P Nicolaidis, NM Fisk, JI Vaughan et al. 1990. Limited role of fetal blood sampling in prediction of outcome in intrauterine growth retardation. *Lancet* 336(8718): 768–772.

Orlandi F, G Damiani, C Jakil, S Lauricella, O Bertolino and A Maggio. 1990. The risks of early cordocentesis (12-21 weeks): analysis of 500 procedures. *Prenat Diagn* 10(7): 425–428.

Overton TG, KR Duncan, M Jolly et al. 2002. Serial aggressive platelet transfusion for fetal alloimmune thrombocytopenia: platelet dynamics and perinatal outcome. *Am J Obstet Gynecol* 186: 826–831.

Pinette MG, Y Pan, SG Pinette and PG Stubblefield. 1993. Treatment of twin-twin transfusion syndrome. *Obstet Gynecol* 82: 841–846.

Pitt C, L Sanchez-Ramos, AM Kaunitz and F Gaudier. 2000. Prophylactic amnioinfusion for intrapartum oligohydramnios: a meta-analysis of randomized controlled trials. *Obstet Gynecol* 96(5 Pt 2): 861–866.

Pryde PG, M Hallak, MR Lauria, L Littman et al. 2000. Severe oligohydramnios with intact membranes: an indication for diagnostic amnioinfusion. *Fetal Diagn Ther* 15(1): 46–49.

Radder CM, A Brand and HHH Kanhai. 2003. Will it ever be possible to balance the risk of intracranial haemorrhage in fetal or neonatal alloimmune thrombocytopenia against the risk of treatment strategies to prevent it? *Vox Sang* 84: 318–325.

Rodeck CH and A Deans.1999. Red cell alloimmunisation. In Rodeck CH and MJ Whittle eds, *Fetal Medicine: Basic Science and Clinical Practice*. London: Churchill Livingstone, 785–804.

Rodeck CH, NM Fisk, DI Fraser and U Nicolini. 1988. Long-term in utero drainage of fetal hydrothorax. *N Engl J Med* 319(17): 1135–1138.

Senat MV, J Deprest, M Boulvain, A Paupe, N Winer and Y Ville. 2004. Endoscopic laser surgery versus serial amnioreduction for severe twin-to-twin transfusion syndrome. *N Engl J Med*. 351:136–144.

Sherer DM and O Langer. 2001. Oligohydramnios: Use and misuse in clinical management. *Ultrasound Obstet Gynaecol* 18: 411–419.

Spitzer A. 1996. The current approach to the assessment of fetal renal function: fact or fiction? *Pediatr Nephrol* 10(2): 230–235.

Sutton LN. 2008. Fetal surgery for neural tube defects. *Best Practice and Research Clinical Obstetrics and Gynaecology*. 22(1): 175–188.

Thilaganathan B, DJ Gloeb, S Sairam and A Tekay. 2000. Sono-endoscopic delineation of the placental vascular equator prior to selective fetoscopic laser ablation in twin-to-twin transfusion syndrome. *Ultrasound Obstet Gynecol* 16: 226–229.

Tiblad E and M Westgren. 2008. Fetal stem-cell transplantation. *Best Practice and Research Clinical Obstetrics and Gynaecology*. 22(1): 189–210.

Touraine JL, D Raudrant, C Royo et al. 1989. In-utero transplantation of stem cells in bare lymphocyte syndrome. *Lancet*. 1:1382.

Trespidi L, C Boschetto, E Caravelli, L Villa, A Kustermann and U Nicolini. 1997. Serial amniocentesis in the management of twin-twin transfusion syndrome: when is it valuable? *Fetal Diagn Ther* 12: 15–20.

Turhan NO and N Atacan. 2002. Antepartum prophylactic transabdominal amnioinfusion in preterm pregnancies complicated by oligohydramnios. *Int J Gynaecol Obstet* 76(1): 15–21.

Ulm MR, D Bettelheim, B Ulm, P Frigo and G Bernaschek. 1997. Fetal bradycardia following cordocentesis. *Prenat Diagn* 17(10): 919–923.

Van den Akker ESA and D Oepkes. 2008. Fetal and neonatal alloimmune thrombocytopenia. *Best Practice and Research Clinical Obstetrics and Gynaecology*. 22(1): 3–14.

Ville Y, K Hecher, A Gagnon, N Sebire, J Hyett and K Nicolaides. 1998. Endoscopic laser coagulation in the management of severe twin-twin transfusion syndrome. *Br J Obstet Gynaecol* 105: 446–453.

Weiner C. 1998. Cordocentesis: technique. In: *Textbook of Perinatal Medicine*. np: Parthenon Publishing. Vol 2: 1061–1064.

Weiner CP, KD Wenstrom, SL Sipes, RA Williamson. 1991. Risk factors for cordocentesis and fetal intravascular transfusion. *Am J Obstet Gynecol* 165(4 Pt 1): 1020–1025.

Wilson JM, JW DiFiore and CA Peters. 1993. Experimental fetal tracheal ligation prevents the pulmonary hypoplasia associated with fetal nephrectomy: possible application for congenital diaphragmatic hernia. *J Pediatr Surg* 28(11): 1433–1439.

Wilson JM and NA Wivel. 1999. Report on the potential use of gene therapy in utero. Gene therapy advisory committee. *Hum Gene Ther* 10: 689–692.

Wilson RD. 2008. Management of fetal tumors. *Best Prac Res Clinical Obstet Gynaecol.* 22(1): 159–173.

40

Controversies in Obstetrics

Vanita Jain | Rashmi Bagga

Management of clinical situations usually varies widely based on opinion and experience and not always on evidence. In this chapter, an evidence-based approach to the management of some of these situations is suggested.

Investigations for Recurrent Pregnancy Loss (RPL)

The diagnostic workup of couples with RPL requires a complete medical history, physical examination and the following investigations:

Assessment of anatomical causes: The anatomical causes of RPL such as septate, bicornuate uterus and uterine myomas can be diagnosed using hysterosalpingography (HSG) or sonohysterography (Goldeberg 1997; Soares 2000). Hysteroscopy, laparoscopy and magnetic resonance imaging (MRI) may also be performed as second-line tests when additional information is required to determine the diagnosis; however, these tests are more expensive or more invasive than sonohysterography. Ultrasonography is particularly useful in pregnant women when the other tests are relatively or absolutely contraindicated.

Anticardiolipin antibodies and lupus anticoagulant: Anticardiolipin antibody (IgG and IgM) and lupus anticoagulant tests should be carried out twice, 6–8 weeks apart, because a low to mid-positive level may be due to a viral illness and it revert to normal when the illness resolves (Stephenson 1996 Vinatier 2001).

Karyotype: The overall prevalence of major chromosomal abnormalities coupled with two or more pregnancy losses was 2.9–4.7%, which is 5–6 times higher than that of the general adult population (Tharapel 1985; de Braekeleer 1990). Because of the low likelihood of an abnormal karyotype in couples with RPL, this is the last test that is carried out and only if the preceding workup yields negative results. Many experts also recommend karyotyping of the abortus or products of conception.

LH and FSH: These tests are carried out in the early follicular phase (Days 2–4).

Thyroid function: There is increased risk of miscarriage in women with subclinical hypothyroidism (Christiansen 2005). Therefore, screening asymptomatic women for subclinical thyroid dysfunction is reasonable.

Additional laboratory tests may be indicated as suggested by history or examination.

Routine Prenatal Thyroid Function Screening

Untreated maternal hypothyroidism may lead to congenital hypothyroidism, which affects 1 in 4000 newborns, and is the most common treatable cause of mental retardation. Therefore, newborn screening programmes in which T4 and TSH levels are measured using a heel-stick blood sample obtained 2–5 days after delivery have been initiated (Rose et al 2006). There is also evidence of an association between maternal subclinical hypothyroidism and adverse pregnancy outcome. Routine prenatal thyroid function screening will help diagnose maternal subclinical hypothyroidism. However, there is uncertainty about the benefits of therapy in subclinical hypothyroidism in preventing these adverse outcomes. Therefore, the controversy between targeted and universal prenatal thyroid function screening continues (Ringel and Mazzaferri 2005).

At present, there is insufficient evidence to recommend or discourage universal prenatal thyroid function screening. Consensus guidelines from an expert panel sponsored by the American Thyroid Association, American Association of Clinical Endocrinologists and The Endocrine Society do not advocate universal prenatal thyroid function screening but recommend testing only high-risk women with a personal history of thyroid or other autoimmune disorders or with a family history of thyroid disorders (Surks et al 2004). However, in a recent trial of 1560 women undergoing universal prenatal thyroid screening, it was observed that targeted screening would have missed 30% of the women with TSH values greater than 4.2 mIU/ml, as they were in the low-risk group (Vaidya et al 2007). Therefore, some experts recommend universal screening for thyroid dysfunction in pregnant women or those attempting to become pregnant (Brent 2007). It is acknowledged that obstetricians are under increasing pressure to screen and treat maternal subclinical hypothyroidism despite uncertainty over whether such therapy would be beneficial, and endocrinology organisations have emphasised the need for large clinical trials to address this issue (Casey and Leveno 2006).

Management of Missed Abortions and Intrauterine Death

Management of Missed Abortions After First Trimester

First trimester missed abortions diagnosed by sonography may be managed surgically, medically or expectantly. In surgical management, dilatation and curettage (D&C) or dilatation and evacuation (D&E) are performed to prevent potential hemorrhagic and infectious complications from the retained products of conception. In medical management, misoprostol is commonly used for uterine evacuation. Its efficacy depends on the dose and route of administration. A higher dose and vaginal administration (as compared to oral) may be more efficacious because of its local effect on the cervix and increased bioavailability (Neilson et al 2006). In expectant management, the women are observed and most of them spontaneously expel the products of conception within two weeks, and some by 3–4 weeks (Banerjee et al 2001). If spontaneous expulsion does not occur by 4 weeks, medical or surgical treatment is offered. In a large series evaluating the outcome of expectant management, 686 women with first trimester incomplete or missed abortions were offered either expectant management or surgical evacuation and were followed up for 4 weeks. Spontaneous expulsion occurred in 81% of the expectantly managed women (in 91% with incomplete abortion, 76% with missed abortions and 66% with anembryonic pregnancies). Complications—infection, severe pain or excessive bleeding—occurred in 1% with expectant and in 2% with surgical management. The authors concluded that expectant management for one month was safe and effective (Luise et al 2002).

Randomised trials and systematic reviews summarised that expectant, medical and surgical management were similarly effective and major complications were infrequent in all options. However, complete evacuation within 48 hours was more likely with surgery followed by medical methods, and was least likely with expectant management (Sotiriadis et al 2005), which was associated with a higher risk of incomplete evacuation, need for unplanned curettage and bleeding, but was found to be reasonable if the woman desired non-intervention (Nanda et al 2006). A randomised trial in 1200 women observed that the risk of infection (2%–3%) was similar with all three methods, but expectant management was less costly than medical or surgical management (Petrou et al 2006; Trinder et al 2006). Another randomised trial noted that women given misoprostol bled for a longer duration and experienced a greater fall in hemoglobin than those who underwent curettage (Davis et al 2007). Thus, any of the three approaches may be used depending on the woman's wishes and the ability to reach a medical facility in an emergency, which may be necessary with expectant or medical management.

Management After Fetal Death in the Second and Third Trimester

Induction vs Waiting for 3–4 Weeks for Spontaneous Labour Induction of labour is usually offered after second or third trimester fetal demise to reduce the mental stress associated with carrying a dead baby, and also to reduce the risk of consumptive coagulopathy in the woman. However, immediate induction is not medically necessary and some women may choose to delay induction or even wait for spontaneous labour. With expectant management, 80–90% of the women have spontaneous onset of labour within two weeks of fetal demise.

Retention of a dead fetus may cause chronic consumptive coagulopathy due to the slow release of thromboplastin from the placenta into maternal circulation; it usually occurs after four weeks, but may occur earlier. The patient's fibrinogen concentration should be determined to detect a potential coagulopathic state developing from retention of a nonviable fetus, which is most common after 20 weeks of gestation and at more than six weeks from actual fetal death. It has been reported in 25% of women who retain a dead fetus for more than a month (Maslow et al 1996). In addition to fibrinogen levels, the platelet count, prothrombin time (PT) and activated partial thromboplastin time (APTT) may also be measured. If these parameters are normal, and the patient shows no obvious signs of bleeding, expectant management is appropriate. If these are abnormal, disseminated intravascular coagulation (DIC) is treated prior to labour induction. This is done by administration of blood products and coagulation factors. Low-dose heparin is given to women with intact circulation to correct hypofibrinogenemia (fibrinogen < 100 mg/dl) prior to labour induction (Lurie et al 2000).

Expectant management is a better option than immediate induction in women with a previous cesarean as they are at a higher risk of intrapartum uterine rupture than women with an unscarred uterus. This risk is higher with induced labour than with spontaneous labour (Lydon-Rochelle et al 2001). For this reason, prostaglandins for cervical ripening and labour induction should be used cautiously or, better still, avoided in women with a scarred uterus. If the cervix is unfavourable, mechanical methods should be used for cervical ripening (Foley's catheter). Careful counselling about the risks and benefits of vaginal birth in women with a scarred uterus must be undertaken and a repeat cesarean may be performed if the patient desires it.

Pregnancy-induced Hypertension (PIH) or Gestational Hypertension

Role of Aspirin and Calcium in Prevention of PIH

Low-dose aspirin Early studies assessing the efficacy of aspirin therapy were performed in women at especially high risk of developing pre-eclampsia. These included the National Institute of Child Health and Human Development Network of Maternal–Fetal Medicine Units Double-blind Study with 2539 women (Caritis 1998) and the Collaborative Low-dose Aspirin Study in Pregnancy (CLASP) trial that included 9364 women at increased risk of pre-eclampsia. Although not statistically significant, a small decrease in the incidence of pre-eclampsia with aspirin therapy was demonstrated in both of these trials. The Cochrane Group analysed the data obtained from 51 trials with over 36,000 women of varying risk statuses (Duley 2004). Use of these drugs was associated with a modest but significant reduction in the rates of pre-eclampsia, preterm birth and perinatal death. Trials in unselected nulliparous women have shown little or no benefit from prophylactic aspirin therapy (Sibai 1993).

The American College of Obstetricians and Gynecologists practice bulletin does not recommend aspirin therapy for women at low risk of developing pre-eclampsia (ACOG 2002). However, no conclusions were reached about moderate- to high-risk women.

Calcium supplementation The role of calcium in the prevention of pre-eclampsia has been a subject of several studies.

A large trial, Calcium for Pre-eclampsia Prevention (CPEP), was performed in the United States on 4589 healthy nulliparous women at 13–21 weeks of gestation. The women were randomly assigned to receive either calcium (2 g/day) or placebo therapy for the rest of their pregnancy. No benefits from calcium supplementation were identified—there was no difference between the two groups in the incidence of pre-eclampsia (6.9% versus 7.3%), pregnancy-associated hypertension or adverse fetal outcome (Levine 1997).

These results are compatible with several meta-analyses of placebo-controlled trials in low-risk women with adequate dietary calcium intake, which showed that calcium supplementation does not prevent pre-eclampsia, in contrast to studies in high-risk, low calcium–intake populations (DerSimonian 1999; Atallah 2002; Hofmeyr 2006).

Thus, there does not appear to be any benefit from routine calcium supplementation for healthy, nulliparous women with adequate baseline dietary calcium intake. There may be some benefit for pre-eclampsia prevention in high-risk populations, but further study is required.

Initiation of Antihypertensive Drugs

Antihypertensive drugs do not alter the course of the disease or diminish perinatal morbidity or mortality in pre-eclampsia; in fact treatment-induced decrease in maternal blood pressure may adversely affect fetal growth (von Dadelszen 2000). Thus, indications for antihypertensive drugs in pre-eclampsia are purely maternal—diastolic pressure ≥105–110 mmHg or systolic pressure ≥160 mmHg, a level at which the risk of cerebral hemorrhage in the mother becomes appreciable (Cunningham 1992; Sibai 1996; Working Group 2000; ACOG 2001; Martin 2005).

Induction of Labour in Mild Gestational Hypertension The definitive treatment of pre-eclampsia is delivery to prevent development of maternal or fetal complications. The decision to deliver the fetus depends on the gestational age, maternal and fetal condition and the severity of pre-eclampsia. Severe pre-eclampsia is generally regarded as an indication for delivery, regardless of gestational age, to minimise the risk of development of maternal and fetal complications. In mild pre-eclampsia, women are induced at term if there are no contraindications to vaginal birth. This minimises the risk of progression to severe disease and its attendant complications. Women who are at at least 37 weeks of gestation and have a favourable cervix (Bishop score >6) should be induced, as even mild pre-eclampsia may possibly be of more risk to the mother and the fetus than the induction. In women with mild pre-eclampsia and firm, closed cervix, the hazards of cesarean section may be more than those of continuing pregnancy under supervision. Alternatively, in women with an unfavourable cervix, cervical ripening agents may be considered. All pre-eclamptic women should be delivered by 40 weeks of gestation (Working Group Report 2000; Sibai 2003; Nicholson 2006).

Gestational Diabetes

Diagnosis: GTT Values during Pregnancy

A three-hour 100 g oral glucose tolerance test (GTT) is routinely performed to diagnose gestational diabetes mellitus (GDM). Two different sets of glucose values have been proposed to diagnose GDM on GTT. The Fourth International Workshop–Conference on Gestational Diabetes GTT values are based on the Carpenter and Coustan modifications to the earlier values of O'Sullivan and Mahan, and their criteria to diagnose GDM are two or more plasma glucose values equal to or more than the following values:

Fasting ≥95 mg/dl one hour ≥180, two hours ≥155 and three hours ≥140 (Carpenter and Coustan 1982; Fourth International Workshop–Conference on Gestational Diabetes Mellitus 1998; Gestational Diabetes Mellitus 2004)

These values are lower than the values proposed by the Expert Committee on the Diagnosis and Classification of Diabetes Mellitus and the National Diabetes Data Group (NDDG), which used cut-off values of 105, 190, 165 and 145 mg/dl, respectively (Report of the Expert Committee on the Diagnosis and Classification of Diabetes Mellitus 2000). The NDDG values are adapted from the O'Sullivan and Mahan criteria, which used the Somogyi–Nelson method of glucose analysis from whole blood (O'Sullivan and Mahan 1964). Currently, the enzymatic (glucose oxidase) method is used for plasma glucose estimation; this gives lower values than the Somogyi–Nelson method. The thresholds derived from the older Somogyi–Nelson method were corrected to account for the enzymatic assays used.

One retrospective review of 8857 pregnant women screened for GDM suggested that the Carpenter and Coustan criteria diagnosed more women with GDM (5% versus 3% with NDDG) without much benefit. The use of the more stringent Carpenter and Coustan criteria would have only reduced the prevalence of infants weighing ≥4000 g from 17.1% to 16.9%, and weighing ≥4500 g from 3.0% to 2.9% (Schwartz et al 1999).

The American College of Obstetricians and Gynecologists (ACOG) considers the use of either the Fourth International Workshop or the NDDG criteria acceptable for diagnosis of GDM (ACOG Practice Bulletin 2001), whereas the American Diabetes Association (ADA) recommends the Fourth International Workshop criteria (Gestational Diabetes Mellitus 2004). This issue may be resolved on the publication of results of the Hyperglycemia and Adverse Pregnancy Outcomes (HAPO) trial sponsored by the National Institutes of Health, USA; this is a seven-year, multi-national, observational study of over 23,000 women. After this, the sixth International Gestational Diabetes Workshop will be held to decide on the appropriate criteria and methods for screening and diagnosis of GDM (Diabetes 2007).

Use of Oral Hypoglycemics in Gestational Diabetes Traditionally, insulin therapy has been considered the gold standard for the management of patients with diabetes not controlled by diet alone. This is because of its efficacy in achieving good blood glucose control, predictability of its response and the fact that it does not cross the placenta. Defects in insulin secretion and resistance are characteristics of GDM; thus, the use of oral hypoglycemic agents to target these defects is of potential interest (Christine et al 2006). However, because of concerns regarding the unpredictability of response, transplacental passage and possibility of teratogenicity and prolonged neonatal hypoglycemia, especially with older sulfonylureas (tolbutamide and chlorpropamide), these agents are avoided during pregnancy (Langer et al 2005). The ADA and the United States Food and Drug Administration (FDA) do not endorse the use of oral anti-hyperglycemic agents during pregnancy (Gestational Diabetes Mellitus 2004). The ACOG also recommends insulin and states that the use of oral agents for control of Type 2 diabetes during pregnancy should be limited and individualised until more data confirming safety and efficacy becomes available (ACOG 2005).

However, after the introduction of glyburide (glibenclamide) and metformin, there has been renewed interest in using these agents in GDM. Glyburide is a long-acting, second generation oral sulfonylurea with lower incidence of side effects and minimal transplacental passage as compared to first generation sulfonylureas. It acts on the pancreatic sulfonylurea receptors and increases the rate of insulin secretion at any glucose concentration. It also slows the hepatic degradation of insulin and sensitises the target tissues to the action of insulin (Tripathy 2003). Langer et al (2005) evaluated glyburide in 404 women with GDM who required medical treatment. The women were randomised to receive either glyburide or insulin between 11 and 33 weeks and both groups had a similar degree of glycemic control and perinatal outcome. Glyburide may be less effective in obese patients or those with marked hyperglycemia earlier in pregnancy but may be a good option in women with mild to moderate degrees of hyperglycemia (Langer et al 2005). Though the use of glyburide in GDM is becoming more prevalent, caution is advised until its safety and efficacy are confirmed.

Metformin, an orally acting biguanide, differs from sulfonylureas as it does not stimulate pancreatic beta cells and does not cause insulin release. It is classified as an anti-hyperglycemic agent, which should be distinguished from a hypoglycemic agent. Possible mechanisms for its anti-hyperglycemic action are

i) suppression of hepatic glucose output,
ii) improvement in insulin-mediated glucose utilisation in peripheral organs,
iii) decrement of fatty acid oxidation
iv) increase in splanchnic glucose turnover.

Further, it counters insulin resistance by decreasing the endogenous or exogenous insulin requirement and reducing basal plasma insulin concentration. It improves the lipid profile and there is no risk of serious hypoglycemia (Denno et al 1994). A meta-analysis of first-trimester exposure to metformin did not find an increased risk of major congenital malformations (Gilbert et al 2006). Being an anti-hyperglycemic agent, metformin may prevent development of GDM in women with polycystic ovary syndrome (PCOS). GDM occurred in only 3% (1 of 33) women with PCOS taking metformin compared to 23% (9 of 39) not taking metformin (Glueck et al 2002).

Hellmuth et al (2001) treated 50 diabetic women with metformin and 68 with tolbutamide during pregnancy. A reference group of 42 diabetic women were treated with insulin during pregnancy. The incidence of pre-eclampsia was significantly higher in the metformin group than in the insulin group (32% against 10%), and in the group treated with metformin in the third trimester, perinatal mortality was significantly increased as compared to women not treated with metformin (11.6 against 1.3%). The increased rate of stillbirths in the metformin group could have been due to the preponderance of obese Type 2 diabetics with poorly controlled glucose levels and elderly mothers in this group. A study of 109 women with PCOS who conceived on and continued with metformin through pregnancy showed that metformin reduced the development of GDM, was not teratogenic and did not adversely affect birth length and weight, growth or motor-social development in the first 18 months of life (Glueck et al 2004). However, more randomised trials are needed to establish maternal and fetal safety, and the efficacy of glyburide and metformin in GDM.

Continuation of Metformin during Pregnancy in Women with PCOS

Treatment of Type 2 diabetes mellitus is the only indication for metformin use approved by the FDA. It is classified as a Category B drug and is not approved for use during pregnancy. After oral administration, high concentrations of metformin are found in jejunal and ileal walls. This leads to its common side effect of abdominal discomfort. Malabsorption can occur as a result of a Ca^{2+} channel effect, or local serosal release of 5HT and other neurotransmitters. High concentration of metformin in the intestinal wall stimulates anaerobic metabolism of glucose with lactate release into the portal vein. This may result in its rare but serious adverse event of lactic acidosis. The situation is aggravated by renal insufficiency, impaired liver function and other conditions that decrease tissue perfusion. Metformin should be taken with meals or immediately before meals to minimise gastrointestinal effects (Tripathi 2003).

Metformin is frequently used in women with PCOS to treat anovulation and infertility. It may be stopped when pregnancy is diagnosed. However, its continuation during pregnancy has been thought to reduce the otherwise high rate of spontaneous abortions associated with PCOS. The spontaneous abortion rate in women with PCOS is 20–40% higher than the baseline in the general obstetric population (Glueck et al 2002). Observational studies have shown that abortions occurred in 62–73% of pregnancies without metformin and in 9–36% of pregnancies in the same women when metformin was continued during pregnancy (Jakubowicz et al 2002; Glueck et al 2001, 2002). Metformin appeared to be effective in reducing spontaneous abortions even when it was stopped at the time of diagnosis of pregnancy (Thatcher et al 2006). A meta-analysis after first-trimester exposure to metformin did not find an increased risk of major malformations (Gilbert et al 2006). A randomised trial is needed to better understand the effect of metformin use during pregnancy on the rate of spontaneous abortions.

Another advantage of continuing metformin during pregnancy may be a reduction in the incidence of GDM. The incidence of GDM is higher in women with PCOS than in the general obstetric population (Thatcher et al 2006). Metformin use throughout pregnancy may reduce this risk (Glueck et al 2002). In 109 women with PCOS who conceived on and continued with metformin throughout pregnancy and 252 women without PCOS who did not take metformin, metformin treatment was associated with a reduced rate of GDM—7.6% against 15.9% in controls (Glueck et al 2004).

Induction of Labour at 38 Weeks or 40 Weeks in Well-controlled GDM Pregnant women with diabetes requiring insulin need intensive surveillance, plasma glucose monitoring and fetal surveillance (biophysical profile and non-stress test, at least twice a week), as data suggests that perinatal mortality may increase by five times for such women as compared to the general population (Graves 2007).

A Cochrane review assessed the effect of elective delivery in diabetic pregnant women on maternal and perinatal outcome. One randomised trial compared active induction of labour at 38 completed weeks to expectant management until 42 weeks in 200 insulin-requiring diabetic women, of whom 187 had GDM and 13 had Type 2 pre-existing diabetes (Class B) (Kjos et al 1993). The risk of cesarean section was not different between the two groups (relative risk 0.81). The risk of macrosomia was reduced in the active induction group (RR 0.56) and three cases of mild shoulder dystocia were reported in the expectant management group. No other perinatal morbidity was reported. However, 50% in the expectant management group ultimately required induction for obstetric indications. The Cochrane reviewers concluded that induction of labour at 38 completed weeks in women with GDM treated with insulin reduces the risk of macrosomia but there was no difference in maternal or neonatal morbidity (Boulvain et al 2001).

In a retrospective study, 143 women with GDM not controlled with diet alone (Class A-2, requiring primarily oral hypoglycemic therapy), who underwent labour induction at 38 weeks were compared with 137 diet-controlled diabetic women (Class A-1) who underwent expectant management at 38 weeks. The study group (elective delivery) was found to be more likely to have an unfavourable cervix (75% against 45%) and require oxytocin (76% against 56%), but early onset meconium was less common (3.5% against 13.1%). Primary cesarean rates were similar in the two groups (12.7% against 11.7%). There was one stillbirth in the control group due to tight nuchal cord encirclement. Mean birth weight and frequency of birth weight >4000 g were also similar. Shoulder dystocia, low Apgar scores and infants needing special neonatal care were infrequent in either group. The authors concluded that routine delivery at 38 weeks in these women was not associated with additional intrapartum morbidity or a greater need for cesarean delivery.

The morbidity from prematurity and failed induction should be weighed against the benefits of early delivery. Respiratory distress syndrome (hyaline membrane disease) is more likely in infants of diabetic mothers delivered early than in infants of non-diabetic mothers, and this risk equalises in the two groups after 38.5 weeks (Robert et al 1976). High fetal insulin levels cause cellular hypertrophy and hyperplasia, but with less cellular maturation, leading to macrosomia and immature lung function (Piper et al 1998).

It is unclear whether women with good glycemic control and reassuring antepartum surveillance are at increased risk of intrauterine demise at term. There is insufficient data to convincingly demonstrate that the risk of fetal demise with modern, intensive perinatal care is increased in these women. There is probably little benefit in continuing pregnancy beyond 39 weeks in diabetic mothers, even with good metabolic control (Molsted-Pedersen et al 1986). Labour induction for these pregnancies by 40 weeks of gestation is suggested (ACOG 2005). However, early induction for suspected fetal macrosomia is not recommended because this intervention has not been proven to improve maternal or fetal outcome, and may increase the cesarean delivery rate (Sanchez-Ramos et al 2002). In contrast, elective induction of appropriately grown fetuses at 38–39 weeks appears to be associated with lower prevalence of macrosomia than in expectant management (Kjos et al 1993). This observation also favours elective induction at 39 completed weeks. In women with an unfavourable cervix, induction may be delayed till 40 weeks provided there is excellent glycemic control, no vascular disease or pre-eclampsia, normal fetal growth, reassuring antepartum fetal surveillance and no history of stillbirth (Rasmussen et al 1992; ACOG 2005). If these criteria are not met or the woman is not compliant, induction is done using safe cervical ripening agents (Rayburn 1989).

Pre-pregnancy Counselling in IDDM Pre-pregnancy evaluation and counselling of women with pre-gestational diabetes mellitus (Type 1 or 2) is important to minimise the risk to the fetus and the mother. The risk of spontaneous abortions and fetal malformations is higher in women with poor glycemic control during the period of organogenesis, which is almost complete by the seventh week after conception (Temple et al 2002). The maternal risks depend on the presence of associated systemic problems like retinopathy, nephropathy, hypertension, neuropathy, cardiovascular disease and thyroid disease.

Pregnancy complications are higher than in the general obstetric population and were reported among 1215 women from Denmark with Type 1 diabetes as macrosomia (63% against 10%), cesarean delivery (56% versus 20%), preterm delivery (42% versus 12%), pre-eclampsia (18% against 6%), neonatal jaundice (18%), respiratory distress syndrome (17%), congenital malformations (5% against 3%) and perinatal mortality (3% versus < 1%) (Jensen et al 2004).

According to the American Diabetes Association, the risk of offspring developing diabetes is as follows:

- If the father has Type 1 diabetes, the risk is 1 in 17
- If the mother has Type 1 diabetes, the risk is 1 in 25 if she is < 25 years of age and 1 in 100 if she is ≥ 25 years
- If both parents have Type 1 diabetes, the risk is between 1 in 10 and 1 in 4
- If one parent has Type 2 diabetes, the risk

to the offspring is between 1 in 13 and 1 in 7; the offspring's risk is greater when the mother is affected
- If both parents have Type 2 diabetes, the risk is 1 in 2 (www.diabetes.org)

Pregnancy is not a risk factor for the development of early nephropathy, retinopathy or neuropathy, but it may worsen these conditions if they are pre-existing (Verier-Mine et al 2005). Pre-conceptional glycemic control reduces the risk of progression of retinopathy during pregnancy. Laser photocoagulation should be carried out in severe pre-proliferative retinopathy. During pregnancy, pre-existing retinopathy may worsen with strict glycemic control, as reduced plasma volume after sudden correction of hyperglycemia leads to closure of some already narrowed retinal blood vessels (Diabetes Control and Complications Trial 1998). Pre-pregnancy serum creatinine, 24-hour urinary protein excretion and creatinine clearance estimation are advised. Progression of nephropathy during pregnancy depends on the degree of renal impairment. The risk is increased if serum creatinine is >2.0 mg/dl, proteinuria is >2 g/day and creatinine clearance is <50 ml/min. Hence, such findings are relative contraindications to pregnancy (Jovanovic-Peterson and Peterson 1984). The blood pressure should be kept at or below 130/80 to prevent cardiovascular disease and minimise the progression of diabetic nephropathy and retinopathy. Alphamethyldopa, nifedipine and labetalol may be used for blood pressure control. Lifestyle modifications like exercise, maintenance of ideal body weight, not smoking and correction of hyperlipidemia help control the condition. Thyroid function tests and screening and treatment of asymptomatic bacteriuria must also be carried out.

Optimum glycemic control, blood glucose monitoring 6 times a day (before and after each meal) and normal HbA1c levels before conception are necessary. Hemoglobin A_{1C} (HbA_{1C}) values reflect the mean blood glucose concentration during the preceding 6–8 weeks (preceding 8 weeks in non-pregnant and 6 weeks in pregnant women because the mean age of red blood cells is shortened due to increased production during pregnancy). An HbA_{1C} level of 6% correlates with an average glucose concentration of 120 mg/dl and each 1% increase in HbA1C reflects a 30 mg/dl increase in average glucose concentration. Pre-conceptional folic acid supplements are advised. Ideally, Type 2 diabetics on oral anti-hyperglycemic agents should be switched to insulin therapy pre-conceptionally, so that their glycemic control is not jeopardised during the process of switching therapies early in pregnancy, which is the period of organogenesis. If a woman conceives on oral hypoglycemic agents, these are to be switched to insulin once pregnancy is diagnosed by a urine test.

Placenta Previa

Diagnosis by Ultrasound and Correlation of os-Placenta Distance with Mode of Delivery The current classification of placenta previa is based on ultrasonography findings and has evolved from the original classification of Types I to IV. According to the Royal College of Obstetricians and Gynaecologists (RCOG), if the placenta lies over the cervical os, it is termed major previa, otherwise, minor previa (RCOG 2005). The ultrasonography-based classification is (Williams Obstetrics 2001) as follows:

Total: The internal os is covered completely by the placenta.

Partial: The internal os is covered partially by the placenta.

Marginal: The edge of the placenta is at the margin of the internal os.

Low-lying: The placenta is implanted in the lower uterine segment (LUS) in such a way that the placental edge does not reach the internal os but is in close proximity to it.

Traditionally, transabdominal sonography (TAS) has been used to diagnose placenta previa, but currently, transvaginal sonography (TVS) is preferred, as it images the cervix precisely and can accurately measure the distance of the leading edge of the placenta to the internal os (os–placenta distance) (Leerentveld et al 1990). Although some studies have correlated the os–placenta distance with the mode of delivery, it is not clear at up to what distance from the internal os a placenta should be to be considered low lying, or the appropriate mode of delivery with respect to this distance (Dawson et al 1996; RCOG 2005). Low-lying placentas are also associated with increased risk of bleeding and adverse perinatal outcome, although less than with true placenta previa. However, what exactly constitutes a low-lying placenta on ultrasonography is not precisely defined and this term is used:

(i) to describe an apparent placenta previa in the second trimester
(ii) to describe a placenta that lies in the LUS, but its exact relationship to the internal os is not determined
(iii) to describe a placental edge that lies within 2–3 cm of the internal os (Oppenheimer et al 1991).

The maximum os–placenta distance for diagnosing a low-lying placenta has been arbitrarily selected as 5.8 cm, 3.0 cm and 3.5 cm by various authors (Dawson et al 1996; Oppenheimer et al 2001; RCOG 2005). A recent study suggested that a placenta located >3.5 cm from the internal os need not be considered as previa (Lahoria et al 2007).

The os–placenta distance has been correlated with the mode of delivery. According to the RCOG, the mode of delivery should be based on clinical judgement supplemented by sonographic information (RCOG 2005). Decisions regarding the mode of delivery should take into account the relation of the fetal head to the pelvic brim (assessed clinically), the relation of the fetal head to the leading edge of the placenta (assessed sonographically) and the os–placenta distance (assessed sonographically). A placental edge less than 2 cm from the internal os is likely to need delivery by cesarean section, especially if it is posterior or thick. A recommendation about the mode of delivery based only on sonography findings is difficult as most of the studies relating to this are observational and often retrospective. These findings should also be interpreted according to the time interval between the last TVS examination and delivery, so that any alteration in the os–placenta distance due to placental migration is accounted for; this is another variable that influences the os–placenta distance. The differential growth of the LUS or progressive unidirectional growth of trophoblastic tissue toward the uterine fundus (trophotropism) results in 'placental migration', which relocates the lower edge of the placenta away from internal os. The length of the LUS may increase from 0.5 cm at 20 weeks to >5 cm at term, and placental migration of 0.54 cm per week in the third trimester has been reported (Oppenheimer et al 2001).

A retrospective analysis of 52 women (who underwent sonography in the third trimester on an average 5 weeks before delivery) observed that 31 women with total previa and 7 with an os–placenta distance of 1.1±0.8 cm (range 0–2 cm) underwent cesarean section, whereas 14 women with an os–placenta distance of 3.1±1.1 cm (range 1.8–5.8 cm) delivered vaginally. The mean os–placenta distance was significantly less in those delivered by cesarean section with a cut-off distance of 2 cm (Oppenheimer et al 1991). Another study observed that vaginal delivery was safe with an os–placenta distance of >2.0 cm, that vaginal delivery was an option with careful monitoring between 1 cm and 2 cm, and that cesarean section was needed if <1 cm; however, these scans were performed on an average of 6 weeks prior to delivery (Dawson et al 1996). A prospective observational study of 63 women demonstrated that in those who delivered vaginally, the os–placenta distance was 2 cm in case of anterior placenta previa and 3 cm in case of posterior previa on TVS performed within two weeks of delivery (Ghourab and Al-Jabari 2000). In a retrospective analysis of 121 women with an average scan-to-delivery interval of 10.5 days, the cesarean rate was 90% and 37% when the os–placenta distance was <2.0 cm and >2.0 cm, respectively (Bhide et al 2003). The thickness of the encroaching tongue of placenta has also been shown to influence outcome—the thicker the placenta (>1 cm), the higher the likelihood of cesarean section (Ghourab 2001).

Management of Asymptomatic Low-lying Placenta Painless bleeding after 20 weeks of gestation occurs in 70–80% women with placenta previa; 10–20% have bleeding associated with contractions; only <10% remain asymptomatic and reach term without bleeding. A Cochrane review to assess the impact of clinical interventions in placenta previa found only three randomised trials and concluded that the data was insufficient to make evidence-based recommendations (Neilson 2003). Women are advised to avoid exercise and decrease physical activities in the third trimester, although this is not based on data from well-designed studies. General principles of management in asymptomatic women are:

- Perform TVS if low-lying placenta is suspected during the anomaly scan (20–24 weeks).
- Confirm persistence of a previously suspected placenta previa sonographically. In asymptomatic major previa, repeat TVS at 32 weeks and in minor previa, at 36 weeks.
- Perform serial sonography every 2–4 weeks to assess placental location and monitor fetal growth.
- Avoid coitus and digital examination.
- Counsel to seek immediate medical attention if the mother has contractions or vaginal bleeding.
- In major previa, hospital admission at 32–34 weeks is advised.
- Provide antenatal advice regarding iron supplementation, correction of anemia and arrangement of blood transfusion facilities in case of emergency.

Asymptomatic Major Placenta Previa

Hospital admission The concern is that the affected women may bleed profusely and suddenly, and require emergency delivery. Hospital admission at around 32–34 weeks is advised. A very select group of women who opt for outpatient care must be counselled carefully and allowed such management only after a fully informed consent is obtained. It must be ascertained that she will be able to reach the hospital in a very short time (15 minutes) and have the constant presence of an adult companion. Studies to assess features associated with the likelihood of antepartum hemorrhage in women with placenta previa suggest that raised serum alphafetoprotein levels at 15–20 weeks (Butler et al 2001), placentas which encroach on the os (Bhide et al 2003; Dola et al 2003) and are thick inferiorly (Ghourab 2001) or show turbulent flow at their lower margin (Saitoh et al 2002) by ultrasound imaging are most associated with antepartum hemorrhage. Sonography should also assess for a morbidly adherent placenta, especially if there is a history of cesarean and anterior placenta previa.

Asymptomatic Marginal or Low-lying Placenta Previa

Hospital admission Women who have never bled are followed-up as outpatients, with activity restrictions. They may be given home management till delivery is planned, with arrangements to be able to reach hospital in a short time if needed, have an adult companion constantly and after an informed consent. They should be reliable and be able to comprehend the nature of their problem, including the possibility of an emergency arising.

Timing and mode of delivery A cesarean delivery at term (after confirming fetal pulmonary maturity) is suggested when the placenta is within 2 cm of the internal os. Alternatively, especially when the placenta is > 2 cm from the os, the woman can be told to reach the hospital as soon as labour begins and be monitored closely for excessive vaginal bleeding. Occasionally, a 'double set-up examination' may be considered if there is diagnostic uncertainty regarding placental localisation. If such an examination demonstrates a low-lying placenta or descent of the fetal head beyond an intact placental edge, vaginal delivery may be considered (Chervenak et al 1984). Facilities for emergency cesarean and blood transfusion should be made available.

Role of Cerclage in Placenta Previa During conservative management in symptomatic placenta previa, cervical cerclage has been used to minimise the early development of LUS, which is thought to promote placental separation, thereby leading to antepartum hemorrhage. There is no clear evidence of its benefit. Although one series (n = 25) noted longer gestations (34.9 against 31.6 weeks) and heavier birth weight (2709 versus 1812 g) with cerclage (Arias 1988), a subsequent randomised trial (n = 36) failed to confirm these benefits (Cobo et al 1998), though there was a reduction in antenatal hospitalisation with cerclage (10 versus 15 days). More trials are needed to determine the benefits of cerclage, if any, and currently, its routine use in placenta previa is not indicated.

Role of Tocolytics in Placenta Previa As part of conservative management (usually carried out in about 75% of symptomatic placenta previa), tocolysis has been used by many centres to eliminate uterine contractions, which are theorised to exacerbate placental detachment and bleeding. Tocolysis may be considered and safely utilised if contractions are present, bleeding is diminishing or has ceased, and delivery is not otherwise mandated by the maternal or fetal condition. Tocolysis is not used in active bleeding.

Tocolysis for treatment of bleeding due to placenta previa may be useful in selected cases. Hemorrhage in placenta previa is due to the development of the LUS and also due to uterine contractions. Conservative aggressive management of placenta previa using cerclage and/or tocolysis has been reported (Cotton et al 1980; Silver et al 1984). A prospective RCT of 60 women who presented with antepartum hemorrhage due to placenta previa between 28 and 34 weeks used tocolysis with 10 mg ritodrine every six hours (intramuscularly) for seven days (Sharma et al 2004). This was compared with no treatment. Tocolysis was associated with prolongation of pregnancy (25.33 ± 17.7 days compared with 14.47 ± 20.33 days; $P < 0.05$) and increased birth weight (2.27 ± 0.59 kg compared with 1.95 ± 0.55 kg). There were no adverse maternal, fetal or neonatal effects. Besinger et al gave tocolysis to 72 women with significant uterine activity among the 112 women with placenta previa who presented with hemorrhage. There was prolongation of the admission-to-delivery interval (39.2 days versus 26.9 days; $P < 0.02$) and increase in birth weight (2.520 kg versus 2.124 kg, $P < 0.03$) with tocolysis when compared to the 40 women who were not given tocolysis (Besinger et al 1995). Towers et al retrospectively reviewed the use of tocolysis in 105 women who presented with bleeding in the third trimester, which included 76 women with placenta previa. These results suggested no increased morbidity or mortality associated with such use in a tertiary care setting (Towers et al 1999). However, prophylactic use of terbutaline to prevent bleeding in women with placenta previa was not beneficial (Magann et al 1993). Most studies on tocolysis in placenta previa have used beta-mimetics, which are associated with significant side effects. Hence, further research on the optimum drug, route and duration of therapy is needed in this area.

Preterm Labor

Role of Bed Rest in Preterm Labour Bed rest has been shown to improve uteroplacental blood flow but its effect on preterm labour is controversial. A randomised trial comparing women who were hospitalised against those sent home after arrested preterm labour showed similar outcomes in both the groups (Yost 2005). Other studies have also shown that bed rest does not decrease the incidence of preterm delivery (Goldenerg 1994). The Cochrane review also concluded that bed rest does not improve the outcome in women with preterm labour (Cochrane Review 2004). On the contrary, it has been shown that bed rest for three or more days increased thromboembolic complications to 16 per 1000 women compared to one per 1000 in the normal population (Kovacevich 2000).

Role of Diagnostic Amniocentesis in PPROM Subclinical intrauterine infection is both a cause and an effect of preterm premature rupture of membranes (PTPROM). The rate of positive cultures obtained by transabdominal amniocentesis at the time of PTPROM is 25–40%, while clinical chorioamnionitis is present on admission in only 1–2% of cases (Cotton 1984; Romero 1988; Asrat 1990; Yoon 1996). Intrauterine infections are closely associated with serious adverse neonatal outcomes and are thus an indication for delivery. Positive amniotic fluid culture is the most definite evidence of infection. In addition, amniotic fluid glucose, WBC and Gram stain are rapid tests for presumptive diagnosis of infection.

The management of PPROM is to deliver the fetus when the risks of prematurity are outweighed by the risks of pregnancy prolongation. Lung maturity assessment could be a useful guide to plan delivery in the 32–34 week interval. Thus, amniocentesis could help determine lung maturity as well as provide evidence of infection. Both, a retrospective study and a randomised trial, support the use of amniocentesis in women with PPROM to aid delivery planning (Cotton 1984; Dudley 1991). The randomised controlled trial showed that when amniocentesis is used aggressively to determine delivery, neonatal period of stay and morbidity are decreased (Cotton 1984). Moreover, amniocentesis is not associated with fetal injury or shorter latency (Yeast 1984).

Thus, amniocentesis is recommended for patients with PPROM to obtain amniotic fluid for culture to evaluate early markers of infection and assessment of lung maturity.

Role of Bed Rest and Nutritional Supplementation in IUGR Nutrient supplementation for the mother has been tried to improve fetal growth when it is impaired. Different nutrients such as carbohydrates and aminoacids have been suggested as treatment for impaired fetal growth. The Cochrane Systematic Review on the subject found three small studies involving 121 women (Cochrane 2000). No difference was detected in the number of small for gestational age infants whose mothers had received nutrients compared to those who did not. The reviewers concluded that there was not enough evidence to evaluate the use of nutrient therapy for suspected impaired fetal growth.

Bed rest in hospital or at home is widely advised for many complications of pregnancy. However, it increases the risk of thrombosis, stress on the pregnant women, as well as the cost to families and health services. A Cochrane Systematic Review assessed the effects of bed rest in hospital for women with suspected impaired fetal growth (Cochrane 2000). Only one randomised trial involving 107 women comparing a policy of bed rest in the hospital with ambulatory management for women with suspected impaired fetal growth was included. The reviewers concluded that there was not enough evidence to evaluate the use of bed rest in the hospital policy for women with suspected impaired fetal growth.

Management of Patients with Previous History of Abruptio placentae The risk of recurrence of abruption placentae in a subsequent pregnancy after one episode is 5–15% and after two consecutive abruptions, the risk of a third rises to 25% (Furuhashi 2002; Toivonen 2004; Tikkanen 2006). Placental abruption may also predict a greater likelihood of other problems in subsequent pregnancies like higher rates of small for gestational age infants, spontaneous preterm birth and pre-eclampsia (Rasmussen 2000).

The subsequent pregnancies should be monitored for fetal growth and blood pressure. Antepartum fetal monitoring tests in women with a history of abruption are not useful since these tests are not predictive of abruption (Seski 1976). Women should be advised to avoid smoking as it is a risk factor for abruption. Thromboprophylaxis may be tried in women with inherited thrombophilias (Oyelese 2006). In some women, such as those with prior perinatal deaths due to abruption, preterm delivery on documentation of fetal lung maturity may be reasonable.

Labour Management

Use of Misoprostol in Scarred Uterus in Second Trimester There is limited data regarding the safety of misoprostol (or other prostaglandins) for second trimester pregnancy termination in women with previous cesarean deliveries. A few small series have reported its use to be safe. Dickinson reviewed 101 women between 14 and 28 weeks of gestation with previous cesarean deliveries who were given misoprostol to induce abortion for a fetal anomaly. Seventy-eight women had at least one prior cesarean, 19 women had 2, and 4 women had 3 prior cesareans. Misoprostol was given in various dose regimens, the most frequent being 400 μg vaginally every 6 hours. There were no uterine ruptures (Dickinson 2005). Bhattacharjee et al used misoprotol vaginally or sublingually (200 μg if >20 weeks, 400 μg if <20 weeks; 6 hourly) for pregnancy termination in 80 women between 16 and 26 weeks and reported no ruptures (Bhattacharjee et al 2007). Daskalakis et al reviewed 108 women with previous cesarean section and 216 women without a uterine scar (control group) who underwent pregnancy termination between 17 and 24 weeks of gestation with 400 μg of oral misoprostol plus 400 μg of intravaginal misoprostol followed by 400 mcg intravaginal misoprostol 6 hourly for a maximum of five doses. Complications such as hemorrhage requiring transfusion, infection, retained placenta and uterine rupture occurred in 15% of women with a previous cesarean and in 12% in the control group. There was one ruptured uterus in the control group.

However, case reports have described uterine rupture in such patients. A woman with two prior cesareans underwent pregnancy termination at 23 weeks gestation by dilation and evacuation. She had laminariae placed a day before, 400 μg misoprostol placed intravaginally at midnight, then 400 μg misoprostol given buccally at 6:00 AM on the day of the procedure. During evacuation, uterine rupture was diagnosed. She underwent emergency laparotomy, and the uterus was repaired (Berghahn et al 2001). A woman with one prior cesarean and one vaginal delivery underwent termination of pregnancy at 17 weeks with misoprostol, which was given vaginally for two days. This resulted in uterine rupture which was repaired by laparotomy (Petri 2003). More data from large studies is needed to determine the magnitude of risk and determine whether it should be used routinely for second trimester pregnancy termination in women with a previous cesarean section.

Misoprostol for Induction of Labour

Administration of misoprostol for cervical ripening and labour induction may be done by the vaginal or the oral route. An earlier meta-analysis reported that when used vaginally, a 50 μg dose was more effective than 25 μg, but the safety of the higher dose could not be adequately evaluated. Therefore, lower doses, such as 25 μg, should be used at a re-dosing interval of 3–6 hours (Sanchez-Ramos et al 2002). Oxytocin may be initiated, if necessary, 4 hours after the final misoprostol dose (Hofmeyr and Gulmezoglu 2003).

Orally administered misoprostol for cervical ripening and labour induction is also being explored (Dodd et al 2006). The concentration of orally administered misoprostol peaks sooner and declines more rapidly than that given vaginally (Khan et al 2004). Most trials have used an oral dose of 50 μg every four hours. In a Cochrane review of 16 trials (3645 participants) comparing oral and vaginal misoprostol, the vaginal delivery and cesarean rates were similar with both routes. There was less uterine hyperstimulation with oral misoprostol (RR 0.37). However, it was associated with increased need for oxytocin augmentation (RR 1.28) and more meconium-stained liquor (RR 1.27). If misoprostol is used orally, the dose should not exceed 50 μg (Alfirevic and Weeks 2006). The regimens for labour induction using 25 μg vaginal misoprostol 4-hourly, 50 μg oral misoprostol 4-hourly or 20 mcg oral misoprostol solution 2-hourly are all safe and effective (Weeks et al 2007).

Intrapartum Monitoring CTG or Manual Intermittent Ascultation The aim of intrapartum FHR monitoring is to identify hypoxemic fetuses in whom timely intervention may prevent birth asphyxia, neurologic injury and death. The two commonly used modalities are continuous electronic FHR monitoring and intermittent auscultation with a stethoscope or a Doppler device used to count the FHR over 1–2 minutes at intervals of 5–30 minutes, depending on the stage of labour. The FHR is checked both during and after a contraction and the lowest rate is recorded. In contrast to continuous cardiotocography, intermittent auscultation does not provide any information about FHR variability, the shape of FHR decelerations or uterine contractions.

There is no definite evidence that any of these techniques reduce asphyxia-related fetal morbidity or mortality, or that any one is better in low-risk pregnancies (Graham et al 2006; Larma et al 2007). A Cochrane review of randomised trials comparing these two techniques showed that the intrapartum fetal death rate was 0.5 per 1000 births with either approach; Apgar scores and neonatal ICU admission rates were similar for both modalities and neither approach reduced the risk of cerebral palsy (Cochrane Database System Review 2006).

Use of electronic FHR monitoring instead of intermittent auscultation has not led to a reduction in the overall risk of perinatal death (RR 0.85) (Cochrane Database System Review 2006). However, the limitation of these results is that a significant decrease in the perinatal death rate would be difficult to demonstrate since perinatal death is a rare outcome and even pooling results from multiple trials lacked sufficient power to provide an answer.

Use of electronic FHR monitoring instead of intermittent auscultation has also not led to a reduction in the prevalence of cerebral palsy (RR 1.74) (Cochrane Database System Review 2006). The absence of reduction in cerebral palsy may be because many of these cases are caused by an antepartum event, rather than intrapartum asphyxia (Nelson et al 1996).

The major benefit of continuous electronic FHR monitoring is a reduction in the frequency of neonatal seizures (RR 0.50) (Cochrane Database System Review 2006).

A disadvantage of continuous electronic FHR monitoring is that it leads to higher cesarean (RR 1.66) and instrumental vaginal delivery rates (RR 1.16) without an associated neonatal benefit (Cochrane Database System Review 2006). The results were similar even in high-risk pregnancies, but data was limited. However, some type of intrapartum FHR monitoring is now routine in most labour units because both patients and clinicians are reassured by normal results and believe there is some value in detecting non-reassuring patterns.

The United States Preventive Services Task Force and the Canadian Task Force on Preventive Health Care state that routine intrapartum electronic FHR monitoring for low-risk women is not recommended, and there is insufficient evidence to recommend for or against intrapartum electronic FHR monitoring for high-risk pregnant women (Canadian Task Force on Preventive Health Care 2005; US Preventive Services Task Force 2005). The American College of Obstetricians and Gynecologists states that either intermittent auscultation or electronic FHR monitoring is appropriate for uncomplicated pregnancies. High-risk pregnancies should be monitored continuously during labour (ACOG Practice Bulletin 2005).

Epidural Analgesia in Labour There is considerable controversy concerning the effects of epidural anesthesia on the length of the first stage of labour, cesarean delivery rate and instrumental delivery rate. It is believed that neuraxial analgesia tends to slow labour and result in increased rates of instrumental and cesarean delivery. A study combining five randomised trials showed that epidural analgesia prolongs labour, increases the need for oxytocin stimulation as well as that for instrumental delivery due to prolonged second stage of labour but does not lead to any adverse neonatal effects (Sharma 2004). However, a meta-analysis of 20 trials concluded that epidural analgesia did not significantly increase the risk of cesarean delivery but was associated with increased risk of instrumental vaginal delivery (Anim-Somuah 2005). Newer low-dose techniques, by achieving sensory block while preserving motor strength, have been shown to decrease the rate of instrumental delivery. Therefore, low-dose techniques should be recommended over traditional epidural administration to reduce the rate of operative vaginal delivery (Thompson 2001). It has been shown that patients with severe pain and protracted, dysfunctional labour are more likely to request or receive epidural analgesia. Thus, it may be falsely concluded that neuraxial techniques are causally related to poor labour outcome, whereas the relationship may simply be an associative one (Hess 200). An ACOG Committee Opinion concluded that "maternal request is sufficient medical indication for pain relief during labor" and that neuraxial anesthesia does not increase the frequency of cesarean delivery (ACOG 2006). Moreover, early administration of neuraxial analgesia does not increase the rates of cesarean or instrumental delivery.

Thus, although an association between regional analgesia and prolonged labour or increased cesarean delivery rates may exist, a cause-and-effect relationship has not been established, except perhaps for an increase in the rate of instrumental deliveries when epidural analgesia is used.

Uncomplicated Breech and Mode of Delivery The options for a woman with uncomplicated breech presentation at term include:

- External cephalic version
- Vaginal delivery
- Cesarean delivery

External cephalic version: The Royal College of Obstetricians and Gynaecologists (1999) and the American College of Obstetricians and Gynecologists (2000) recommend that all women near term with breech presentation should be offered an attempt at external cephalic version if they have no contraindications to the procedure. A systematic review showed that ECV significantly reduces incidence of breech births and cesarean deliveries (Hofmeyr 2000). ECV also appears to be a safe option for women who present in labour with breech presentation, intact membranes and no contraindications. The advantages of ECV during labour are that the maximum time for spontaneous version has been allowed, the fetal condition can be monitored continuously until delivery and cesarean delivery can be performed expeditiously if required. The disadvantages are that the opportunity for ECV may be lost due to ruptured membranes or rapid labour.

Vaginal delivery versus cesarean delivery: A large multicentre trial, Term Breech Trial, compared planned cesarean delivery with planned vaginal delivery in women with breech presentation (Hannah 2000).The results showed lower rates of perinatal and neonatal death and short-term neonatal morbidity in babies delivered by cesarean section and a modest increase in short-term maternal morbidity. Outcomes of children from the Term Breech Trial at two years after delivery have subsequently reported that although neonatal morbidity and mortality were reduced in the first six weeks of life by planned cesarean delivery, at two years of age there was no significant difference in the combined risk of death/ neurodevelopmental delay between the planned vaginal and planned cesarean groups (Whyte 2004). These trials indicate that a policy of planned cesarean delivery for term breech presentation is associated with reduced perinatal mortality and short-term morbidity, but not long-term morbidity. Similar results were shown by a systematic review (Hofmeyr 2003).

However, these results should be applied with due consideration to specific healthcare environments and individual women. In terms of short-term outcomes, the results favour a policy of planned cesarean delivery. However, this policy may not be affordable or feasible in resource-poor settings and there may be clinical situations in which the risks of cesarean section to the mother or the mother's desire to avoid cesarean delivery may outweigh the risks of vaginal birth to the baby. Moreover, a few studies have shown no difference in perinatal outcome where breech was delivered by vaginal routes in one-fourth to half of the patients (Giuliani 2002; Alarab 2004). The ACOG Committee on Obstetric Practice recommended the use of external cephalic version and planned cesarean delivery for persistent singleton breech presentation at term (2001). However, they subsequently allowed that planned vaginal delivery of a term singleton breech may be reasonable with detailed patient informed consent, under hospital-specific protocol guidelines and by a healthcare provider experienced in vaginal breech delivery (2006). Vaginal delivery, if selected, should be performed by an experienced healthcare provider.

References

Alfirevic Z and A Weeks. 2006. Oral misoprostol for induction of labour. *Cochrane Database Syst Rev* (2): CD001338.

American College of Obstetricians and Gynecologists. 2000. External cephalic version. ACOG Practice Bulletin No. 13.

American College of Obstetricians and Gynecologists. 2001. ACOG Committee Opinion No. 265. Mode of term single breech delivery. *Obstet Gynecol* 98:1189.

American College of Obstetricians and Gynecologists. 2001. ACOG Practice Bulletin No. 30. Clinical management guidelines for obstetrician-gynecologists (replaces Technical Bulletin No. 200, 1994). Gestational diabetes. *Obstet Gynecol* 98:525.

American College of Obstetricians and Gynecologists. 2001. Chronic hypertension in pregnancy. ACOG Practice Bulletin No. 29.

American College of Obstetricians and Gynecologists. 2001. Gestational Diabetes. ACOG Practice Bulletin No. 30. ACOG.

American College of Obstetricians and Gynecologists. 2002. Diagnosis and management of preeclampsia and eclampsia. ACOG Practice Bulletin No. 33. Washington, DC: ACOG.

American College of Obstetricians and Gynecologists. 2005. ACOG Practice Bulletin No. 70.

Intrapartum fetal heart rate monitoring. *Obstet Gynecol* 106:1453.

American College of Obstetricians and Gynecologists. 2005. ACOG Practice Bulletin No 60. Pregestational diabetes mellitus. *Obstet Gynecol* 105:675.

American College of Obstetricians and Gynecologists. 2006. ACOG Committee Opinion No 339. Analgesia and cesarean delivery rates. *Obstet Gynecol* 107:1487.

American College of Obstetricians and Gynecologists. 2006. ACOG Committee Opinion No 340. Mode of term singleton breech delivery. *Obstet Gynecol* 108:235.

Anim-Somuah M, R Smyth, C Howell. 2005. Epidural versus non-epidural or no analgesia in labour. *Cochrane Database Syst Rev* 19:CD00033.

Arias F. 1998. Cervical cerclage for the temporary treatment of patients with placenta previa. *Obstet Gynecol* 71:545.

Asrat T, MP Nageotte, TJ Garite et al. 1990. Gram stain results from amniocentesis in patients with preterm premature rupture of membranes - comparison of maternal and fetal characteristics. *Am J Obstet Gynecol* 163:887–889.

Atallah AN, GJ Hofmeyr, L Duley. 2002. Calcium supplementation during pregnancy for preventing hypertensive disorders and related problems (Cochrane review). *Cochrane Database Syst Rev* 1: CD001059.

Banerjee S, N Aslam, B Woelfer et al. 2001. Expectant management of early pregnancies of unknown location: A prospective evaluation of methods to predict spontaneous resolution of pregnancy. *Br J Obstet Gynaecol* 108:158.

Berghahn L, D Christensen, S Droste. 2001. Uterine rupture during second-trimester abortion associated with misoprostol. *Obstet Gynecol* 98:976–977.

Besinger RE, CW Moniak, LS Paskiewicz, SG Fishes, PG Tomich. 1995. The effect of tocolytic use in the management of symptomatic placenta previa. *Am J Obstet Gynecol* 172:1770–1778.

Bhattacharjee N, RP Ganguly, SP Saha. 2007. Misoprostol for termination of mid-trimester post-cesarean pregnancy. *Aust NZ J Obstet Gynaecol.* 47:23–25.

Bhide A, F Prefumo, J Moore, B Hollis, B Thilaganathan. 2003. Placenta edge to internal os distance in the late third trimester and mode of delivery in placenta previa. *Br J Obstet Gynaecol* 110:860–864.

Boulvain M, C Stan, O Irion. 2001. Elective delivery in diabetic pregnant women. *Cochrane Database Syst Rev* (2):CD001997.

Brent GA. 2007. Diagnosing thyroid dysfunction in pregnant women: Is case finding enough? *J Clin Endocrinol Metab* 92:39.

Butler EL, JS Dasheand, RM Ramus. 2001. Association between maternal serum alpha-fetoprotein and adverse outcomes in pregnancies with placenta previa. *Obstet Gynecol* 97:35–38.

Canadian Task Force on Preventive Health Care. 2005. www.ctfphc.org

Caritis S, B Sibai, J Hauth et al. 1998. Low-dose aspirin to prevent pre-eclampsia in women at high risk. *N Engl J Med* 338:701.

Carpenter MW and DR Coustan. 1982. Criteria for screening tests for gestational diabetes. *Am J Obstet Gynecol* 144:768.

Casey BM and KJ Leveno. 2006. Thyroid disease in pregnancy. *Obstet Gynecol* 108:1283–1292.

Chervenak FA, Y Lee, MA Hendler, RF Monoson, RL Berkowitz. 1984. Role of attempted vaginal delivery in the management of placenta previa. *Obstet Gynecol* 64: 798.

Christiansen OB, AM Nybo Andersen, E Bosch et al. 2005. Evidence-based investigations and treatments of recurrent pregnancy loss. *Fertil Steril* 83:821.

Christine A, D Home, M Lumsden. 2006. Diabetes. In *High risk pregnancy management options*, 3rd ed. 986–1004. Eds James DK, PJ Steer, CP Weiner and B Gonik. Philadelphia: Elsevier.

CLASP (Collaborative Low-dose Aspirin Study in Pregnancy) Collaborative Group. 1994. CLASP: A randomised trial of low-dose aspirin for the prevention and treatment of pre-eclampsia among 9364 pregnant women. *Lancet* 343:619.

Cobo E, DJ Conde-Agudelo, H Canaval, A Congote. 1998. Cervical cerclage: An alternative for the management of placenta previa? *Am J Obstet Gynecol* 179:122.

Cotton DB, B Gonik, SF Bottoms. 1984. Conservative versus aggressive management of preterm rupture of membranes. A randomized trial of amniocentesis. *Am J Perinatol* 1:322–324.

Cotton DB, JA Read, RH Paul, EJ Quilligan. 1980. The conservative aggressive management of placenta previa. *Am J Obstet Gynecol* 137:687.

Cunningham FG and MD Lindheimer. 1992. Hypertension in pregnancy. *N Engl J Med* 326:927.

Cunningham FG, NF Gant, KJ Leveno, LC Gilstrap, JC Hauth, KD Wenstrom. 2001. *Williams Obstetrics*, 21st ed. New York: McGraw Hill.

Daskalakis GJ, SA Mesogitis, NE Papantoniou, GG Moulopoulos, AA Papapanagiotou, AJ Antsaklis. 2005. Misoprostol for second trimester pregnancy termination in women with prior cesarean section. *Br J Obstet Gynaecol* 112:97–99.

Davis AR, SK Hendish, C Westhoff et al. 2007. Bleeding patterns after misoprostol versus surgical treatment of early pregnancy failure: results from a randomised trial. *Am J Obstet Gynecol* 196:31.

Dawson WB, MD Dumas, WM Romano, R Gagnon, RJ Gratton, RD Mowbray. 1996. Translabial ultrasonography and placenta previa: does measurement of the os–placenta distance predict outcome? *J Ultrasound Med* 15:441–446.

De Braekeleer M and TN Dao. 1990. Cytogenetic studies in couples experiencing repeated pregnancy losses. *Hum Reprod* 5:519.

Denno KM and TW Sadler. 1994. Effects of the biguanide class of oral hypoglycemic agents on mouse embryogenesis. *Teratology* 49:260–266.

DerSimonian R and RJ Levine. 1999. Resolving discrepancies between a meta-analysis and a subsequent large controlled trial. *JAMA* 282:664.

Dickinson JE. 2005. Misoprostol for second-trimester pregnancy termination in women with a prior cesarean delivery. *Obstet Gynecol* 105:352–356.

Dodd JM, CA Crowther, JS Robinson. 2006. Oral misoprostol for induction of labour at term: Randomised controlled trial. *Br Med J* 332:509.

Dola CP, TJ Garite, DD Dowling, D Friend, D Ahdoot, T Asrat. 2003. Placenta previa: does its type affect pregnancy outcome? *Am J Perinatol* 20:353–360.

Dudley J, G Malcolm and D Ellwood. 1991. Amniocentesis in the management of preterm premature rupture of the membranes. *Aust NZ J Obstet Gynaecol* 31:331–336.

Duley L, D Henderson-Smart, M Knight, J King. 2004. Antiplatelet agents for preventing pre-eclampsia and its complications. *Cochrane Database Syst Rev* 1:CD004659.

Early worsening of diabetic retinopathy in the Diabetes Control and Complications Trial. 1998. *Arch Ophthalmol* 116:874.

Fourth International Workshop-Conference on Gestational Diabetes Mellitus. 1998. Diabetes Care Suppl 2.

Furuhashi M, O Kurauchi and N Suganuma. 2002. Pregnancy following placental abruption. *Arch Gynecol Obstet* 267:11.

Gestational diabetes mellitus. 2004. Diabetes Care 27; Suppl 1:S88.

Ghourab S and A Al-Jabari. 2000. Placental migration and mode of delivery in placenta previa: Transvaginal sonographic assessment during the third trimester. *Ann Saudi Med* 20:382–385.

Ghourab S. 2001.Third trimester transvaginal ultrasonography in placenta previa: does the shape of the lower placental edge predict clinical outcome? *Ultrasound Obstet Gynecol* 18:103–118.

Gilbert C, M Valois, G Koren. 2006. Pregnancy outcome after first-trimester exposure to metformin: a meta-analysis. *Fertil Steril* 86:658.

Giuliani A, WMJ Scholl, A Basver et al. 2002. Mode of delivery and outcome of 699 term singleton breech deliveries at a single center. *Am J Obstet Gynecol* 187:1694.

Glueck CJ, H Phillips, D Cameron et al. 2001. Continuing metformin throughout pregnancy in women with polycystic ovary syndrome appears to safely reduce first-trimester spontaneous abortion: A pilot study. *Fertil Steril* 75:46.

Glueck CJ, N Goldenberg, J Pranikoff, M Loftspring, L Sieve, P Wang. 2004. Height, weight, and motor, social development during the first 18 months of life in 126 infants born to 109 mothers with polycystic ovary syndrome who conceived on and continued metformin through pregnancy. *Hum Reprod* 19:1323–1330.

Glueck CJ, P Wang, N Goldenberg and L Sieve-Smith. 2002. Pregnancy outcomes among women with polycystic ovary syndrome treated with metformin. *Hum Reprod* 17:2858.

Glueck CJ, P Wang, S Kobayashi et al. 2002. Metformin therapy throughout pregnancy reduces the development of gestational diabetes in women with polycystic ovary syndrome. *Fertil Steril* 77:520.

Goldberg JM, T Falcone, M Attaran. 1997. Sonohysterographic evaluation of uterine abnormalities noted on hysterosalpingography. *Hum Reprod* 12:2151.

Goldenberg RL, SP Cliver, J Bronstein, GR Cutter, WW Andrews, ST Mennemeyer. 1994. Bed rest in pregnancy. *Obstet Gynecol* 84:131.

Graham EM, SM Petersen, DK Christo, HE Fox. 2006. Intrapartum electronic fetal heart rate monitoring and the prevention of perinatal brain injury. *Obstet Gynecol* 108: 656.

Graves CR. 2007. Antepartum fetal surveillance and timing of delivery in the pregnancy complicated by diabetes mellitus. *Clin Obstet Gynecol* 50:1007–1013.

Gulmezoglu AM and GJ Hofmeyr 2000. Bed rest in hospital for suspected impaired fetal growth. *Cochrane Database Syst Rev* CD000034.

Gulmezoglu AM and GJ Hofmeyr. 2000. Maternal nutrient supplementation for suspected impaired fetal growth. *Cochrane Database Syst Rev* CD000148.

Hannah ME, WJ Hannah, SA Hewson, ED Hodnett. 2000. Planned caesarean section versus planned vaginal birth for breech presentation at term: A randomised multicentre trial. Term Breech Trial Collaborative Group. *Lancet* 356:1375.

Hellmuth E, P Damm, L Molsted-Pedersen. 2001. Oral hypoglycaemic agents in 118 diabetic pregnancies. *Diabet Med* 18:604–605.

Hess PE, SD Pratt, AK Soni et al. 2000. An association between severe labour pain and cesarean delivery. *Anesth Analg* 90:881.

Hofmeyr GJ and AM Gulmezoglu. 2003. Vaginal misoprostol for cervical ripening and induction of labour. *Cochrane Database Syst Rev* CD000941.

Hofmeyr GJ and ME Hannah. 2003. Planned caesarean section for term breech delivery. *Cochrane Database Syst Rev*: CD000166.

Hofmeyr GJ and R Kulier. 2000. External cephalic version for breech presentation at term. *Cochrane Database Syst Rev* CD000083.

Hofmeyr GJ, AN Atallah and L Duley. 2006. Calcium supplementation during pregnancy for preventing hypertensive disorders and related problems. Cochrane Database Syst Rev 3:CD001059.

Jakubowicz DJ, MJ Iuorno, S Jakubowicz et al. 2002. Effects of metformin on early pregnancy loss in the polycystic ovary syndrome. *J Clin Endocrinol Metab* 87:524.

Jensen DM, P Damm, L Moelsted-Pedersen et al. 2004. Outcomes in type 1 diabetic pregnancies: a nationwide, population-based study. *Diabetes Care* 27:2819.

Jovanovic-Peterson L and CM Peterson. 1984. Is pregnancy contraindicated in women with diabetes mellitus? Diabet Nephrop 3:36.

Khan RU, H El-Refaey, S Sharma et al. 2004. Oral, rectal and vaginal pharmacokinetics of misoprostol. *Obstet Gynecol* 103:866.

Kjos SL, OA Henry, M Montoro, TA Buchanan and JH Mestman. 1993. Insulin-requiring diabetes in pregnancy: a randomized trial of active induction of labor and expectant management. *Am J Obstet Gynecol* 169:611–615.

Kovacevich GJ, SA Gaich, JP Lavin et al. 2000. The prevalence of thromboembolic events among women with extended bed rest prescribed as part of the treatment for premature labour or preterm premature rupture of membranes. *Am J Obstet Gynecol* 182:1089.

Kraemer J, J Klein, A Lubetsky and G Koren. 2006. Perfusion studies of glyburide transfer across the human placenta: implications for fetal safety. *Am J Obstet Gynecol* 195:270.

Lahoria K, S Malhotra and R Bagga. 2007. Transabdominal and transvaginal ultrasonography of placenta previa. *Int J Gynecol Obstet* 98: 258–259.

Langer O, Y Yogev, FM Xenakis, B Rosenn. 2005. Insulin and glyburide: Therapy, dosage, severity level of GDM and pregnancy outcome. *Am J Gynecol* 192:134–139.

Larma JD, AM Silva, CJ Holcroft et al. 2007. Intrapartum electronic fetal heart rate monitoring and the identification of metabolic acidosis and hypoxic-ischemic encephalopathy. *Am J Obstet Gynecol* 197:301.

Leerentveld RA, EC Gilberts, MJ Arnold and JW Wladimiroff. 1990. Accuracy and safety of transvaginal sonographic placental localisation. *Obstet Gynecol* 76:759–762.

Levine RJ, JC Hauth, LB Curet et al. 1997. Trial of calcium to prevent pre-eclampsia. *N Engl J Med* 337:69.

Luise C, K Jermy, C May et al. 2002. Outcome of expectant management of spontaneous first trimester miscarriage: Observational study. *Br Med J* 324:873.

Lurie S, M Feinstein, Y Mamet. 2000. Disseminated intravascular coagulopathy in pregnancy: Thorough comprehension of etiology and management reduces obstetricians' stress. *Arch Gynecol Obstet* 263:126.

Lydon-Rochelle M, VL Holt, TR Easterling, DP Martin. 2001. Risk of uterine rupture during labour among women with a prior cesarean delivery. *N Engl J Med* 345:3.

Magann EF, CA Johnson, KS Gookin, WE Roberts, RW Martin, JC Morrison. 1993. Placenta previa: Does uterine activity cause bleeding? *Aust NZ J Obstet Gynaecol* 33:22–24.

Martin JN Jr, BD Thigpen, RC Moore et al. 2005. Stroke and severe preeclampsia and eclampsia: A paradigm shift focusing on systolic blood pressure. *Obstet Gynecol* 105:246.

Maslow AD, TW Breen, MC Sarna et al. 1996. Prevalence of coagulation abnormalities associated with intrauterine fetal death. *Can J Anaesth* 43:1237.

Molsted-Pedersen L and C Kuhl. 1986. Obstetrical management in diabetic pregnancy: The Copenhagen experience. *Diabetologia* 29:13.

Nanda K, A Peloggia, D Grimes et al. 2006. Expectant care versus surgical treatment for miscarriage. *Cochrane Database Syst Rev* CD003518.

National Institutes of Health. 2000. Working group report on high blood pressure in pregnancy. Washington, DC:NIH.

Neilson J, M Hickey, J Vazquez. 2006. Medical treatment for early fetal death (less than 24 weeks). *Cochrane Database Syst Rev* 3:CD002253.

Neilson JP. 2003. Interventions for suspected placenta previa. *Cochrane Database Syst Rev* CD001998.

Nelson KB, JM Dambrosia, TY Ting, JK Grether. 1996. Uncertain value of electronic fetal monitoring in predicting cerebral palsy. *N Engl J Med* 334:613.

Nicholson JM, LC Kellar, GM Kellar. 2006. The impact of the interaction between increasing gestational age and obstetrical risk on birth outcomes: evidence of a varying optimal time of delivery. *J Perinatol* 26:392.

Oppenheimer L, P Holmes, P Simpson, N Holmes, A Dabrowski. 2001. Diagnosis of low-lying placenta: can migration in the third trimester predict outcome? *Ultrasound Obstet Gynecol* 18:100–102.

Oppenheimer LW, D Farine, JW Ritchie, RM Lewinsky, J Telford and LA Fairbanks. 1991. What is a low-lying placenta? *Am J Obstet Gynecol* 165:1036–1038.

O'Sullivan JB and CM Mahan. 1964. Criteria for the oral glucose tolerance test in pregnancy. *Diabetes* 13:278–285.

Oyelese Y and CV Ananth. 2006. Placental abruption. *Obstet Gynecol* 108:1005.

Petri AL. 2003. Uterine rupture during second trimester abortion induced with misoprostol. *Ugeskr Laeger* 165:2894–5.

Petrou S, J Trinder, P Brocklehurst, L Smith. 2006. Economic evaluation of alternative management methods of first-trimester miscarriage based on results from the MIST trial. *Br J Obstet Gynaecol* 113:879.

Piper JM, EM Xenakis, O Langer. 1998. Delayed appearance of pulmonary maturation markers is associated with poor glucose control in diabetic pregnancies. *J Matern Fetal Med* 7:148.

Rasmussen MJ, R Firth, M Foley and JM Stronge. 1992. The timing of delivery in diabetic pregnancy: a 10-year review. *Aust NZ J Obstet Gynaecol* 32:313.

Rasmussen S, LM Irgens, K Dalaker. 2000. Outcome of pregnancies subsequent to placental abruption: a risk assessment. *Acta Obstet Gynecol Scand* 79:496.

Rayburn WF. 1989. Prostaglandin E2 gel for cervical ripening and induction of labor: A critical analysis. *Am J Obstet Gynecol* 160:529.

RCOG Green Top Guidelines: The Management of Breech Presentation. 1999. Guideline No 20. London:RCOG.

RCOG Guideline Number 27. 2005. Placenta previa and placenta previa accreta: Diagnosis and management. RCOG.

Report of the Expert Committee on the Diagnosis and Classification of Diabetes Mellitus. 2000. Diabetes Care 23 Suppl 1:S4.

Report of the National BP Education Programme. 2000. Working group report on high blood pressure in pregnancy. *Am J Obstet Gynecol* 183:511–522.

Ringel MD and EL Mazzaferri. 2005. Subclinical thyroid dysfunction—can there be a consensus about the consensus? *J Clin Endocrinol Metab* 90:588–590.

Robert MF, RK Neff, JP Hubbell, JP, HW Taeusch, ME Avery. 1976. Association between maternal diabetes and the respiratory-distress syndrome in the newborn. *N Engl J Med* 294:357.

Romero R, R Quintero, E Oyarzun et al. 1988. Intraamniotic infection and the onset of labor in preterm premature rupture of the membranes. *Am J Obstet Gynecol* 159:661–666.

Rose SR, RS Brown, T Foley, PB Kaplowitz, CL Kaye, S Sundararajan, SK Varma. 2006. Update of newborn screening and therapy for congenital hypothyroidism. *Pediatrics* 117:2290–2303.

Saitoh M, K Ishihara, T Sekiya, T Araki. 2002. Anticipation of uterine bleeding in placenta previa based on vaginal sonographic evaluation. *Gynecol Obstet Invest* 54:37–42.

Sanchez-Ramos L, AM Kaunitz, I Delke. 2002. Labour induction with 25 µg versus 50 µg intravaginal misoprostol: A systematic review. *Obstet Gynecol* 99:145.

Sanchez-Ramos L, S Bernstein, AM Kaunitz. 2002. Expectant management versus labor induction for suspected fetal macrosomia: A systematic review. *Obstet Gynecol* 100:997.

Schwartz ML, WN Ray, SL Lubarsky. 1999. The diagnosis and classification of gestational diabetes mellitus: Is it time to change our tune? *Am J Obstet Gynecol* 180:1560.

Seski JC and Compton AA. 1976. Abruptio placentae following a negative oxytocin challenge test. *Am J Obstet Gynecol* 125:276.

Sharma A, V Suri , I Gupta. 2004. Tocolytic therapy in conservative management of symptomatic placenta previa. *Int J Gynecol Obstetn* 84:109–113.

Sharma SK, DD McIntire, J Wiley et al. 2004. Labour analgesia and cesarean delivery. An individual patient meta-analysis of nulliparous women. *Anesthesiology* 100:142.

Sibai B, S Caritis, E Thom et al. 1993. Prevention of preeclampsia with low-dose aspirin in healthy nulliparous pregnant women. *N Engl J Med* 329:1213.

Sibai BM. 1996. Treatment of hypertension in pregnant women. *N Engl J Med* 335:257.

Sibai BM. 2003. Diagnosis and management of gestational hypertension and preeclampsia. *Obstet Gynecol* 102:181.

Silver R, R Depp, RE Sabbagha, SL Dooley, ML Socol and RK Tamura. 1984. Placenta previa: aggressive expectant management. *Am J Obstet Gynecol* 150:15–22.

Soares SR, MMB Barbosa dos Reis, AF Camargos. 2000. Diagnostic accuracy of sonohysterography, transvaginal sonography, and hysterosalpingography in patients with uterine cavity diseases. *Fertil Steril* 73:406.

Sosa C, F Althabe, J Belizan, E Bergel. 2004. Bed rest in singleton pregnancies for preventing preterm birth. *Cochrane Database Syst Rev* CD003581.

Sotiriadis A, G Makrydimas, S Papatheodorou, JP Ioannidis. 2005. Expectant, medical or surgical management of first-trimester miscarriage: a meta-analysis. *Obstet Gynecol* 105:1104.

Stephenson MD. 1996. Frequency of factors associated with habitual abortion in 197 couples. *Fertil Steril* 66:24.

Surks MI, E Ortiz, GH Daniels, CT Sawin, NF Col, RH Cobin et al. 2004. Subclinical thyroid disease: scientific review and guidelines for diagnosis and management. *JAMA* 291:228–238.

Temple R, V Aldridge, R Greenwood et al. 2002. Association between outcome of pregnancy and glycaemic control in early pregnancy in type 1 diabetes: Population based study. *Br Med J* 325:1275.

Tharapel AT, SA Tharapel, RM Bannerman. 1985. Recurrent pregnancy losses and parental chromosome abnormalities: a review. *Br J Obstet Gynaecol* 92:899.

Thatcher SS and EM Jackson. 2006. Pregnancy outcome in infertile patients with polycystic ovary syndrome who were treated with metformin. *Fertil Steril* 85:1002.

The 67th Annual Scientific Sessions of the American Diabetes Association, Chicago. 2007. Diabetes Yale University School of Medicine, Department of Internal Medicine, From the Section of Endocrinology Volume 15 (3):5.

Thornton JG and G Capogna. 2001. Reducing likelihood of instrumental delivery with epidural anaesthesia. *Lancet* 358:2.

Tikkanen M, M Nuutila, V Hiilesmaa et al. 2006. Prepregnancy risk factors for placental abruption. *Acta Obstet Gynecol Scand* 85:40.

Toivonen S, S Heinonen, M Anttila et al. 2004. Obstetric prognosis after placental abruption. *Fetal Diagn Ther* 19:336.

Towers CV, RA Pircon and M Heppard. 1999. Is tocolysis safe in the management of third trimester bleeding? *Am J Obstet Gynecol* 180:1572–1578.

Trinder J, P Brocklehurst, R Porter et al. 2006. Management of miscarriage: expectant, medical or surgical? Results of randomised controlled trial (miscarriage treatment (MIST) trial). *Br Med J* 332:1235.

Tripathi KD. 2003. Insulin, oral hypoglycemic drugs and glucagons. In *Essentials of medical pharmacology*, 5th ed, 235–253. New Delhi:Jaypee Publishers.

US Preventive Services Task Force. 2005. Intrapartum Electronic Fetal Monitoring. www.ahcpr.gov/clinic/uspstf/uspsiefm.htm

Vaidya B, S Anthony, M Bilous, B Shields, J Drury, S Hutchison, R Bilous. 2007. Detection of thyroid dysfunction in early pregnancy: Universal screening or targeted high-risk case finding? *J Clin Endocrinol Metab* 92:203.

Verier-Mine O, N Chaturvedi, D Webb, JH Fuller. 2005. Is pregnancy a risk factor for microvascular complications? The EURODIAB Prospective Complications Study. *Diabet Med* 22:1503.

Vinatier D, P Dufour, M Cosson, JL Houpeau. 2001. Antiphospholipid syndrome and recurrent miscarriages. *Eur J Obstet Gynecol Reprod Biol* 96:37.

von Dadelszen P, MP Ornstein, SB Bull et al. 2000. Fall in mean arterial pressure and fetal growth restriction in pregnancy hypertension: a meta-analysis. *Lancet* 355:87.

Weeks A, Z Alfirevic, A Faúndes, GJ Hofmeyr, P Safar, D Wing. 2007. Misoprostol for induction of labour with a live fetus. *Int J Gynaecol Obstet* 99:S194–197.

Whyte H, ME Hannah, S Saigal et al. 2004. Outcomes of children at two years after planned cesarean birth versus planned vaginal birth for breech presentation at term: The international randomized Term Breech Trial. *Am J Obstet Gynecol* 191:864.

Yeast JD, TJ Garite, W Dorchester. 1984. The risks of amniocentesis in the management of premature rupture of the membranes. *Am J Obstet Gynecol* 149:505–508.
Yoon BH, JK Jun, KH Park et al. 1996. Serum C-reactive protein, white blood cell count and amniotic fluid white blood cell count in women with preterm premature rupture of membranes. *Obstet Gynecol* 88:1034–1040.
Yost NP, SL Bloom, DD McIntire and KJ Leveno. 2005. Hospitalization for women with arrested preterm labor: A randomized trial. *Obstet Gynecol* 106:14.

Index

I

J

K

L